PROGRESS IN BRAIN RESEARCH

VOLUME 51

DEVELOPMENT AND CHEMICAL SPECIFICITY OF NEURONS

Recent volumes in PROGRESS IN BRAIN RESEARCH

Volume 44: Understanding the Stretch Reflex, by H. Homma (Ed.) – 1976

Volume 45: Perspectives in Brain Research, by M. A. Corner and D. F. Swaab (Eds.) – 1976

Volume 46: Membrane Morphology of the Vertebrate Nervous System. A Study with Freeze-etch Technique, by C. Sandri, J. M. Van Buren and K. Akert – 1977

Volume 47: Hypertension and Brain Mechanisms, by W. De Jong, A. P. Provoost and A. P. Shapiro (Eds.) – 1977

Volume 48: Maturation of the Nervous System, by M. A. Corner, R. E. Baker, N. E. Van der Pol, D. F. Swaab and H. B. U. Uylings (Eds.) – 1978

Volume 49: The Cholinergic Synapse, by S. Tuček (Ed.) – 1979

Volume 50: Reflex Control of Posture and Movement, by R. Granit and O. Pompeiano (Eds.) – 1979

Volume 51: Development and Chemical Specificity of Neurons, by M. Cuénod, G. W. Kreutzberg and F. Bloom (Eds.) – 1979

Volume 52: The Pineal Gland of Vertebrates including Man, by J. Ariëns Kappers and P. Pévet (Eds.) – 1979

PROGRESS IN BRAIN RESEARCH

VOLUME 51

DEVELOPMENT AND CHEMICAL SPECIFICITY OF NEURONS

Proceedings of the Schatzalp Symposium, September 1978

EDITED BY

M. CUÉNOD

Brain Research Institute, University of Zurich, CH-8029 Zurich (Switzerland)

G. W. KREUTZBERG

Max-Planck Institute for Psychiatry, 8000 Munich 40 (G.F.R.)

AND

F. E. BLOOM

Arthur Vining Davis Center for Behavioral Neurobiology, The Salk Institute, San Diego, Calif. 92112 (U.S.A.)

ELSEVIER/NORTH-HOLLAND BIOMEDICAL PRESS
AMSTERDAM/NEW YORK/OXFORD
1979

PUBLISHED BY:
ELSEVIER/NORTH-HOLLAND BIOMEDICAL PRESS
335 JAN VAN GALENSTRAAT, P.O. BOX 211
AMSTERDAM, THE NETHERLANDS

SOLE DISTRIBUTORS FROM THE U.S.A. AND CANADA:
ELSEVIER NORTH-HOLLAND INC.
52 VANDERBILT AVENUE
NEW YORK, NY 10017, U.S.A.

ISBN 0–444–80104–9 (SERIES)
ISBN 0–444–80128–6 (VOL. 51)

Library of Congress Cataloging in Publication Data

Main entry under title:

Development and chemical specificity of neurons.

(Progress in brain research ; v. 51)
Bibliography: p.
Includes index.
1. Brain--Congresses. 2. Neurons--Congresses.
3. Brain chemistry--Congresses. 4. Neuro-
transmitters--Congresses. I. Cuénod, M.
II. Kreutzberg, Georg W. III. Bloom, Floyd E.,
1936- IV. Series.
QP376.P7 vol 51 612'.82'08s [599'.01'88]
ISBN 0-444-80128-6 79-19246

WITH 210 ILLUSTRATIONS AND 25 TABLES

PRINTED IN THE NETHERLANDS

List of Contributors

P. ANDERSEN, Institute of Neurophysiology, University of Oslo, Karl Johansgatan 47, Oslo 1, Norway.

R. E. BAKER, Netherlands Institute for Brain Research, IJdijk 28, Amsterdam-O., The Netherlands.

R. BALÁZS, M.R.C. Developmental Neurobiology Unit, Institute of Neurology, 33 John's Mews, London WC1N 2NS, Great Britain.

Y.-A. BARDE, Max-Planck-Institut für Psychiatrie, Abteilung Neurochemie, Am Klopferspitz 18a, 8033 Martinsried bei München, G.F.R.

C. BLAKEMORE, The Physiological Laboratory, Cambridge CB2 3EG, Great Britain.

F. E. BLOOM, Arthur Vining Davis Center for Behavioral Neurobiology, The Salk Institute, P.O. Box 1809, San Diego, Calif. 92112, U.S.A.

W. BOMMELI, Federal Vaccinal Institute of Basle, Basle, Switzerland.

B. B. BOYCOTT, M.R.C. Cell Biophysics Unit, King's College, 26–29 Drury Lane, London WC2B 5RL, Great Britain.

J. P. BROCKES, Medical Research Council Neuroimmunology Project, Zoology Department, University College London, London WC1E 6BT, Great Britain.

V. CHAN-PALAY, Department of Neurobiology, Harvard Medical School, 25 Shattuck Street, Boston, Mass. 02115, U.S.A.

M. A. CORNER, Netherlands Institute for Brain Research, IJdijk 28, Amsterdam-O., The Netherlands.

C. W. COTMAN, Department of Psychobiology, University of California, Irvine, Calif. 92717, U.S.A.

H. D. COULTER, Department of Anatomy, University of Minnesota, Minneapolis, Minn. 55455, U.S.A.

M. CUÉNOD, Brain Research Institute, University of Zurich, August-Forel-Strasse 1, Postfach, CH-8029 Zurich, Switzerland.

W. DAMES, Max Planck Institute for Biophysical Chemistry, Department of Neurobiology/Neuroanatomy, Göttingen, G.F.R.

N. DE LANEROLLE, Department of Psychiatry, Yale University, New Haven, Conn. 06510, U.S.A.

M. DOLIVO, Department of Physiology, University of Lausanne, Lausanne, Switzerland.

J. J. DREIFUSS, Department of Physiology, University of Geneva Medical School, Geneva, Switzerland.

M. J. DRIAN, Laboratoire de Culture de Tissu Nerveux, INSERM U106, 42, rue Desbassyns de Richemont, 92150 Suresnes, France.

J. C. ECCLES, Max-Planck-Institut für biophysikalische Chemie, Abteilung für Neurobiologie, Göttingen, G.F.R.

D. EDGAR, Max-Planck-Institut für Psychiatrie, Abteilung Neurochemie, Am Klopferspitz 18a, 8033 Martinsried bei München, G.F.R.

R. ELDE, Department of Anatomy, 262 Jackson Hall, 321 Church Street S.E., University of Minnesota, Minneapolis, Minn. 55455, U.S.A.

A. FAIRÉN, Sección de Neuroanatomía Comparada, Instituto Cajal, C.S.I.C., Velázquez 144, Madrid 6, Spain.

M. FAUQUET, Institut d'Embryologie du C.N.R.S. et du Collège de France, 49 bis, Avenue de la Belle-Gabrielle, 94130 Nogent-sur-Marne, France.

K. L. FIELDS, Medical Research Council Neuroimmunology Project, Zoology Department, University College London, London WC1E 6BT, Great Britain.

F. FONNUM, Norwegian Defence Research Establishment, Division for Toxicology, N-2007 Kjeller, Norway.

B. H. GÄHWILER, Biological and Medical Research Division, Sandoz Ltd., Basle, Switzerland.
L. J. GAREY, Institut d'Anatomie, Université de Lausanne, Rue du Bugnon 9, CH-1011 Lausanne, Switzerland.
C. GEORGE, Department of Physiology, University of Lausanne, Lausanne, Switzerland.
G. GERISCH, Biozentrum der Universität Basel, Klingelbergstrasse 70, 4056 Basel, Switzerland.
A. M. GRAYBIEL, Department of Psychology and Brain Science, Massachusetts Institute of Technology, Cambridge, Mass. 02139, U.S.A.
R. GUGGENHEIM, Laboratory of Scanning Electron Microscopy, Universität Basel, Bernoullistrasse 32, 4056 Basel, Switzerland.
R. W. GUILLERY, Department of Pharmacological and Physiological Sciences, University of Chicago, 947 East 58th Street, Chicago, Ill. 60637, U.S.A.
H. HATANAKA, Max-Planck-Institut für Psychiatrie, Abteilung Neurochemie, Am Klopferspitz 18a, 8033 Martinsried bei München, G.F.R.
T. HATTORI, Kinsmen Laboratory of Neurological Research, Department of Psychiatry, University of British Columbia, Vancouver, B.C. V6T 1W5, Canada.
H. HENKE, Brain Research Institute, University of Zurich, August-Forel-Strasse 1, Postfach, CH-8092 Zurich, Switzerland.
R. HO, Department of Anatomy, Ohio State University, Columbus, Ohio 43210, U.S.A.
T. HÖKFELT, Department of Histology, Karolinska Institute, Stockholm, Sweden.
P. HONEGGER, Department of Physiology, University of Lausanne, Lausanne, Switzerland.
G. M. INNOCENTI, Institute of Anatomy, University of Lausanne, Rue du Bugnon 9, CH-1011 Lausanne CHUV, Switzerland.
G. ISENBERG, Max Planck Institute for Psychiatry, Kraepelinstrasse 2, 8000 Munich 40, G.F.R.
F. JOÓ, Laboratory of Molecular Neurobiology, Institute of Biophysics, Biological Research Center, Szeged, Hungary.
J.-K. KIM, Department of Physiology, Catholic Medical College, Seoul 110, Korea.
M. KIRALY, Department of Physiology, University of Lausanne, Lausanne, Switzerland.
G. W. KREUTZBERG, Max Planck Institute for Psychiatry, Kraepelinstrasse 2, 8000 Munich 40, G.F.R.
N. M. LE DOUARIN, Institut d'Embryologie du C.N.R.S. et du Collège de France, 49 bis, Avenue de la Belle-Gabrielle, 94130 Nogent-sur-Marne, France.
R. LLINÁS, Departments of Physiology and Biophysics, New York University Medical Center, 550 First Avenue, New York, N.Y. 10016, U.S.A.
R. LUND KARLSEN, Norwegian Defence Research Establishment, Division for Toxicology, N-2007 Kjeller, Norway.
D. MALTHE-SØRENSEN, Norwegian Defence Research Establishment, Division for Toxicology, N-2007 Kjeller, Norway.
A. M. MARSON, Laboratoire de Culture de Tissu Nerveux, INSERM U106, 42, rue Desbassyns de Richemont, 92150 Suresnes, France.
M. F. MAYLIÉ-PFENNINGER, Department of Anatomy, Columbia University College of Physicians and Surgeons, New York, N.Y., U.S.A.
E. G. McGEER, Kinsmen Laboratory of Neurological Research, Department of Psychiatry, University of British Columbia, Vancouver, B.C. V6T 1W5, Canada.
P. L. McGEER, Kinsmen Laboratory of Neurological Research, Department of Psychiatry, University of British Columbia, Vancouver, B.C. V6T 1W5, Canada.
P. MICEVYCH, Department of Anatomy, University of Minnesota, Minneapolis, Minn. 55455, U.S.A.
R. MIRSKY, Medical Research Council Neuroimmunology Project, Zoology Department, University College London, London WC1E 6BT, Great Britain.
C. NITSCH, Neurobiologische Abteilung, Max-Planck-Institut für Hirnforschung, Deutschordenstrasse 46, D-6000 Frankfurt/M. 71, G.F.R.
U. OTTEN, Max-Planck-Institut für Psychiatrie, Abteilung Neurochemie, Am Klopferspitz 18a, 8033 Martinsried bei München, G.F.R.
P. H. PATTERSON, Harvard Medical School, Department of Neurobiology, Boston, Mass., U.S.A.
L. PEICHL, Friedrich-Miescher-Laboratorium, Max-Planck-Gesellschaft, Spemannstrasse 37–39, D-74 Tübingen, G.F.R.
K. H. PFENNINGER, Department of Anatomy, Columbia University College of Physicians and Surgeons, New York, N.Y., U.S.A.
A. PRIVAT, Laboratoire de Culture de Tissu Nerveux, INSERM U106, 42, rue Desbassyns de Richemont, 92150 Suresnes, France.

M. C. RAFF, Medical Research Council Neuroimmunology Project, Zoology Department, University College London, London WC1E 6BT, Great Britain.

G. RAGER, Department of Neurobiology, Max Planck Institute for Biophysical Chemistry, Am Fassberg, 3400 Göttingen, G.F.R.

U. RAGER, Department of Neurobiology, Max Planck Institute for Biophysical Chemistry, Am Fassberg, 3400 Göttingen, G.F.R.

C. W. RAGSDALE, Jr., Department of Psychology and Brain Science, Massachusetts Institute of Technology, Cambridge, Mass. 02139, U.S.A.

M. REDDINGTON, Max Planck Institute for Psychiatry, Kraepelinstrasse 2, 8000 Munich 40, G.F.R.

J. C. REUBI, Brain Research Institute, University of Zurich, August-Forel-Strasse 1, Postfach, CH-8029 Zurich, Switzerland.

M. SCHACHNER, Department of Neurobiology, Heidelberg University, Im Neuenheimer Feld 347, D-6900 Heidelberg, G.F.R.

P. SCHUBERT, Max Planck Institute for Psychiatry, Kraepelinstrasse 2, 8000 Munich 40, G.F.R.

M. SCHWAB, Max-Planck-Institut für Psychiatrie, Abteilung Neurochemie, Am Klopferspitz 18a, 8033 Martinsried bei München, G.F.R.

V. SEYBOLD, Department of Anatomy, University of Minnesota, Minneapolis, Minn. 55455, U.S.A.

C. SHIMADA, Department of Neurochemistry, Tokyo Metropolitan Institute for Neurosciences, Fuchu-shi, Tokyo, Japan.

W. SINGER, Max-Planck-Institut für Psychiatrie, Kraepelinstrasse 2, 8000 Munich 40, G.F.R.

K. K. SKREDE, Norwegian Defence Research Establishment, Division for Toxicology, N-2007 Kjeller, Norway.

J.V. SMALL, Institute for Molecular Biology, Austrian Academy of Sciences, Salzburg, Austria.

J. SMITH, Institut d'Embryologie du C.N.R.S. et du Collège de France, 49 bis, Avenue de la Belle-Gabrielle, 94130 Nogent-sur-Marne, France.

P. STREIT, Brain Research Institute, University of Zurich, August-Forel-Strasse 1, Postfach, CH-8029 Zurich, Switzerland.

M. SUGIMORI, Departments of Physiology and Biophysics, New York University Medical Center, 550 First Avenue, New York, N.Y. 10016, U.S.A.

H. THOENEN, Max-Planck-Institut für Psychiatrie, Abteilung Neurochemie, Am Klopferspitz 18a, 8033 Martinsried bei München, G.F.R.

F. VALVERDE, Sección de Neuroanatomía Comparada, Instituto Cajal, C.S.I.C., Velázquez 144, Madrid 6, Spain.

F. VITAL-DURAND, Laboratoire de Neuropsychologie Expérimentale, INSERM U. 94, 16 Avenue du Doyen-Lépine, 69500 Bron, France.

M. J. VOADEN, Department of Visual Science, Institute of Ophthalmology, Judd Street, London WC1H 9QS, Great Britain.

I. WALAAS, Norwegian Defence Research Establishment, Division for Toxicology, N-2007 Kjeller, Norway.

H. WÄSSLE, Friedrich-Miescher-Laboratorium, Max-Planck-Gesellschaft, Spemannstrasse 37–39, D-74 Tübingen, G.F.R.

M. WILLINGER, Department of Neuroscience, Children's Hospital Medical Center, Boston, Mass. 02115, U.S.A.

M. WOLFENSBERGER, Brain Research Institute, University of Zurich, August-Forel-Strasse 1, Postfach, CH-8029 Zurich, Switzerland.

J. R. WOLFF, Max Planck Institute for Biophysical Chemistry, Department of Neurobiology/Neuroanatomy, Göttingen, G.F.R.

C. ZILLER, Institut d'Embryologie du C.N.R.S. et du Collège de France, 49 bis, Avenue de la Belle-Gabrielle, 94130 Nogent-sur-Marne, France.

Preface

This volume includes the proceedings of the Symposium on "Development and Chemical Specificity of Neurons" held at Schatzalp/Davos, Switzerland, from September 11 to 15, 1978. It was both an EMBO Meeting and the 8th International Neurobiology Society Meeting. The organizing committee consisted of Drs. Konrad Akert (Zurich), Günter Baumgartner (Zurich), Floyd Bloom (San Diego, Calif.), M. Cuénod (Zurich) and Georg Kreutzberg (Munich). About 140 participants from 16 countries attended the meeting. We should particularly like to thank the members of the Brain Research Institute in Zurich who assisted in the organization of the symposium, especially Drs. Peter Streit and Hermann Henke, and Miss Myrtha Jäckli, who as secretary of the meeting contributed much to its success.

The first part of the symposium was devoted to the basic biological mechanisms underlying cell growth, cell contacts and chemical interactions, including transmitters in the nervous tissue. The second part was concerned with the application of the basic principles to some specific circuits in the vertebrate brain. Four systems have been selected for discussion of morphological, physiological and biochemical parameters: the hippocampus, the basal ganglia, the cerebellum and the visual system. The present proceedings cover the invited main lectures and a few communications selected by the editors of the volume.

The meeting could not have been held without the generous support of a number of organizations. It is a pleasure to acknowledge, with gratitude, the financial assistance given by the following:

Dr. Eric Slack-Gyr-Foundation, Zurich, Switzerland
European Molecular Biology Organization (EMBO), Heidelberg, G.F.R.
European Training Programme in Brain and Behaviour Research (ETP), Rijswijk, The Netherlands
Interpharma (Ciba-Geigy AG, F. Hoffmann-La Roche + Co. AG, Sandoz AG), Basel, Switzerland
Kontron AG, Zurich, Switzerland
Kurverein, Davos, Switzerland
Migros-Genossenschafts-Bund, Zurich, Switzerland
National Foundation March of Dimes, White Plains, N. Y., U.S.A.
Schweizerische Naturforschende Gesellschaft, Berne, Switzerland
Schweizerische Rückversicherungs-Gesellschaft, Zurich, Switzerland
Swiss National Science Foundation, Berne, Switzerland

Michel Cuénod – Georg Kreutzberg – Floyd Bloom

Zurich, September 1979

Dedication
to
Konrad Akert
In honour of his 60th birthday

Contents

Part II–Organization of Neural Ensembles

PART I

CELLULAR PROPERTIES OF NEURAL FUNCTION

Cell Communication and Specific Adhesion in the Microorganism *Dictyostelium*

GÜNTHER GERISCH and RICHARD GUGGENHEIM

Biozentrum der Universität Basel, Klingelbergstrasse 70, 4056 Basel, and Laboratory of Scanning Electron Microscopy, Universität Basel, Bernoullistrasse 32, 4056 Basel (Switzerland)

The abilities to generate signals and to respond to them are by no means peculiarities of neurons and of the target cells connected to them. Hormones control cellular activities not only in the adult but also in the developing organism. A host of probably chemical signal systems, those mediating cell communication during early embryogenesis, are still little understood. It is an idea expressed already in the twenties by Child (1924) that neurotransmitters and the morphogenetic signals acting during embryogenesis may have a common origin. It can be supposed that spatio-temporal signal patterns underly the organisation of an embryo, and that these patterns share basic features with patterns of neuronal activities in the central nervous system. With these possibilities in mind it may be justified to discuss in a volume devoted to neurobiology the signal system that guides the development of a micro-organism which, in a sense, behaves like a "free-living brain".

Cells of *Dictyostelium discoideum* feed and divide as single amoeboid cells. Within several hours after the end of their growth phase they become able to communicate with each other (Fig. 1). As a result they aggregate into a multicellular body where the cells finally differentiate into two types, stalk cells and spores, which constitute a fruiting body. The transmitter released from aggregating cells is cyclic AMP (Konijn et al., 1967). It exerts its function by interaction with cell surface receptors. In this primitive system the whole intercellular space replaces the synaptic cleft. Pre- and postsynaptic cells are not distinguished: signal generation and reception are temporally separated functions of the same cells. In analogy to neural signal transmission cAMP can be released periodically, but the periods have the length of minutes. cAMP-phosphodiesterase is present on the cell surface and has the same function as the esterase in a cholinergic synapse. Aggregating cells are excitable. They propagate periodic signals in form of waves travelling in a dense cell layer with a speed of about 40 μm/min. This indicates a signal output to input delay of about 15 sec (Fig. 2).

The main function of cAMP in aggregating cells of *D.discoideum* is that of a chemotactic agent. In certain strains cAMP does not only orientate aggregating cells towards centers, but also affects cell development from the growth phase to the aggregation competent stage. This means that full development of the signal system functioning in aggregation is established by its early, still rudimentary activity. One constituent of the cell membrane which is controlled by cAMP signals is a specific glycoprotein. It is probably involved in cell adhesion which is one requirement for the association of aggregating cells into a tissue-like assembly.

The following is a survey on the biochemical changes observed in signalling and responding cells, and on the resulting changes of cell shape and behavior.

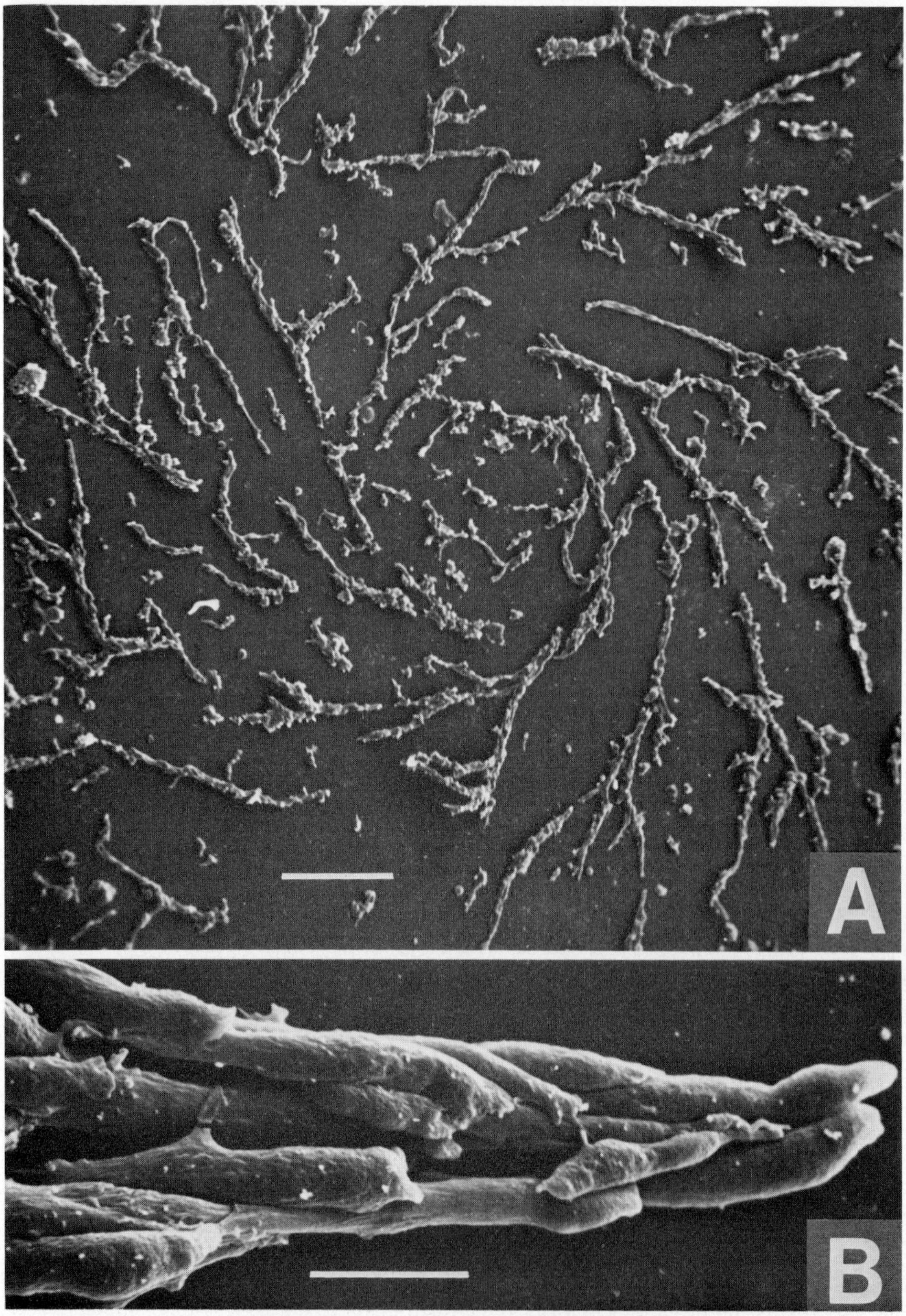

Fig. 1. Cell aggregation in *Dictyostelium discoideum.* A: cells harvested from a suspension culture in the aggregation competent stage assemble into streams of cohering cells which become aligned by chemotactic orientation into patterns which often are of whirl-like structure. In the central region of such a whirl the cells will usually condense into a solid aggregation center. B: part of a stream showing the elongation which is typical of aggregating cells, as well as their adhesion end-to-end and also side-by-side. The bar indicates 100 μm in A and 10 μm in B.

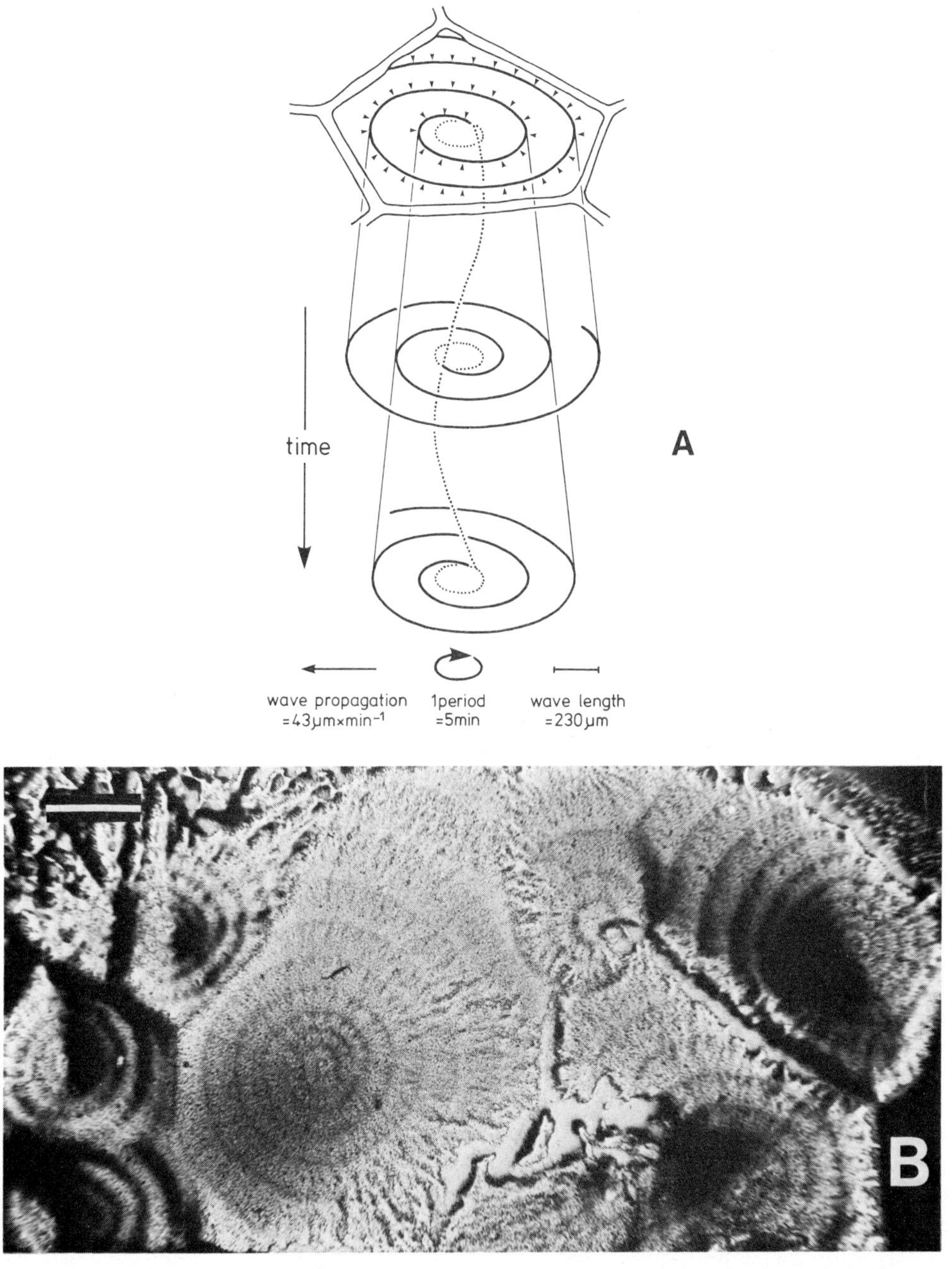

Fig. 2. Spatio-temporal pattern of chemotactic activity in an early aggregation stage. If cells cultivated in suspension are spread on a surface, the almost uniform layer is organized into systems of excitation waves which often have the shape of spirals. The sharp boundaries of the territories are formed where the waves meet each other. At the stage shown, waves rarely spread into another territory, obviously because signalling is followed by relative refractoriness. A: data on wave propagation were obtained from time lapse movies and apply to dense layers of cells (Gerisch, 1965). In more dispersed cell populations the speed of wave propagation is higher (Alcantara and Monk, 1974). The arrows indicate the site and direction of chemotactic orientation. By responding to local concentration profiles the cells move towards the aggregation center. From Gerisch (1978). B: photograph of wave patterns in a cell layer on agar. The bar indicates 1 mm. From Gerisch (1971).

CHEMOTAXIS

Aggregating cells of *D.discoideum* and related species orientate in concentration gradients of cAMP. They recognize a concentration difference as small as $\frac{\Delta c}{c} = 0.01$. This means that a concentration difference of 1% over the length of a cell of about 10 μm is sufficient for orientation (Mato et al., 1975). The direction of cell motion is determined by the location of a front of pseudopods which in orientated cells points towards the source of the gradient. The cells can be locally stimulated from microcapillaries filled with cAMP (Gerisch et al., 1975a). This way a front of pseudopods can be elicited within about 5 sec from every part of the cell surface, indicating that the about 5×10^5 cAMP receptors present on an aggregating cell are distributed over its whole surface. A second conclusion is that these cells do not have a stable polarity. Every part of the cell is a potential tip.

Like granulocytes and unlike chemotactic bacteria, *Dictyostelium* cells move along a gradient in more or less straight lines. There are two principal possibilities how an amoeboid cell can translate the direction of an external concentration gradient into orientated motion. First, the cell can evaluate the distribution of occupied receptors over its surface. Second, it senses the gradient by a temporal response mechanism: the cell can use pseudopods extending into arbitary directions (Fig. 3) in order to discover the direction of a gradient by measuring, with these sensors, an increase of concentration in time (Gerisch et al., 1975a).

The observation of intracellular biochemical changes accompanying chemotactic orientation is difficult. The second of the above possibilities led to experiments in which suspended cells were stimulated under stirring by pulses of cAMP. Under these conditions the whole cell surface is uniformly exposed to cAMP, and biochemical changes in response to an increase of the attractant concentration with time can easily be measured. Two changes have been found which occur within a few seconds after stimulation, i.e. fast enough to be potential steps in the signal processing pathway for chemotaxis. These changes are uptake of Ca^{2+} (Wick et al., 1978) and increase of the cyclic GMP concentration (Mato et al., 1977; Wurster et al., 1977, 1978). The latter has been observed in cells of *D.discoideum* or related species stimulated by any of the chemotactic agents known. This is cAMP in aggregating cells of *D.discoideum,* folic acid in pre-aggregative cells of the same species, a factor which is probably an oligopeptide in *Polysphondylium violaceum,* and a chemically yet undefined chemotactic factor in *D.lacteum.* In *D.discoideum* it has been established that the rise of cGMP is due to the activation of guanylate cyclase (Mato and Malchow, 1978).

Cells of *D.discoideum* contain a cGMP binding protein whose activation presumably represents the next step in signal processing (Rahmsdorf and Gerisch, 1978; Mato et al., 1978). The function of this protein is still unknown. The final step in the chemotactic pathway must be the local control of contractility. It has been shown that stimulation of the cells with cAMP causes an increase of ^{32}P incorporation from γ-^{32}P-ATP into myosin heavy chains (Rahmsdorf et al., 1978). Since in other cells the phosphorylation of either myosin light chains or heavy chains results in an increase of the actin-activated ATPase activity of myosin (Maruta and Korn, 1977; Adelstein, 1978), the modulation of myosin phosphorylation is an attractive candidate for the mechanism by which a chemotactic agent exerts its control over cell motion.

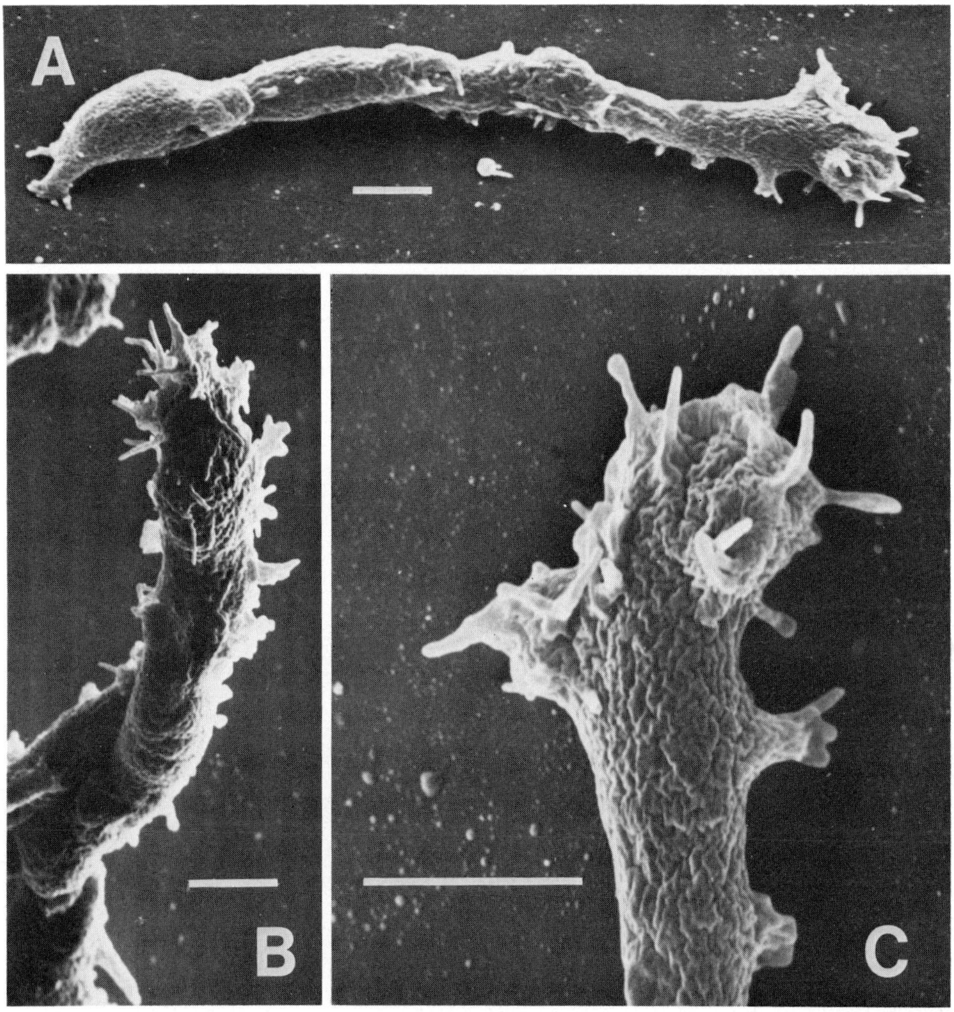

Fig. 3. Morphological correlates of chemotactic orientation. A: a short chain of end-to-end assembled cells with the leader cell showing a number of filopodia which are suppressed in the followers. B: another terminal cell from a stream, covered by numerous extensions of its surface. C: the terminal cell from A. The bars indicate 5 μm.

SIGNAL RELAY

In cells which are able to propagate chemotactic signals, the release of cAMP must be coupled to excitation by cAMP. Pulses of cAMP in fact trigger the release of cAMP (Gerisch et al., 1975a; Shaffer, 1975). The cells can amplify the signals by two orders of magnitude (Roos et al., 1975). The major part of the cAMP released is newly synthesized after stimulation. Thus in contrast to neurotransmitter release, the generation of cAMP signals has to be preceded by a period of raised net synthesis of cAMP. The determination of adenylate cyclase activity in homogenates of unstimulated and stimulated cells has provided direct evidence for the short-term activation of this enzyme in response to cAMP pulses (Roos and Gerisch, 1976). Then, within 2 min after stimulation, the adenylate cyclase activity declines to the basal level of resting cells even under conditions where the concentration of the stimulant is kept at a constant elevated level (Fig. 4). This indicates rapid adaptation of the response system to steady stimuli. The adaptation limits the duration of the response, and phosphodiesterase limits the lifetime of cAMP in the extracellular space. Both together determine the shape of the cAMP pulses.

The mechanism of adenylate cyclase activation through cAMP receptors on the cell surface is unknown. Accompanying events are an increase of the intracellular cGMP concentration, which precedes the rise of cAMP, and an increase of the extracellular proton concentration (Malchow et al., 1978a).

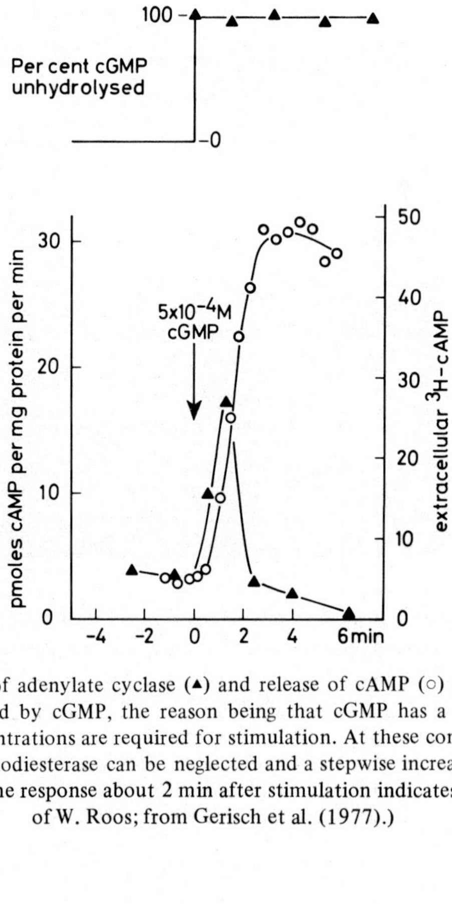

Fig. 4. Transient activation of adenylate cyclase (▲) and release of cAMP (○) from stimulated cells. As a stimulant cAMP was replaced by cGMP, the reason being that cGMP has a low affinity to the cAMP receptors so that high concentrations are required for stimulation. At these concentrations the amount of cGMP hydrolysed by phosphodiesterase can be neglected and a stepwise increase followed by a plateau is the result (top). Decline of the response about 2 min after stimulation indicates adaptation. (Experiments of W. Roos; from Gerisch et al. (1977).)

PERIODICITY OF ADENYLATE CYCLASE ACTIVATION

The propagated pulses of chemotactic signals are generated in aggregation centers. In early aggregates the waves often have the shape of spirals with a rotating origin (Fig. 2).

Later on established aggregation centers usually pulse as a whole, thus giving rise to concentric waves. Autonomous periodicity of cAMP production is also obtained in stirred cell suspensions (Gerisch and Hess, 1974; Gerisch and Wick, 1975). If cells are in the right developmental stage, they start spontaneously in suspension to generate cAMP signals almost synchronously and continue to do so in periods of about 8 min (Fig. 5). cAMP itself acts via its cell surface receptors as a synchronizing agent. This is indicated by the fact that exogenous cAMP pulses of 5 or 10 nM amplitude shift the phase of the oscillator (Fig. 6). Sign and degree of the phase shifts depend on the phase of the cycle in which the disturbing pulse is given (Malchow et al., 1978b).

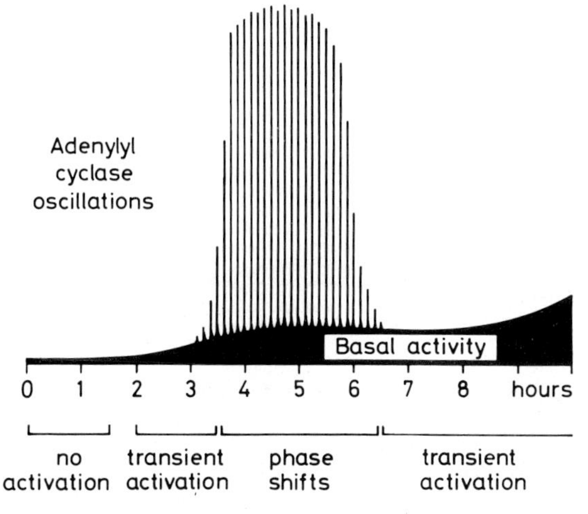

Fig. 5. Diagram of activity changes of adenylate cyclase during development in cell suspensions. The increase of basal activity is measured in homogenates of unstimulated cells (Klein, 1976). Oscillations of activity are superimposed to the changes of basal activity (Roos et al., 1977a). Before and after the stage in which autonomous oscillations are observed, the adenylate cyclase can be transiently activated by pulses of extracellular cAMP. From Gerisch et al. (1977).

Autonomous periodicity of cAMP production is based on oscillatory changes of adenylate cyclase activity (Roos et al., 1977a). This does not necessarily mean that the cyclase is an essential part of the "clock". Oscillations of cellular activities may continue in the absence of detectable changes of cAMP concentrations or of adenylate cyclase activities. Thus the possibility that the adenylate cyclase is only coupled to the basic oscillator rather than being indispensable for its function has to be taken into consideration.

Autonomous cAMP pulses, like induced ones, are preceded by an increase of the cGMP concentration and are accompanied by a fall of the extracellular pH (Malchow et al., 1978b).

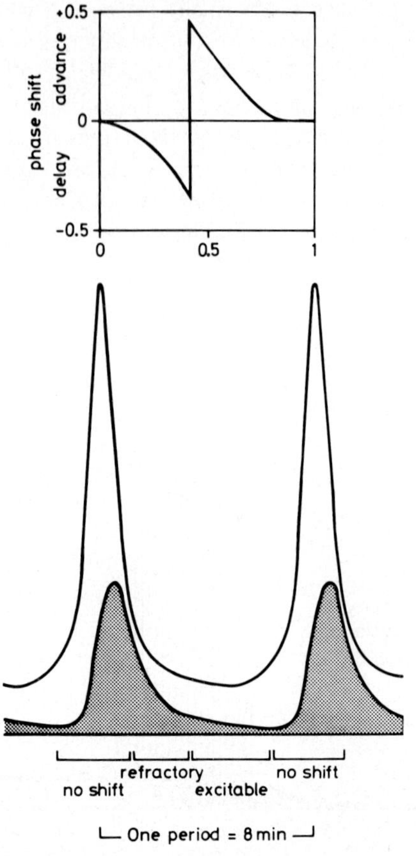

Fig. 6. Phases of spontaneous oscillations and the disturbances caused by small pulses of 5–10 nM cAMP. Bottom: changes of intracellular (open area) and extracellular (shaded) cAMP concentrations in cell suspensions according to experiments of U. Wick. Top: phase response curve showing the shifts caused by cAMP pulses applied at different phases of a cycle. When a stimulus causes an advanced entry into the signalling phase, the autonomously oscillating cells are called excitable. Phase delay is considered as being equivalent to refractoriness. From Gerisch et al. (1977).

DEVELOPMENT OF THE SIGNAL SYSTEM IS STIMULATED BY cAMP PULSES

The biochemical oscillator which is responsible for periodic cAMP production becomes functional during cell differentiation from the growth phase to the aggregation competent stage. Known components of the cAMP signal system which change during that period are cAMP receptors on the cell surface, adenylate cyclase and cell surface cAMP-phosphodiesterase. These 3 components increase in either activity or number, and this increase is accentuated in certain strains of *D.discoideum* by stimulation of the cells by cAMP pulses (Roos et al., 1977b). Periodic cAMP application also accelerates the onset of autonomous oscillations (Gerisch and Hess, 1974). These results show that the development of the cAMP signal and response system is facilitated by its own function, and that multiple loops of positive feedback are implemented in the control of cell differentiation (Fig. 7).

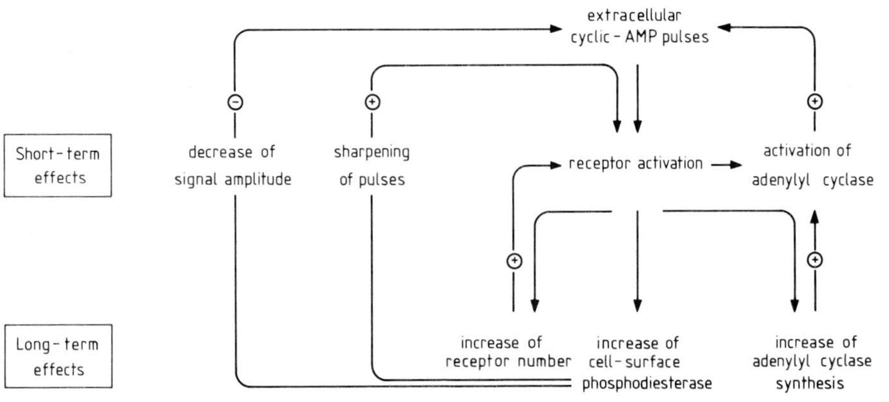

Fig. 7. Network controlling the development of the cyclic AMP signal system. Short-term controls imply the activity changes elicited by a single pulse of cAMP, and also the comparable changes occurring during one period of autonomous oscillations. cAMP binds to cell surface receptors and thus transiently activates the adenylate cyclase. The synthesized cAMP is released into the extracellular space where it is hydrolysed by phosphodiesterase. Long-term controls are those regulatory effects of cAMP pulses which are manifested after several hours of stimulation: the increase of basal adenylate cyclase activity, of cAMP-phosphodiesterase activity on the cell surface, and of the number of cAMP binding sites on the surface. These effects probably involve the regulation of de novo synthesis of the corresponding proteins. From Roos et al. (1977b).

DEVELOPMENTAL CONTROL OF CELL ADHESION

The effects of cAMP pulses on cell development are also manifested as changes of cell shape and behavior. Cells stimulated repeatedly by cAMP pulses acquire the ability to elongate and to associate into stream-like aggregates earlier than control cells (Fig. 8). Typical for aggregating cells is their end-to-end adhesion which is largely resistant to EDTA. Previous work in which cell adhesion was blocked by Fab against different cell surface antigens has revealed two classes of target sites of adhesion blocking Fab, called contact sites (Beug et al., 1973). One class, contact sites B, is already present on the surface of growth phase cells and is maintained during development. Blockage of these sites eliminates the side-by-side adhesion of aggregating cells. The other class, contact sites A, is developmentally regulated and virtually absent from growth phase cells. Blockage of contact sites A by Fab specifically inhibits the end-to-end adhesion. Blockage of either one class of contact sites does not block the function of the other, indicating that they represent two independent adhesion systems (Fig. 9). Antibodies against contact sites of *D.discoideum* do not cross-react with those of another species, *Polysphondylium pallidum.* Specificity of the action of contact sites might be a basis for species-specific sorting out of aggregation competent cells (Bozzaro and Gerisch, 1978; Nicol and Garrod, 1978).

The blocking activity of Fab directed against contact sites A is neutralized by a single concanavalin A binding glycoprotein which has been recently purified (Müller and Gerisch, 1978). Carbohydrate binding proteins are also present on the surface of *D.discoideum* cells and have been suggested to play a role in cell adhesion (Reitherman et al., 1975; Siu et al., 1976). The purified glycoprotein is free of these lectins, called discoidin I and II, and a functional relationship remains to be demonstrated.

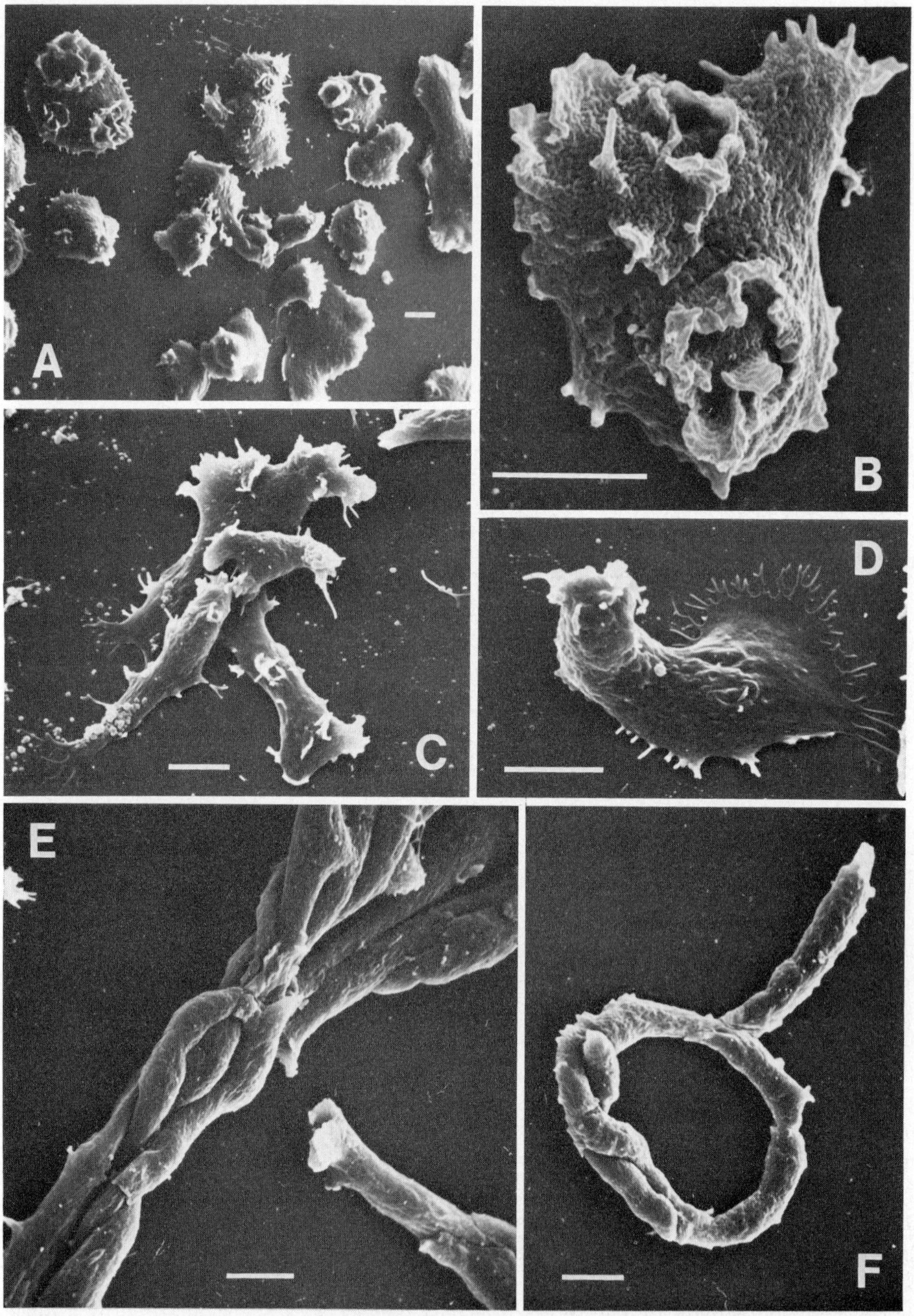

Fig. 8. Changes of cell shape during development from the growth phase to the aggregation competent stage, and the enhancement of these changes by pulsatile cyclic AMP stimuli. A, B: growth phase cells are of irregular shape, typically with crown-like surface extensions. C, D: after 6 h of development the cells are at an intermediate stage of transformation into elongating, aggregation competent cells. E, F: parallel to B, but cells stimulated with pulses of 10^{-7} M cAMP every 6 min. After having washed the cells free of added cAMP they were plated on coverslips and allowed to aggregate for 30 min. Elongation and strong end-to-end adhesion indicate the advanced state of development of the stimulated cells as compared to the control shown in C and D. The end-to-end adhesion often leads to closed rings to which cells from the outside can attach (F). The bars indicate 5 μm.

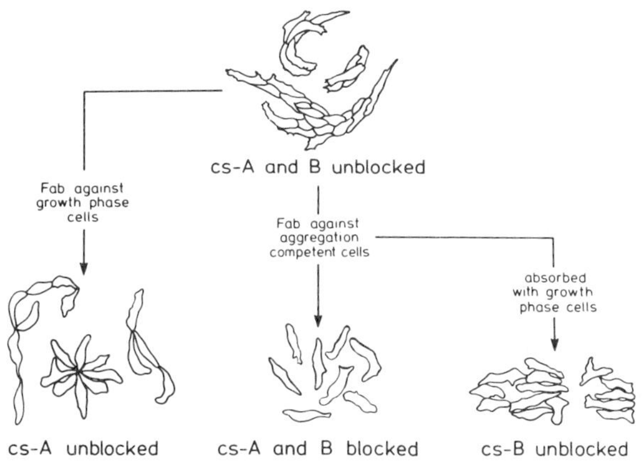

Fig. 9. Analysis of the cell adhesion system in *D.discoideum* by the use of Fab. Cells aggregate into streams where they adhere to each other end-to-end as well as side-by-side. Polyspecific Fab prepared from antisera raised against membranes of aggregation competent cells completely dissociates the cells (middle). After absorption of this Fab preparation with membrane antigens of growth phase cells, only the blocking activity for the end-to-end adhesion is retained (right). By contrast, Fab specific for antigens of growth phase cells blocks only side-by-side adhesion (left). The conclusions are that (1) side-by-side adhesion is blocked by Fab directed against antigen(s) present both on growth phase and aggregation competent cells, and (2) the target antigen of Fab that blocks end-to-end adhesion is expressed between the end of growth and the beginning of aggregation. Data of Beug et al. (1973), reproduced from Müller and Gerisch (1978).

The expression of contact sites A on the cell surface is strongly stimulated by cAMP pulses (Darmon et al., 1975; Gerisch et al., 1975b). The purified glycoprotein appears to be the cell surface antigen which is expressed in response to cAMP pulses.

SUMMARY

Dictyostelium discoideum is a microorganism which during its development from a unicellular to a multicellular state releases cyclic AMP as a chemotactic agent and a transmitter of propagated stimuli. The transmitter is generated periodically by virtue of oscillatory regulation of the synthesizing enzyme, and its lifetime in the intercellular space is limited by a hydrolyzing enzyme, cyclic AMP-phosphodiesterase. Development of the signal system is enhanced by its function. Association of the cells into a tissue-like assembly is mediated by a duplicate cell adhesion system. One component is a specific cell membrane glycoprotein. Its control by pulses of cAMP links the full expression of the adhesion system to this transmitter and to its recognition by cell surface receptors.

ACKNOWLEDGEMENTS

Our work was supported by the Schweizerischer Nationalfonds.
We thank Mr. H. Guiliani and Mr. J. Beltzer for valuable cooperation.

REFERENCES

Adelstein, R. S. (1978) Myosin phosphorylation, cell motility and smooth muscle contraction. *Trends Biochem. Sci.*, 3: 27–30.

Alcantara, F. and Monk, M. (1974) Signal propagation in the cellular slime mould *Dictyostelium discoideum. J. gen. Microbiol.*, 85: 321–324.

Beug, H., Katz, F. E. and Gerisch, G. (1973) Dynamics of antigenic membrane sites relating to cell aggregation in *Dictyostelium discoideum. J. Cell Biol.*, 56: 647–658.

Bozzaro, S. and Gerisch, G. (1978) Contact sites in aggregating cells of *Polysphondylium pallidum. J. molec. Biol.*, 120: 265–279.

Child, C. M. (1924) *Physiological Foundations of Behavior.* Holt, New York.

Darmon, M., Brachet, P. and Pereira da Silva, L. H. (1975) Chemotactic signals induce cell differentiation in *Dictyostelium discoideum. Proc. nat. Acad. Sci. (Wash.)*, 72: 3163–3166.

Gerisch, G. (1965) Stadienspezifische Aggregationsmuster bei *Dictyostelium discoideum. Roux' Arch. Entwickl.-Mech.*, 156: 127–144.

Gerisch, G. (1971) Periodische Signale steuern die Musterbildung in Zellverbänden. *Naturwissenschaften*, 58: 430–438.

Gerisch, G. (1978) Cell interactions by cyclic AMP in *Dictyostelium. Biol. Cell.*, 32: 61–68.

Gerisch, G. and Hess, B. (1974) Cyclic-AMP controlled oscillations in suspended *Dictyostelium* cells: their relation to morphogenetic cell interactions. *Proc. nat. Acad. Sci. (Wash.)*, 71: 2118–2122.

Gerisch, G. and Wick, U. (1975) Intracellular oscillations and release of cyclic AMP from *Dictyostelium* cells. *Biochem. biophys. Res. Commun.*, 65: 364–370.

Gerisch, G., Hülser, D., Malchow, D. and Wick, U. (1975a) Cell communication by periodic cyclic-AMP pulses. *Phil. Trans. B*, 272: 181–192.

Gerisch, G., Fromm, H., Huesgen, A. and Wick, U. (1975b) Control of cell-contact sites by cyclic AMP pulses in differentiating *Dictyostelium* cells. *Nature (Lond.)*, 255: 547–549.

Gerisch, G., Maeda, Y., Malchow, D., Roos, W., Wick, U. and Wurster, B. (1977) Cyclic AMP signals and the control of cell aggregation in *Dictyostelium discoideum.* In *Proceedings of the EMBO Workshop on Development and Differentiation in Cellular Slime Moulds,* P. Cappuccinelli and J. M. Ashworth (Eds.), Elsevier/North-Holland Biomedical Press, Amsterdam, pp. 105–124.

Klein, C. (1976) Adenylate cyclase activity in *Dictyostelium discoideum* amoebae and its changes during differentiation. *FEBS Lett.*, 68: 125–128.

Konijn, T. M., Van de Meene, J. G. C., Bonner, J. T. and Barkley, D. S. (1967) The acrasin activity of adenosine-3′,5′-cyclic phosphate. *Proc. nat. Acad. Sci. (Wash.)*, 58: 1152–1154.

Malchow, D., Nanjundiah, V., Wurster, B., Eckstein, F. and Gerisch, G. (1978a) Cyclic-AMP induced pH-changes in *Dictyostelium discoideum* and their control by calcium. *Biochim. biophys. Acta (Amst.)*, 538: 473–480.

Malchow, D., Nanjundiah, V. and Gerisch, G. (1978b) pH-oscillations in cell suspensions of *Dictyostelium discoideum:* their relation to cyclic-AMP signals. *J. Cell Sci.*, 30: 319–330.

Maruta, H. and Korn, E. D. (1977) Purification from *Acanthamoeba castellanii* of proteins that induce gelation and syneresis of F-actin. *J. biol. Chem.*, 252: 399–402.

Mato, J. M. and Malchow, D. (1978) Guanylate cyclase activation in response to chemotactic stimulation in *Dictyostelium discoideum. FEBS Lett.*, 90: 119–122.

Mato, J. M., Losada, A., Nanjundiah, V. and Konijn, T. M. (1975) The signal input for a chemotactic response in the cellular slime mold *Dictyostelium discoideum. Proc. nat. Acad. Sci. (Wash.)*, 72: 4991–4993.

Mato, J. M., Krens, F. A., Van Haastert, P. J. M. and Konijn, T. M. (1977) 3′:5′-cyclic AMP-dependent 3′:5′-cyclic GMP accumulation in *Dictyostelium discoideum. Proc. nat. Acad. Sci. (Wash.)*, 74: 2348–2351.

Mato, J. M., Woelders, H., Van Haastert, P. J. M. and Konijn, T. M. (1978) Cyclic GMP binding activity in *Dictyostelium discoideum. FEBS Lett.*, 90: 261–264.

Müller, K. and Gerisch, G. (1978) A specific glycoprotein as the target site of adhesion blocking Fab in aggregating *Dictyostelium* cells. *Nature (Lond.)*, 274: 445–449.

Nicol, A. and Garrod, D. R. (1978) Mutual cohesion and cell sorting-out among four species of cellular slime moulds. *J. Cell Sci.*, 32: 377–387.

Rahmsdorf, H. J. and Gerisch, G. (1978) Specific binding proteins for cyclic AMP and cyclic GMP in *Dictyostelium discoideum. Cell Diff.*, 7: 249–257.

Rahmsdorf, H. J., Malchow, D. and Gerisch, G. (1978) Cyclic AMP-induced phosphorylation in *Dictyostelium* of a polypeptide comigrating with myosin heavy chains. *FEBS Lett.*, 88: 322–326.

Reitherman, R. W., Rosen, S. D., Frazier, W. A. and Barondes, S. H. (1975) Cell surface species-specific high affinity receptors for discoidin: developmental regulation in *Dictyostelium discoideum. Proc. nat. Acad. Sci. (Wash.)*, 72: 3541–3545.

Roos, W. and Gerisch, G. (1976) Receptor-mediated adenylate cyclase activation in *Dictyostelium discoideum. FEBS Lett.*, 68: 170–172.

Roos, W., Nanjundiah, V., Malchow, D. and Gerisch, G. (1975) Amplification of cyclic-AMP signals in aggregating cells of *Dictyostelium discoideum. FEBS Lett.*, 53: 139–142.

Roos, W., Scheidegger, C. and Gerisch, G. (1977a) Adenylate cyclase activity oscillations as signals for cell aggregation in *Dictyostelium discoideum. Nature (Lond.)*, 266: 259–261.

Roos, W., Malchow, D. and Gerisch, G. (1977b) Adenylyl cyclase and the control of cell differentiation in *Dictyostelium discoideum. Cell Diff.*, 6: 229–239.

Shaffer, B. M. (1975) Secretion of cyclic AMP induced by cyclic AMP in the cellular slime mould *Dictyostelium discoideum. Nature (Lond.)*, 255: 549–552.

Siu, C.-H., Lerner, R. A., Ma, G., Firtel, R. A. and Loomis, W. F. (1976) Developmentally regulated proteins of the plasma membrane of *Dictyostelium discoideum.* The carbohydrate-binding protein. *J. molec. Biol.*, 100: 157–178.

Wick, U., Malchow, D. and Gerisch, G. (1978) Cyclic-AMP stimulated calcium influx into aggregating cells of *Dictyostelium discoideum. Cell Biol. Int. Rep.*, 2: 71–79.

Wurster, B., Schubiger, K., Wick, U. and Gerisch, G. (1977) Cyclic GMP in *Dictyostelium discoideum:* oscillations and pulses in response to folic acid and cyclic AMP signals. *FEBS Lett.*, 76: 141–144.

Wurster, B., Bozzaro, S. and Gerisch, G. (1978) Cyclic GMP regulation and responses of *Polysphondylium violaceum* to chemoattractants. *Cell Biol. Int. Resp.*, 2: 61–69.

Neural Cell Markers: the End of the Beginning

MARTIN C. RAFF, JEREMY P. BROCKES, KAY L. FIELDS and RHONA MIRSKY

Medical Research Council, Neuroimmunology Project, Zoology Department, University College London, London WC1E 6BT (Great Britain)

In order to understand the molecular details of how neural cells interact with each other in the developing and mature nervous system, one will ultimately need to study homogeneous populations of neural cells interacting in vitro. In principle, there are two ways of achieving this: one is to study established neural cell lines, while the other is to find ways of purifying normal neural cells that can be maintained and studied in culture. We have been pursuing the latter approach and have followed the lead of the immunologists who have made use of cell type-specific surface markers for dissecting the cellular complexity of the immune system. Such markers have underpinned the explosive advances in cellular immunology of the last 10 years.

RAT NEURAL ANTIGEN-1 (Ran-1): A SCHWANN CELL-SPECIFIC SURFACE ANTIGEN IN RATS

We began our search for cell type-specific neural markers by inducing a large number of neural tumours in inbred rats with the carcinogen ethylnitrosourea (ENU). When injected into perinatal rats, ENU induces tumours of the central and peripheral nervous system in the majority of animals. We established in vitro cell lines from many of these tumours and attempted to define neural-specific cell surface antigens by raising antibodies in rabbits and mice against the various tumours and cell lines. The remarkable outcome of these immunizations was that most of the antibodies produced reacted with all types of neural and non-neural tissues: not only were the antibodies unable to distinguish between different types of neural cells, they were unable to distinguish neural cells from lymphocytes or liver cells!

Fortunately, one type of antiserum raised in certain strains of mice against a particular cell line (derived from a tumour which arose in the spinal cord and adjacent nerve roots) proved to be interesting (Fields et al., 1975). After adsorption with a variety of non-neural tissues, it reacted with a cell surface antigen that was present on all of the neural tumours, including gliomas, Schwannomas and neuroblastomas but not with non-neural tumours. Moreover, the antigen was present in normal central and peripheral neural tissues but not in significant amounts in non-neural tissues. For this reason it was called rat neural antigen-1, or Ran-1.

In order to determine which normal neural cells expressed Ran-1, we studied its distribution in the simplest of neural cultures – dissociated cells from newborn rat sciatic nerve. In principle, there should be only two major cell types in such cultures – Schwann cells and fibroblasts. To identify the fibroblasts, we used antibody against the Thy-1 cell surface antigen, which was originally defined as an antigen of thymocytes, brain and nerve (Reif and Allen, 1964) and only later was found to be on a variety of other cell types including fibroblasts (Stern, 1973). In indirect immunofluorescence studies with rabbit anti-Thy-1 followed by goat antibody against rabbit immunoglobulin conjugated to fluorescein, we found that approximately 50% of the cells were fluorescent, and all of these looked like fibroblasts. Using mouse anti-Ran-1 followed by goat anti-mouse immunoglobulin conjugated to rhodamine, we again found that about 50% of the cells were labelled, but now most of the labelled cells had the typical bipolar morphology of Schwann cells. When both antisera and conjugates were used together, it was found that all of the cells in the cultures were labelled with either anti-Thy-1 (and fluoresced green) or anti-Ran-1 (and fluoresced red) but never with both. Thus, there are only two cell types in these cultures – Thy-1^+, Ran-1^- fibroblasts and Ran-1^+, Thy-1^- Schwann cells (Brockes et al., 1977).

As we shall see, Ran-1 appears to be present only on Schwann cells and not any other neural or non-neural cell type so far studied. This is surprising since it is present on all types of ENU-induced neural tumours of glial and neuronal origin (Fields et al., 1975). This points up the danger of extrapolating from results with tumours and cell lines to normal cells.

TETANUS TOXIN: A CELL SURFACE MARKER FOR NEURONAL CELLS IN CULTURE

Tetanus toxin has been shown to bind principally to neurones in a variety of peripheral and central neural cultures (Dimpfel et al., 1975; Mirsky et al., 1978). When used in double immunofluorescence assays together with anti-Thy-1 and anti-Ran-1 antibodies on dissociated cell cultures of rat dorsal root ganglia (DRG), it was found that the neurones were tetanus toxin$^+$, Thy-1^+, Ran-1^-, the Schwann cells were Ran-1^+, Thy-1^-, tetanus toxin$^-$, and the fibroblasts were Thy-1^+, tetanus toxin$^-$, Ran-1^-. Thus, by using 3 cell surface markers, the 3 major cell types in DRG cultures can be unambiguously identified (Fields et al., 1978).

While it is clear that the great majority of neurones in cultures of peripheral and central neural tissues in various species are labelled by tetanus toxin, it is not certain whether all neurones label with tetanus toxin. As we shall see, most glial cells and fibroblasts are not labelled by tetanus toxin; however, some fibrous astrocytes in dissociated cell cultures of rat optic nerve are weakly labelled by tetanus toxin, although this is not the case for astrocytes in various other cultures (Raff et al., 1979). Therefore, one must be cautious in using tetanus toxin as a neuronal marker, particularly since some preparations of tetanus toxin label various cell types "non-specifically". In general, this problem can be avoided by purifying the toxin by gel filtration on a G-150 Sephadex column and by high-speed centrifugation prior to use.

GLIAL FIBRILLARY ACIDIC PROTEIN (GFAP): AN INTRACELLULAR MARKER FOR ASTROCYTES

GFAP has been shown to be associated with glial filaments (Schachner et al., 1977) and to be astrocyte-specific in immunofluorescent and immunoperoxidase studies on frozen sections of brain in a variety of species including man (Bignami et al., 1972; Ludwin et al.,

1976). To determine its specificity in neural cells in culture, we have studied its distribution in dissociated cell cultures of various rat neural tissues by indirect immunofluorescence (Raff et al., 1978a); since GFAP is an intracellular antigen, cells must be prefixed in alcohol or acetone in order for the anti-GFAP antibodies to penetrate the cell. We began with optic nerve cultures from 1-week-old rats as these are the simplest central neural cultures, being devoid of neurones.

There are two major morphological cell types in such optic nerve cultures: (i) fibroblastic cells, which are large and flat and have large vesicular nuclei, and (ii) process-bearing cells, which are smaller and darker and have processes which can be long and/or branched. Approximately 20% of the fibroblastic cells and 75% of the process-bearing cells are labelled by anti-GFAP antibody. It seems likely that the former are protoplasmic astrocytes (found mainly in grey matter in vivo) while the latter are fibrous astrocytes (found mainly in white matter). Consistent with this view is the fact that about 50% of GFAP$^+$ cells in cultures of white matter (optic nerve and corpus callosum) are process-bearing, while such cells are rarely seen in cultures of grey matter (such as cerebral cortex).

GFAP$^+$ cells are not found in sciatic nerve or DRG cultures. Moreover, tetanus toxin$^+$ neurones are GFAP$^-$. Thus, it seems probable that GFAP is found only in astrocytes and can be used to identify both fibrous and protoplasmic astrocytes in culture (Raff et al., 1978a).

GALACTOCEREBROSIDE: A CELL SURFACE MARKER FOR OLIGODENDROCYTES

In optic nerve cultures, approximately 25% of the process-bearing cells are GFAP$^-$. Since there are no tetanus toxin$^+$ neurones in these cultures, it seemed likely that such GFAP$^-$ process-bearing cells are oligodendrocytes. That this is the case is suggested by experiments in which antibody against galactocerebroside is used simultaneously in double fluorochrome immunofluorescence assays with anti-GFAP antibody (Raff et al., 1978a). Galactocerebroside is the major glycolipid in myelin (Norton and Autilio, 1966; O'Brien et al., 1967); in fact, whereas the lipid bilayers of most plasma membranes contain only a small amount of glycolipid ($< 5\%$) and at most only trace amounts of galactocerebroside, myelin membrane consists of $> 20\%$ galactocerebroside. In such double labelling experiments, $\sim$ 25% of process-bearing cells in optic nerve cultures label intensely with anti-galactocerebroside and none of these are GFAP$^+$. Since galactocerebroside$^+$ cells are generally not found in cultures of peripheral nervous tissue or non-neural tissue, and tetanus toxin$^+$ neurones are unlabelled by anti-galactocerebroside antibody, it seems likely that galactocerebroside can be used as a specific cell surface marker for oligodendrocytes (Raff et al., 1978a).

Since galactocerebroside is a major lipid in peripheral as well as central myelin, it was surprising to find that cultured Schwann cells were not labelled by anti-galactocerebroside antibody. This may be an in vitro artifact, as Schwann cells freshly isolated from newborn or 9-day-old rat sciatic nerve are galactocerebroside$^+$ but become negative after 24 hr in culture. Why Schwann cells lose their ability to express galactocerebroside in culture while oligodendrocytes do not is unknown.

MICROGLIAL CELLS CAN BE IDENTIFIED BY THEIR Fc RECEPTORS AND PHAGOCYTIC PROPERTIES

Approximately 2% of cells in central neural cultures are labelled in a characteristic vesicular pattern by any fluorescent antibody, including fluorescein-conjugated normal IgG. All such cells are actively phagocytic as judged by their ability to ingest latex beads. If fluorescent antibodies are digested with pepsin to produce $F(ab')_2$ fragments devoid of Fc regions, they no longer label these phagocytic cells, suggesting that the binding of undigested antibody to these cells is mediated by Fc receptors. In these and other properties, such cells are indistinguishable from macrophages found in other tissues. Schwann cells, neurones, astrocytes and oligodendrocytes do not appear to be phagocytic or to have Fc receptors in these assays (Raff et al., 1979b).

STUDYING THE PROPERTIES OF MARKED NEURAL CELL TYPES

Although the morphologies of some neural cell types are, at times, sufficiently distinctive to allow identification by this criterion alone, this is usually not the case. Having markers for the major neural cell types allows one for the first time to unambiguously study some of the properties of these cells in culture. For example, one can study their antigens and glycolipids in double labelling experiments, using one fluorochrome to distinguish the cell type-specific marker and the other to assay for another antigen or a glycolipid. In this way it has been found that (Raff et al., 1979b): (i) Ran-1 is expressed only by Schwann cells and not by other glial or neuronal cells; (ii) Thy-1 is expressed by some neurones but not Schwann cells or oligodendrocytes, while astrocytes are Thy-1^- in cultures less than 7 days old, some of them become Thy-1^+ in longer term cultures (R. Pruss, unpublished); (iii) no neural cells make detectable amounts of the large external transformation-sensitive (LETS) protein in culture; (iv) most neurones and oligodendrocytes have large amounts of GM_1 on their surfaces, while $\sim$ 50% of most other cell types express this ganglioside; (v) the ganglioside GM_3 is found on all oligodendrocytes but not on other neural cell types.

USING ANTIBODIES TO PURIFY SCHWANN CELLS

As has been demonstrated so successfully in immunology, cell surface markers can be used not only for cell identification but also for cell separation. In principle, this can be done by either positive or negative selection. Thus far, negative selection procedures (where cells carrying a specific cell surface marker are eliminated from a mixed population of cells) have been most widely used. We have used this approach to purify Schwann cells.

When dissociated primary cultures of newborn rat sciatic nerve are examined after 1–3 days, approximately half of the cells are Thy-1^+ fibroblasts and half are Ran-1^+ Schwann cells. After 1 week in culture, more than 90% of the cells are fibroblasts. The explanation for this is apparent when one exposes such cultures to [^{3}H]thymidine and combines autoradiography with two fluorochrome immunofluorescence: whereas the great majority of fibroblasts are found to be dividing in such assays, the great majority of Schwann cells are not (Brockes et al., 1977). If these cultures are exposed to a mitotic poison (such as cytosine arabinoside), the majority of fibroblasts are killed while most Schwann cells survive; at the end of 1 week, $\sim$ 85% of cells are now Schwann cells, compared to $<$ 10% in cultures not exposed to cytosine arabinoside. To eliminate the residual 15% of fibroblasts in cytosine arabinoside-treated cultures, cells are removed from the culture dish and treated with anti-Thy-1 antiserum and complement, which kills the fibroblasts but does not affect the Schwann cells, which are Thy-1$^-$. In this way, cultures can be reproducibly obtained which contain ≥ 99.5% Ran-1$^+$ Schwann cells (Brockes et al., 1979). These purified Schwann cells can be maintained in culture for more than 5 months.

In order to obtain large numbers of purified Schwann cells it was necessary to find ways of inducing these cells to divide. We have found that crude extracts of bovine brain or pituitary are potent mitogens for Schwann cells in vitro (Raff et al., 1979a). Moreover, any manoeuvre which elevates cyclic AMP in these cells stimulates them to divide (Raff et al., 1978b). The combination of cholera toxin (which irreversibly activates adenyl cyclase and hence raises intracellular cyclic AMP levels) and pituitary extract has a striking synergistic effect in stimulating Schwann cell proliferation so that these cells double their numbers every 36 h or so, compared to a doubling time of 8–10 days for unstimulated Schwann cells (Raff et al., 1979a). In this way, we have been able to obtain large numbers of purified Schwann cells for biochemical and cell biological studies.

THE FUTURE

Having the major neural cell populations specifically marked is not the end of the neural cell marker story. Nor is it the beginning of the end. If anything, it is the end of the beginning. One can anticipate using these and new markers to purify astrocytes, oligodendrocytes and neurones. New markers may well subdivide the major glial cell types into functional subclasses. Perhaps more importantly, antibodies or other ligands should someday be able to subdivide and separate all neurones according to their different neurotransmitters.

If one can extrapolate from the history of immunology in the last 10 years, then cellular neurobiology is in the process of a revolution. The ability to study purified neural cells in culture should mark the beginning of a new era in neurobiology.

REFERENCES

Bignami, A., Eng, L. F., Dahl, D. and Uyeda, C. T. (1972) Localization of the glial fibrillary acidic protein in astrocytes by immunofluorescence. *Brain Res.*, 43: 429–435.

Brockes, J. P., Fields, K. L. and Raff, M. C. (1977) A surface antigenic marker for rat Schwann cells. *Nature (Lond.)*, 266: 364–366.

Brockes, J. P., Fields, K. L. and Raff, M. C. (1979) Studies on cultured rat Schwann cells. I. Establishment of purified populations from cultures of peripheral nerve. *Brain Res.*, 165: 105–118.

Dimpfel, W., Neale, J. H. and Habermann, E. (1975) ^{125}I-labelled tetanus toxin as a neuronal marker in tissue cultures derived from embryonic CNS. *Naunyn-Schmiedeberg's Arch. exp. Path. Pharmak.*, 290: 329–333.

Fields, K. L., Gosling, C., Megson, M. and Stern, P. L. (1975) New cell surface antigens in rat defined by tumours of the nervous system. *Proc. nat. Acad. Sci. (Wash.)*, 72: 1286–1300.

Fields, K. L., Brockes, J. P., Mirsky, R. and Wendon, L. M. B. (1978) Cell surface markers for distinguishing different types of rat dorsal root ganglion cells in culture. *Cell*, 14: 43–51.

Ludwin, S. K., Kosek, J. C. and Eng, L. F. (1976) The topographical distribution of S-100 and GFA proteins in the adult rat brain: an immunohistochemical study using horseradish peroxidase-labelled antibodies. *J. comp. Neurol.*, 165: 197–208.

Mirsky, R., Wendon, L. M. B., Black, P., Stolkin, C. and Bray, D. (1978) Tetanus toxin: a cell surface marker for neurons in culture. *Brain Res.*, 148: 251–259.

Norton, W. T. and Autilio, L. A. (1966) The lipid composition of purified bovine brain myelin. *J. Neurochem.,* 13: 213–222.

O'Brien, J. S., Sampson, E. L. and Stern, M. B. (1967) Lipid composition of myelin from the peripheral nervous system. *J. Neurochem.,* 14: 357–365.

Raff, M. C., Mirsky, R., Fields, K. L., Lisak, R. P., Dorfman, S. H., Silberberg, D. H., Gregson, N. A., Liebowitz, S. and Kennedy, M. (1978a) Galactocerebroside: a specific cell surface antigen marker for oligodendrocytes in culture. *Nature (Lond.),* 274: 813–816.

Raff, M. C., Hornby-Smith, A. and Brockes, J. P. (1978b) Cyclic AMP as a mitogenic signal for cultured rat Schwann cells. *Nature (Lond.),* 273: 672–674.

Raff, M. C., Abney, E., Brockes, J. P. and Hornby-Smith, A. (1979a) Schwann cell growth factors. *Cell,* 15: 813–822.

Raff, M. C., Fields, K. L., Mirsky, R., Pruss, R. M. and Winter, J. (1979b) Studies on marker-identified rat glial and neuronal cells in culture: antigens, bacterial toxin-binding properties and glycolipids. *Brain Res.,* in press.

Reif, A. E. and Allen, J. M. V. (1964) The AKR thymic antigen and its distribution in leukemias and nervous tissues. *J. exp. Med.,* 120: 413–433.

Schachner, M., Hedley-Whyte, E. T., Hsu, D. W., Schoonmaker, G. and Bignami, A. (1977) Ultrastructural localization of glial fibrillary acidic protein in mouse cerebellum by immuno-peroxidase labelling. *J. Cell Biol.,* 75: 67–73.

Stern, P. L. (1973) Theta alloantigen on mouse and rat fibroblasts. *Nature New Biol.,* 246: 76–78.

Cell Type-Specific Cell Surface Antigens in the Cerebellum

M. SCHACHNER and M. WILLINGER

Department of Neurobiology, Heidelberg University, 6900 Heidelberg (G.F.R.) and Department of Neuroscience, Children's Hospital Medical Center, Boston, Mass. 02115 (U.S.A.)

INTRODUCTION

Cell-cell interactions have been developed to a high degree of precision in the nervous system, since no other organ, to our knowledge, displays a similar wealth of cellular connections diverging and converging from one cell to another in time and space. The coordinations of these cell interactions are important events during the formation of multicellular organisms and may be due to genetic and epigenetic mechanisms. The molecular strategies underlying these phenomena have remained largely obscure, but it is assumed that cells migrate and differentiate by means of diffusible signals (Wolpert, 1969; Gierer and Meinhardt, 1972; Lawrence et al., 1972; McMahon, 1974) or specific cell surface contacts between neighbouring cells (Barbera et al., 1973; Cauldwell et al., 1973; Weinbaum and Burger, 1973; Balsamo and Lilien, 1974; Gottlieb et al., 1974; Hausman and Moscona, 1976; Rutishauser et al., 1976; Barondes, 1978). The question which mechanism might be favoured at particular phases during development will remain one of the intriguing problems for future neurobiological research.

Of the many disparate regions of the central nervous system the cerebellar cortex offers special advantages in the study of cell rearrangements and synaptogenesis (Eccles et al., 1967; Llinás, 1969; Palay and Chan-Palay, 1973). It contains relatively few cell types. The 5 neuronal cell types are granule, Purkinje, Golgi type II, basket and stellate cells. These cell types are organized in relatively simple geometric arrays repeated throughout the cerebellum and are remarkably constant from vertebrate species to species. The major glial cell populations consist of astroglia and oligodendroglia. Astroglia assume two anatomically distinct forms, Golgi epithelial cells with radial processes traversing the molecular layer and fibrous astrocytes in white matter. Accessory cell populations are meningeal, ependymal and endothelial cells, microglia, macrophages and fibroblasts. In mammals some major events in neurone formation and migration as well as overt synaptogenesis take place postnatally so they become easily amenable to experimental analysis. Also, a possible malignant counterpart of cerebellar external granule cells, the medulloblastoma, has been described which may retain some of the properties of normal granule cells (Kadin et al., 1970) and may be propagated in vivo or in vitro as an apparently homogeneous cell population in sufficient quantities for cell biological, biochemical and immunological analysis. In addition, a selective loss of granule cells can be induced by X-irradiation (Altman et al., 1969; Altman and Anderson, 1972), drug injection (Matsumoto et al., 1972; Nathanson et al., 1969) and infection with viruses (Herndon et al., 1971). In the mouse, a number of mutants show selective neuronal death in the cerebellum, perhaps based on developmental abnormalities in cell-cell interaction (Sidman et al., 1965; Sidman, 1972; Rakic and Sidman, 1973; Privat et al., 1979).

Crucial to the investigation of cell-cell interactions in the cerebellar cortex is the availability of preparative amounts of isolated populations of a particular cell type with a high degree of homogeneity and morphological integrity. Methods have been described for the separation and enrichment of classes of cerebellar cell types by sedimentation and centrifugation techniques (Barkley et al., 1973; Sellinger et al., 1974; Cohen et al., 1978). However, cell populations which meet the criteria of morphological, biochemical and pharmacological homogeneity are not achieved by these methods. Several reasons led to the assumption that a combination of immunological and molecular biological techniques could achieve this aim.

Immunological tools have been shown to be sensitive and specific probes for the composition of cell surfaces in various differentiative systems, the most well characterized of which is the mouse lymphoid system in its normal and malignant states (see for instance Boyse and Old, 1969). The serological approach to the investigation of neural cell surfaces was attempted in our laboratory to search for cell surface components not only unique to nervous tissue, but also to a particular cell class and a particular developmental event. This approach is potentially a very versatile one, and its possibilities can be summarized as follows:

(1) Antibodies permit identification and immunological characterization of new and sometimes minor cell surface constituents which are expressed in the developing and adult nervous system.

(2) Antibodies may serve as assay reagents to analyze the molecular nature of the corresponding antigens characterized initially by purely immunological methods (see (1)). These antigens can then be isolated and purified by affinity chromatography by means of antibody coupled to solid-state carriers.

(3) When coupled to visual tags (fluorescein, ferritin, peroxidase, gold, and others) antibodies can be used to define the cellular and subcellular distribution of antigens in histological sections. In view of the fact that nerve cells are organized in specialized domains of functional and structural properties (for instance, pre- and postsynaptic sites, axon, dendrite, cell body) visually labelled antibodies are of particular value in probing for the topographical distribution of antigens.

(4) Cell type-specific antibodies can be used to isolate antigen-positive and -negative cell types from their mixtures, provided that cells can be obtained as single cell suspensions. The unique advantage of surface antigens is that antibody can bind to live cells without destroying their integrity and viability. In contrast, intracellular antigens only become accessible to antibody after disrupting the plasma membrane for instance by aldehyde fixation or lipid extraction. After such treatment cells are naturally of reduced value for structural and functional characterization.

(5) Antibodies may serve as modifiers of functional properties of the molecules they combine with (Gluecksohn-Waelsch, 1957; Brent, 1966; Williams, 1969; DeRobertis et al., 1971; Köhler and Melchers, 1972; Menge et al., 1974; Rutishauser et al., 1976; Brackenbury et al., 1977; Kemler et al., 1977; Thiery et al., 1977). Since the influence of antibodies on cell surface constituents can be monitored on intact cells, various physiological and cell biological functions can be assayed in vitro and even in vivo. Of particular interest in regard to the study of cell surface interactions is the adhesion and aggregation behaviour of dissociated neural cells (Moscona, 1965; Roth, 1968; Walther et al., 1973; Gottlieb et al., 1974; Brackenbury et al., 1977; Stallcup, 1977; Thiery et al., 1977).

In the past, antisera were raised for these purposes by immunization with whole cells or crude membrane fractions and, less frequently, with purified proteins. Even in the fortunate cases, when highly purified compounds are used as antigens, the antiserum's specificity for only a single molecular species cannot be guaranteed. Recently, a novel refinement in the production of highly specific antisera has been introduced by Köhler and Milstein (1975, 1976). The approach is based on the fact that a single, immunocompetent cell committed to synthesize a single immunoglobulin species can be made immortal by somatic cell genetic manipulations: a normal lymphoid cell committed to specific antibody production against a particular antigen can be induced to proliferate and continuously synthesize this particular immunoglobulin by fusion with a myeloma cell, the malignant counterpart of antibody secreting cells. The normal lymphoid cell has been primed in vivo by active immunisation. The myeloma partner in the fusion hybrid can be selected such that it is inhibited from secreting functional immunoglobulins, but does not suppress the synthesis of the normal cell's specific immunoglobulins. Since a normal antibody synthesizing cell is designed to produce only one single kind of antibody molecule with an immutable amino acid sequence and protein structure, monoclonal and furthermore monospecific antibodies can be obtained, even if complex mixtures of antigens, like whole cells or brain parts are used. These antibodies do not only react with a single molecular species but may also distinguish between different haptenic sites on a particular molecule. The application of this methodology will usher an unprecedented improvement of precision in neuroimmunology, which has hitherto not been attained with conventionally prepared antisera.

LIST OF CELL TYPE-SPECIFIC CEREBELLAR ANTIGENS

In spite of the expected limited usefulness of conventionally prepared antisera in the detection of differences among neural cell types, several antigenic cell surface markers have been identified which distinguish among cerebellar cell populations.

Several methods were used to characterize the cell type specificity of cell surface markers. Cell surface localization of the markers is unequivocally identified by the complement dependent cytotoxicity test using live single cells as the antigen carrying targets (see for instance Schachner et al., 1975). Visually, these markers can also be detected by labelling the antisera with fluorescein, peroxidase or gold which can be recognized at the light or electron microscopic levels. These visual labels can be applied to single cells freshly dispersed from the intact cerebellar tissue, to cells cultured in vitro under monolayer conditions or to tissue sections, where correlation between label and cell type can be achieved. Another approach is to physically isolate cerebellar cells by virtue of a particular cell surface marker and assaying the isolated cell populations for expression of independent biochemical markers such as S-100 (Moore, 1965; Moore and Perez, 1968), glial fibrillary acidic protein (Eng et al., 1971; Bignami et al., 1972), neurofilament protein (Shelanski et al., 1971; Davison and Winslow, 1974; Schlaepfer and Lynch, 1977; Schachner et al., 1978a) or enzymes known to be restricted to certain cell types.

By a combination of these methods several cell surface antigens have been attributed to the glial and neuronal populations in the cerebellum (Tables I and II). Oligodendrocytes are characterized by the presence of NS-1 antigen (Schachner, 1974; Schachner and Willinger, 1979), galactocerebroside (Rapport and Graf, 1969; Schachner and Willinger, 1979), "corpus callosum antigen" (Schachner et al., 1977), antigens detected by serum from animals with experimental allergic encephalomyelitis (EAE) (Schachner and Willinger, 1979) and the

TABLE I

CELLULAR DISTRIBUTION OF ANTIGENS IN TISSUE SECTIONS OF 8-DAY-OLD AND ADULT CEREBELLUM

	NS-1	*Galacto-cerebroside*	*Myelin basic protein*	*Corpus callosum antigen*	*NS-4*	*Cholera toxin binding site (G_{M1} ganglio-side)*	*Tetanus toxin binding site (G_{D1b} and G_{T1} gangliosides)*	*LETS*
Neurone	–	–	–	–	+	+	+	–
Astrocyte	–	–	–	+	–	–	–	–
Oligodendro-cyte	+	+	+	+	–	–	–	–
Meninges	–	–	–	–	–	–	–	+
Choroid plexus	–	–	–	–	–	–	–	+

cholera toxin binding site which is identified as G_{M1} ganglioside. "Corpus callosum antigen" is also expressed on cell surfaces of astroglia and is therefore a marker for all macroglia. All classes of neuronal cells are characterized by the presence of cholera toxin and tetanus toxin binding sites which represent G_{M1} ganglioside (Cuatrecasas, 1973; Holmgren et al., 1975; Mullin et al., 1976) and gangliosides G_{D1b} and G_{T1} (Van Heyningen, 1963), respectively. NS-4 antigen can also be taken as neuronal marker since, like some of the other markers listed above, it seems to be represented more on neuronal than on glial cells. A distinction between the neuronal cell types, granule, Purkinje, Golgi type II, stellate and basket cells has so far not been possible by immunological methods.

Endothelial cells, choroid epithelial cells, leptomeningeal cells and fibroblasts are characterized in tissue sections by the presence of LETS (large external transformation sensitive protein) on their surfaces (Schachner et al., 1978b). In vitro the protein is confined to cells with epithelioid and fibroblastic morphology.

TABLE II

CELLULAR DISTRIBUTION OF ANTIGENS IN MONOLAYER CULTURES OF 7-DAY-OLD CEREBELLUM

+++ = strongly positive immunofluorescence; ++ = moderately positive immunofluorescence; + = weakly positive immunofluorescence; – = undetectable immunofluorescence

	NS-1	*Galacto-cerebroside*	*Myelin basic protein*	*Corpus callosum antigen*	*NS-4*	*Cholera toxin binding site (G_{M1} ganglio-side)*	*Tetanus toxin binding site (G_{D1b} and G_{T1} gangliosides)*	*LETS*
Neurone	–	–	–	–	+++	+++	+++	–
Astrocyte	–	–	–	++	++	++ (only few astrocytes are positive)	+	–
Oligodendro-cyte	+++	+++	–	+++	++	+++	–	–
Fibroblast	–	–	–	–	–	–	–	+++

It is interesting that the distribution of cell surface markers among cell types is not the same when assayed at several stages of development with cerebellar cells under monolayer conditions in vitro or in tissue sections. These differences can be recognized by comparing Tables I and II. Particularly salient is the finding that several neuronal markers (gangliosides G_{M1}, G_{D1b}, G_{T1} and NS-4 antigen) are not detectable on glial cells in histological sections, although in vitro they can be detected on some but not all glial cells.

The evidence for these findings will be described and discussed in the following paragraphs.

GLIAL MARKER

The oligodendroglial marker NS-1 antigen was the first of several neural cell surface antigens described in this laboratory (Table II). A glial tumour of putative oligodendrocytic origin was used as source of antigen. We and others (Akeson and Herschman, 1974; Martin, 1974; Fields et al., 1975; Raff et al., 1979) have turned to the use of tumours as sources of antigens because they may retain some properties characteristic of normal cells, because they grow in relatively homogeneous form, and because the cells are available in preparative amounts. It was hoped that tumours would circumvent a major difficulty in delineating antigenic surface components that distinguish among classes of brain cells because populations of normal neural cells are not pure. Indeed, one is caught in a vicious circle since very pure cell populations would be needed as antigens in order to raise specific antisera, while at the same time the immunological approach itself is expected to provide the desired cell separations. NS-1 is expressed on malignant as well as normal oligodendroglia, but not expressed on non-neural cells, astroglia or neurones. Other cell surface antigens, for instance NS-3, NS-6 and NS-7 are not differentially expressed among cell types, while NS-2 and NS-5 antigens have not yet been characterized completely with respect to their cell type specificity.

In the adult cerebellum NS-1 is localized exclusively in white matter tracts (Fig. 1). At the end of a cerebellar folium the antigen can be visualized in fine finger-like tracts, probably corresponding to myelinated fibres, which extend into the adjacent granular layer. In cultures of cerebellar cells obtained by enzymatic dispersion of the solid tissue and maintained under monolayer conditions for several days in vitro, a particular cell type constituting between 3–5% of the total cell population is antigen-positive. This particular cell type displays several distinct morphological characteristics. Cell bodies are surrounded by an extensive network of cellular processes which extend concentrically around the cell body. Cellular processes emerge from the cell body as rather thin fibres or as broader flattened processes which elongate into thin web-like structures. Often, a cell elaborates out of this web a single process leaving the concentric network to seek, as it seems, a cellular target around which another network of multiple fine and short fibres is developed. Cell body and cellular processes express antigen in comparable amounts. To prove that the antibody reaction is antigen specific absorption of anti-NS-1 antiserum with cells of oligodendroglioma G26, the tumour carrying NS-1 antigen, and with NS-1 antigen-negative tissues like liver, spleen and thymus are carried out. Only oligodendroglioma G26 absorbs antiserum activity removing all positive immunofluorescence of the labelled cells.

Another antibody, anti-cholera toxin antibody, was applied to cerebellar cell cultures after a short incubation with cholera toxin, to localize the cholera toxin binding site, G_{M1} ganglioside. When these antibodies absorbed onto colloid gold are used, the "hairy eye ball"

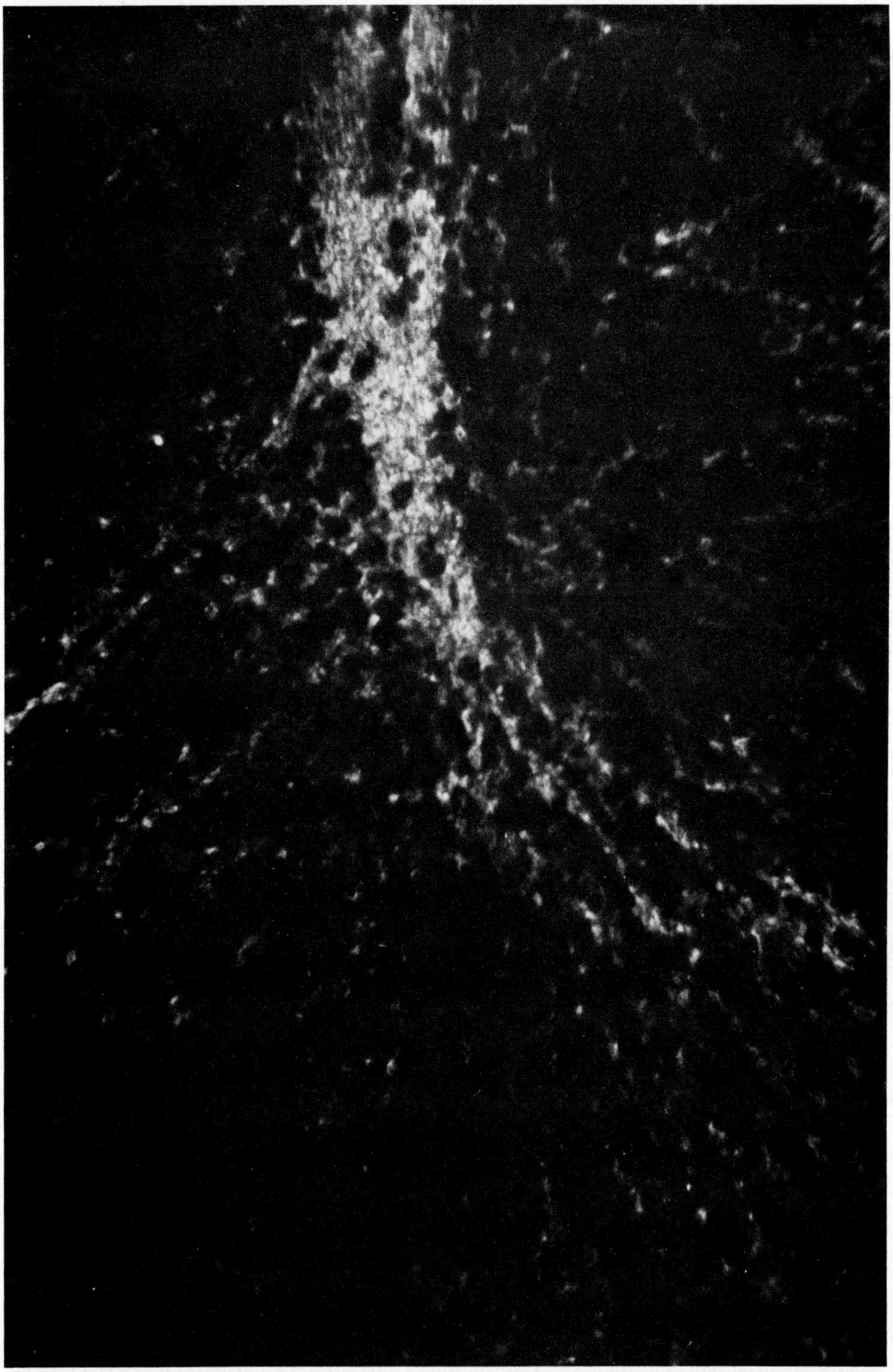

Fig. 1. Immunohistological localization of NS-1 antigen. Sagittal sections of fresh frozen adult mouse cerebellum were incubated with anti-NS-1 serum and then with goat anti-mouse immunoglobulin coupled to fluorescein isothiocyanate (GAM-FITC). Fluorescence is only visible in white matter tracts. Molecular, granular and Purkinje cell layers are antigen-negative.

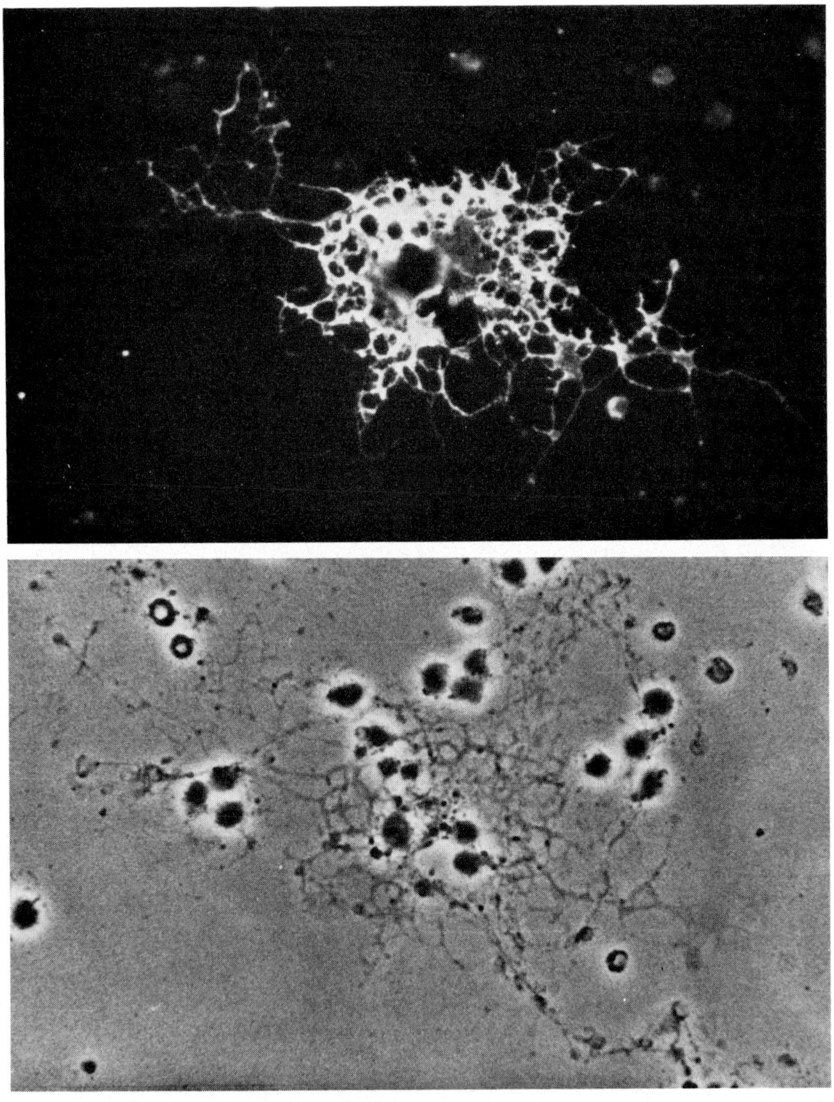

Fig. 2. Localization of NS-1 antigen on the cell surface of an oligodendrocyte in culture. Indirect immunofluorescence was carried out as described under Fig. 1. Specific labelling of a particular cell type, the "hairy eye ball" cell, is also seen with anti-galactocerebroside (a gift of Dr. M. M. Rapport) serum and serum from an animal with experimental allergic encephalomyelitis.

cell can be simultaneously examined for subcellular distribution of antigen on the cell surface and intracellular cytological features (Fig. 3). The particular cell in Fig. 3 is characterized by a rather small cell body which is almost completely filled with a cell nucleus leaving scanty cytoplasm characteristic of oligodendrocytes in vivo. It is noteworthy, however, that the cytoplasm lacks the characteristic electron-dense textures found in tissue sections. Also, these cells which are presumably oligodendrocytes carry many processes, contrary to the suggestion inherent in the name oligodendrocyte, a cell with a small number of extensions. NS-1 is a differentiation antigen (Boyse and Old, 1969) since it has not been detected in peri- or prenatal cerebellum.

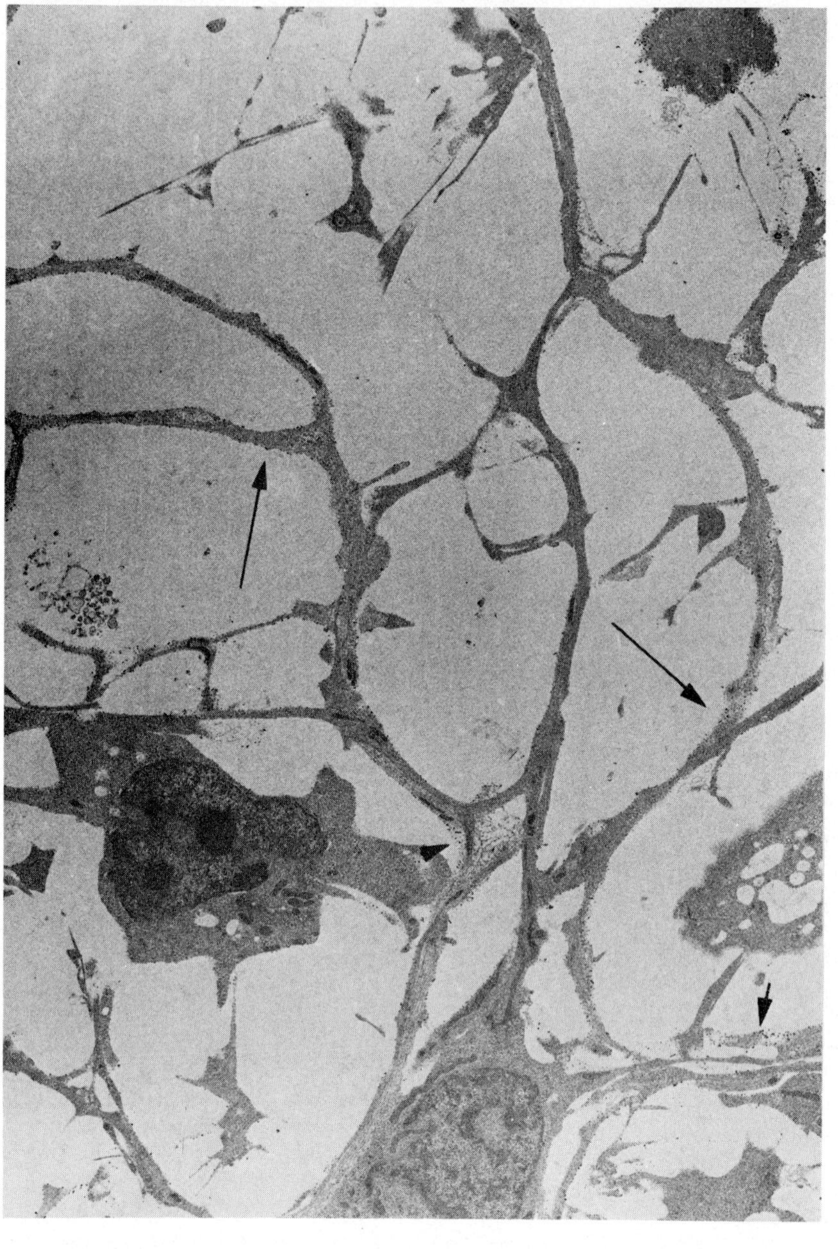

Fig. 3. Transmission electron micrograph of oligodendrocyte stained for the presence of cholera toxin binding sites. Cerebellar cells from postnatal day 6 mice were cultured for 48 hr on a polylysine substrate. They were incubated with 25 μg/ml choleragenoid (a gift of Dr. R. A. Finkelstein), fixed and reacted with rabbit anti-cholera toxin (a gift of Dr. V. R. Zurawski, Jr.), followed by goat IgG directed against rabbit IgG coupled to colloidal gold particles (20 nm in diameter). Note the particles (arrows) coating the fine extensions of this presumptive oligodendrocyte. Magn., × 6000.

Two other cell surface components, galactocerebroside and antigens detected by serum from animals with experimental allergic encephalomyelitis (EAE), show labelling patterns identical with NS-1 antigen (Schachner and Willinger, 1979). In tissue sections of adult and early postnatal cerebellum these antigens are confined exclusively to white matters tracts with no label seen in astroglia. Between 3–5% of cells freshly dispersed or maintained in culture for several days express the two antigens. As in the case of NS-1 the antigen-positive cell is characterized by a "hairy eye ball" morphology. Specificity of the reaction is proven by absorption of the two sera with galactocerebroside mixed together with the appropriate auxiliary lipids; gangliosides or oligodendroglioma G26 are not effective in removing antiserum activity.

Galactocerebroside is known to be uniquely expressed by oligodendrocytes in vivo. It is part of the myelin sheath which is elaborated during development and contributes to the adult physiological properties of the neurone (Davidson and Peters, 1970). Serum from a rabbit who showed clinical signs of EAE (Kies and Alvord, 1959) with degeneration of myelin and oligodendroglia, but no other cell types, also shows this preference for oligodendroglia. Since all 3 antigens, NS-1, galactocerebroside and EAE, show the same labelling pattern it is likely that they react with the same cell type, the oligodendrocyte.

"Corpus callosum" antigen is a cell surface antigen detected by an antiserum from rabbits injected with white matter dissected from bovine corpus callosum (Schachner et al., 1977). The antiserum recognizes an antigen or set of antigens shared by oligodendrocytes and astrocytes but by no other organ in the mouse. In histological sections of adult cerebellum a predominant labelling of myelin tracts is seen by immunofluorescence, while Golgi epithelial cells and their processes, the Bergmann fibres, are only faintly visible. In the young postnatal cerebellum and at prenatal ages from embryonic day 14 onwards these two glial cell types express the antigen in quantities comparable to the adult cerebellum. In contrast to NS-1 and galactocerebroside the corpus callosum antigen is therefore not only present on differentiating or differentiated glial cells, but also on their precursors. In freshly dissociated early postnatal cerebellar cell populations and cultured cells, both oligodendrocytes and astroglia display the antigen on their cell surfaces. When double labelling experiments are performed with anti-glial fibrillary acidic protein antibody (Schachner et al., 1978a) specific for astrocytes (labelled with rhodamine) and corpus callosum antibody (labelled with fluorescein), no cell is easily distinguished which is labelled by only one of these antisera. A similar situation holds true when rhodamine-labelled NS-1 antiserum is used as second marker specific for oligodendroglia. Again, the "hairy eye ball" cell type appears labelled with the two dyes.

Corpus callosum antiserum has been used to separate oligodendro- and astroglia from neurones in freshly dispersed cells from 10-day-old mouse cerebellum (Campbell et al., 1977). The isolation of glial cells was achieved by the fluorescence activated cell sorting apparatus (FACS). Cells were separated on a single cell basis using a fluorescence signal associated with a particular cell as the parameter which allows a physical isolation from non-fluorescent cells. Cerebellar cells labelled by indirect immunofluorescence with corpus callosum antiserum were processed by the sorting machine and two cell populations were obtained, one carrying the fluorescent label to more than 99% purity, indicating a high degree of fidelity in the sorting process, and an antigen- and therefore fluorescence-negative, cell population, also with a purity of more than 99%. Both cell populations are viable by two criteria: that of trypan blue exclusion, with more than 90% of the sorted cells excluding the dye, and that of survival in culture for up to a week, when sorting was carried out under sterile conditions. A plating efficiency of 30–50% is observed for the antigen-negative and antigen-positive cell fractions,

TABLE III

	NS-1 *Mouse anti-glioma G26*	*NS-2* *Rabbit anti-glioblastoma*	*NS-3* *Rabbit anti-neuroblastoma*	*NS-4* *Rabbit anti-cerebellum*	*NS-5* *Mouse anti-cerebellum*	*NS-6* *Mouse anti-MUNTAD**	*NS-7* *Rabbit anti-MUNTAD**
Reference	(Schachner, 1974)	(Schachner and Carnow, 1975; Yuan et al., 1977)	(Schachner and Wortham, 1975; Doyle et al., 1977)	(Schachner, 1974; Schachner et al., 1976, 1977; Goridis et al., 1978a, b)	(Zimmermann and Schachner, 1976; Zimmermann et al., 1976)	(Chaffee and Schachner, 1978a)	(Chaffee and Schachner, 1978b)
Brain							
Adult	+	+	+	+	+	+	+
Foetal	–	–	–	+	+	+	+
Retina	–	–	+	+	+	+	+
Kidney	–	–	+	– (+)**	+	+	+
Sperm	–	–	–	+	+	+	+
Other tissues	–	–	–	–	–	–	–

* MUNTAD = mouse undifferentiated tumour adenovirus induced.
** Sera from some, but not all rabbits react with kidney.

respectively. These results compare favourably with unfractionated cells where we observe a plating efficiency of ± 50%. The antigen-positive cells carrying antibody on their cell surfaces shed these antibodies within 16 hr in vitro by metabolic turnover of the corresponding antigens, as has been observed before with other cell types.

In addition to preserving the viability of the sorted cells the sorter does not preferentially select for a particular cell type during the sorting process. This can be shown by comparing the per cent of antigen-positive cells in the total cell population before and after sorting. In both cases does the antigen-positive cell fraction amount to about 7% of the total cell population.

Since debris and cell clumps in the cell suspension to be sorted can clog the cell sorting machinery, considerable attention has to be paid to avoid these. To achieve removal of dead cells, cellular debris and cell clumps a bovine serum albumin (BSA) step gradient was introduced which by itself already achieves an enrichment of cell classes of the cerebellum (Campbell et al., 1977). A dual purpose is therefore effected by the BSA step gradient procedure which increases both efficiency and rate of sorting, especially in cases where minor cell populations are to be isolated.

To prove that the "corpus callosum" antigen-positive cell fraction is indeed enriched in properties known to be specific for oligodendro- and astroglia, a biochemical analysis of the non-separated fraction (fraction C in Table IV) and the separated cell populations was carried out. CNPase (2′,3′-cyclic nucleotidophosphohydrolase) was chosen as a marker, because it is present in oligodendrocytes in very high levels. S-100 and glial fibrillary acidic protein were used as markers for astrocytes. An enrichment of these 3 markers in the antigen-positive cell population was in fact observed (Table IV). If sorting would be carried out using rhodamine as a label for oligodendroglia in addition to the fluorescein-labelled anti-corpus callosum serum, the isolation of pure astro- and oligodendroglial cell populations could be envisaged.

TABLE IV

DETERMINATION OF CNPase ACTIVITY, S-100 AND GFA PROTEIN IN CEREBELLAR CELL POPULATIONS SORTED WITH ANTI-CORPUS CALLOSUM ANTISERUM

Values for sorted cells represent the average from two experiments. (From Campbell et al., 1977.)

	CNPase (*μmoles/hr/10⁶ cells*)	*GFA protein* (*% positive cells*)	*S-100 protein* (*% positive cells*)
Antigen-positive fraction	0.27	27.5	12.0
Antigen-negative fraction	0.05	0	0
Fraction C	0.12	< 1	< 1

LETS ANTIGEN AS A MARKER FOR NON-NEURAL CELLS

Before discussing the neuronal markers, cell populations present in the cerebellum which do not belong to the glial or neuronal cell types will be briefly described. LETS (large external transformation sensitive) protein has shown to be a particularly useful cell surface marker for these populations (Schachner et al., 1978b). In histological sections of developing

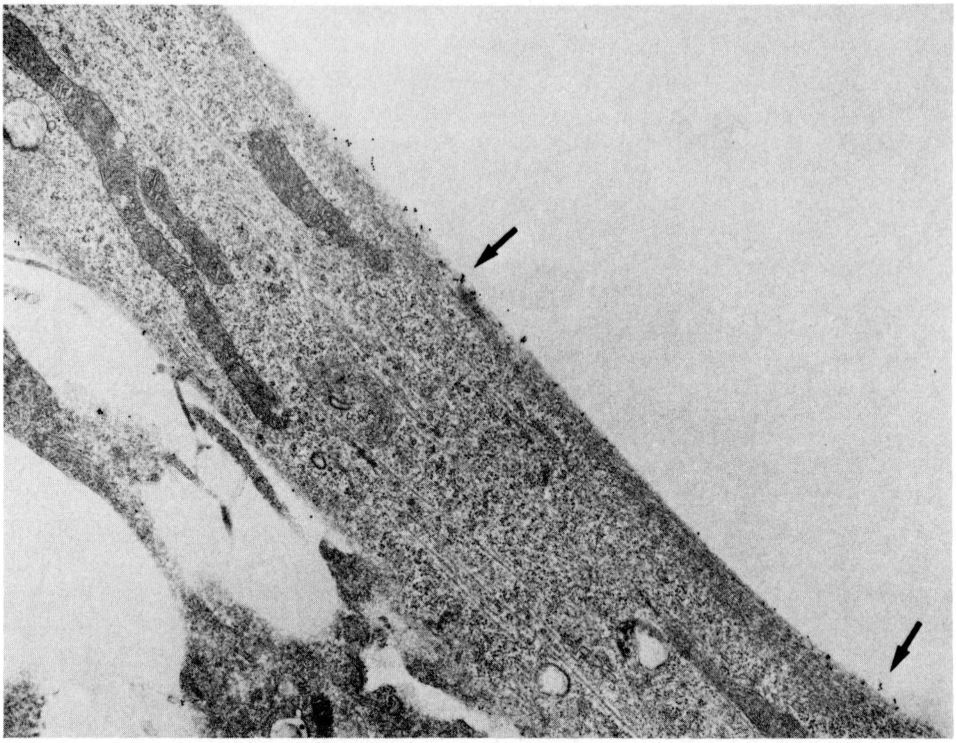

Fig. 4. Transmission electron micrograph of fibroblast stained for LETS protein. Cerebellar cells from postnatal day 6 mice were cultured for 48 hr on a polylysine substrate. They were fixed with 3.5% paraformaldehyde and reacted with rabbit anti-LETS protein (a gift of Dr. R. Hynes) followed by goat IgG directed against rabbit IgG coupled to colloidal gold particles (20 nm in diameter). Note the patches of gold along the surface of the fibroblast (arrows). Magn., × 24,000.

and adult cerebellum LETS has been localized on endothelial cells, choroid epithelial cells, leptomeningeal cells and fibroblasts. Furthermore, in vitro neither glial nor neuronal cells express LETS protein when dissociated cerebellar cells are cultured under monolayer conditions. LETS-positive cell populations cannot be distinguished from each other in vitro by purely morphological criteria. All seem to appear with a fibroblastic and epithelioid morphology and can amount to a sizeable percentage of the total cells depending on the cell preparation and timespan elapsed after plating in vitro. Ultrastructurally these epithelioid cells are all LETS-positive and show the cytological characteristics of fibroblasts (Fig. 4).

The fact that anti-LETS serum uniquely stains these fibroblast-like cells can again be exploited for cell isolation. Since LETS protein is enzymatically removed from cells by trypsin treatment carried out to disperse cerebellar cells, time has to be allowed in culture for LETS protein to regenerate on the cell surface. After 16–24 hr in vitro LETS is expressed again on fibroblasts. If anti-LETS serum is then used in the presence of complement these cells are selectively killed and cellular remainders removed by short trypsinisation. After two cycles of a combination of cytotoxic kill and trypsinisation at intervals of 16–24 hr all fibroblasts can be removed from the culture and thus do not constitute a contaminating and quickly proliferating cell population in cerebellar cultures.

Macrophages, a cell population not easily detectable under normal conditions in histological sections, are recognizable in vitro by their distinct ultrastructural characteristics. All immunoglobulins of the IgG class attach to the macrophage's cell surface by virtue of the Fc receptor. Therefore all macrophages bind immunoglobulins and appear labelled by the indirect immunofluorescence method. When indirect methods are used in complement-mediated immunocytolysis, macrophages are automatically removed.

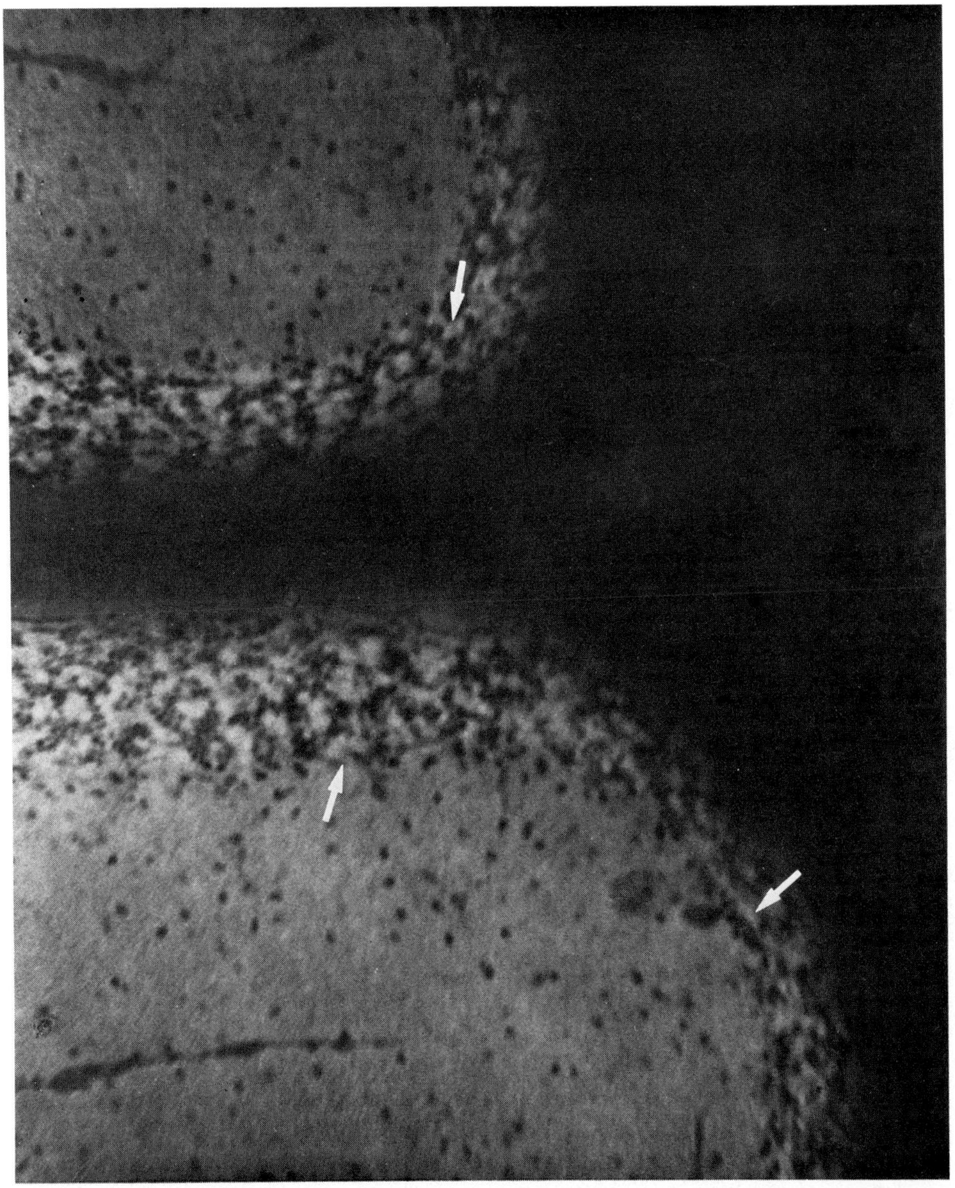

Fig. 5. Fluorescence micrograph of NS-4 antigen in sagittal section of adult mouse cerebellum. Indirect immunofluorescence shows no label in white matter. Molecular, granular and Purkinje cell layers are antigen-positive. Synaptic glomeruli in the granular layer are strongly labelled (arrows).

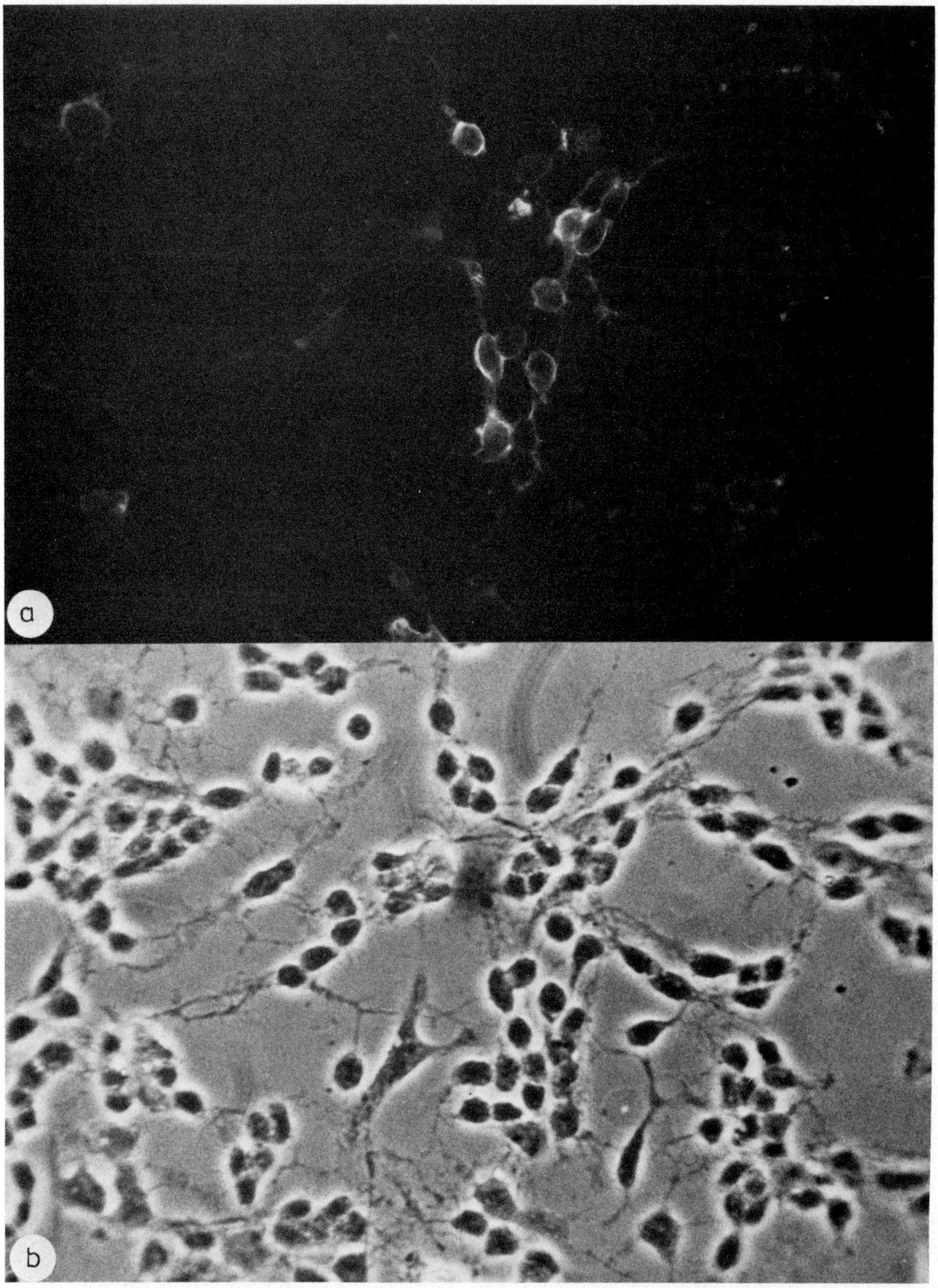

Fig. 6. Cultured cerebellar cells stained for the presence of G_{M1} ganglioside. Cerebellar cells from 6-day-old mice were cultured 24 hr, incubated with choleragenoid and fixed. Choleragenoid was detected on the cell surface by indirect immunofluorescence. Granule cells stain with varying intensity while fibroblasts and astroglia are devoid of stain. (a) fluorescence; (b) phase contrast.

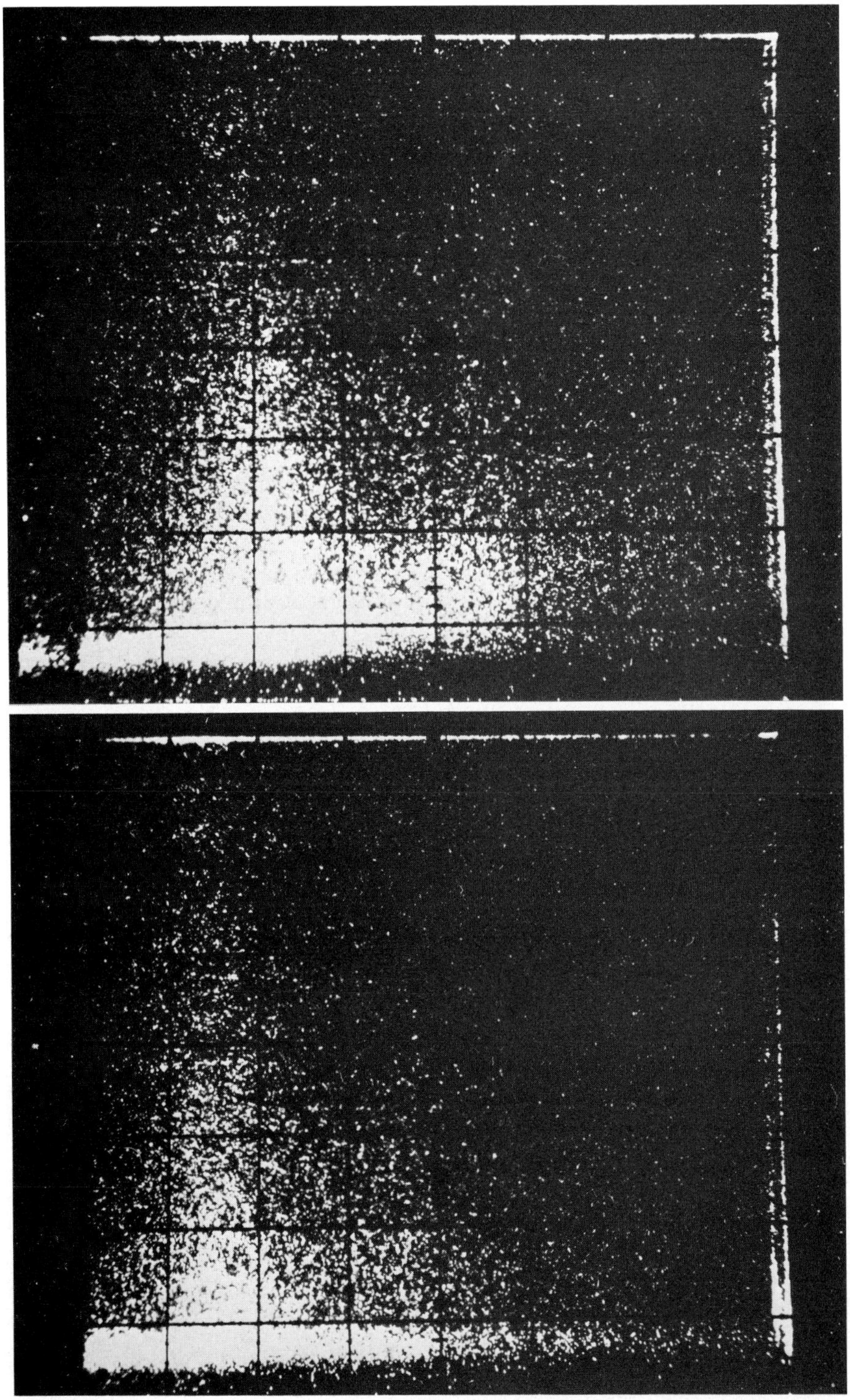

Fig. 7. Cytofluorograph display of dissociated cerebellar cells incubated with cholera toxin, anti-toxin and FITC-goat IgG anti-rabbit IgG. A sample of 50,000 cells, each dot representing a cell, is plotted as a function of fluorescence intensity (ordinate) vs. light scatter (abscissa). Upper panel: cerebellar cells from 7-day-old mouse. Lower panel: cerebellar cells from a newborn mouse.

NEURONAL MARKERS

In this section cell surface antigens and constituents will be described which are uniquely localized on neuronal cells when assayed for in histological sections. NS-4 antigen and gangliosides G_{M1}, G_{D1b} and G_{T1} have been investigated in these respects. Some representation on glial cell is apparent, however, when these cell surface components are tested in vitro. Although these cell surface components are present to some extent on non-neuronal cells, and cannot be called neuronal markers in a strict sense, they have served for practical purposes a worthwhile role in the isolation of pure cerebellar cell populations.

NS-4 (see Table III, also for references) is an antigen present in higher amounts in foetal than in adult brain. The antiserum is obtained by injecting rabbits with crude particulate fractions of cerebellum from 4-day-old C57BL6/J mice. The antigen is present in all brain parts, but cerebellum and retina express relatively higher levels. Other adult tissues are negative, except egg, sperm and kidney. In our first characterization of NS-4 antigen (Schachner et al., 1975) kidney was found to be antigen-negative and this clearly distinguished it from NS-5 which was recognized by an antiserum similarly prepared in C3H.SW/Sn mice (Zimmermann and Schachner, 1976). However, subsequent immunizations in 8 rabbits have shown that kidney is positive for NS-4 antigen with antisera from some rabbits but not from others. This aspect will need further investigation using monoclonal antibodies.

The presence of NS-4 antigen in developing neuroectoderm was traced back to embryonic day 9. At cleavage and trophoblast stages NS-4 is surprisingly found to be present on all cells of the early mouse embryo (Solter and Schachner, 1976). It is also expressed on the unfertilized egg and sperm. A line of primitive teratocarcinoma cells also carries specificities shared with NS-4 (Goridis et al., 1978b). The biochemical characterization of NS-4 antigen from cerebellar cells reveals two polypeptides of approximately 200,000 and 145,000 daltons which can be labelled by the lactoperoxidase catalysed radioiodination reaction and which are degraded by exposing live cells to low concentrations of trypsin (Goridis et al., 1978a).

In histological sections of the adult cerebellum NS-4 is completely confined to the molecular, Purkinje and granule cell layers (Fig. 5) (Schachner et al., 1976). Granule and Purkinje cell bodies are distinctly outlined as antigen-positive. More strikingly, the molecular layer consisting of granule cell processes and the synaptic glomeruli are highly antigen-positive. A remarkable feature of the developing cerebellum is that non-differentiated granule cells in the external granular layer carry less NS-4 antigen than differentiated post-mitotic granule cells in the internal granular layer, when examined in histological sections of 8-day-old cerebellum. Monolayer cultures of 8-day-old cerebellum show a preferred labelling of neuronal cells over glial cells, while fibroblast-like cells appear completely antigen-negative. Both, astro- and oligodendroglia are weakly labelled by anti-NS-4 antiserum while neuronal cell types carry higher levels of the antigen.

Cholera toxin has also been shown to attach selectively to particular cerebellar cell types (Willinger and Schachner, 1978). The G_{M1} binding subunit of cholera toxin, choleragenoid, has been used in our experiments to rule out any interaction with adenylate cyclase. Toxin binding sites were detected by incubating the target tissue with toxin, then with anti-toxin antibody and finally with fluorescent anti-immunoglobulin label. As has been observed by others (De Baecque et al., 1976) G_{M1} ganglioside is localized only on neuronal cells.

However, G_{M1} has also been detected on glial cells in histological sections of other brain parts (Manuelidis and Manuelidis, 1976; Hansson et al., 1977). In cultures of 7-day-old cerebellum, some astrocytes as specified by their expression of glial fibrillary acidic protein carry G_{M1} ganglioside. Oligodendroglia are highly G_{M1}-positive, while fibroblasts are completely antigen-negative. In general, granule cells are antigen-positive but, after 24 hr in vitro some granule cells (Fig. 6) are labelled more intensely than others. This differential labelling intensity is also observed when freshly trypsinized and mono-disperse cerebellar cells of two different ages, postnatal day 0 and day 7 are tested for quantity of G_{M1} on the cell surface as a function of light scatter (Fig. 7). At day 0 a class of fluorescent cells is visible as shown by the lower frequency profile in Fig. 7. Each white dot represents a fluorescent cell in a total cell population of 50,000 measured cells. At postnatal day 7 (upper profile in Fig. 7) the quantity of choleragenoid binding sites is increased on the major cell population, and a second population appears which is less fluorescent than the major population. This population may represent immature granule cells since a burst of neuroblast division occurs at this time. Two additional lines of evidence support the concept that G_{M1} increases on the cell surface with granule cell differentiation. Examination of histological sections incubated with choleragenoid followed by indirect immunofluorescence reveals that the external side of the external granule cell layer of 8-day-old cerebellum is relatively unstained compared with the internal half, consisting of postmitotic cells ready to migrate to the internal granule cell layer. Postmitotic granule cells were shown to acquire G_{M1} ganglioside by a more definitive technique. Mice were injected with [^{3}H]thymidine and sacrificed 3 hr or 3 days later. In the former case only the external matrix cells are labelled; in the latter cells in the external layer and most in the internal layer are labelled with the internal granule cells having the most label. Cerebellar cells are cultured from mice injected in this manner and scored simultaneously for the presence of [^{3}H]thymidine by autoradiography and ganglioside by immunofluorescence. None of the external matrix cells (cells labelled for 3 hr) possesses cholera toxin binding sites. On the other hand, 70% of the toxin-positive cells of the animal injected 3 days earlier contain [^{3}H]thymidine. Therefore the differential labelling of granule cells observed in dissociated cell preparations and at early times in vitro probably reflects in vivo development (Willinger and Schachner, 1979).

TABLE V

IMMUNOLYSIS OF CEREBELLAR CELLS WHICH CONTAIN G_{M1} GANGLIOSIDE

The number of cells containing glial fibrillary acidic protein divided by the total numbers of cells. Immunolysis was performed on P8 cerebellar cells cultured 44 hr. The residual cells are fibroblasts.

Treatment	*Astroglial cells (%)*
1. BSA + anti-toxin + complement	7.2
2. Choleragenoid + complement	6.25
3. Choleragenoid + Anti-toxin	5.6
4. Choleragenoid + anti-toxin + complement	69.0

Antiserum to cholera toxin can be cytotoxic for the toxin-positive cells in the presence of complement and after exposure to choleragenoid (Table V). Cells carrying toxin binding sites can be drastically reduced in culture and a 10-fold enrichment of astroglial cells is achieved.

Similar to choleragenoid tetanus toxin was observed by us in vitro not only on neurones, but also on glia (Tables I and II); however, the difference in apparent concentration of toxin binding sites is more pronounced for tetanus than for cholera toxin. It is therefore possible that tetanus toxin may serve as an additional neuronal marker for immunocytolysis in the cerebellum, as it was shown to be in other parts of the nervous system (Dimpfel et al., 1977; Fields et al., 1978; Mirsky et al., 1978).

CONCLUSIONS AND OUTLOOK

Several surface antigens of neural cells have been characterized which allow the distinction between the major cell types in the cerebellum: neurones, astro- and oligodendroglia, and mesodermally derived accessory populations, such as fibroblasts, endothelial and meningeal cells. The physical isolation of these cells is possible through the use of immunoselective methods including complement-dependent cytolysis eliminating the antigen-positive cell class, and fluorescence activated cell sorting which allows the simultaneous collection of both antigen-negative and -positive populations. The isolated cells are viable and can be maintained in vitro under conditions which permit growth of cellular extensions and, in the case of non-neuronal cells, cell division.

It is conceivable that with the advent of more refined immunological tools in the form of monoclonal antibodies a more selective detection of even more specific and minor cell surface markers will be possible which are not only unique to particular cell classes and subcellular components in the cerebellum, but to particular developmental events.

ACKNOWLEDGEMENTS

The authors thank G. Schoonmaker, K. A. Wortham and E. Sawadski for excellent assistance.

This work was supported by NIH Grant NS 12659, Deutsche Forschungsgemeinschaft, Hertie Stiftung and Stiftung Volkswagenwerk. M. Willinger is supported by a postdoctoral fellowship from NIH.

REFERENCES

Akeson, R. and Herschman, H. (1974) Modulation of cell-surface antigens of a murine neuroblastoma. *Proc. nat. Acad. Sci. (Wash.)*, 71: 187–191.

Altman, J. and Anderson, W. J. (1972) Experimental reorganization of the cerebellar cortex. I. Morphological effects of elimination of all microneurons with prolonged X-irradation started at birth. *J. comp. Neurol.*, 146: 355–406.

Altman, J., Anderson, W. J. and Wright, K. A. (1969) Early effects of X-irradation of the cerebellum in infant rats: decimation and reconstruction of the granular layer. *Exp. Neurol.*, 24: 196–216.

Balsamo, J. and Lilien, J. (1974) Functional identification of three components which mediate tissue-type specific embryonic cell adhesion. *Nature (Lond.)*, 251:522–524.

Barbera, A. J., Marchase, R. B. and Roth, S. (1973) Adhesive recognition and retinotectal specificity. *Proc. nat. Acad. Sci. (Wash.)*, 70: 2482–2486.

Barkley, D. S., Rakic, L. L., Chaffee, J. K. and Wong, D. L. (1973) Cell separation by velocity sedimentation of postnatal mouse cerebellum. *J. Cell Physiol.*, 28: 271–280.

Barondes, S. H. (1978) Developmentally regulated slime mold lectins and specific cell cohesion. In *Molecular Basis of Cell-Cell Interaction*, R. A. Lerner and D. Bergsma (Eds.), Alan R. Liss Inc., New York, pp. 491–497.

Bignami, A., Eng, L. F., Dahl, D. and Uyeda, C. T. (1972) Localization of the glial fibrillary acidic protein in astrocytes by immunofluorescence. *Brain Res.*, 43: 429–435.

Boyse, E. A. and Old, L. J. (1969) Some aspects of normal and abnormal cell surface genetics. *Ann. Rev. Genet.*, 3: 269–291.

Brackenbury, R., Thiery, J.-P., Rutishauser, U. and Edelman, G. M. (1977) Adhesion among neural cells of the chick embryo. I. An immunological assay for molecules involved in cell-cell binding. *J. biol. Chem.*, 232: 6835–6840.

Brent, R. L. (1966) The production of congenital malformations using tissue antisera. IV. Evaluation of the mechanism of teratogenesis by varying the route and time of administration of anti-rat kidney antiserum. *Amer. J. Anat.*, 119: 555–562.

Campbell, G. LeM., Schachner, M. and Sharrow, S. O. (1977) Isolation of glial cell-enriched and -depleted populations from mouse cerebellum by density gradient centrifugation and electronic cell sorting. *Brain Res.*, 127: 69–86.

Cauldwell, C. B., Herkart, P. and Humphreys, T. (1973) Physical properties of sponge aggregation factor. A unique proteoglycan complex. *Biochemistry*, 12: 3051–3055.

Chaffee, J. K. and Schachner, M. (1978a) NS-6 (nervous system antigen-6), a new cell surface antigen of brain, kidney and spermatozoa. *Develop. Biol.*, 62: 173–184.

Chaffee, J. K. and Schachner, M. (1978b) NS-7 (nervous system antigen-7), a cell surface antigen of mature brain, kidney and spermatozoa shared by embryonal tissues and transformed cells. *Develop. Biol.*, 62: 185–192.

Cohen, J., Balázs, R., Hajós, F., Currie, D. N. and Dutton, G. R. (1978) Separation of cell types from the developing cerebellum. *Brain Res.*, 148: 313–331.

Cuatrecasas, P. (1973) Gangliosides and membrane receptors for cholera toxin. *Biochemistry*, 12: 3558–3566.

Davidson, A. N. and Peters, A. (1970) *Myelination*. Thomas, Springfield, Ill.

Davison, F. P. and Winslow, B. (1974) The protein subunit of calf brain neurofilament. *J. Neurobiol.*, 5: 119–133.

De Baecque, C., Johnson, A. B., Naiki, M., Schwarting, G. and Marcus, D. M. (1976) Ganglioside localization in cerebellar cortex: an immunoperoxidase study with antibody to G_{M1} ganglioside. *Brain Res.*, 114: 117–122.

DeRobertis, E., Wald, F. and Lapetina, E. G. (1971) Ultrastructural and bioelectrical effects of antisera against subcellular particles from brain. In: *Immunological Disorders of the Nervous System*, L. P. Rowland (Ed.), Williams and Wilkins, Baltimore, Md., pp. 8–26.

Dimpfel, W., Huang, R. T. C. and Habermann, E. (1977) Gangliosides in nervous tissue and binding of ^{125}I-labelled tetanus toxin, a neuronal marker. *J. Neurochem.*, 29: 329–334.

Doyle, J. M., Schachner, M. and Davidson, R. L. (1977) Expression of nervous system antigen-3 by lines of mouse fibroblasts and kidney cells and continued expression in hybrid cells. *J. Cell Physiol.*, 93: 197–204.

Eccles, J., Ito, M. and Szentágothai, J. (1967) *The Cerebellum as a Neuronal Machine*. Springer, Berlin.

Eng, L. F., Vanderhaeghen, J. J., Bignami, A. and Gerstl, B. (1971) An acidic protein isolated from fibrous astrocytes. *Brain Res.*, 28: 351–354.

Fields, K. L., Gosling, C., Megson, M. and Stern, P. L. (1975) New cell surface antigens in rat defined by tumors of the nervous system. *Proc. nat. Acad. Sci. (Wash.)*, 72: 1296–1300.

Fields, K. L., Brockes, J. P., Mirsky, R. and Wendon, L. M. B. (1978) Cell surface markers for distinguishing different types of rat dorsal root ganglion cells in culture. *Cell*, 14: 43–51.

Gierer, A. and Meinhardt, H. (1972) A theory of biological pattern formation. *Kybernetik*, 12: 30–39.

Gluecksohn-Waelsch, S. (1957) The effect of maternal immunization against organ tissues on embryonic differentiation in the mouse. *J. Embryol. exp. Morph.*, 5: 83–92.

Goridis, C., Joher, J. A., Hirsch, M. and Schachner, M. (1978a) Cell surface proteins of cultured brain cells and their recognition by anti-cerebellum (anti NS-4) antiserum. *J. Neurochem.*, 31: 531–539.

Goridis, C., Artzt, K., Wortham, K. A. and Schachner, M. (1978b) Brain cell surface antigens on embryonal carcinoma cells. *Develop. Biol.*, 65: 238–243.

Gottlieb, D. I., Merrell, R. and Glaser, L. (1974) Temporal changes in embryo cell surface recognition. *Proc. nat. Acad. Sci. (Wash.)*, 71: 1800–1802.

Hansson, H.-A., Holmgren, J. and Svennerholm, L. (1977) Ultrastructural localization of cell membrane G_{M1} ganglioside by cholera toxin. *Proc. nat. Acad. Sci. (Wash.)*, 74: 3782–3786.

Hausman, R. E. and Moscona, A. A. (1976) Isolation of retina-specific cell-aggregation factor from membranes of embryonic neural retina tissue. *Proc. nat. Acad. Sci. (Wash.)*, 73: 3594–3598.

Herndon, R. M., Margolis, G. and Kilham, L. (1971) The synaptic organization of the malformed cerebellum induced by prenatal infection with feline leukopenia virus. *J. Neuropath. exp. Neurol.*, 30: 557–570.

Holmgren, J., Lönnroth, I., Mansson, J. E. and Svennerholm, L. (1975) Interaction of cholera toxin and membrane G_{M1} ganglioside of small intestine. *Proc. nat. Acad. Sci. (Wash.)*, 72: 2520–2524.

Kadin, M. E., Rubinstein, L. J. and Nelson, J. S. (1970) Neonatal cerebellar medulloblastoma originating from the fetal external granular layer. *J. Neuropath. exp. Neurol.*, 29: 583–600.

Kemler, R., Babinet, C., Eisen, H. and Jacob, F. (1977) Surface antigen in early differentiation. *Proc. nat. Acad. Sci. (Wash.)*, 74: 4449–4452.

Kies, M. W. and Alvord, Jr., E. C. (Eds.) (1959) *Allergic Encephalomyelitis.* Thomas, Springfield, Ill.

Köhler, G. and Melchers, F. (1972) Isoelectric focusing spectra of antibodies which activate mutant β-galactosidases. *Europ. J. Immunol.*, 2: 453–456.

Köhler, G. and Milstein, C. (1975) Continuous cultures of fused cells secreting antibody of predefined specificity. *Nature (Lond.)*, 256: 495–497.

Köhler, G. and Milstein, C. (1976) Derivation of specific antibody-producing tissue culture and tumor lines by cell fusion. *Europ. J. Immunol.*, 6: 511–519.

Lawrence, P. A., Crick, F. H. C. and Munro, M. (1972) A gradient of positional information in an insect, Rhodnius. *J. Cell Sci.*, 11: 815–853.

Llinás, R. (1969) *Neurobiology of Cerebellar Evolution and Development, Proc. First Int. Symp.* Inst. Biomed. Res. Amer. Med. Ass. Educ. Res. Found., Chicago, Ill.

Manuelidis, L. and Manuelidis, E. E. (1976) Ultrastructural study of plasma membrane G_{M1} in neuroectodermal cells using cholera-peroxidase. *J. Neurocytol.*, 5: 575–589.

Martin, S. E. (1974) Mouse brain antigen detected by rat anti-C1300 antiserum. *Nature (Lond.)*, 249: 71–73.

Matsumoto, H., Spatz, M. and Laqueur, G. L. (1972) Quantitative changes with age in the DNA content of methylazoxymethanol-induced microencephalic rat brain. *J. Neurochem.*, 19: 297–306.

McMahon, D. (1974) Chemical messengers in development: a hypothesis. Science, 185: 1012–1021.

Menge, A. C., Rosenberg, A. and Burkons, D. M. (1974) Effects of uterine fluids and immunoglobulins from serum-immunized rabbits on rabbit embryos cultured in vitro. *Proc. Soc. exp. Biol. Med. (N.Y.)*, 145: 371–378.

Mirsky, R., Wendon, L., Black, P., Stolkin, C. and Bray, D. (1978) Tetanus toxin: a cell surface marker for neurones in culture. *Brain Res.*, 148: 251–259.

Moore, B. W. (1965) A soluble protein characteristic of the nervous system. *Biochem. biophys. Res. Commun.*, 19: 739–344.

Moore, B. W. and Perez, V. J. (1968) Specific acidic proteins of the nervous system. In *Physiological and Biochemical Aspects of Nervous Integration,* F. D. Carlson (Ed.), Prentice-Hall, Englewood Cliffs, N.J., pp. 343–359.

Moscona, A. A. (1965) Recombination of dissociated cells and the development of cell aggregates. In *Cells and Tissues in Culture,* E. N. Willmer (Ed.), Academic Press, New York, pp. 498–529.

Mullin, B. R., Aloj, S. M., Fishman, P. H., Lee, G., Kohn, L. D. and Brady, R. O. (1976) Cholera toxin interactions with thyrotropin receptors on thyroid plasma membrane. *Proc. nat. Acad. Sci. (Wash.)*, 73: 1679–1683.

Nathanson, N., Cole, G. A. and Van der Loos, H. (1969) Heterotopic cerebellar granule cells following administration of cyclophosphamide to suckling rats. *Brain Res.*, 5: 532–536.

Palay, S. and Chan-Palay, V. (1973) *Cerebellar Cortex Cytology and Organization.* Springer, New York.

Privat, A., Marson, A. M. and Drian, M. J. (1979) In vitro models of neural growth and differentiation. In *Development and Chemical Specificity of Neurons, Progress in Brain Research, Vol. 51,* M. Cuénod, G. Kreutzberg and F. Bloom (Eds.), Elsevier/North-Holland, Amsterdam, pp. 335–356.

Raff, M. C., Brockes, J. P., Fields, K. L. and Mirsky, R. (1979) Neural cell markers: the end of the beginning. In *Development and Chemical Specificity of Neurons, Progress in Brain Research, Vol. 51,* M. Cuénod, G. Kreutzberg and F. Bloom (Eds.), Elsevier/North-Holland, Amsterdam, pp. 17–22.

Rakic, P. and Sidman, R. L. (1973) Weaver mutant mouse cerebellum: defective neuronal migration secondary to specific abnormality of Bergmann glia. *Proc. nat. Acad. Sci. (Wash.),* 70: 240–244.

Rapport, M. M. and Graf, L. (1969) Immunochemical reactions of lipids. *Progr. Allergy,* 13: 273–331.

Roth, S. (1968) Studies on intercellular adhesive selectivity. *Develop. Biol.,* 18: 602–631.

Rutishauser, U., Thiery, J.-P., Brackenbury, R., Sela, B.-A. and Edelman, G. M. (1976) Mechanism of adhesion among cells from neural retina of chick embryo. *Proc. nat. Acad. Sci. (Wash.),* 73: 577–581.

Schachner, M. (1974) NS-1 (nervous system antigen-1), a glial cell specific antigenic component of the surface membrane. *Proc. nat. Acad. Sci. (Wash.),* 71: 1795–1799.

Schachner, M. and Carnow, T. B. (1975) Nervous system antigen (NS-2), an antigenic cell surface component expressed on a murine glioblastoma. *Brain Res.,* 88: 394–402.

Schachner, M. and Willinger, M. (1979) Developmental expression of oligodendrocyte-specific cell surface markers: NS-1 (nervous system antigen-1), cerebroside, and basic protein of myelin. In *The Menarini Series on Immunopathology,* P. A. Miescher (Ed.), Schwabe, Basel, in press.

Schachner, M. and Wortham, K. A. (1975) Nervous system antigen-3 (NS-3), an antigenic cell surface component expressed on neuroblastoma C1300. *Brain Res.,* 99: 201–208.

Schachner, M., Wortham, K. A., Carter, L. D. and Chaffee, J. K. (1975) NS-4 (nervous system antigen-4), a cell surface antigen of developing and adult mouse brain and mature sperm. *Develop. Biol.,* 44: 313–325.

Schachner, M., Ruberg, M. Z. and Carnow, T. B. (1976) Histological localization of nervous system antigens in the cerebellum by immunoperoxidase labeling. *Brain Res. Bull.,* 1: 367–377.

Schachner, M. Wortham, K. A., Ruberg, M. Z., Dorfman, S. and Campbell, G. LeM. (1977) Brain cell surface antigens detected by anti-corpus callosum antiserum. *Brain Res.,* 127: 87–97.

Schachner, M., Smith, C. and Schoonmaker, G. (1978a) Immunological distinction between neurofilament and glial fibrillary acidic proteins by mouse antisera and their immunohistological distribution. *Develop. Neurosci.,* 1: 1–14.

Schachner, M., Schoonmaker, G. and Hynes, R. O. (1978b) Cellular and subcellular localization of LETS protein in the nervous system. *Brain Res.,* 158: 149–158.

Schlaepfer, W. W. and Lynch, R. G. (1977) Immunofluorescence studies of neurofilaments in the rat and human peripheral and central nervous system. *J. Cell Biol.,* 74: 241–250.

Sellinger, O. Z., Legrand, J., Clos, J. and Ohlsson, W. G. (1974) Unequal patterns of succinate-dehydrogenase and acetylcholinesterase in Purkinje cell bodies and granule cells isolated in bulk from the cerebellar cortex of the immature rat. *J. Neurochem.;* 23: 1137–1144.

Shelanski, M. L., Albert, S., DeVries, G. H. and Norton, W. T. (1971) Isolation of filaments from brain. *Science,* 174: 1242–1245.

Sidman, R. L. (1972) Cell interactions in developing mammalian central nervous system. In *Cell Interactions, Proceedings of the Third Lepetit Colloquium,* L. G. Silvestri (Ed.), North-Holland, Amsterdam, pp. 1–13.

Sidman, R. L., Green, M. C. and Appel, S. H. (1965) *Catalog of the Neurological Mutants of the Mouse.* Harvard University Press, Cambridge, Mass.

Solter, D. and Schachner, M. (1976) Brain and sperm cell surface antigen (NS-4) on preimplantation mouse embryos. *Develop. Biol.,* 52: 98–104.

Stallcup, W. B. (1977) Specificity of adhesion between cloned neural cell lines. *Brain Res.,* 126: 475–486.

Thiery, J.-P., Brackenbury, R., Rutishauser, U. and Edelman, G. M. (1977) Adhesion among neural cells of the chick embryo. II. Purification and characterization of a cell adhesion molecule from neural retina. *J. biol. Chem.,* 252: 6841–6845.

Van Heyningen, W. E. (1963) The fixation of tetanus toxin, strychnine, serotonin and other substances by ganglioside. *J. gen. Microbiol.,* 31: 375–387.

Walther, B. T., Ohman, R. and Roseman, S. (1973) A quantitative assay for intercellular adhesion. *Proc. nat. Acad. Sci. (Wash.),* 70: 1569–1573.

Weinbaum, G. and Burger, M. M. (1973) Two component systems for surface guided reassociation of animal cells. *Nature (Lond.),* 244: 510–512.

Williams, R. M. (1969) Antibodies to acetylcholinesterase. *Proc. nat. Acad. Sci. (Wash.),* 62: 1175–1180.

Willinger, M. and Schachner, M. (1978) Distribution of G_{M1} ganglioside in developing cerebellum. *J. supramol. Struct.*, 2 (Suppl.): 128.

Willinger, M. and Schachner, M. (1979) G_{M1} ganglioside as a marker for neuronal differentiation in mouse cerebellum. In preparation.

Wolpert, L. (1969) Positional information and the spatial pattern of cellular differentiation. *J. theoret. Biol.*, 25: 1–47.

Yuan, D., Vitetta, E. S. and Schachner, M. (1977) Partial characterization of murine nervous system specific cell surface antigens. *J. Immunol.*, 118: 551–557.

Zimmermann, A. and Schachner, M. (1976) Nervous system antigen-5, an antigenic cell surface component of neuroectodermal origin. *Brain Res.*, 115: 297–310.

Zimmermann, A., Schachner, M. and Press, J. L. (1976) Central nervous system antigen (NS-5) and its presence during murine ontogenesis. *J. supramol. Struct.*, 5: 417–429.

The Cytoskeleton and its Influence on Shape, Motility and Receptor Segregation in Neuroblastoma Cells

G. ISENBERG, J. V. SMALL and G. W. KREUTZBERG

Max Planck Institute for Psychiatry, Munich (G.F.R.) and (J.V.S.) Institute for Molecular Biology, Austrian Academy of Sciences, Salzburg (Austria)

INTRODUCTION

The unique architecture of the neuron with its long axonal and dendritic extensions requires intracellular mechanisms for maintaining stability and controlling motility. The cytoskeleton is believed to serve both functions by providing a stiffening backbone as well as a structure on which force-generating mechanisms for directed movements or transport can be attached.

The most prominent constituents of the cytoskeleton are the microtubules, the microfilaments, and the 10 nm filaments which in the neuron are referred to as neurofilaments. Their role in cellular motility and intracellular transport processes in the developing and mature neuron is generally accepted, although the interaction between the various cytoskeletal structures is poorly understood. The main constituents of the cytoskeletal structures are well defined. Actin, tubulin and 10 nm filament protein are ubiquitous and are especially prominent in brain tissue. Their biochemistry and subcellular organization have been reviewed for a variety of non-muscle systems (Pollard and Weihing, 1974; Perry et al., 1976; Korn, 1978; Trifaro, 1978).

Neuronal and neuroblastoma cells in culture are widely used as a model, since, in spite of marked differences in properties compared with nerve cells in vivo, they may resemble in many respects the developing nerve cell. In the neuroblastoma cell the distribution of actin, tubulin and 10 nm filament protein was investigated with immunofluorescence techniques (Jorgensen et al., 1976; Isenberg et al., 1977). As had been shown earlier in ultrastructural studies (Chang and Goldman, 1973; Ross et al., 1975) actin was found to underly the plasma membrane and to constitute the leading edges of the cell (lamellipodia). On the basis of improved methods for the visualization of the cytoskeleton using Triton-extracted, negatively stained cell monolayers (Isenberg and Small, 1978; Small and Celis, 1978), it was demonstrated that actin shows at least two supramolecular aggregation states: a planar filament meshwork and paracrystalline-like filament bundles, partly corresponding to the microspikes. Further, decoration with myosin subfragment-1 (S-1) revealed that the actin filaments in this area are singly polarized towards the cell body. This unipolar organization of actin is a characteristic feature of the advancing lamellae of cultured cells, not only in microspikes but also in the interconnecting meshwork of actin filaments (Isenberg and Small, 1978; Small et al., 1978). Microtubules and 10 nm filaments are found to arise from the cell center around the nucleus and to display a continuous organization pattern up to the end of neuronal extensions (Fig. 2).

Based on the detailed knowledge of the cytoskeletal arrangement in neuroblastoma cells, the mobility of cell surface constituents and their possible transmembranous control by cytoplasmic elements were studied. Such control would be of crucial interest for cell recognition, contact phenomena and cellular communication.

RESULTS AND DISCUSSION

The two-step process of clustering and patch formation of ligand-receptor complexes and their subsequent accumulation at one pole of the cell surface has been termed capping (Taylor et al., 1971; De Petris and Raff, 1972). Submembranous cytoskeletal elements have also been shown to be involved in this process, since the patching and capping of receptors are associated with the redistribution of actin and myosin (for literature see Poste and Nicolson, 1977). This raises the question as to whether microfilaments *directly* influence receptor movement on the cell surface.

Studying the redistribution of receptors which bind concanavalin A (Con A) (Isenberg et al., 1978) it was found that neuroblastoma cells undergo marked morphological changes in response to Con A treatment (100 μg/ml). These involve the retraction of neurites and the induction of broad and extensive lamellae regions around the cell periphery (Fig. 3). The rapid retraction is induced specifically by Con A in neuroblastoma cells. Vinblastine and col-

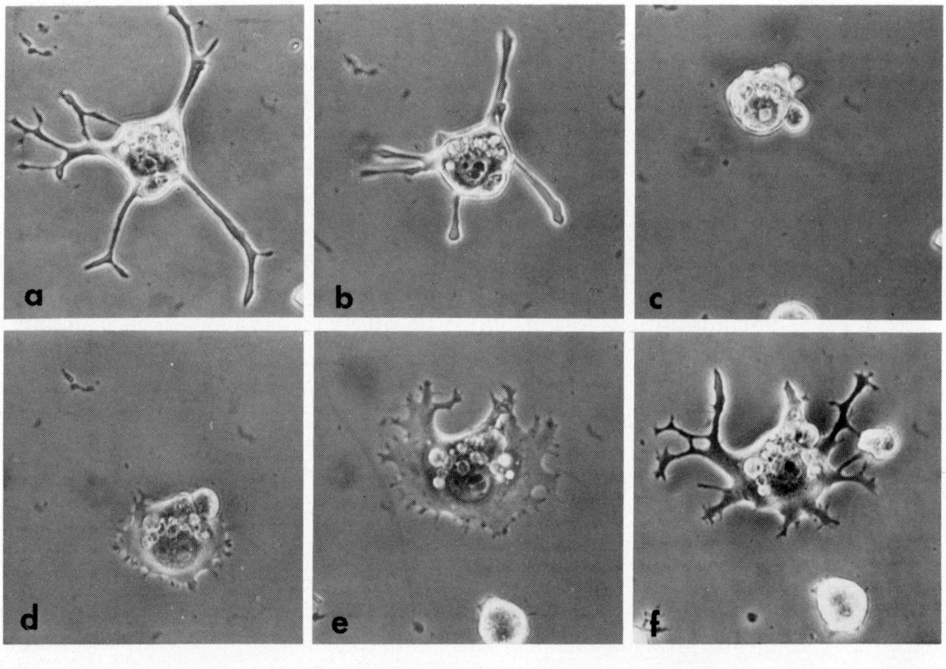

Fig. 1. The shape-changing capacity of neuroblastoma (N18) cells demonstrated after treatment with 10 ng/ml vinblastine. Neurites (a = 0 min) are gradually disintegrated (b = 20 min, c = 60 min) and reconstitute after removal of the drug during a time period of d = 120 min, e = 180 min and f = 240 min. Phase contrast, × 300.

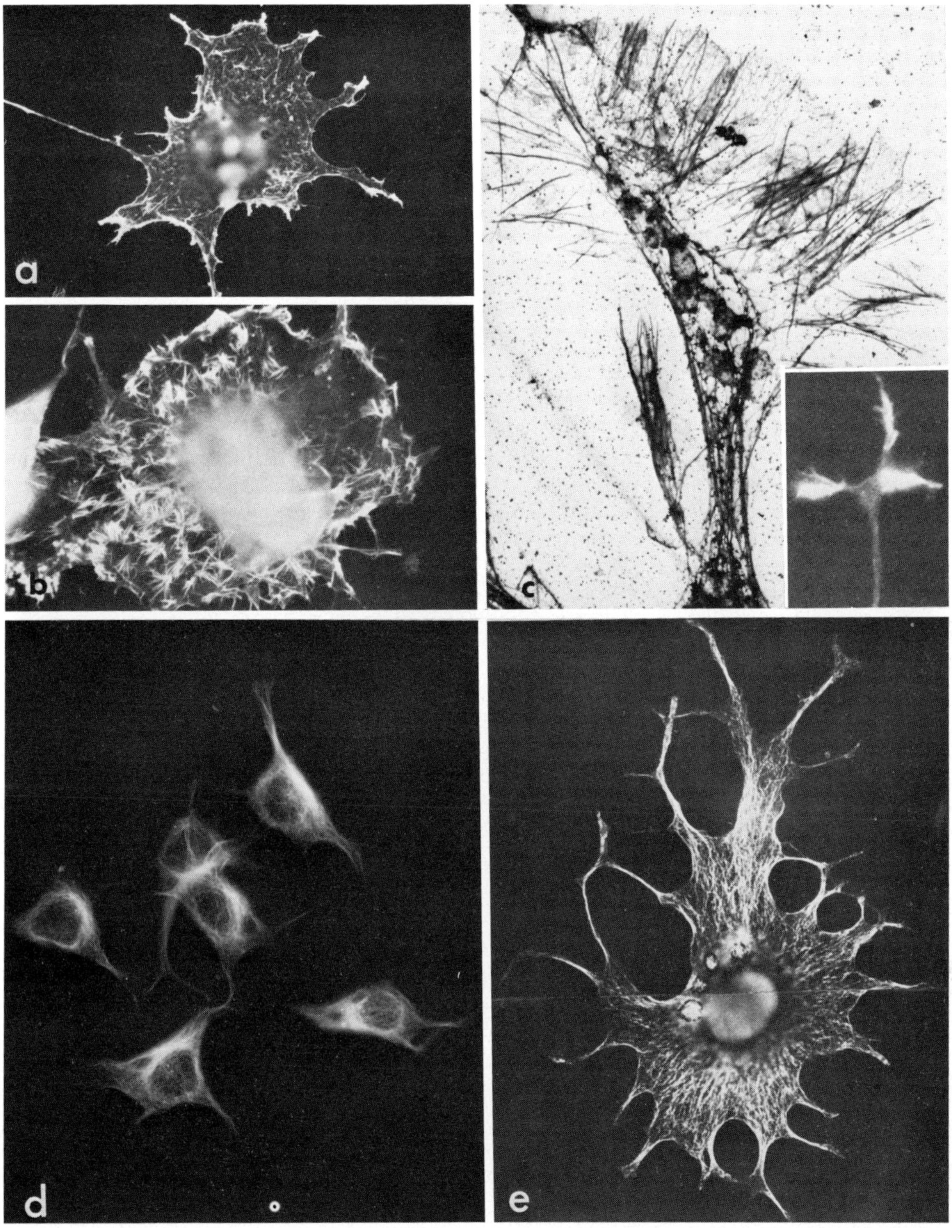

Fig. 2. The distribution of actin and tubulin in neuroblastoma (N18) cells. a + b: immunofluorescent staining with anti-actin antibody showing actin predominantly located beneath the plasma membrane (a), in microspikes (b) and in the tips of growing extensions (growth cones) (a and c inset). This corresponds to the location of a filamentous actin meshwork and paracrystalline actin bundles in the growth cone as revealed in Triton-extracted, negatively stained cells (c). Immunofluorescent staining with anti-tubulin (d + e). Tubulin is concentrated perinuclear in the initial phase of the formation of processes (d). A widely spread, very large cell with many extensions shows microtubules radiating from the cytocenter and running up to the tips of neurites (e). Magnifications: (a) × 200, (b) × 330, (c) × 3500, inset × 400, (d) × 200, (e) × 150.

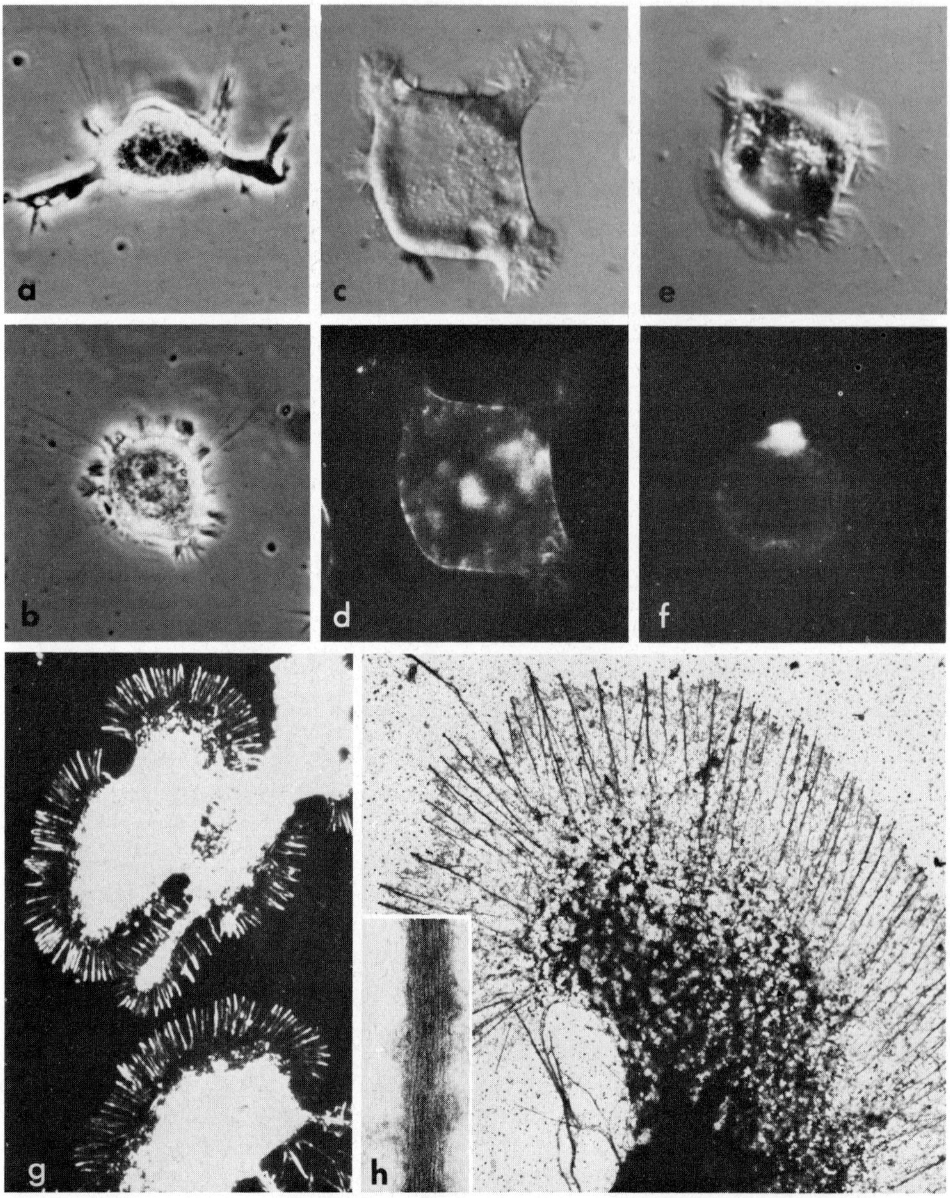

Fig. 3. Correlation of actin polymerization and receptor segregation in neuroblastoma (N18) cells. a + b: stages of the morphological reaction after treatment with 100 μg/ml concanavalin A. Neurites are retracted within a few minutes (a) followed by the formation of cytoplasmic lamellae around the cell perimeter (b). c–f: sequential stages of two different cells incubated for increasing times in the presence of FITC-Con A. The same cell is viewed in Nomarski (c + e) and fluorescent optics (d + f). Fluorescence is absent from lamellar regions (d). Note that the final cap of surface receptors (f) is located over a peripheral region devoid of lamellar cytoplasm. g + h: stages of lamellipodia formation as observed by dark-field microscopy of acetone-extracted, myosin subfragment-1 labeled, air dried cells (g) and after Triton extraction and negative staining (h). Cytoplasmic lamellae show regularly arranged, radiating filament bundles composed of co-linear arranged actin filaments (h, inset). Magnifications: (a + b) × 500, (c + d) × 1000, (e + f) × 550, (g) × 520, (h) × 3800, inset × 200,000.

chicine both cause gradual disintegration of neurites but were found to have no inducing effect on lamellae formation in comparable time periods (cf. Fig. 1).

After Triton extraction, labelling with myosin subfragment-1 and drying in air, lamellar regions may be more clearly visualized and details become apparent even with light microscopical techniques. This results from the binding of S-1 to the actin filaments in the leading edge. With longer time after Con A treatment, intralamellar bundle and microspike formation are increasing. Treatment of neuroblastoma cells with Con A coupled to fluoroisothiocyanate (FITC-Con A) reveals at first a uniform distribution of fluorescent label followed by a patchy accumulation of the ligand. In the subsequent period of lamellae formation, the label is restricted to the cell body and cannot be detected under these conditions in the forming lamellipodia. When the lamellae are observed around the major part of the cell perimeter, small patches of fluorescence occur on the cell surface. Finally, when aggregates or caps form at the cell periphery, their position coincides with areas free of lamellae (Fig. 3).

The examination of Triton-extracted, negatively stained cells at this stage reveals the lamellae showing a large number of regularly spaced and radially arranged paracrystalline-like actin bundles. As described above, the thin filaments, when decorated with myosin subfragment-1, show a single polarization towards the cell body. Since the polymerization of actin occurs in a direction opposite to that pointed to by the arrowheads, this bundle formation of paracrystalline actin can be regarded as a force-generating mechanism for the establishment of cytoplasmic lamellae. The formation of these lamellae around nearly the whole cell perimeter can thus be correlated with: (1) the unidirectional polymerization of actin bundles, and (2) a concomitant segregation of surface receptors between the cell body and the lamellae regions. This resulting polarity is also clearly visible in normal thin sections. On one-half of the cell, cytoplasmic protrusions, presumed to be components of the lamellae, form in response to Con A. Cell organelles are absent from this region and accumulate at the other pole of the cell. Numerous vacuoles can also be seen here. Since these accumulated vacuoles are not observed in untreated cells, it is possible that they arise as a result of the internalization of Con A receptors by endocytosis.

It has been claimed that receptor patches are actively collected into a cap since actin accumulates submembranously in the region undergoing patching, capping and finally receptor endocytosis. During these processes, receptor-linked actin filaments are supposed to participate in an actin-myosin contraction mechanism (Bourguignon and Singer, 1977). While the data currently available point to an involvement of actin in receptor movement, there exists so far no conclusive evidence that receptors in the surface plane are moved by microfilaments via a direct linkage. Indeed, more recent data suggest that actin (Oliver et al., 1977) and myosin (Pollard, personal communication) may be, but must not necessarily be, co-capped with receptors.

In neuroblastoma cells receptor complexes are segregated in regions away from areas of actin filament organization, i.e. away from peripheral lamellae. In this respect it is noteworthy that, when terminal caps were observed, these form at poles of cells which are free of lamellar cytoplasm. From the fact that in Con A-treated neuroblastoma cells, receptor complexes are segregated on the cell surface simultaneously as actin filaments polymerize in the opposite direction, it is concluded that actin may influence receptor movement even without a direct linkage, possibly by previously suggested countercurrent membrane flow (De Petris and Raff, 1972).

ACKNOWLEDGEMENTS

We thank Dr. K. Weber for the generous gift of antibodies. N18 cells orginally provided by Dr. B. Hamprecht were kindly supplied by Dr. E. Rieske.

REFERENCES

Bourguignon, L. Y. W. and Singer, S. J. (1977) Transmembrane interactions and the mechanism of capping of surface receptors by their specific ligands. *Proc. nat. Acad. Sci. (Wash.)*, 74: 5031–5035.

Chang, C. M. and Goldman, R. D. (1973) The localization of actin-like fibers in cultured neuroblastoma cells as revealed by heavy meromyosin binding. *J. Cell Biol.*, 57: 867–874.

De Petris, S. and Raff, M. C. (1972) Distribution of immunoglobulin on the surface of mouse lymphoid cells as determined by immunoferritin electron microscopy. Antibody-induced, temperature-dependent redistribution and its implications for membrane structure. *Europ. J. Immunol.*, 2: 523–535.

De Petris, S. and Raff, M. C. (1973) Fluidity of the plasma membrane and its implications for cell movement. In *Locomotion of Tissue Cells (CIBA Foundation Symposium No. 14)*, R. Porter and D. W. Fitzsimmons (Eds.), Excerpta Medica, Amsterdam, pp. 27–41.

Isenberg, G. and Small, J. V. (1978) Filamentous actin, 100 A filaments and microtubules in neuroblastoma cells – their distribution in relation to sites of movement and neuronal transport. *Cytobiologie*, 16: 326–344.

Isenberg, G., Rieske, E. and Kreutzberg, G. W. (1977) Distribution of actin and tubulin in neuroblastoma cells. *Cytobiologie*, 15: 382–389.

Isenberg, G., Small, J. V. and Kreutzberg, G. W. (1978) Correlation between actin polymerization and surface receptor segregation in neuroblastoma cells treated with concanavalin A. *J. Neurocytol.*, 7: 649–661.

Jorgensen, A. O., Subrahmanyan, L., Turnbull, C. and Kalnins, V. I. (1976) Localization of the neurofilament protein in neuroblastoma cells by immunofluorescent staining. *Proc. nat. Acad. Sci. (Wash.)*, 73: 3192–3196.

Korn, E. D. (1978) Biochemistry of actomyosin-dependent cell motility. *Proc. nat. Acad. Sci. (Wash.)*, 75: 588–599.

Oliver, J. M., Lalchandani, R. and Becker, E. L. (1977) Actin redistribution during concanavalin A cap formation in rabbit neutrophils. *J. Reticuloendothel. Soc.*, 21: 359–364.

Perry, S. V., Margreth, A. and Adelstein, R. S. (1976) *Contractile Systems in Non-muscle Tissues*. North-Holland Publ., Amsterdam.

Pollard, T. D. and Weihing, R. R. (1974) Actin and myosin and cell movement. *CRC Crit. Rev. Biochem.*, 2: 1–65.

Poste, G. and Nicolson, G. L. (1977) *Dynamic Aspects of Cell Surface Organization. Cell Surface Reviews, Vol. 3*, North-Holland Publ., Amsterdam.

Ross, J., Olmsted, J. B. and Rosenbaum, J. L.. (1975) The ultrastructure of mouse neuroblastoma cells in tissue culture. *Tissue Cell*, 7: 107–136.

Small, J. V. and Celis, J. E. (1978) Filament arrangements in negatively stained cultured cells. I. The organization of actin. *Cytobiologie*, 16: 308–325.

Small, J. V., Isenberg, G. and Celis, J. E. (1978) Polarity of actin at the leading edge of cultured cells. *Nature (Lond.)*, 272: 638–639.

Taylor, R. B., Duffus, W. P. H., Raff, M. C. and De Petris, S. (1971) Redistribution and pinocytosis of lymphocyte surface immunoglobulin molecules induced by anti-immunoglobulin antibody. *Nature New Biol.*, 233: 225–229.

Trifaro, J. M. (1978) Contractile proteins in tissues originating in the neural crest. *Neuroscience*, 3: 1–24.

Enzymatic Activity, Ultrastructure and Function in Ganglia Infected with a Neurotropic Virus

M. DOLIVO, P. HONEGGER, C. GEORGE, M. KIRALY and W. BOMMELI

Department of Physiology, University of Lausanne, Lausanne, and (W.B.) Federal Vaccine Institute of Basle, Basle (Switzerland)

INTRODUCTION

The infection of nervous tissue with neurotropic viruses raises many problems which necessitate interdisciplinary research in both neurobiology and microbiology. This paper attempts to answer some of the remaining questions, namely: how do the viruses reach the neurons, what are the alterations that they impose on the neuronal machinery, and what are the consequences of these alterations on the function of the infected neurons.

The virus used for this research was the pseudorabies, strain Aujeszky (Hurst, 1933). After their inoculation into the anterior chamber of one eye of the rat, the virus was found for the next 40 hr solely in the superior cervical ganglion and in the ganglion of the fifth nerve on the ipsilateral side of the inoculation. Thus, the superior cervical ganglion can be taken as a model for the infection of the nervous tissue, more so, since the functional responses related to the ultrastructure of this tissue as well as its metabolism in vitro and in vivo have been extensively studied (Larrabee, 1961; Dolivo, 1974; McBride and Klingman, 1974).

METHODS

Wistar rats, anesthetized with ether, were inoculated with 10 μl of a suspension of pseudorabies virus, by injection into the anterior chamber of the eye. At various intervals after the inoculation the following examinations were performed:

(1) Morphology

(a) Virus isolation from various excised organs in tissue culture.

(b) Ultrastructural examinations.

(c) Staining for indirect immunofluorescence.

(2) Biochemistry

(a) Total protein (Lowry et al., 1951).

(b) Activity of the following enzymes: TOH (Nagatsu et al., 1964; Richelson and Nirenberg, 1974; Shiman et al., 1971), CHE (Reed et al., 1966; Wilson et al., 1972), CHAT (Schrier and Shuster, 1967; Wilson et al., 1972).

(c) ACh content of the non-incubated ganglion.

(3) Electrophysiology

(a) Recording of the electrophysiological activity on the post- and preganglionic nerves (Dolivo et al., 1978).

(b) Measurement of the membrane potential using intracellular microelectrodes (Perri et al., 1970).

Abbreviations used

TOH = tyrosine 3-monooxygenase (EC 1.14.16.2) (tyrosine hydroxylase); AChE = acetylcholinesterase (EC 3.1.1.7); CHAT = cholineacetyltransferase (EC 2.3.1.6); ACh = acetylcholine.

RESULTS

(1) Transport of the virus from the eye to the superior cervical ganglion

The virus particles, in their enveloped form, can be detected in the unmyelinated postganglionic fibers of the superior cervical ganglion, where they are frequently seen surrounded by smooth endoplasmic reticulum (Fig. 1), suggesting that the particles are transported by retrograde axonal flow (Droz, 1975; Droz, personal communication). The first neurons to be infected are located near the origin of the postganglionic nerve. If a ligature is placed on the postganglionic nerve, virus particles accumulate in front of it. No infection of the ganglionic neurons occurs if the virus is inoculated after the postganglionic fibers have been cut (axotomy). Finally, if 10 μl colchicine (75 mM) is injected into the eye 12 hr before the inoculation, the infection of the superior cervical ganglion is delayed by at least 3 days.

In the neurons the virus can be found in the nucleus as nucleocapsids, either dispersed in isolated form or assembled in pseudocrystalline aggregates. In the cytoplasm it is in its enveloped form. The virus has never been observed in the presynaptic fibers: since it appears to be unable to cross the synapses (Dolivo et al., 1978). From the above observations we conclude that the virus particles are transported from the eye to the superior cervical ganglion by retrograde axonal flow.

(2) Metabolic alterations imposed on the infected neurons

The genome of the virus modifies the cells' metabolism in such a way that synthesis of viral nucleic acid takes place. This leads to the coding and production of proteins for the capsid (which stabilizes the viral DNA) as well as for the envelope. Indeed, the determination of the total protein content per ganglion showed a marked increase in the infected ganglion (Fig. 2). In addition, electron microscopic observations of infected cells often revealed an abnormally high content of membranes in the cytoplasm (Dolivo et al., 1978). Another aspect of the metabolic alterations associated with the viral infection is an increase in the activity of two enzymes involved in neuronal activity, TOH and CHAT (Fig. 3). No change could be measured in AChE. The acetylcholine content of the ganglion was also increased (Fig. 4).

If the preganglionic nerve is cut 8–10 days before inoculation (decentralization), no increase in CHAT or ACh takes place, demonstrating that the observed metabolic alteration is of presynaptic origin (Figs. 3 and 4). If the postganglionic nerve is cut (axotomy) there are no changes in enzymatic activity of acetylcholine content as the virus does not reach the neurons (Figs. 3 and 4). These results indicate that in the infected ganglion there is a transsynaptic induction of enzymatic activity. The messenger for this induction has not yet been identified.

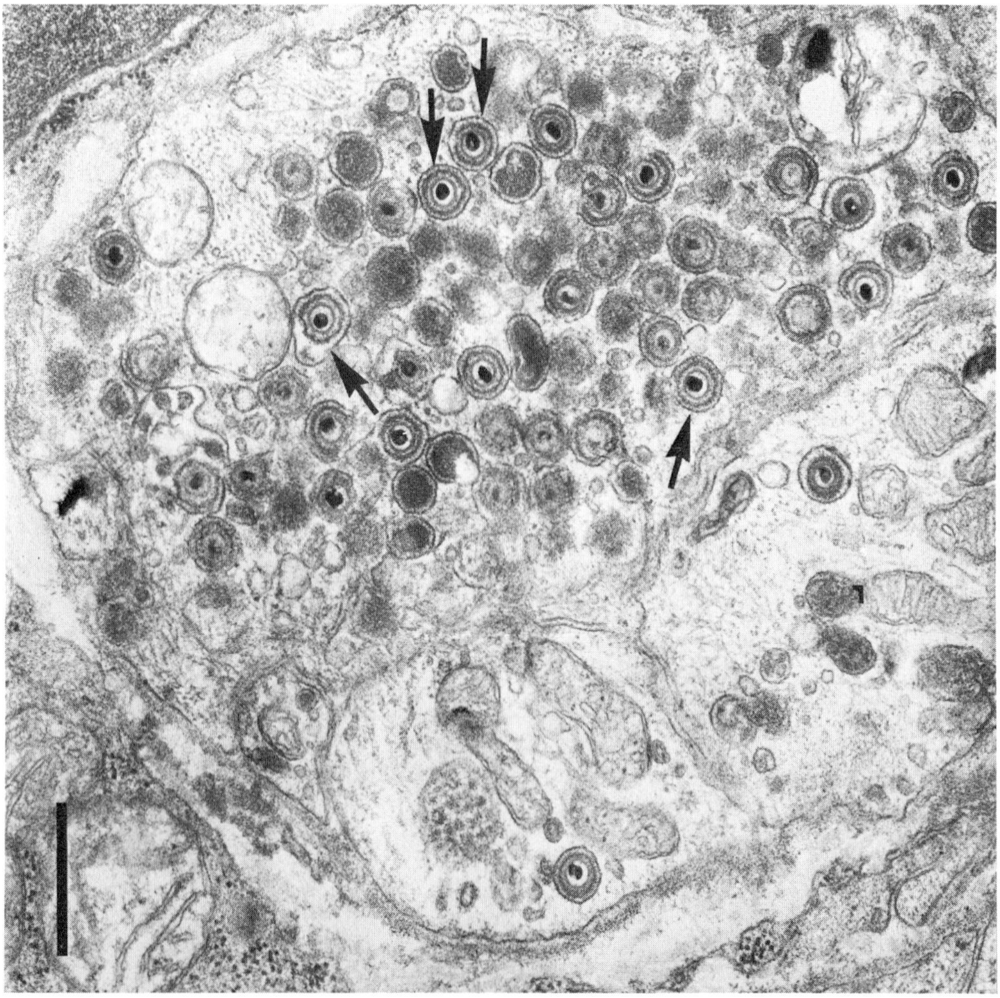

Fig. 1. Pseudorabies virus particles in a postganglionic fiber of the superior cervical ganglion of the rat. The arrows show the reticulum in which the virus particles – in their enveloped form – are transported by retrograde axonal flow. The line indicates 0.5 μm.

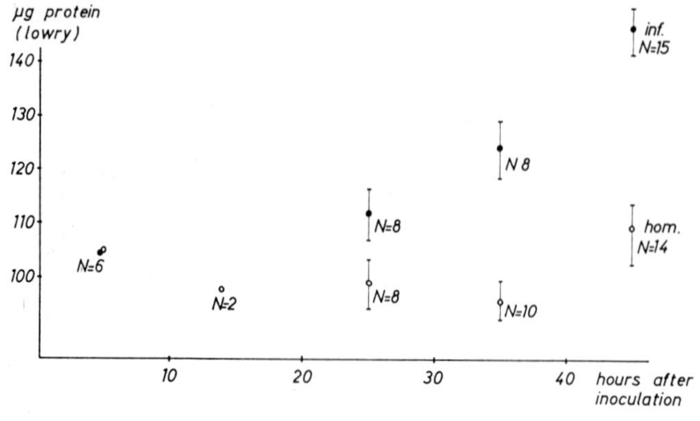

Fig. 2. Ordinate: total amount of proteins per ganglion. Abscissa: time after inoculation. Filled circle: ganglia excised from the side where the inoculation into the eye took place (inf.). Opened circle: ganglia from the contralateral side of the same animal (hom.). 40 hr after the inoculation virus particles may be found in the ganglion opposite the inoculated side.

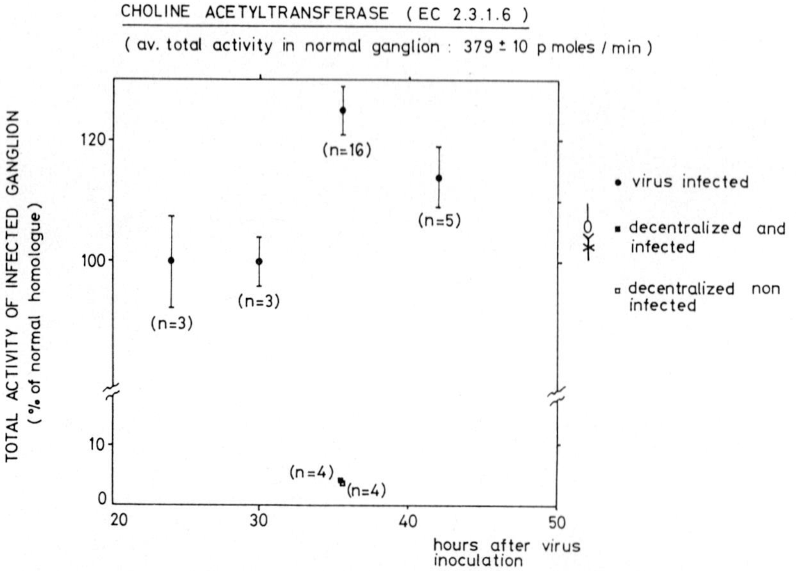

Fig. 3. Ordinate: total activity of the cholineacetyltransferase (CHAT) in infected ganglia, expressed as % of the normal activity. Abscissa: time after the inoculation, 36 hr after the inoculation the activity of the CHAT is increased by 25%. In decentralized ganglia, the activity is decreased by 95% in the normal as well as in the infected tissue due to the degeneration of the preganglionic fibers.

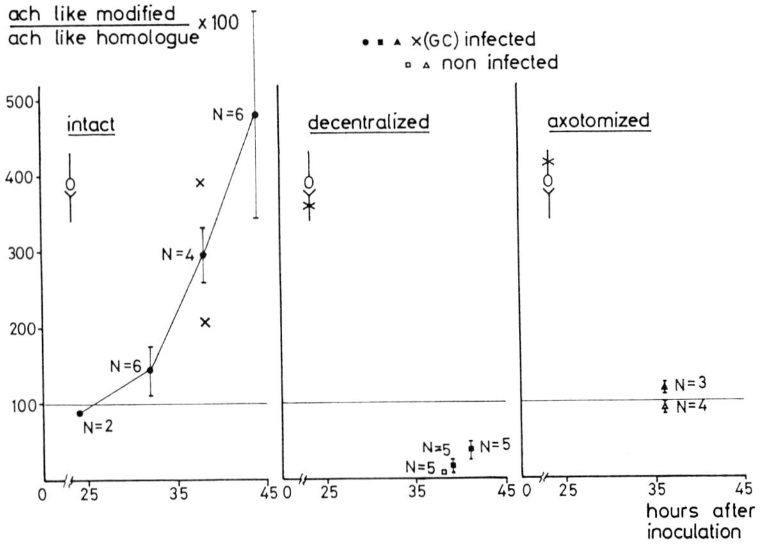

Fig. 4. Ordinate: acetylcholine content of the infected ganglia as compared to the content in the homologous non-infected ganglia. Abscissa: time after inoculation. Acetylcholine contents were determined by a bioassay except for the points indicated by GC (gas chromatography). In decentralized ganglia the amount of acetylcholine is almost not measurable both in the normal and in the infected ganglia as the preganglionic nerves are degenerated. In axotomized ganglia the amount of acetylcholine is normal because the virus could not reach the ganglion.

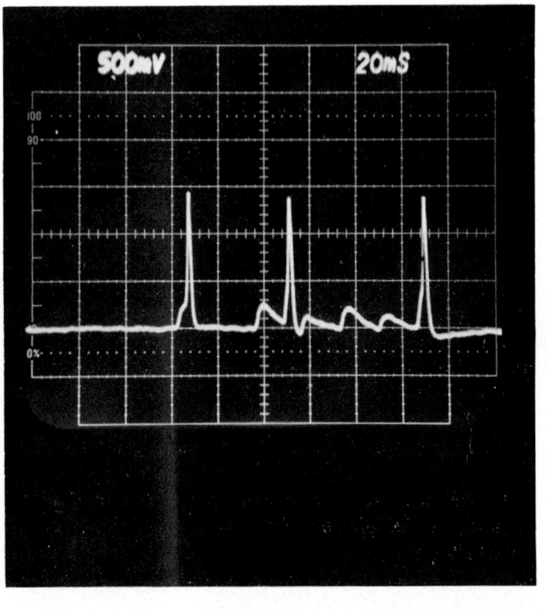

Fig. 5. Intracellular electrophysiological recording in a neuron of an infected sympathetic ganglion. All the recorded spontaneous discharges are on the top of excitatory postsynaptic potentials. This observation indicates the presynaptic origin of this abnormal electrical activity.

(3) Functional alterations of the infected ganglion

It has been shown that spontaneous electrical activity appears on the post- and pre-ganglionic nerves of the excised infected ganglion incubated in standard Krebs solution (Dolivo et al., 1978). Such bursts of activity have never been recorded on normal excised ganglia. Spontaneous discharges have also been observed using intracellular microelectrodes. As shown in Fig. 5 no pacemaker potentials could be recorded: the action potentials appear on the top of excitatory postsynaptic potentials. The spontaneous activity is of cholinergic origin, since it is reversibly blocked by D-tubocurarine.

For the time being, the origin of these discharges as well as of the spontaneous activity recorded on the preganglionic nerve remains unknown. It is also not yet possible to determine if the increased enzymatic activity is caused by the virus or by the spontaneous electrophysiological activity that they induce.

SUMMARY

Pseudorabies virus is transported from the eye to the superior cervical ganglion by retrograde axonal flow. In the sympathetic neurons the virus induces an increased protein synthesis and tyrosine 3-monooxygenase activity, a transsynaptic increased activity of the cholineacetyltransferase and a great rise in the acetylcholine content. Finally, the virus also causes an abnormal spontaneous electrophysiological activity, which also seems to be of presynaptic origin, despite the fact that the virus never crossed the synaptic cleft.

ACKNOWLEDGEMENTS

The present investigation was supported by the grant 3.510.075 from the Swiss National Research Foundation.

We wish to express our gratitude to Mrs. Martin-Meurant for her constant and skilful technical assistance.

REFERENCES

Dolivo, M. (1974) Metabolism of mammalian sympathetic ganglia. *Fed. Proc.*, 33: 1043–1048.

Dolivo, M., Beretta, E., Bonifas, V. and Foroglou, C. (1978) Ultrastructure and function in sympathetic ganglia isolated from rats infected with pseudorabies virus. *Brain Res.*, 140: 111–123.

Droz, B. (1975) Synthetic machinery and axoplasmic transport: maintenance of neuronal connectivity. In *The Nervous System, Vol. 1, The Basic Neurosciences,* D. B. Tower (Ed.), Raven Press, New York.

Hurst, E. W. (1933) Studies on pseudorabies (infectious bulbar paralysis; mad itch). *J. exp. Med.*, 58: 415–433.

Larrabee, M. G. (1961) Glucose metabolism in ganglia and nerves. In *Biophysics of Physiological and Pharmacological Actions,* A. M. Shanes (Ed.), Amer. Ass. for Advancement of Science Publ., Washington, D.C., pp. 199–213.

Lowry, O. H., Rosebrough, N. J., Farr, A. L. and Randall, R. J. (1951) Protein measurement with the Folin phenol reagent. *J. biol. Chem.*, 193: 265–275.

McBride, W. J. and Klingman, J. D. (1974) Effects of excitation on the metabolism of a simple neuronal system: the mammalian sympathetic ganglion. In *Progress in Neurobiology, Vol. 3,* G. A. Kerkut and J. W. Philips (Eds.), Pergamon, Oxford, pp. 253–287.

Nagatsu, T., Levitt, M. and Udenfriend, S. (1964) A rapid and simple radioassay for tyrosine hydroxylase activity. *Anal. Biochem.*, 9: 122–126.

Perri, V., Sacchi, O. and Casella, C. (1970) Electrical properties and synaptic connections of the sympathetic neurons in the rat and guinea-pig superior cervical ganglion. *Pflügers Arch. ges. Physiol.*, 314: 40–54.

Reed, D. J., Goto, K. and Wang, C. H. (1966) A direct radioisotopic assay for acetylcholinesterase. *Anal. Biochem.*, 16: 59–64.

Richelson, E. and Nirenberg, M. W. (1974) Tyrosine hydroxylase (EC 1.14.3a) assay. In *Methods in Enzymology, Vol. 32, part B,* S. Fleischer and L. Packer (Eds.), Academic Press, New York, pp. 785–788.

Schrier, B. K. and Shuster, L. (1967) A simplified radiochemical assay for choline acetyltransferase. *J. Neurochem.*, 14: 977–985.

Shiman, R., Akino, M. and Kaufman, S. (1971) Solubilization and partial purification of tyrosine hydroxylase from bovine adrenal medulla. *J. biol. Chem.*, 246: 1330–1340.

Wilson, S. H., Schrier, B. K., Farber, J. L., Thompson, E. J., Rosenberg, R. N., Blume, A. J. and Nirenberg, M. W. (1972) Markers for gene expression in cultured cells from the nervous system. *J. biol. Chem.*, 247: 3159–3169.

Environmentally Directed Nerve Cell Differentiation: In Vivo and In Vitro Studies

C. ZILLER, J. SMITH, M. FAUQUET and N. M. LE DOUARIN

Institut d'Embryologie du CNRS et du Collège de France, 49bis, Avenue de la Belle-Gabrielle, 94130 Nogent-sur-Marne (France)

INTRODUCTION

The differentiation of autonomic neurons has recently been shown to be highly dependent on the microenvironment to which the neuroblasts are subjected at the early stages of their development. This is based primarily on the results of two kinds of technique: the in vitro culture of differentiating autonomic ganglia (see Patterson (1978) for a review) and the in vivo transplantation of the neural crest, the embryonic primordium from which these structures originate.

Isotopic and isochronic transplantation of neural primordium fragments between quail and chick embryos has enabled our group to demonstrate a heterogeneity of the neural axis with regard to the developmental fate of the autonomic ganglion cells that are derived from it. In essence, one region gives rise exclusively to cholinergic enteric ganglion cells, a second to neurons of the sympathetic chain and also to paraganglion cells of the adrenomedulla, while both adrenergic and cholinergic neurons develop from two other levels. This regionalization of the neural crest, which has been precisely established (Le Douarin and Teillet, 1973; Le Douarin, 1976, 1977; Fig. 1), does not correspond to an early determination, for we were able to show, by experimentally changing the normal pattern of crest cell migration, that the potentialities to give rise to cholinergic neurons and to adrenergic ganglion or paraganglion cells exist throughout the entire neural axis. Thus, transplantation of the "adrenergic" region of the crest to the "vagal" level results in the appearance of graft-derived cholinergic ganglia in the gut and, conversely, the mesencephalic neural crest, grafted at the level of the neural primordium from which the adrenal medulla normally originates, provides cells that colonize the suprarenal glands and differentiate into adrenomedullary-like cells (Le Douarin and Teillet, 1974; Le Douarin et al., 1975). These data suggest the existence at a given level of the developing embryo of preferential migration pathways along which the neural crest cells reach their final destination. Thereafter, their differentiation proceeds according to the local environmental conditions that they encounter.

Whether the environment exerts an instructive influence on pluripotent cells or merely selects among a heterogeneous set of already determined ganglioblasts cannot be decided on the basis of these experiments, since the transplantation of cell populations, rather than single cells, was involved. However, experiments by other workers, using a different

---

Abbreviations used: ACh, acetylcholine; CA, catecholamine(s); CAT, choline acetyltransferase; FIF, formaldehyde-induced fluorescence; SRA, Schmidt-Ruppin strain of Rous sarcoma virus.

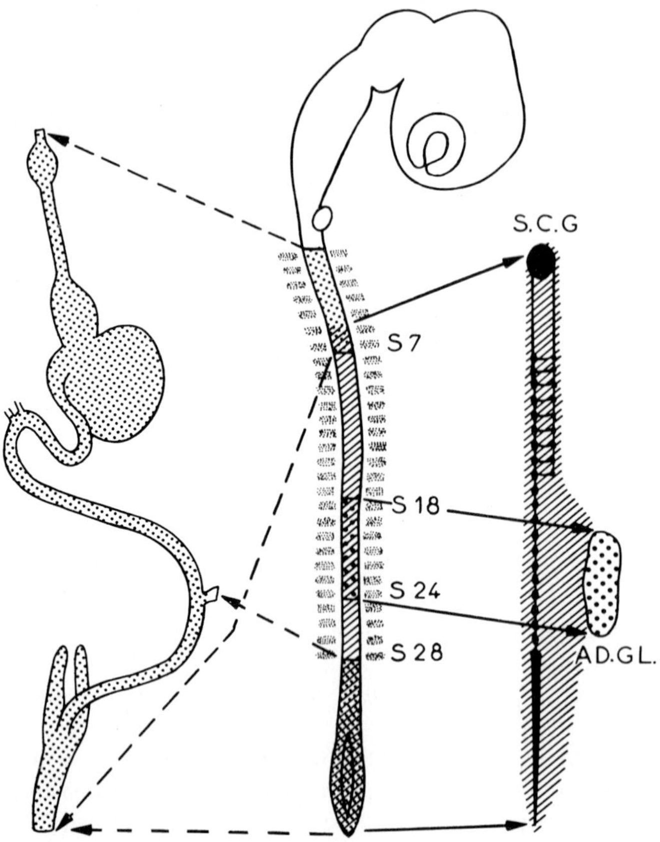

Fig. 1. Levels of origin on the neural axis of the autonomic neurons and adrenomedullary cells. The vagal level of the neural crest (from somites 1–7) provides all the enteric ganglia of the preumbilical gut and contributes to the innervation of the postumbilical gut. The lumbosacral level of the neural crest gives rise to the ganglion of Remak (RG) and some ganglion cells of the postumbilical gut. The orthosympathetic chain is derived from the level of the neural crest posterior to the 5th somite and the adrenomedullary cells originate from the level of somites 18–24. ADGL, suprarenal gland; SCG, superior cervical ganglion; S, somite.

methodological approach, have shown that cells from the superior cervical ganglion (SCG) of the newborn rat have a dual potentiality for neurotransmitter synthesis in vitro. These studies have demonstrated the experimental convertibility of the adrenergic to the cholinergic phenotype in cultures of postmitotic neuroblasts (Patterson et al., 1975; Johnson et al., 1976; Patterson and Chun, 1977a, b) and even, in certain neurons, the simultaneous exhibition of cholinergic and adrenergic properties (Furshpan et al., 1976; Landis, 1976; Reichardt and Patterson, 1977). Consequently, it seems likely that a similar bipotentiality exists at an even earlier developmental stage, i.e., in presumptive neuroblasts of the neural crest. In such an event, environmental influences would be decisive in the expression of the definitive phenotype.

It seemed interesting to see whether developing neuronal cells could be influenced to change their normal differentiative fate, not only in vitro but also in vivo, by experimental modification of their cellular environment. To examine this possibility, ciliary ganglia from

4–13-day quail embryos were grafted into 2-day chicks. The results of these experiments, some of which have already been reported (Le Douarin et al., 1978), are described below.

In addition, and as a complement to our transplantation studies, we are currently examining the developmental capacities of primary cultures of neural crest cells in vitro. The remainder of this article presents the first conclusions that we are able to draw from these experiments.

(I) IN VIVO TRANSPLANTATION OF THE CILIARY GANGLION

The ciliary ganglion, which has been extensively studied in the chick (Ehinger, 1967; Landmesser and Pilar, 1972, 1974a, b; Cantino and Mugnaini, 1974; Chiappinelli et al., 1976), is a cholinergic parasympathetic ganglion in which adrenergic perikarya are absent in all the species so far studied. Acetylcholine (ACh) synthesis is detectable a few hours after

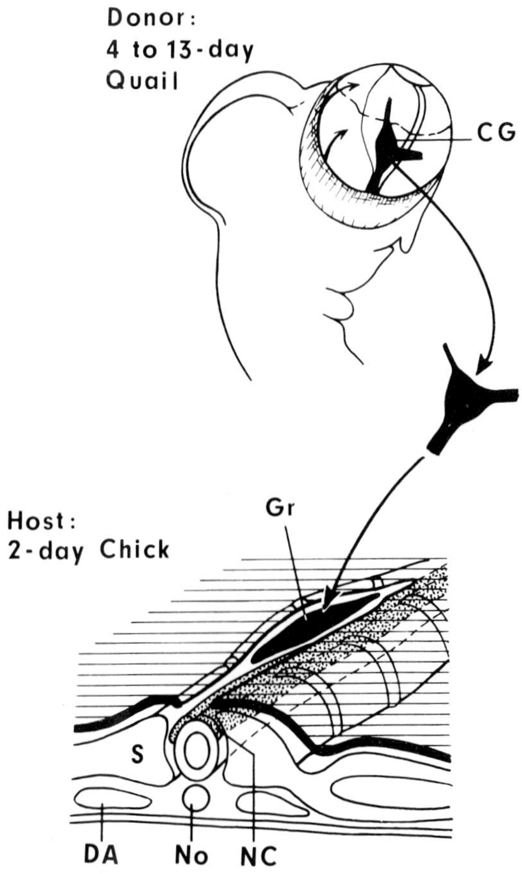

Fig. 2. Experimental design for back-transplantation of the differentiating cholinergic ciliary ganglion from 4–13-day quail donor embryos into 2-day chick hosts. The ganglion (CG) is dissected out and grafted into a slit made between the neural primordium and the somites (S) at the level of somites 18–24 ("adrenomedullary" level) of 24–26 somite chick embryos. Ganglia taken at 4–6 days are grafted in toto. From 6 to 13 days, only pieces of them are implanted. DA, dorsal aorta; Gr, graft; NC, neural crest; No, notochord.

TABLE I

LOCALIZATION OF GRAFTED CILIARY GANGLION CELLS, AS A FUNCTION OF THE AGE OF THE DONOR

+++, structures entirely or mainly made up of grafted quail cells; ++, structures mostly made up of grafted quail cells; +, structures containing some grafted quail cells; –, structures devoid of grafted quail cells.

	Age of donor (days)				
Localization of grafted cells	*4–5*	*6*	*8*	*11*	*13*
Sympathetic ganglion chain	+++	++	+	+	+
Aortic plexus and suprarenal gland	++	++	–	–	–
Remak ganglion	+	–	–	–	–
Enteric ganglia	+	–	–	–	–

the neural crest cells have stopped migrating and begun to form the ganglionic anlagen: as early as 4 days of incubation in the quail embryo, the isolated ciliary ganglion is able to convert [^{3}H]choline to ACh in vitro and this ability increases rapidly during the next few days (Le Douarin et al., 1978). The principle of our experiment was to subject the developing ganglion to the influence of the dorsal trunk of a 2-day embryo, i.e. a region that has been shown to be able to promote adrenergic differentiation in neural crest cells (Cohen, 1972; Norr, 1973; Le Douarin, 1977; Le Douarin et al., 1977). The method is represented and described in Fig. 2.

The operated embryos were taken 4–8 days after grafting and sections cut in appropriate regions were treated to detect both CA content and the quail nuclear marker (see Le Douarin et al. (1978) for technical details). One of the most striking results was that, after transplantation, ciliary ganglion cells were found to be dispersed throughout the host embryo, thus indicating that the integrity of the explant was not maintained after the graft. Furthermore, the localization of the quail cells was strictly limited to the sites in which neural crest cells normally stop. Their distribution varied according to the age of the donor embryo (Table I) and, in addition, the younger the donor the more quail cells there were in each site of arrest. It is noteworthy that, while neural crest cells originating from the 18–24 somite level do not, in the course of normal development, migrate into the mesentery and the gut wall, cells from the grafted ciliary ganglion did so and gave rise to neurons of the ganglion of Remak and of the myenteric plexuses. In contrast, no quail cells were ever detected in the sensory ganglia of the host.

The other interesting result concerned the nature of the neurotransmitter found in the ciliary ganglion cells that had become redistributed in the host. Application of the formaldehyde-induced fluorescence (FIF) technique revealed numerous fluorescent cells in the sympathetic ganglia, the suprarenal glands and the aortic plexus at the level of the graft. Non-fluorescent glial cells with the quail nucleolar marker also occurred in these structures and along the rachidian and sympathetic nerves (Fig. 3). However, in all cases where the ciliary cells colonized the enteric plexuses and the ganglion of Remak, they did not show any fluorescence: consequently, they had probably differentiated into cholinergic neurons.

Identical findings were obtained after comparable grafts of the cholinergic part of the ganglion of Remak (Le Douarin et al., 1978; Teillet, 1978).

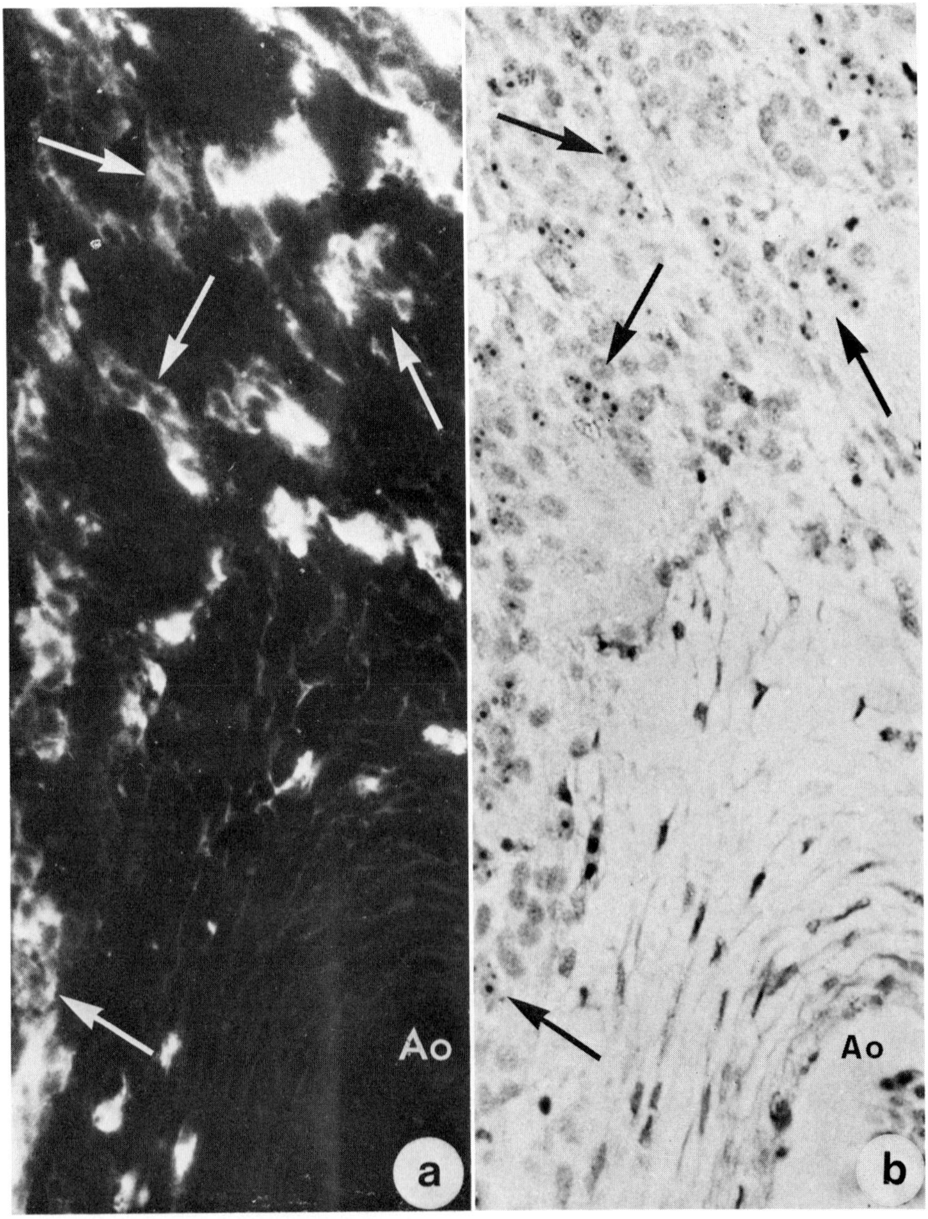

Fig. 3. Suprarenal gland and aortic plexus of a 9-day chick embryo in which the ciliary ganglion of a 4-day quail has been grafted. a: section photographed in UV light after application of the FIF technique showing cords of fluorescent catecholamine-containing cells (× 400). b: the same section, post-stained by the Feulgen-Rossenbeck technique. Clumps of fluorescent cells (arrows) have the quail nuclear marker with a large DNA mass in the center of the nucleus and thus are derived from the grafted ciliary ganglion. Ao, aorta.

These results indicate that developing ganglion cells, back-transplanted into a young embryo, retain (or can reacquire) certain properties of neural crest cells, in particular the ability to migrate and to recognize the sites in which crest cells normally settle. Subsequent events are consistent with the idea that the neurotransmitter metabolism of the differentiating neuroblasts is still unstable at the developmental stages considered and is consolidated or modified according to the nature of the surrounding mesenchymal structures: as in the case of neural crest, cells from the cholinergic ganglion differentiate along the catecholaminergic pathway in the dorsal trunk mesenchyma and into cholinergic neurons in the mesenchyma derived from the splanchnopleure.

(II) IN VITRO STUDIES OF NEURONAL DIFFERENTIATION

(A) Development of primary cultures of normal neural crest cells

This series of studies was undertaken with the aim of seeing whether the tissue interactions that control the differentiation of neural crest cells in vivo and determine the phenotype expressed by autonomic neuroblasts can be mimicked in vitro. If this were indeed the case, the examination of the mechanism involved in nerve cell differentiation would be greatly facilitated.

Since the transplantation studies described earlier have led to the conclusion that the two major classes of autonomic neurons can arise from any region of the neural axis in vivo, it seemed of particular interest to determine whether both adrenergic and cholinergic cells can differentiate in vitro from a given region of the neural crest, and whether particular culture conditions are required for the selective promotion of one or the other metabolic pathway. Recent reports in the literature have already provided indications on these questions. It has been shown by Greenberg and Schrier (1977) that cephalic neural crest can differentiate into cholinergic neurons in culture in the presence of horse serum (but not when the medium contained fetal calf serum), and Cohen (1977) has described the development of FIF-positive cells in cultures of truncal crest of the quail. In both these experiments, the technique used to explant the neural crest cells involved the transplantation of fragments of the neural tube, followed by a 24–48 hr culture period during which the crest cells migrate away from the tube, which can then be removed manually. Since our purpose was to study the developmental capacities of the neural crest cells alone, such a technique was open to criticism for two reasons: first, cells arising from the sectioned surfaces of the neural tube spread over the explant, mingle with the neural crest cells and remain on the dish after removal of the bulk of the tube following the first 48 hr of culture; second, the results of organotypic culture experiments have suggested that the neural tube has a positive influence on adrenergic cell differentiation (Norr, 1973). Therefore, the introduction of neural tube explants in neural crest cell cultures must be avoided if the ability of the crest to differentiate autonomously is to be investigated.

We have therefore directed our efforts towards the isolation from the embryo of pure explants of neural crest. Two regions have been used for these experiments, the mesencephalic crest, from which the ciliary ganglion normally arises (Le Lièvre, 1976), and the truncal crest, corresponding to the presumptive purely adrenergic area (see Fig. 1). At both levels, the tip of the neural fold is excised, before closure of the neural tube, with the aid of steel needles sharpened to fine cutting edges. That the crest so removed is essentially free of neural tube fragments has been confirmed by implanting excised quail crest into the trunk of 2-day chick embryos (according to the technique described in Fig. 2). If some neural tube was included in the implants, it developed as epithelial vesicular structures. In contrast, when the crest alone was taken, such epithelial structures were absent and only crest cell derivatives, dispersed in the host tissues, could be recognized. Epithelial vesicles were found in only 3 out of a total of 20 grafts, showing that the technique that we use to remove the crest is reliable.

Cultures of mesencephalic neural fold were derived from quail embryos of developmental stages equivalent to chick stages 8–9 of Hamburger and Hamilton (1951), i.e. 5–7 somites; truncal crest was taken from embryos of 12–18 somites. For each type of culture, 10–20 fragments were placed in 35 mm plastic dishes containing Dulbecco's modified MEM supplemented with embryo extract and 10% horse serum (replaced by fetal calf serum in some series) and incubated at 37°C in a humidified atmosphere of 5% CO_2 in air.

For the mesencephalic neural crest, another method of explantation was also used. At the 8–12 somite stage, the mesencephalic vesicle has already formed and the crest, abundant at this level, can be distinctly seen as two bands under the ectoderm, migrating laterally away from the tube (Fig. 4). After dissection of this "migrating" neural crest (together with the overlying ectoderm), the fragments (10–16 explants per dish) were cultured under the conditions described above.

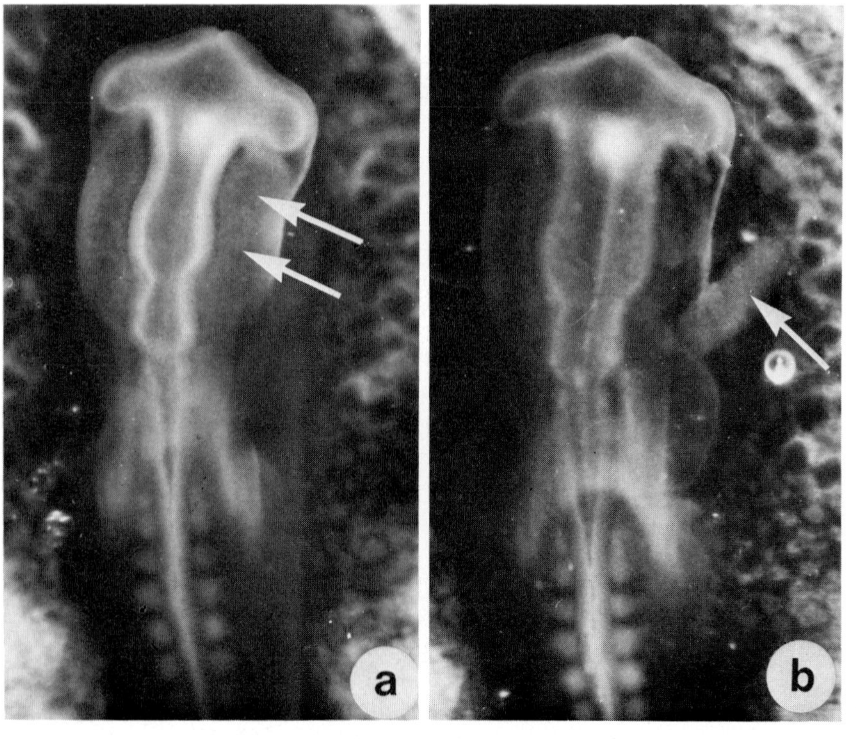

Fig. 4. Quail embryo at 10 somite stage (a) on which the "migrating" neural crest is taken (b) for cultivation. The migrating mesencephalic crest (arrows) appears as a dense sheet of cells underneath the ectoderm that can be selectively removed as shown in (b). × 35.

In some series, both mesencephalic and truncal "crest" cultures were obtained after initial explantation of the entire neural primordium, which was later removed according to the technique employed by Cohen and Konigsberg (1975).

In addition to morphological considerations and cytochemical studies involving the application of the FIF procedure, the appearance of neuronal cells in culture may be monitored by examining the ability of the cells to synthesize and accumulate ACh and CA when provided with [^{3}H]choline and [^{3}H]tyrosine respectively (Mains and Patterson, 1973) and we have routinely employed this method to test the neural crest cultures after 7 days in vitro. In a number of cases, CAT (choline acetyltransferase, EC 2.3.1.6) activity was also assayed to provide an additional criterion of cholinergic differentiation.

(a) Morphological appearance

During the first 3–4 days of culture, the aspect of truncal and mesencephalic cells was the same, i.e. that of small, undifferentiated stellate cells migrating away from the explant. Subsequent differentiation depended on the type of serum used and revealed marked differences between truncal and mesencephalic crest.

In the presence of fetal calf serum, truncal crest cultures contained isolated melanocytes after 4–5 days and developed numerous large pigmented areas after a further 2–3 days. In

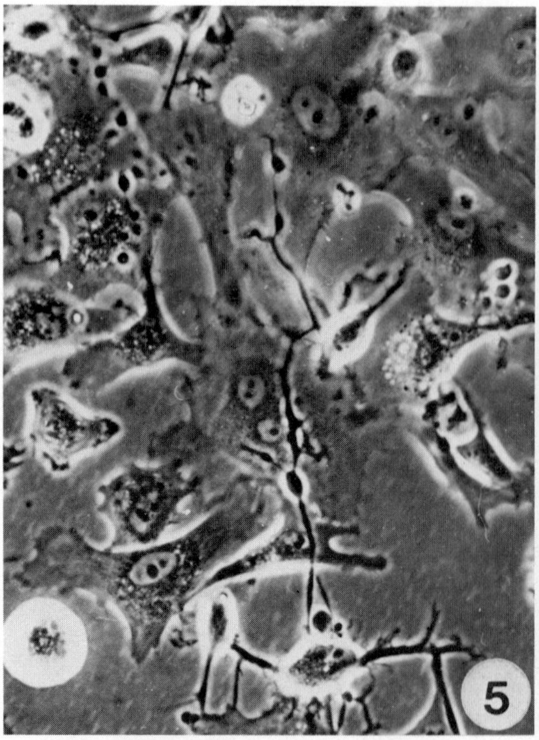

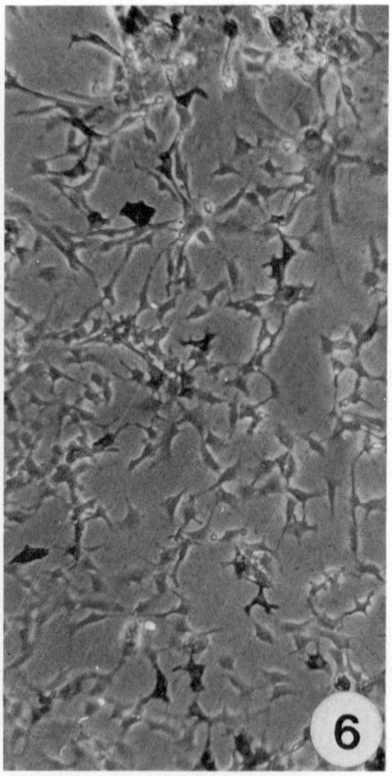

Fig. 5. Neuron-like cells in a culture of the mesencephalic neural fold after 3 weeks in the presence of fetal calf serum. × 300.

Fig. 6. Glial-like cells and melanocytes in a 7-day mesencephalic neural crest culture, in the presence of horse serum. The culture has been prepared from "migrating" crest (see Fig. 4). × 120.

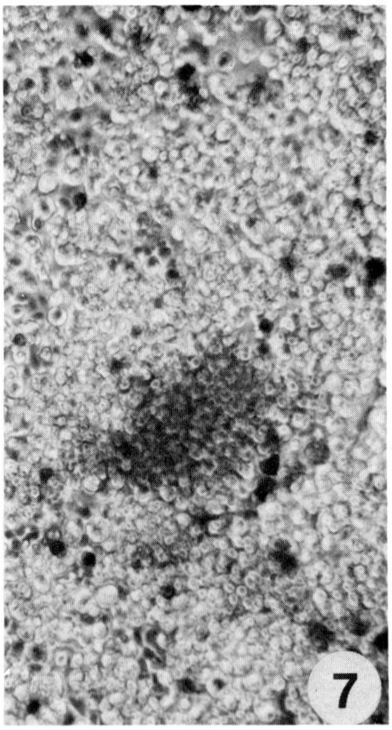

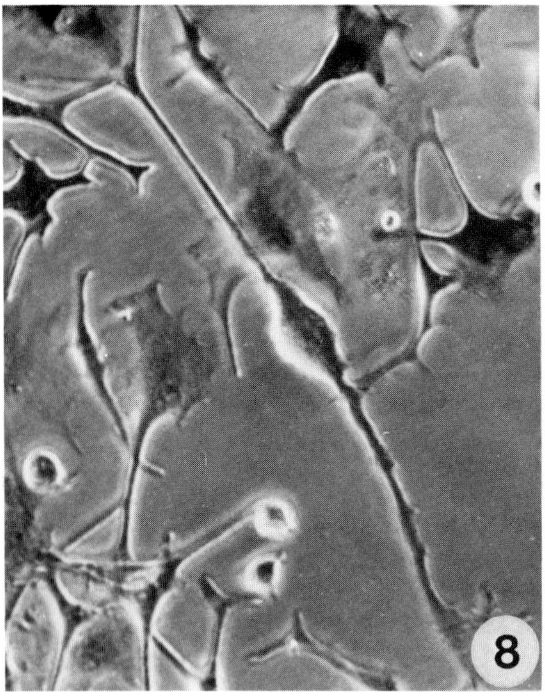

Fig. 7. Actively dividing truncal neural crest cells 3 weeks after transformation by Rous sarcoma virus. The culture has been set up from trunk neural fold taken behind the level of the 15th somite in a 16 somite quail embryo. × 120.

Fig. 8. Same type of culture as in Fig. 7. Melanocytes and neuron-like cells are seen after 3 weeks in vitro; they coexist with cells actively dividing, like those represented in Fig. 7. × 300.

contrast, under the same conditions, mesencephalic crest cultures contained very few pigment cells, but produced large numbers of mesenchymal, fibroblast-like cells, which formed dense multilayered sheets. In both types of culture, glial-like cells, with short, thin processes, and neuron-like cells (Fig. 5) could be observed.

When grown in medium supplemented with horse serum, the differentiation of both types of cultures was more rapid and, in this case, numerous melanocytes were also produced by mesencephalic crest (Fig. 6).

Although cells grown in the presence of fetal calf serum could be maintained in vitro for several weeks, it was found difficult to preserve cultures in medium containing horse serum for more than 7–10 days.

(b) Biochemical differentiation

Mesencephalic crest. Freshly excised, non-cultured mesencephalic neural crest contained no measurable CAT activity; however, after 7 days in medium containing horse serum, significant enzyme levels were found in both "non-migrating" (neural fold) and "migrating" crest cells (Table II). In contrast, in cells cultured in the presence of fetal calf serum, the activity was extremely low (undetectable in 2 out of 4 cases). This bears out the report of

TABLE II

CHOLINE ACETYLTRANSFERASE IN MESENCEPHALIC NEURAL CREST

CAT activity in extracts of neural crest cells was determined by measuring the conversion in vitro of [^{14}C]acetyl CoA to [^{14}C]acetylcholine, the product being separated from unused precursor by electrophoresis at pH 1.9 (Hildebrand et al., 1971). Activities are expressed as the mean ± S.E.M. Protein measurement was carried out according to the technique of Lowry et al. (1951). HS, horse serum; CS, fetal calf serum. Number of experiments in parentheses.

Source of enzyme	*Culture medium*	*CAT activity (ACh formed)*	
		pmol/dish/hr	*nmol/100 mg protein/hr*
"Migrating" neural crest	non-cultured	0 (3)	0 (3)
Neural folds	MEM/HS	37 ± 26 (2)	167 ± 115 (2)
"Migrating" neural crest	MEM/HS	52 ± 12 (5)	116 ± 29 (5)
"Migrating" neural crest	MEM/CS	3 ± 2 (4)	6 ± 4 (4)

TABLE III

SYNTHESIS AND ACCUMULATION OF NEUROTRANSMITTERS BY THE MESENCEPHALIC NEURAL CREST AFTER 7 DAYS IN CULTURE

Neural crest explants (12–15/culture) grown in the media indicated were subsequently incubated with 1 ml of L-15 lacking choline, folic acid, tyrosine and phenylalanine and containing 10 μCi each of methyl [^{3}H]choline and L-[3,5-^{3}H]-tyrosine (specific activities 13 Ci/mmol and 41 Ci/mmol respectively), 40 μg eserine salicylate and 25 μg ascorbate. After 4 hr at 37°C, the cells were scraped off the dish and disrupted ultrasonically. Neurotransmitters were analyzed electrophoretically as described by Hildebrand et al. (1971) and radioactivity in the spots corresponding to acetylcholine and catecholamines (noradrenaline + dopamine) was measured. Synthesis is expressed as fmol produced/dish/4 hr incorporation period. Number of experiments in parentheses

Source of explants	*Culture medium*	*[^{3}H]acetylcholine synthesized (fmol)*	*[^{3}H]catecholamines synthesized (fmol)*
"Migrating" neural crest	MEM/HS	21 ± 8 (4)	0 (4)
"Migrating" neural crest	MEM/CS	0 (1)	0 (1)

TABLE IV

CAT ACTIVITY AND NEUROTRANSMITTER SYNTHESIS AND ACCUMULATION BY 7-DAY CULTURES OF TRUNCAL NEURAL CREST

All cultures (7–10 explants/dish) were grown in MEM/HS. Experiments were performed as described in the legends to Tables II and III.

CAT activity (ACh formed)			
pmol/dish/hr	*nmol/100 mg protein/hr*	*[^{3}H]ACh synthesized (fmol)*	*[^{3}H]CA synthesized (fmol)*
8 ± 3 (4)	37 ± 19 (4)	–	–
–	–	15 ± 9 (3)	0 (3)

Greenberg and Schrier (1977) of the necessity for horse serum in the development of CAT activity in cultures of neural crest cells.

The appearance of cholinergic metabolic pathways in mesencephalic neural crest grown in medium containing horse serum was confirmed by the demonstration of the conversion of [^{3}H]choline to [^{3}H]ACh by intact cells in vitro (Table III). On the other hand, we were not able to detect synthesis of CA in any of the cultures studied, irrespective of the nature of serum used.

Truncal neural crest. These cultures contained relatively low levels of CAT compared with mesencephalic crest cell cultures, but the appearance of cholinergic cells after 7 days in vitro was confirmed by their synthesis of [^{3}H]ACh (Table IV). No CA synthesis was observed. In addition to the cases shown in Table IV, 10 other cultures of truncal crest (or neural tube + crest) were examined for their ability to convert [^{3}H]tyrosine to CA: all were negative.

In conclusion, we demonstrate the capacity of cells both from cephalic and truncal neural crest to undergo cholinergic differentiation in vitro and this maturation does not require even the momentary presence in culture of the neural tube. In contrast, we have been unable to detect adrenergic differentiation by either region of the crest under the same conditions. This result is in contradiction with that obtained by Cohen (1977) and Sieber-Blum and Cohen (1978), who observed fluorescent cells after the application of the FIF technique to cultures of trunk crest.

We have performed several assays with the FIF method on cultures both of trunk and mesencephalic neural crest, with and without preculture with the neural tube. In no case could any fluorescent cells be detected. At the present time we ascribe this discrepancy to subtle differences in culture conditions, perhaps originating from the method used to prepare the embryo extract added to the medium. This question is currently under study.

(B) Development of neural crest cells transformed by Rous sarcoma virus

The relatively small number of potential neuroblasts present in the neural crest (particularly from the trunk level) is an obstacle to the biochemical analysis of their differentiation; in an attempt to overcome this difficulty, we are at present trying to establish cell lines after viral transformation in vitro of crest cells. Explants of mesencephalic and truncal neural crest, obtained as described earlier, were cultured in MEM supplemented with fetal calf serum. Twenty-four hours later, when most of the crest cells had spread out over the dish, the cultures were infected with a suspension of Rous sarcoma virus SRA (a gift from Drs. B. Pessac and G. Calothy).

(a) Morphological appearance

The first signs of rapid cell multiplication could be observed about 5 days after injection and, after 3–4 weeks, most of the cells in the culture appeared to be dividing. Starting from explants containing a few hundred cells, the cultures reached confluence (10^6 cells) in 20–30 days. The proliferation was often so intense that clusters of cells formed (Fig. 7), a phenomenon that never occurred in non-infected cultures.

The actively dividing cells were roughly spherical in shape and detached easily from the dish. In other areas of the culture, the usual cell types characteristic of neural crest cultures could also be observed, i.e. glial-like cells, melanocytes, fibroblasts and neuron-like cells (Fig. 8).

A number of infected cultures were examined for their ability to synthesize neurotransmitters; the results are summarized in Table V.

(b) Biochemical differentiation

Mesencephalic crest. Unlike normal crest, not all transformed cultures synthesized ACh (5 out of 12), and, in the case of the neural fold, the amount of labeled transmitter formed was at the limit of detection. Positive "migrating" crest cultures produced rather more, but the most interesting result was the finding that certain cultures produced limited quantities of CA and one culture was able to synthesize both types of neurotransmitter.

Truncal crest. Transformed cultures of truncal crest synthesized ACh more often (8 cases out of 11) and in somewhat greater quantities than cultures derived from the cephalic region. The same was true for their capacity to synthesise CA and, in addition, 6 cultures produced both types of neurotransmitter simultaneously.

TABLE V

SYNTHESIS AND ACCUMULATION OF NEUROTRANSMITTERS BY TRANSFORMED CULTURES OF MESENCEPHALIC AND TRUNCAL NEURAL CREST

Neurotransmitter synthesis was determined in 2–8-week-old cultures of transformed neural crest cells as described in the legend to Table III.

Source of cultures	*No. experiments*	*No. cultures synthesizing*		
		ACh	*CA*	*ACh + CA*
Neural fold	4	2 (4–5 fmol)	1 (3 fmol)	0
"Migrating" mesencephalic crest	8	3 (5–13 fmol)	3 (3–9 fmol)	1
Truncal crest (derived from neural tube in vitro)	8	6 (5–25 fmol)	6 (3–22 fmol)	4
Excised truncal crest	3	2 (12–18 fmol)	2 (10–12 fmol)	2

CONCLUSIONS AND DISCUSSION

The double potentiality of the neural crest cell population to provide both cholinergic and adrenergic neurons is unequivocally demonstrated by a number of experimental data reported in several previous articles (Le Douarin and Teillet, 1974; Le Douarin et al., 1975, 1977; Le Douarin, 1977; Smith et al., 1977). The ability of differentiating postmitotic neurons from the rat SCG to switch from CA to ACh synthesis (Patterson, 1978), together with evidence for the existence of a class of neurons displaying adrenergic and cholinergic properties simultaneously (Furshpan et al., 1976; Landis, 1976) strongly suggest that a presumptive autonomic ganglioblast is not strictly determined to develop into a sympathetic adrenergic neuron rather than a parasympathetic cholinergic neuron and vice versa. Our recent data concerning the in vivo back transplantation of cholinergic ganglia into 2-day host embryos indicate that the metabolic changes induced in vitro by Patterson and coworkers do not represent merely an unphysiological response to artificial culture conditions but correspond to a real instability of nerve cell determination. According to the findings of Ross et al. (1977) and Patterson and Chun (1977b) this lability is age-dependent and disappears progressively: definitive transmitter function is acquired along with the establishment of functional neuronal activity (Walicke et al., 1977). Although our results support the idea of a certain age dependence of neuroblast instability (Table I), it is nevertheless striking that cell migration and adrenergic differentiation can still be observed with grafted ciliary ganglia up to 13 days old, especially as this age corresponds to a stage where (in the chick) the large number of "surplus" neurons present in the developing ganglion has been eliminated by the massive wave of cell death occurring between 9 and 12 days of incubation (Landmesser and Pilar, 1974b).

Furthermore, our results clearly show that the tissue environment in which the neurons develop determines their final phenotype and is responsible for the observed distribution of catecholaminergic cells in the dorsal trunk structures and cholinergic cells in the splanchnopleural derivatives. As to the nature of the regulatory mechanisms involved, it has recently been demonstrated that conditioned medium from cultures of various cell types (glial, cardiac and certain fibroblasts) acts as a "cholinergizing" agent for adrenergic SCG cells in culture (Patterson and Chun, 1977a). In contrast, the "adrenergizing" influence of the dorsal trunk structures appears to arise predominantly from the notochord (Teillet et al., 1978).

It is of obvious interest to attempt to analyze the factors, whether genetic or epigenetic, controlling autonomic cell differentiation, in order to obtain a clear picture of the events leading from the undetermined to the fully differentiated state. Such a study is problematical in vivo and for this reason we have turned to in vitro systems, with the aim of examining, not differentiating neurons but neural crest cells. Although the experiments reported in this article are only preliminary, a number of results have been obtained which enable future perspectives to be envisaged with a certain optimism. First, the culture of pure crest cells, which is described here for the first time, to our knowledge, has enabled us to show that autonomic nerve cell differentiation from crest cells can occur without any need for interactions with non-neuronal mesodermal cells: this strengthens the idea that an "autonomic cell" population is genetically determined at an early stage. Moreover, the fact that either cholinergic or catecholaminergic phenotypes are expressed according to the culture conditions (cf. our results with truncal crest cultures and those of Cohen (1977)) lends weight to the previous findings that the type of neurotransmitter synthesized is highly dependent on environmental conditions. Although, under the conditions we normally employ, the synthesis of radioactive neurotransmitters is not quantitative, it should be emphasized that the amount produced in our cultures is small and certainly represents only a fraction of the potential synthetic capacity of the crest cell derivatives. One reason for this is undoubtedly the much lower degree of cell proliferation in vitro than in vivo, but, in addition, specific signals are probably required in order to develop this potential fully. Experiments to study this question are already under way.

The results provided by virus-infected cultures show that transformation can allow certain differentiating capabilities to be expressed under conditions in which they do not occur in normal cells. Clonal isolation of neurons with adrenergic, cholinergic and, possibly, dual capacities would certainly be useful for future investigations.

SUMMARY

By using the quail-chick marker system to follow the migration and differentiation of neural crest cells, we have previously shown that the neural axis is regionalized at an early stage into "adrenergic" and "cholinergic" sections, from which arise respectively the sympathetic and parasympathetic/enteric ganglioblasts of the autonomic nervous system. This regionalization does not correspond to an irreversible determination of the crest cells since, under certain experimental conditions, cholinergic neurons can develop from the "adrenergic" region of the crest and vice versa. The phenotypic expression of the presumptive ganglion cells appears to be responsive to the environmental conditions they encounter during and/or after their migration.

Furthermore, the development of parasympathetic ganglion cells that have stopped migrating and at least some of which have begun to differentiate into cholinergic neurons can be profoundly modified if they are transplanted into the trunk of a younger embryo. This is exemplified by experiments in which the ciliary ganglion from 4–13-day quail embryos is grafted into a 2-day chick embryo. The cells from the grafted ganglion are found to migrate to the sites normally colonized by neural crest cells (with the exception of the sensory ganglia). Their subsequent differentiation depends on their new localization: when situated in the adrenergic ganglia and in the suprarenal glands, they synthesize catecholamines, whereas they develop into non-fluorescent, silver-staining ganglion cells if they migrate into the gut wall. Thus, the differentiation of autonomic neurons depends on tissue interactions even after the neural crest cells have grouped to form ganglionic structures in which terminal biochemical differentiation is already in progress.

A study of the nature of the factors required to obtain cholinergic and/or adrenergic differentiation has been undertaken by culturing explants of "pure" neural crest (i.e. free from neural tube) from both "cholinergic" and "adrenergic" regions of the neural axis. The results show that, whereas freshly excised neural crest is biochemically undifferentiated with respect to neurotransmitter metabolism, after 7 days in vitro the cultures contain a number of morphologically distinguishable cell types, possess a significant choline acetyltransferase activity and can synthesize acetylcholine from labeled choline. These cholinergic features are dependent on the presence of horse serum in the medium. No evidence for adrenergic differentiation has been obtained under these conditions, nor after replacement of the horse serum with fetal calf serum. However, after infection with Rous sarcoma virus (SRA), the cells proliferate intensively and give rise to cultures that are, in a number of cases, able to synthesize both acetylcholine and catecholamines from their precursors.

ACKNOWLEDGEMENTS

This work was supported by the Centre National de la Recherche Scientifique, the Délégation Générale à la Recherche Scientifique et Technique, and by a Research Grant from the U.S. National Institutes of Health RO1 DEO 42 57 01 C BY.

REFERENCES

Cantino, D. and Mugnaini, E. (1974) Adrenergic innervation of the parasympathetic ciliary ganglion in the chick. *Science,* 185: 279–281.

Chiappinelli, V., Giacobini, E., Pilar, G. and Uchimura, H. (1976) Induction of cholinergic enzymes in chick ciliary ganglion and iris muscle cells during synapse formation. *J. Physiol. (Lond.),* 257: 749–766.

Cohen, A. M. (1972) Factors directing the expression of sympathetic nerve traits in cells of neural crest origin. *J. exp. Zool.,* 179: 167–182.

Cohen, A. M. (1977) Independent expression of the adrenergic phenotype by neural crest cells in vitro. *Proc. nat. Acad. Sci. (Wash.),* 74: 2899–2903.

Cohen, A. M. and Konigsberg, I. R. (1975) A clonal approach to the problem of neural crest determination. *Develop. Biol.,* 46: 262–280.

Ehinger, B. (1967) Adrenergic nerves in the avian ciliary ganglion. *Z. Zellforsch.,* 82: 577–588.

Furshpan, E. J., MacLeish, P. R., O'Lague, P. H. and Potter, D. D. (1976) Chemical transmission between rat sympathetic neurons and cardiac myocytes developing in microcultures: evidence for cholinergic, adrenergic, and dual-function neurons. *Proc. nat. Acad. Sci. (Wash.),* 73: 4225–4229.

Greenberg, J. H. and Schrier, B. K. (1977) Development of choline acetyltransferase activity in chick cranial neural crest cells in culture. *Develop. Biol.,* 61: 86–93.

Hamburger, V. and Hamilton, H. L. (1951) A series of normal stages in the development of the chick embryo. *J. Morph.,* 88: 49–92.

Hildebrand, J. G., Barker, D. L., Herbert, E. and Kravitz, E. A. (1971) Screening for neurotransmitters: a rapid radiochemical procedure. *J. Neurobiol.,* 2: 231–246.

Johnson, M., Ross, D., Meyers, M., Rees, R., Bunge, R., Walkshull, E. and Burton, H. (1976) Synaptic vesicle cytochemistry changes when cultured sympathetic neurones develop cholinergic interactions. *Nature (Lond.),* 262: 308–310.

Landis, S. C. (1976) Rat sympathetic neurons and cardiac myocytes developing in microcultures: correlation of the fine structure of endings with neurotransmitter function in single neurons. *Proc. nat. Acad. Sci. (Wash.),* 73: 4220–4224.

Landmesser, L. and Pilar, G. (1972) The onset and development of transmission in the chick ciliary ganglion. *J. Physiol. (Lond),* 222: 691–713.

Landmesser, L. and Pilar, G. (1974a) Synapse formation during embryogenesis on ganglion cells lacking a periphery. *J. Physiol. (Lond.),* 241: 715–736.

Landmesser, L. and Pilar, G. (1974b) Synaptic transmission and cell death during normal ganglionic development. *J. Physiol. (Lond.),* 241: 737–749.

Le Douarin, N. (1976) Cell migration in early vertebrate development studied in interspecific chimaeras. In *Embryogenesis in Mammals, Ciba Foundation Symposium,* Elsevier-Excerpta Medica-North-Holland, Amsterdam, pp. 71–101.

Le Douarin, N. (1977) The differentiation of the ganglioblasts of the autonomic nervous system studied in chimeric avian embryos. In *Cell Interactions in Differentiation,* M. Karkinen-Jääskeläinen (Ed.), Academic Press, London, pp. 171–190.

Le Douarin, N. and Teillet, M. A. (1973) The migration of neural crest cells to the wall of the digestive tract in avian embryo. *J. Embryol. exp. Morph.,* 30: 31–48.

Le Douarin, N. M. and Teillet, M. A. (1974) Experimental analysis of the migration and differentiation of neuroblasts of the autonomic nervous system and of neurectodermal mesenchymal derivatives, using a biological cell marking technique. *Develop. Biol.,* 41: 162–184.

Le Douarin, N., Renaud, D., Teillet, M. A. and Le Douarin, G. (1975) Cholinergic differentiation of presumptive adrenergic neuroblasts in interspecific chimaeras after heterotopic transplantations. *Proc. nat. Acad. Sci. (Wash.),* 72: 728–732.

Le Douarin, N. M., Teillet, M. A. and Le Lièvre, C. (1977) Influence of the tissue environment on the differentiation of neural crest cells. In *Cell and Tissue Interactions (30th Annual Meeting of the Society of General Physiologists)*, J. W. Lash and M. Burger (Eds.), Raven Press, New York, pp. 11–27.

Le Douarin, N. M., Teillet, M. A., Ziller, C. and Smith, J. (1978) Adrenergic differentiation of cells of the cholinergic ciliary and Remak ganglia in avian embryo after in vivo transplantation. *Proc. nat. Acad. Sci. (Wash.)*, 75: 2030–2034.

Le Lièvre, C. (1976) *Contribution des Crêtes Neurales à la Genèse des Structures Céphaliques et Cervicales chez les Oiseaux*. Thèse d'Etat, Nantes.

Lowry, O. H., Rosebrough, N. J., Farr, A. L. and Randall, R. J. (1951) Protein measurement with the Folin phenol reagent. *J. biol. Chem.*, 193: 265–275.

Mains, R. E. and Patterson, P. H. (1973) Primary cultures of dissociated sympathetic neurons. I. Establishment of long-term growth in culture and studies of differentiated properties. *J. Cell Biol.*, 59: 329–345.

Norr, S. C. (1973) In vitro analysis of sympathetic neuron differentiation from chick neural crest cells. *Develop. Biol.*, 34: 16–38.

Patterson, P. H. (1978) Environmental determination of autonomic neurotransmitter functions. *Ann. Rev. Neurosci.*, 1: 1–17.

Patterson, P. H. and Chun, L. L. Y. (1977a) The induction of acetylcholine synthesis in primary cultures of dissociated rat sympathetic neurons. I. Effects of conditioned medium. *Develop. Biol.*, 56: 263–280.

Patterson, P. H. and Chun, L. L. Y. (1977b) The induction of acetylcholine synthesis in primary cultures of dissociated rat sympathetic neurons. II. Developmental aspects. *Develop. Biol.*, 60: 473–481.

Patterson, P. H., Reichardt, L. F. and Chun, L. L. Y. (1975) Biochemical studies on the development of primary sympathetic neurons in cell culture. *Cold Spr. Harb. Symp. quant. Biol.*, 40: 389–397.

Reichardt, L. F. and Patterson, P. H. (1977) Neurotransmitter synthesis and uptake by individual rat sympathetic neurons developing in microcultures. *Nature (Lond.)*, 270: 147–151.

Ross, D., Johnson, M. and Bunge, R. (1977) Evidence that development of cholinergic characteristics in adrenergic neurons is age dependent. *Nature (Lond.)*, 267: 536–539.

Sieber-Blum, M. and Cohen, A. M. (1978) Lectin binding to neural crest cells. Changes of the cell surface during differentiation in vitro. *J. Cell Biol.*, 76: 628–638.

Smith, J., Cochard, P. and Le Douarin, N. M. (1977) Development of choline acetyltransferase and cholinesterase activities in enteric ganglia derived from presumptive adrenergic and cholinergic levels of the neural crest. *Cell Diff.*, 6: 199–216.

Teillet, M. A. (1978) Evolution of the lumbo-sacral neural crest in the avian embryo: origin and differentiation of the ganglionated nerve of Remak studied in interspecific quail-chick chimaerae. *Roux's Arch. Develop. Biol.*, 184: 251–268.

Teillet, M. A., Cochard, P. and Le Douarin, N. M. (1978) Relative roles of the mesenchymal tissues and of the complex neural tube-notochord on the expression of adrenergic metabolism in neural crest cells. *Zoon*, 6: 115–122.

Walicke, P. A., Campenot, R. B. and Patterson, P. H. (1977) Determination of transmitter function by neuronal activity. *Proc. nat. Acad. Sci. (Wash.)*, 74: 5767–5771.

Environmental Determination of Neurotransmitter Functions in Developing Sympathetic Neurons

PAUL H. PATTERSON

Harvard Medical School, Department of Neurobiology, Boston, Mass. (U.S.A.)

One area of neuronal development which is particularly interesting is the interaction between cells and their environment as they migrate and differentiate. One of the techniques which has proven useful in studies of such interactions is cell culture, because of the opportunity to control both the fluid and cellular environments surrounding developing neurons. In fact, it is the ability to grow dissociated neurons in culture, either in the virtual absence of other cell types, or in the presence of any of a variety of known types of non-neuronal cells that enables us to control the type of transmitter produced and type of synapse formed by developing sympathetic neurons in culture. These neurons are capable of producing either catecholamines (CA) or acetylcholine (ACh) and forming adrenergic or cholinergic synapses. This, of course, is a choice that neurons in the autonomic system normally have to make, and it is a very critical decision functionally because most autonomic target organs respond to both CA and ACh, but usually in opposite ways; norepinephrine speeds the heart beat while ACh inhibits it.

The cells of the superior cervical ganglion of the neonatal rat can be mechanically dissociated (Bray, 1970) and plated into culture media which are (i) non-permissive for the survival and proliferation of non-neuronal cells or (ii) permissive for co-culture of the neuronal and non-neuronal cells (Mains and Patterson, 1973; Patterson and Chun, 1977a). In the former situation, the neuron-alone cultures can develop many of the properties expected of mature adrenergic cells (Mains and Patterson, 1973a, b, c; Claude, 1973; Rees and Bunge, 1974; O'Lague et al., 1974; Burton and Bunge, 1975).

In contrast to the development in the absence of non-neuronal cells, when sympathetic neurons are co-cultured with appropriate (see below) non-neuronal cells, they develop striking cholinergic properties: they synthesize and store large amounts of acetylcholine (ACh) (Patterson and Chun, 1974) and use it at functional cholinergic synapses with a number of targets (O'Lague et al., 1974, 1975; Nurse and O'Lague, 1975; Furshpan et al., 1976; Johnson et al., 1976; Ko et al., 1976). Furthermore, this cholinergic induction caused by non-neuronal cells can be mediated by a diffusible factor (Patterson et al., 1975, Patterson and Chun, 1977a). Neurons grown in culture medium that has been conditioned by incubation on cultures of appropriate non-neuronal cells (CM) also causes dramatic increases in (i) choline acetyltransferase activity (CAT) as measured in neuronal extracts (Patterson and Chun, 1977a), (ii) ACh synthesis and accumulation from [^{3}H]choline by living cells (Patterson et al., 1975; Patterson and Chun, 1977a), and (iii) cholinergic synapse formation between the neurons (Landis et al., 1976; MacLeish, 1976). At the same time, however, growth in CM causes a marked reduction in adrenergic properties: catecholamine (CA) synthesis and the proportion of synaptic vesicles containing small dense cores following permanganate fixation are considerably lower than controls (Landis et al., 1976; Patterson and Chun, 1977a, b). Similarly, co-culture with appropriate non-neuronal cells reduces the proportion of small granular vesicles observed after loading with exogenous CA (Johnson et al., 1976). In addition, the CM effects are graded. A higher proportion of CM (Landis et al., 1976; Patterson and Chun, 1977a) or a greater number of non-neuronal cells (MacLeish, 1976) gives a higher ratio of ACh to CA synthesis, a higher incidence of cholinergic transmission, and a higher proportion of synapses that lack small granular vesicles and appear cholinergic. Thus the presence of certain non-neuronal cells, or a medium conditioned by them, has a profound effect on the type of transmitter chosen by the sympathetic neurons.

These effects of CM are rather specific. Doses of CM that increase the ratio of ACh to CA production 100–1000-fold do not appreciably affect neuronal survival or growth (as monitored by number of somas and total neuronal protein and lipid) (Patterson and Chun, 1977a). This constancy in survival and growth is not because only a few neurons in the population are involved in these transmitter changes: single cell experiments have shown that most if not all of the neurons are influenced in this manner by the culture environment. We have developed methods for growth of single neurons in microcultures containing various concentrations of CM or non-neuronal cells (Reichardt et al., 1976); as many as 80–90% of individual neurons grown on heart or skeletal muscle can be cholinergic, while as few as 0% are cholinergic under "control" conditions (Nurse, 1977; Reichardt and Patterson, 1977). Furthermore, by growing cultures in various concentrations of CM it is possible to obtain populations of single cells in which almost every cell synthesizes CA or in which a high proportion of cells synthesize ACh (Reichardt and Patterson, 1977). Finally, we obtained no evidence for a significant population of "silent" neurons that make no transmitter under these conditions (Reichardt and Patterson, 1977). These observations and the constancy in neuronal number and growth in the mass cultures suggest that CM affects the choice of transmitter and type of synapse formed by individual sympathetic neurons and does not select certain predetermined cell types for survival. Preliminary characterization of this interesting developmental signal suggests that it is a basic glycoprotein with an apparent molecular weight of 50,000 on Sephadex chromatography (M. Weber and P. Patterson, unpublished).

What is the developmental time course of appearance of adrenergic and cholinergic properties? Present information about normal development in the rat superior cervical ganglion suggests that most of the neurons express adrenergic functions (at relatively low levels) before birth, that is, before the neurons are put into culture (Champlain et al., 1970; Eränkö, 1972a, b). In fact, sympathetic neuroblasts can contain CA even before they cease mitosis (Cohen, 1974; Rothman et al., 1977). Moreover, the cultured neurons synthesize CA during the first week in vitro (Mains and Patterson, 1973a), and all their varicosities contain high proportions of small granular vesicles at one week (Johnson et al., 1976), even when grown in CM from day one (S. Landis, in preparation). These observations suggest that most, if not all, of the neurons are adrenergic when initially placed in culture and, as previously discussed, they can either continue to develop adrenergically or, in the presence of CM, become cholinergic. Since most, if not all, of the neurons can become cholinergic (see above), many can reverse their differentiative fate after beginning to express another phenotype. It is possible that a similar sequence may occur in vivo in embryonic gut. CA-containing cells have been seen in the area of the myenteric plexus and subsequently disappear

(Cochard et al., 1978). It is not yet clear if these same cells later become cholinergic neurons, however.

Under certain conditions, mass neuronal cultures produce both ACh and CA, and the question arises whether individual neurons can display both transmitter functions simultaneously. Electrophysiological (Furshpan et al., 1976) and electron microscopic (Landis, 1976) observations on young single neurons grown in microcultures on rat cardiac myocytes for about 2 weeks indicate that this is possible. Three categories of neurons were identified: (i) neurons that formed hexamethonium-sensitive cholinergic synapses (with no small granular vesicles) on their own somas and elicited atropine-sensitive cholinergic responses in the heart cells, (ii) neurons that elicited propranolol-sensitive adrenergic responses in the heart cells and had neuronal varicosities containing high proportions of small granular vesicles, and (iii) neurons that where of "dual function"; they elicited first a cholinergic response and then an adrenergic response in beating myocytes, and their varicosities contained only occasional small granular vesicles. The incidence of these dual-function neurons has not yet been determined satisfactorily, but they are not exceedingly rare (Furshpan et al., 1976). On the other hand, our biochemical assays of transmitter production on older (3–5 weeks) single neurons have provided few if any examples of dual-function cells (Reichardt and Patterson, 1977); the vast majority of neurons made detectable amounts of either CA or ACh, depending on the culture conditions. The difference between the electrophysiological and biochemical results with respect to dual-function neurons may reflect an inability of the biochemical methods to detect a low level of one of the two transmitters in cells that were actually bifunctional. Alternatively, the young dual-function neurons detected electrophysiologically may have been passing through a transient stage that leads to one of the two differentiated states observed in the older cells with biochemical methods. It will clearly be of interest to study a single neuron over time and see if it can be shifted from one transmitter function to another by addition or withdrawal of CM at various intervals.

After 3–5 weeks, when the cells have matured either cholinergically or adrenergically, do the neurons still have the capacity to reverse their phenotype? Since ganglionic explants develop CAT activity and form cholinergic synapses in vitro (Crain and Peterson, 1974; Purves et al., 1974; Hill et al., 1976), it is possible to assay the development of CAT and adrenergic enzymes in explants from rats of various ages. Recent findings show that CAT develops in vitro only in explants taken from young rats; explants from older animals develop only adrenergic enzymes (Hill and Hendry, 1977; Ross et al., 1977). Thus, after full adrenergic maturation the neurons may not respond to cholinergic cues. We have obtained similar results with the dissociated cell cultures (Patterson et al., 1977; Patterson and Chun, 1977b). These experiments demonstrate that (i) the neurons become more refractory to induction of ACh synthesis by CM as they mature adrenergically, and (ii) they become more refractory to induction of adrenergic function by CM withdrawal as they mature cholinergically. Therefore, the cholinergic-adrenergic decision appears to be a function of the developmental stage. Young neurons can respond to available cues and can differentiate to become either adrenergic or cholinergic (or sometimes both). They can alter their decision even after beginning to express such functions, but they become less plastic as they mature. This may represent a third and final stage in which the decision to produce a particular transmitter is not easily reversible but where its production can be quantitatively modulated by various stimuli (Thoenen, 1975).

Given that it is possible in culture to influence virtually all of the neurons to become cholinergic, why then in vivo are only a small proportion of the neurons in sympathetic ganglia cholinergic (Sjöqvist, 1963; Aiken and Reit, 1969)? One possibility is that the cholinergic signal in vivo is highly localized, perhaps in a target tissue such as the sweat gland which contains cholinergic sympathetic endings. In this situation, most of the neurons would not receive the signal and thus remain adrenergic. One useful way to ask if this is the case would be to develop a radioimmune assay for that factor and assay different tissues in the developing rat. Since this assay is not yet available, only indirect experiments have been done. We have asked what tissues in culture can produce the CM factor and we found earlier on that a glial cell line and ganglionic non-neuronal cells can induce neuronal ACh production (Patterson and Chun, 1974). Subsequently we observed that cells cultured from a variety of tissues taken from the newborn rat can induce cholinergic changes (Patterson and Chun, 1977a). Large quantitative differences were observed in the ability of cells from the various non-neuronal sources to induce cholinergic functions, and some of these differences are intriguing. Targets that receive cholinergic or mixed innervation, such as skeletal and heart muscle, are excellent inducers whereas targets that receive only adrenergic innervation, such as brown fat (Cottle, 1970) and liver (Forssman and Ito, 1977) are relatively poor inducers. There is also the interesting possibility that cues from targets may play a role in the development of other parts of the nervous system. For instance, spinal cord cells cultured with skeletal muscle cells, or CM from them, show increased CAT activity (Giller et al., 1973, 1977), whereas some spinal cord cells cultured with liver display adrenergic properties (Bird and James, 1975). Although the concept that a target organ can modify the transmitter used by its innervation is an interesting one, it is still too early to evaluate its merits. Several types of cells which are effective medium-conditioners are not normally innervated, in the sense of receiving synapses. Among these cells are primary embryonic fibroblasts (Patterson and Chun, 1977a) and the previously mentioned glioma and ganglionic non-neuronal cells. Evidently, a complete explanation of the choice of transmitter will include factors in addition to those discussed thus far. Two additional factors known to be important in the development of sympathetic neurons are nerve growth factor (NGF) and the acquisition of the normal preganglionic input from the spinal cord. Do these factors influence the choice of transmitter?

NGF is essential for the survival, growth and differentiation of adrenergic sympathetic neurons (Levi-Montalcini and Angeletti, 1968). What then is the role of NGF in the development of the sympathetic cholinergic neurons? Recently we have compared the role of NGF in the development of sympathetic neurons grown in the absence of non-neuronal cells under conditions where the vast majority of the neurons are adrenergic (0% CM) or cholinergic (62% CM). Immature neurons (< 2 weeks old) in both types of cultures have an absolute requirement for NGF; in its absence all the neurons die, and NGF causes a dose-dependent increase in survival. Both types of culture become less dependent on NGF with time (Chun and Patterson, 1977a, b, c; see also Lazarus et al., 1976). NGF also increases, in a dose-dependent fashion, the ability of the neurons in adrenergic cultures to produce catecholamines (Chun and Patterson, 1977a). This increase is not simply a consequence of the effect of NGF on neuronal survival or growth, because it is seen even when the CA production is expressed per neuron, or per total neuronal protein or lipid phosphate (Chun and Patterson, 1977a). Therefore, as in earlier in vivo experiments (Thoenen et al., 1971), NGF stimulates not only survival and growth, but enhances adrenergic differentiation in a dose-dependent manner. Perhaps unexpectedly, NGF also stimulates the differentiation of cholinergic cultures. ACh production per neuron increases as the NGF concentration is raised (Chun and Patterson, 1977c; see also Hill and Hendry, 1977). In fact, NGF stimulates the production of both transmitters to the same extent. That is, the ratio of ACh to CA, which is a reflection of the relative rates of the synthesis of these transmitters, remains constant over a wide range of

NGF concentrations for both adrenergic (ACh/CA = 0.02) and cholinergic (ACh/CA = 200) cultures (Chun and Patterson, 1977c). Thus, with respect to transmitter production, NGF is permissive rather than instructive in that it is necessary for survival and stimulates growth and differentiation but does not tell the neurons which transmitter to produce. That NGF does not determine what transmitter a cell will make is further suggested by the fact that dorsal root ganglion cells that are sensitive to NGF for certain periods of embryonic life do not appear to produce significant levels of CA or ACh.

To summarize these observations, NGF appears to enhance the differentiation of immature sympathetic neurons along either adrenergic or cholinergic paths. In fact, at least at young ages, some cultured neurons appear to secrete both transmitters simultaneously. The particular phenotype chosen depends on other developmental cues. CM produced by certain types of non-neuronal cells can direct the neurons in the cholinergic direction. CM is a qualitatively different developmental signal from NGF because it is not necessary for neuronal survival and does not appreciably stimulate neuronal growth. By analogy, there would be another cue for adrenergic function, which is not NGF. This factor may be produced by a combination of neural tube, somitic mesenchyma, and perhaps notochord (see Le Douarin, this volume). It is not yet clear whether these embryonic tissues actively signal the crest cells or merely provide a permissive environment for the expression of a previously determined phenotype. However, even if cells have been previously instructed as to neurotransmitter synthesis, this order can be countermanded in young neurons in culture (and also in vivo; Le Douarin et al., 1978). This reversal can occur after ganglion formation in vivo and initial differentiation in vitro has begun. Thus the question raised earlier still remains, why is it that non-neuronal cells or CM can cause almost all the neurons to become cholinergic in culture, yet only a few sympathetic neurons become cholinergic in vivo, even in the presence of an abundance of non-neuronal cells? One possibility, already discussed, is that the cholinergic signal is selectively localized so that most of the sympathetic neurons are not affected by it. The problems with this idea were already considered. Another possibility is that many, or all of the neurons receive the cholinergic signal in vivo, but most are prevented from responding to it by a factor that is absent from the cultures.

One obvious factor missing from the sympathetic cultures is the preganglionic input from the spinal cord. In fact, it is already known that if the preganglionic input to sympathetic ganglia of young mice is cut, further development of adrenergic properties is prevented (Black, 1978). These observations raised the question whether electrical activity imposed on postganglionic neurons as they acquire their preganglionic input during the first 3 postnatal weeks plays a role in the choice of transmitter.

We have tested the consequences on the adrenergic-cholinergic decision of mimicking the electrical effects of spinal cord innervation by depolarizing the cultured sympathetic neurons (Walicke et al., 1977). The depolarization was done either chronically with elevated K^+ or veratridine or intermittently, with direct electrical stimulation. These treatments, either before or during CM application, caused as much as a 300-fold depression in the ACh/CA ratio, leaving the cultures primarily adrenergic. Elevated K^+ and veratridine produced this effect on cholinergic development without significantly altering neuronal survival. It did not appear that neuronal activity directly inhibited ACh synthesis because pretreatment with elevated K^+, veratridine, or electrical stimulation all reduced the ACh/CA ratios of cultures subsequently exposed to CM in the absence of these depolarizing agents. It is as if increased activity in the neurons stabilizes their prenatal instruction to become adrenergic and curtails their plasticity with respect to transmitter choice. This failure of the cells to respond to cholinergic induction by CM suggests that the onset of activity is a signal for final determination of transmitter choice. Since depolarization causes Ca^{2+} entry in a number of cell types, the effects of several Ca^{2+} antagonists were investigated. In the presence of Mg^{2+} or D600, K^+ did not prevent the induction of cholinergic properties by CM (Walicke et al., 1977). Thus depolarization, either steady or accompanying activity, is one of the factors determining whether cultured sympathetic neurons become adrenergic or cholinergic, and this effect may be mediated by the entry of Ca^{2+}. Our more recent work suggests that cyclic nucleotides may be involved in the depolarization effect. That is, addition of cyclic nucleotide derivatives themselves or effectors that raise intracellular cyclic AMP levels (adenosine, PGE_1 or cholera toxin) can mimic the depolarization effect on transmitter development (Walicke and Patterson, 1978). We are currently assaying the effects of elevated K^+ and CM on neuronal cyclic nucleotide levels.

These observations raise the possibility that in vivo the majority of sympathetic neurons are preserved in their prenatal adrenergic condition, in spite of the presence of ganglionic or other non-neuronal cells, by activity imposed on the neurons when they acquire their preganglionic innervation from the spinal cord. A corollary hypothesis is that the minority of neurons destined to become cholinergic (and to innervate certain blood vessels and sweat glands) acquires its preganglionic input only after it has been affected by non-neuronal cells. An interesting possibility is inherent in such a mechanism. Perhaps the selective formation of synapses between given preganglionic axons and particular neurons in the ganglion (Nja and Purves, 1977) not only determines circuitry, but also influences the type of neuron that individual sympathetic cells will become. This idea emphasizes the potential importance of neuronal activity in the development of the nervous system.

REFERENCES

Aiken, J. W. and Reit, E. (1969) A comparison of the sensitivity to chemical stimuli of adrenergic and cholinergic neurons in the cat stellate ganglion. *J. Pharmacol. exp. Ther.*, 169: 211–223.

Bird, M. and James, D. (1975) The culture of previously dissociated embryonic chick spinal cord cells on feeder layers of liver and kidney, and the development of paraformaldehyde-induced fluorescence upon the former. *J. Neurocytol.*, 4: 633–646.

Black, I. B. (1978) Regulation of autonomic development. *Ann. Rev. Neurosci.*, 1: 183–214.

Bray, D. (1970) Surface movements during the growth of single explanted neurons. *Proc. nat. Acad. Sci. (Wash.)*, 65: 905–910.

Burton, H. and Bunge, R. P. (1975) A comparison of the uptake and release of [^{3}H]norepinephrine in rat autonomic and sensory ganglia in tissue culture. *Brain Res.*, 97: 157–162.

Champlain, J. de, Malmfors, T., Olson, L. and Sachs, C. (1970) Ontogenesis of peripheral adrenergic neurons in the rat: pre- and postnatal observations. *Acta physiol. scand.*, 80: 276–288.

Chun, L. L. Y. and Patterson, P. H. (1977a) The role of nerve growth factor in the development of rat sympathetic neurons in vitro. I. Survival, growth and differentiation of catecholamine production. *J. Cell Biol.*, 75: 694–704.

Chun, L. L. Y. and Patterson, P. H. (1977b) The role of nerve growth factor in the development of rat sympathetic neurons in vitro. II. Developmental studies. *J. Cell Biol.*, 75: 705–711.

Chun, L. L. Y. and Patterson, P. H. (1977c) The role of nerve growth factor in the development of rat sympathetic neurons in vitro. III. Effect on acetylcholine production. *J. Cell Biol.*, 75: 712–718.

Claude, P. (1973) Electron microscopy of dissociated rat sympathetic neurons in vitro. *J. Cell Biol.*, 59: 57A.

Cochard, P., Goldstein, M. and Black, I. B. (1978) Ontogenetic appearance and disappearance of tyrosine hydroxylase and catecholamines in the rat embryo. *Proc. nat. Acad. Sci. (Wash.)*, 75: 2986–2990.

Cohen, A. M. (1974) DNA synthesis and cell division in differentiating avian adrenergic neuroblasts. In *Dynamics of Degeneration and Growth in Neurons*, K. Fuxe, L. Olson and Y. Zotterman (Eds.), Pergamon Press, New York, pp. 359–370.

Cottle, W. H. (1970) The innervation of brown adipose tissue. In *Brown Adipose Tissue*, O. Lindberg (Ed.), Elsevier, New York, pp. 155–178.

Crain, S. M. and Peterson, E. R. (1974) Development of neural connections in culture. *Ann. N.Y. Acad. Sci.*, 228: 6–33.

Eränkö, L. (1972a) Ultrastructure of the developing sympathetic nerve cell and the storage of catecholamines. *Brain Res.*, 46: 159–175.

Eränkö, L. (1972b) Postnatal development of histochemically demonstrable catecholamines in the superior cervical ganglion of the rat. *Histochem. J.*, 4: 225–236.

Forssman, W. G. and Ito, S. (1977) Morphology of efferent liver innervation in primates. *J. Cell Biol.*, 74: 299–314.

Furshpan, E. J., MacLeish, P. R., O'Lague, P. H. and Potter, D. D. (1976) Chemical transmission between rat sympathetic neurons and cardiac myocytes developing in microcultures: evidence for cholinergic, adrenergic, and dual-function neurons. *Proc. nat. Acad. Sci. (Wash.)*, 73: 4225–4229.

Giller, E. L., Schrier, B. K., Shainberg, A., Fisk, H. R. and Nelson, P. G. (1973) Choline acetyltransferase activity is increased in combined cultures of spinal cord and muscle cells from mice. *Science*, 182: 588–589.

Giller, E. L., Neale, J. H., Bullock, P. N., Schrier, B. K. and Nelson, P. G. (1977) Choline acetyltransferase activity of spinal cord cell cultures increased by co-culture with muscle and by muscle-conditioned medium. *J. Cell Biol.*, 74: 16–29.

Hill, C. E. and Hendry, A. I. (1977) Development of neurons synthesizing noradrenaline and acetylcholine in the superior cervical ganglion of the rat in vivo and in vitro. *Neuroscience*, 2: 741–749.

Hill, C. E., Purves, R. D., Watanabe, H. and Burnstock, G. (1976) Specificity of innervation of iris musculature by sympathetic nerve fibers in tissue culture. *Pfluegers Arch. ges. Physiol.*, 361: 127–134.

Johnson, M., Ross, D., Meyers, M., Rees, R., Bunge, R., Wakshull, E. and Burton, H. (1976) Synaptic vesicle cytochemistry changes when cultured sympathetic neurons develop cholinergic interactions. *Nature (Lond.)*, 262: 308–310.

Ko, C.-P., Burton, H., Johnson, M. I. and Bunge, R. P. (1976) Synaptic transmission between rat superior cervical ganglion neurons in dissociated cell cultures. *Brain Res.*, 117: 461–485.

Landis, S. C. (1976) Rat sympathetic neurons and cardiac myocytes developing in microcultures: correlation of the fine structure of endings with neurotransmitter function in single neurons. *Proc. nat. Acad. Sci. (Wash.)*, 73: 4220–4224.

Landis, S. C., MacLeish, P. R., Potter, D. D., Furshpan, E. J. and Patterson, P. H. (1976) Synapses formed between dissociated neurons: the influence of conditioned medium. *Sixth Ann. Soc. Neurosci.*, Abstr. 280, p. 197.

Lazarus, K. J., Bradshaw, R. A., West, N. R. and Bunge, R. P. (1976) Adaptive survival of rat sympathetic neurons cultured without supporting cells or exogenous nerve growth factor. *Brain Res.*, 113: 159–164.

Le Douarin, N. M., Teillet, M. A., Ziller, C. and Smith, J. (1978) Adrenergic differentiation of cells of the cholinergic ciliary and Remak ganglion in avian embryo after in vivo transplantation. *Proc. nat. Acad. Sci. (Wash.)*, 75: 2030–2034.

Levi-Montalcini, R. and Angeletti, P. U. (1968) Nerve growth factor. *Physiol. Rev.*, 48: 534–569.

MacLeish, P. R. (1976) *Synapse Formation in Cultures of Dissociated Rat Sympathetic Neurons grown on Dissociated Rat Heart Cells.* Ph.D. Thesis, Harvard Univ., Cambridge, Mass., 142 pp.

Mains, R. E. and Patterson, P. H. (1973a) Primary cultures of dissociated sympathetic neurons. I. Establishment of long-term growth in culture and studies of differentiated properties. *J. Cell Biol.*, 59: 329–345.

Mains, R. E. and Patterson, P. H. (1973b) Primary cultures of dissociated sympathetic neurons. II. Initial studies on catecholamine metabolism. *J. Cell Biol.*, 59: 346–360.

Mains, R. E. and Patterson, P. H. (1973c) Primary cultures of dissociated sympathetic neurons. III. Changes in metabolism with age in culture. *J. Cell Biol.*, 59: 361–366.

Nja, A. and Purves, D. (1977) Specific innervation of guinea pig superior cervical ganglion cells by preganglionic fibers arising from different levels of the spinal cord. *J. Physiol. (Lond.)*, 264: 565–583.

Nurse, C. A. (1977) *The Formation of Cholinergic Synapses between Dissociated Rat Sympathetic Neurons and Skeletal Myotubes in Cell Culture.* Ph.D. Thesis, Harvard Univ., Cambridge, Mass., 124 pp.

Nurse, C. A. and O'Lague, P. H. (1975) Formation of cholinergic synapses between dissociated sympathetic neurons and skeletal myotubes of the rat in cell culture. *Proc. nat. Acad. Sci. (Wash.)*, 72: 1955–1959.

O'Lague, P. H., Obata, K., Claude, P., Furshpan, E. J. and Potter, D. D. (1974) Evidence for cholinergic synapses between dissociated rat sympathetic neurons in cell culture. *Proc. nat. Acad. Sci. (Wash.)*, 71: 3602–3606.

O' Lague, P. H., MacLeish, P. R., Nurse, C. A., Claude, P., Furshpan, E. J. and Potter, D. D. (1975) Physiological and morphological studies on developing sympathetic neurons in dissociated cell culture. *Cold Spr. Harb. Symp. quant. Biol.*, 40: 399–407.

Patterson, P. H. and Chun, L. L. Y. (1974) The influence of nonneuronal cells on catecholamine and acetylcholine synthesis and accumulation in cultures of dissociated sympathetic neurons. *Proc. nat. Acad. Sci. (Wash.)*, 71: 3607–3610.

Patterson, P. H. and Chun, L. L. Y. (1977a) The induction of acetylcholine synthesis in primary cultures of dissociated rat sympathetic neurons. I. Effects of conditioned medium. *Develop. Biol.*, 56: 263–280.

Patterson, P. H. and Chun, L. L. Y. (1977b) The induction of acetylcholine synthesis in primary cultures of dissociated rat sympathetic neurons. II. Developmental aspects. *Develop. Biol.*, 60: 473–481.

Patterson, P. H., Reichardt, L. F. and Chun, L. L. Y. (1975) Biochemical studies on the development of primary sympathetic neurons in cell culture. *Cold Spr. Harb. Symp. quant. Biol.*, 40: 389–397.

Patterson, P. H., Chun, L. L. Y. and Reichardt, L. F. (1977) The role of nonneuronal cells in the development of sympathetically-derived neurons. In *Cellular Neurobiology*, Z. Hall, R. Kelly and F. Fox (Eds.), Liss, New York, pp. 94–104.

Purves, R. D., Hill, C. E., Chamley, J. H., Mark, G. E., Fry, D. M. and Burnstock, G. (1974) Functional autonomic neuromuscular junctions in tissue culture. *Pfluegers Arch. ges. Physiol.*, 350: 1–7.

Rees, R. and Bunge, R. P. (1974) Morphological and cytochemical studies of synapses formed in culture between isolated rat superior cervical ganglion neurons. *J. comp. Neurol.*, 157: 1–11.

Reichardt, L. F. and Patterson, P. H. (1977) Neurotransmitter synthesis and uptake by individual rat sympathetic neurons developing in microculture. *Nature (Lond.)*, 270: 147–151.

Reichardt, L. F., Patterson, P. H. and Chun, L. L. Y. (1976) Norepinephrine and acetylcholine synthesis by individual sympathetic neurons under various culture conditions. *Sixth. Ann. Soc. Neurosci.*, Abstr. 327, p. 197.

Ross, D., Johnson, M. and Bunge, R. (1977) Evidence that development of cholinergic characteristics in adrenergic neurons is age dependent. *Nature (Lond.)*, 267: 536–539.

Rothman, T. P., Gershon, M. D. and Holtzer, H. (1977) Cell division in the development of adrenergic neurons. *7th Ann. Soc. Neurosci.*, Abstr. 820, p. 259.

Sjöqvist, F. (1963) The correlation between the occurrence and localization of acetylcholinesterase-rich cell bodies in the stellate ganglion and the outflow of cholinergic sweat secretory fibres to the forepaw of the cat. *Acta physiol. scand.*, 57: 339–351.

Thoenen, H. (1975) Transsynaptic regulation of neuronal enzyme synthesis. In *Handbood of Psychopharmacology*, L. Iversen, S. D. Iversen and S. H. Snyder (Eds.), Plenum, New York, pp. 443–475.

Thoenen, H., Angeletti, P. U., Levi-Montalcini, R. and Kettler, R. (1971) Selective induction by nerve growth factor of tyrosine hydroxylase and dopamine-β-hydroxylase in the rat superior cervical ganglion. *Proc. nat. Acad. Sci. (Wash.)*, 68: 1598–1602.

Walicke, P. A. and Patterson, P. H. (1978) Effects of neuronal activity and cyclic nucleotide derivatives on the development of transmitter function in cultured sympathetic neurons. *8th Ann. Soc. Neurosci.*, Abstr. 394, p. 129.

Walicke, P. A., Campenot, R. B. and Patterson, P. H. (1977) Determination of transmitter function by neuronal activity. *Proc. nat. Acad. Sci. (Wash.)*, 74: 5767–5771.

Properties and Dynamics of Plasmalemmal Glycoconjugates in Growing Neurites

K. H. PFENNINGER and M. F. MAYLIÉ-PFENNINGER

Department of Anatomy, Columbia University College of Physicians and Surgeons, New York, N.Y. (U.S.A.)

INTRODUCTION

The development of higher vertebrate and invertebrate nervous systems necessitates the operation of cellular mechanisms which introduce order at two levels of organization: at first, a widespread morphogenetic phenomenon, which might be called the *grouping event,* leads to the formation of the proper cellular arrays. The grouping step regulates the establishment of specific cytoarchitectonics in certain brain regions, the formation of brain nuclei, peripheral ganglia, etc. A second organizing process is needed, however, to join together appropriate neurons and target cells, i.e., to form the intricate neuritic network which characterizes the mature brain. This second ordering phenomenon, which is unique to the nervous system, may be called the *linkage event.* Linkage involves at least two steps, guidance of the outgrowing neurite into the target region and recognition of appropriate target cells, the step which triggers synapse formation. The organizing mechanisms that lead to proper grouping and linkage are still completely unknown. We can assume, however, at least in the form of a working hypothesis, that neither neuronal perikarya (grouping) nor neurites (linkage) can reach their proper destination or address themselves to the appropriate target without selective interaction with their immediate environment. In other words, feedback from the microenvironment regarding the position of a cell and recognition of its neighbors appear to be crucial developmental determinants in neural (as in non-neural) tissues. The necessary clues may occur in at least 3 different forms which are not mutually exclusive: (1) diffusible or humoral factors – their concentration or mere presence; (2) intercellular matrix – its properties, such as the nature and concentration of glycosaminoglycans; (3) cell surfaces – properties of molecules which are part of the plasma membrane and extend into the extracellular space. Today's experimental evidence makes the cell surface appear particularly attractive as a governing factor in development (see e.g., Moscona, 1974). Many studies have shown that alteration of the chemical properties of the plasmalemmal surface, or interaction of ligands with some of its components, may lead to changes in cellular behavior (e.g., Edelman, 1976; Glaser et al., 1977; Moscona and Hausman, 1977; Rutishauser et al., 1978). The chief components involved in such phenomena seem to be *plasmalemmal glycoconjugates* which are anchored in the hydrophobic portion of the membrane but extend a hydrophilic peptide and/or carbohydrate segment into the intercellular space. The importance of glycoconjugates is further emphasized by the finding of plasmalemmal glycosyltransferases (Roth et al., 1971) and carbohydrate-binding proteins, the so-called endogenous lectins (Den et al.,

1976; DeWaard et al., 1976; Nowak et al., 1976). These latter membrane components could act as receptors for complex surface carbohydrates in cellular interaction.

In this article, we will describe localization and partial characterization of plasmalemmal glycoconjugates in various anatomical regions of the developing neuron and at different stages of differentiation. We will first try to deal with the sparse information available that may pertain to some of the mechanisms involved in the process of neurulation, an event at the grouping level. Considerably more is known about glycoconjugates during the neurite-forming phase of neuronal differentiation. These data may be relevant to organizational mechanisms occurring at the linkage level and will be discussed in the second part of this paper. Last, we will briefly discuss some of the changes in plasmalemmal glycoconjugates that occur during synaptogenesis, the process which leads to full neuronal maturity.

NEURULATION

During mammalian neurulation, a central region of the ectoderm of the embryonic disk becomes thickened and forms the neural plate. Subsequently this neural ectoderm is indented, thus generating the neural groove which runs in rostro-caudal direction. As neuro-ectodermal invagination advances the ectodermal rims are joined together, a change in configuration that results eventually in the formation of the neural tube and its sequestration from the surface ectoderm. During this process, however, the ectodermal cells that have formed the ridges on either side of the groove, the neural crest cells, dissociate themselves from both surface ectoderm and neural tube, and migrate out into various body regions to form the peripheral nervous system, melanocytes, head mesenchyma, etc. How does the highly selected group of future crest cells realize that it has to embark on a differentiative pathway which departs from that of the remaining ectodermal and tube cells? Undoubtedly, neural crest cells must acquire positional information from their microenvironment. Similar clues are very likely to guide the formation of the neural tube, but proof for this hypothesis is not available at present.

The study of plasmalemmal glycoconjugates in surface-ectodermal, crest, and tube cells, and their derivatives may shed some light onto this cell grouping phenomenon. Quantitative lectin labeling (see, e.g., Sharon and Lis, 1975) of different types of process-forming neurons (see below) has indicated that the surfaces of such cells from the peripheral nervous system are quite distinctive from those from the central nervous system (Pfenninger and Maylié-Pfenninger, 1978). In other words, process-forming neurons derived from neural tube and neural crest bear different sets of sugar moieties on their surfaces. One can therefore ask specifically at what time in neural development this distinction in cell surface properties becomes apparent, and whether such cell surface differentiation is related to the grouping events that occur during neurulation.

Other authors (O'Dell et al., 1974) have found with light microscopic labeling studies with fluorescent concanavalin A, that this lectin binds differentially to surface ectoderm and neural plate, especially its ridges, very early on, i.e., when they still reside in the embryonic ectoderm. We have chosen a similar approach to examine cell surfaces during neurulation, but utilize as probes for carbohydrate a variety of lectins conjugated to ferritin in a ratio of approximately one-to-one. Thus, lectin binding can be assessed quantitatively at the electron microscope level by counting membrane-bound ferritin particles (Fig. 1; Currie et al., 1978; Pfenninger and Maylié-Pfenninger, 1978; Maylié-Pfenninger and Jamieson, 1979). Prior to the labeling step, the microdissected dorsal region of the embryo is treated with collagenase

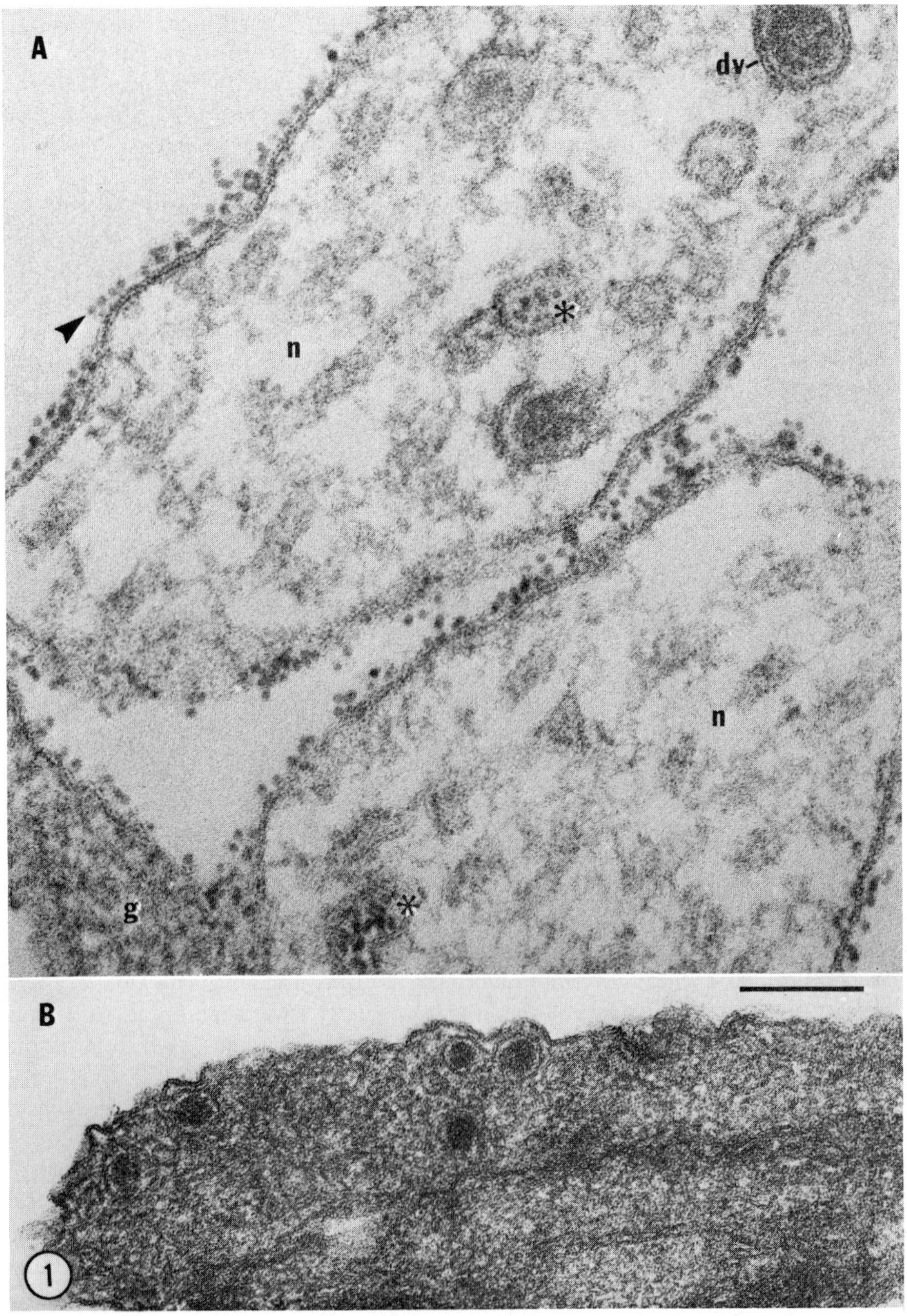

Fig. 1. The labeling of cell surfaces with ferritin-conjugated lectins. A: neurites (n) of a rat superior cervical ganglion culture labeled live with ferritin-wheat germ agglutinin. Note the layer of electron-dense ferritin particles (arrowhead) on the surface of plasma membranes. Some of the label has been internalized (asterisks). B.: control experiments in which the labeling was carried out in the presence of the hapten sugar, 0.2 M N-acetyl-glucosamine. Note the absence of surface marker. g, glial process; dv, large dense-core vesicle. Calibration bar, 0.1 μm for A, 0.2 μm for B.

and hyaluronidase and carefully rinsed in order to remove non-membrane glycoproteins from cell surfaces. Our results confirm and extend in the rat the results obtained in *Xenopus* by O'Dell et al. (1974). Indeed, even as early as 10 days of gestation, in areas where neural groove closure has not yet occurred (11th somite level), the apical plasma membranes of surface ectoderm, crest, and tube cells can be distinguished in their binding of ferritin-conjugates of *Ricinus communis* agglutinin I (RCA I, specific for galactosyl residues) and of wheat germ agglutinin (WGA, specific for N-acetyl-glucosaminyl moieties; Currie et al., 1978). However, the density of lectin binding sites found on the dorsally exposed surface of ectodermal cells in the open neural groove is several times as high as the density of lectin receptors in the process-forming neuron derived from the respective ectodermal region. The glycocalyx-like, thick carbohydrate layer on tube and crest cells disappears gradually as the neural tube closes in rostro-caudal direction. That way, both crest- and tube-derived neural cells undergo with cytodifferentiation a gradual transformation of surface properties to acquire, at a time point presently unknown, the plasmalemmal carbohydrate composition observed in the process-forming neuron.

NEURITIC GROWTH

As pointed out in the Introduction, particularly important in neuronal differentiation is the phase when neurites are formed for the generation of neuronal networks and the establishment of neuron-target cell connectivity. These linkage events usually occur when grouping events have already established the cellular order, and, for the neurons involved, the cell cycle has been arrested. Here again, the role of cell surface components in the two major steps of the linkage process, neuritic guidance and target recognition, are being investigated.

The plasma membrane of the growing neurite is a relatively well characterized membrane of the neuron due to its accessibility in tissue culture systems (Pfenninger and Rees, 1976; Estridge and Bunge, 1978; Pfenninger and Maylié-Pfenninger, 1978). Explants of embryonic nerve tissue or dissociated neurons can be cultured in vitro where, under appropriate conditions, they will form rapidly growing neurites within a few days. The newly formed, naked nerve fibers can be labeled with various biochemical markers and then analyzed in different ways, e.g., electron microscopically, the avenue which we have taken so far. As described above, various plant lectins, specific for different carbohydrates and linked to ferritin in a ratio of approximately one-to-one, were applied to aldehyde-prefixed or live nerve tissue cultures. The labeled cultures were then processed for electron optical analysis (Fig. 1A and B). Several important observations could be made in the course of this work.

The *distribution of receptors for various lectins* in the plasmalemma of rat spinal cord and superior cervical ganglion principal neurons appears to be uniform and of equal density throughout the neurite-forming phase, as least within the limitations of our labeling experiments (Pfenninger and Maylié-Pfenninger, 1975, 1978). This finding is somewhat surprising because one might expect the leading edge of the growing neurite, the growth cone, to exhibit a distinctive set of sugar moieties on its surface. However, it is also possible that our plant lectin probes are not suitable for revealing very subtle differences in plasmalemmal glycoconjugate composition. Such differences might still exist between the various anatomical regions of the growing neuron (see below).

Comparison of lectin binding properties of neurites from different types of neuron has indicated that there exists a wide range of receptor densities for the various lectins in dif-

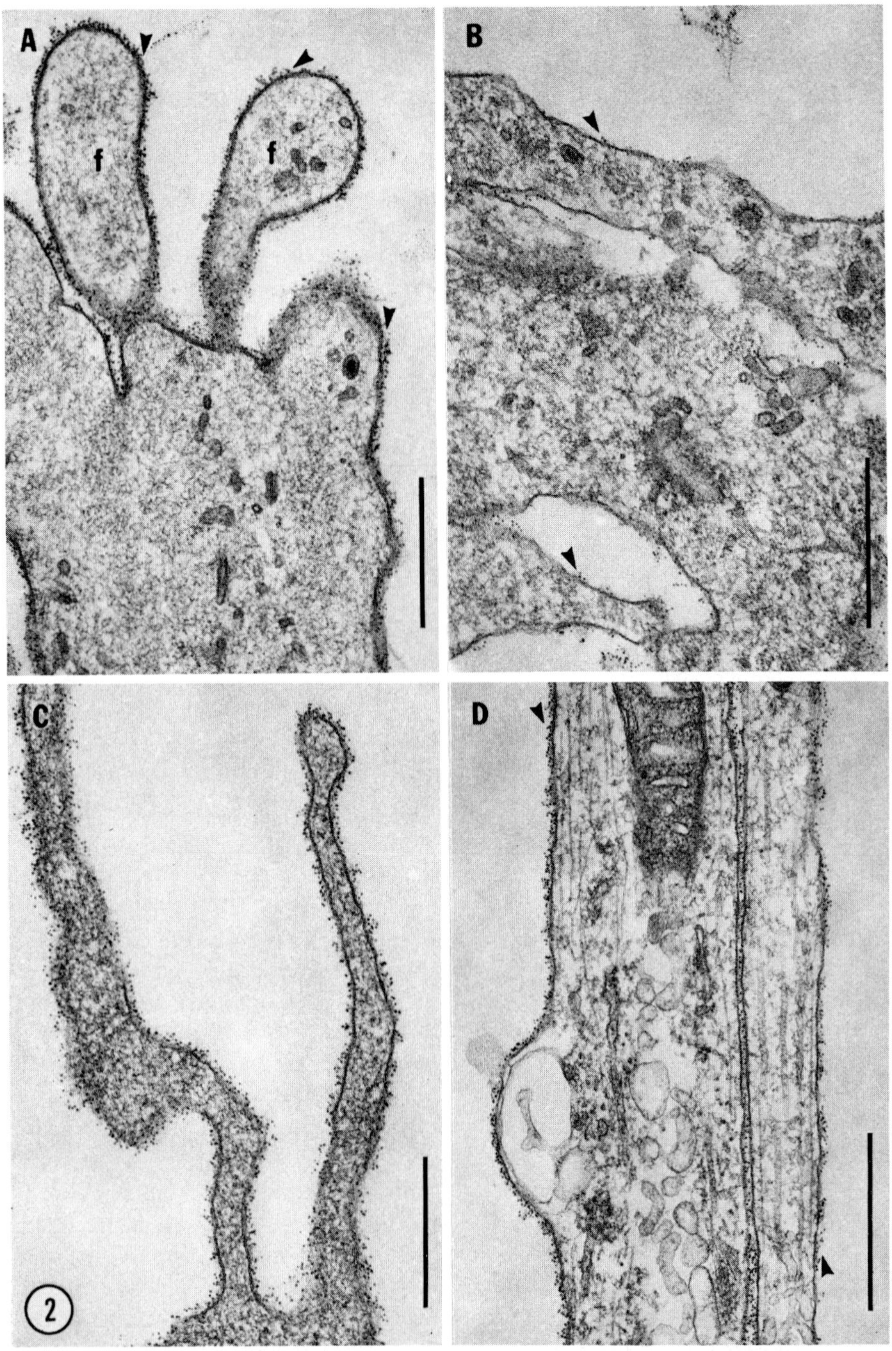

Fig. 2. Differential labeling of neural cells with ferritin-conjugate of *Ricinus communis* agglutinin I. Process-forming neurons of the superior cervical ganglion bear a high density of binding sites (arrowheads) on their surfaces as shown on a growth cone in A. By contrast, the distal portion of a neurite from a cerebellar neuron (B) is only very sparsely labeled. A non-neuronal process (probably glial) in the same cerebellar culture (C) exhibits much more lectin binding than the neuritic elements. However, if cerebellar neurites are fixed first, neuraminidase-digested, and then exposed to the marker (D), a dramatic increase in lectin labeling can be observed (cf. B and D). For discussion, see text. Fetal rat tissues grown for 3–7 days in vitro. f, filopodia. Calibration in all parts, 0.5 μm.

TABLE I

LECTIN RECEPTOR DENSITIES ON DEVELOPING NEURITES OF DIFFERENT ORIGIN

Binding sites/μm^2 of plasma membrane. Key: SCG, superior cervical ganglion; DRG, dorsal root ganglion; SC, spinal cord; CBL, cerebellum; OB, olfactory bulb (fetal rat tissues); Con A, concanavalin A; WGA, wheat germ agglutinin; RCA I, *Ricinus communis* agglutinin I; neuramin., neuraminidase treatment before labeling; SBA, soybean agglutinin; UEA, *Ulex europeus* agglutinin; LTA, *Lotus tetragonolobus* agglutinin. Preliminary data; figures in parentheses are estimated values. nd, not done. (From: Pfenninger and Maylié-Pfenninger, 1978.)

	Con A *glc/man*	*WGA* *glcNAc*	*RCA I* *gal*	*Neuramin.* *RCA I*	*SBA* *galNAc*	*LTA/UEA* *fucose*
SCG	(1400)	2740	1440	nd	(1400)	0
DRG	(1800)	2220	(2200)	nd		0
SC	(800)	910	210	(2200)	0	0
CBL		530	560	2210	0	0
OB	(600)	1830	0	1950		0

ferent neurons (Fig. 2A, B). Furthermore, especially when comparing the binding of more than one lectin, e.g., WGA (specific for glcNAc) and RCA I (specific for gal), each neuron type analyzed so far bears its own characteristic set of lectin receptors (Table I). In other words, neurons carry a carbohydrate signature on their surface at the time of neurite formation (Pfenninger and Maylié-Pfenninger, 1976, 1978; cf. Hatten and Sidman, 1977; McLaughlin and Wood, 1977; Sieber-Blum and Cohen, 1978).

Closer examination of the lectin binding data just described reveals that there are *two major groups of neurons* characterized by either high densities of lectin receptors (neurons from superior cervical and dorsal root ganglia, Figs. 1A, 2A) or relatively modest numbers of lectin binding sites (spinal cord, olfactory bulb, cerebellum; Fig. 2B, Table I). Interestingly, these cell surface classes of neurons are derived from neural crest and neural tube, respectively (Pfenninger and Maylié-Pfenninger, 1978). If tube derivatives are first digested with neuraminidase, an enzyme which cleaves terminal sialic acid, before labeling with RCA I, this results in a tremendous increase in RCA I binding, probably by uncovering previously hidden galactosyl residues (Fig. 2B, D). This experiment suggests that a main feature distinguishing the surfaces of peripheral and central neurons consists of the density and distribution of terminal sialic acid residues.

The lectin labeling data just described are incomplete without consideration of the *dynamics of membrane components* in the growing neurite. As a consequence of neurite elongation, the plasma membrane has to be expanded at a very rapid rate, up to approximately 1 μm^2/min in the mammalian sympathetic neuron. Early work by Hughes (1953) and by Bray (1970, 1973) has suggested that the insertion of new membrane takes place primarily in the most distal part of the growing neurite. We have studied the problem of neuritic membrane expansion in a series of pulse-chase experiments with both unconjugated and ferritin-labeled lectins in order to reveal the relative movement of pre-existing lectin receptors and the appearance of new lectin receptors during plasmalemmal growth (Pfenninger and Maylié-Pfenninger, 1977, 1978; cf. Abercrombie et al., 1972; Brown and Revel, 1976). In the most critical experiment, the existing plasmalemmal lectin receptors are first saturated

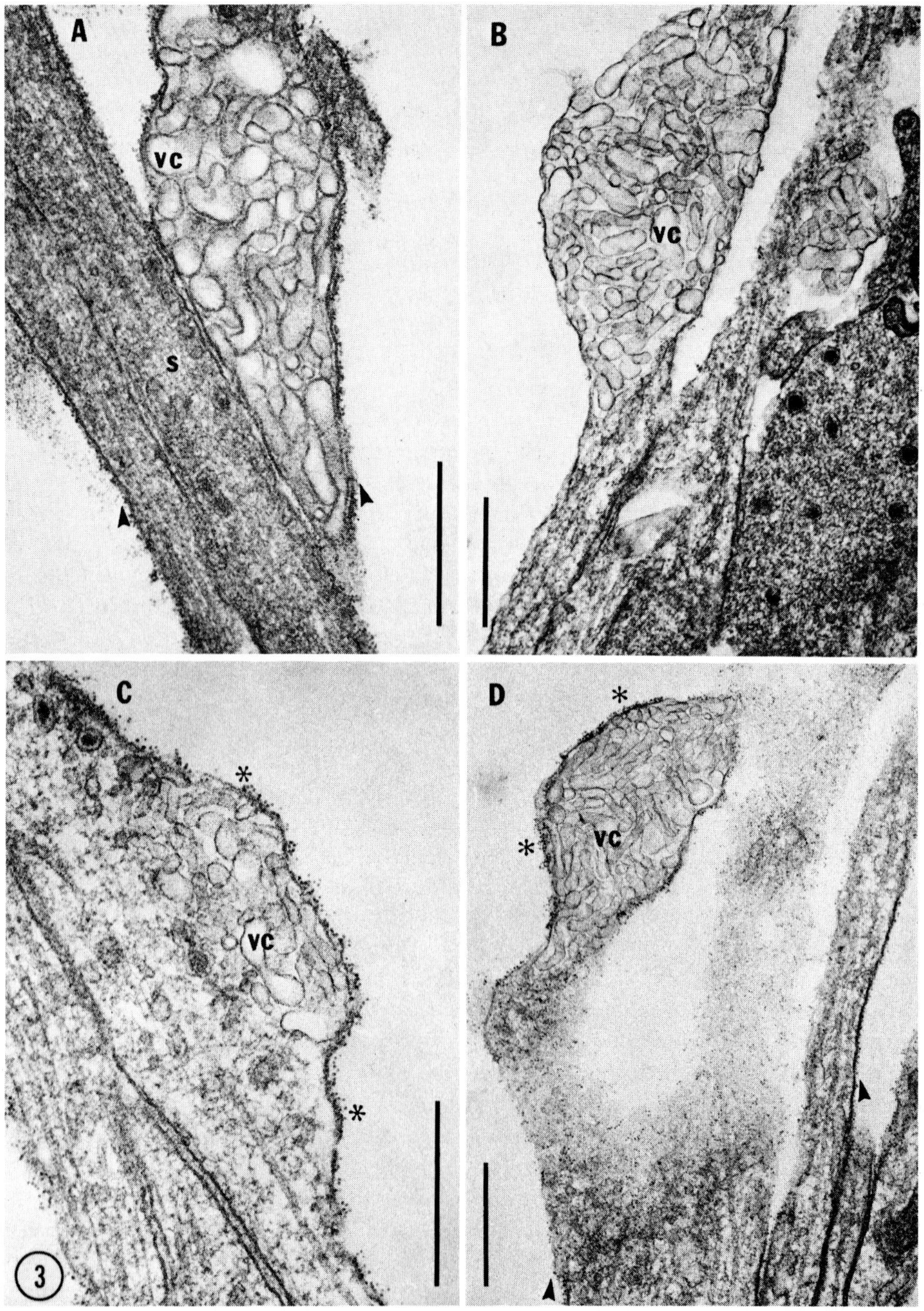

Fig. 3. Lectin labeling of the plasmalemma over clusters of clear vesicles (vc), presumed areas of insertion of new membrane. A: prefixed neuritic shafts (s) and surface of vesicle cluster are evenly labeled (arrowheads) with wheat germ agglutinin. B: neurites labeled with agglutinin II of *Ricinus communis* at 0°C, fixed, and then labeled with the ferritin conjugate of the same lectin. No bound ferritin is visible. C: labeling with *Ricinus communis* agglutinin I at 36°C, 3 min chase, aldehyde fixation, and then labeling with the ferritin conjugate of this lectin. D: same experiment, but carried out with wheat germ agglutinin and its ferritin conjugate. Note in C and in D the selective, dense labeling of patches of plasma membrane over the vesicle clusters (asterisks). The results are very similar for various lectins. This result can be interpreted as the consequence of insertion of new plasma membrane components. Rat superior cervical ganglion cultures. Calibration in all parts, 0.5 μm.

with the invisible unconjugated label (WGA, RCA I, or RCA II, which is specific for galNAc); then the cultures are grown for several minutes in the absence of the marker before being fixed in aldehyde and relabeled with the ferritin conjugate of the same lectin. In this experiment only those lectin receptors which have appeared on the cell surface during the chase period are marked with ferritin. Thus, this experiment should demonstrate, as a function of membrane growth, where new glycoconjugates are inserted in to the plasmalemma. We have observed the appearance of new lectin receptors within periods of 3–20 min primarily in the growth cone region, especially on the surface of cytoplasmic protrusions which are filled with large clear vesicles (Fig. 3A, C, D). From there, the label seems to spread into adjacent plasmalemmal regions, mainly the surface of the filopodia. In a control experiment, carried out in the cold where no growth can occur, no labeling with lectin-ferritin conjugate is observed (Fig. 3B). We still cannot fully exclude the possibility that, during the experiment, cell surface components have been rearranged in the presumed regions of insertion of new membrane components. Such a rearrangement in the plane of the membrane could have uncovered pre-existing, but previously buried, receptors for the same lectin. However, saturation of receptors is carried out with a large excess of the smaller, unconjugated lectin while relabeling is done with a two to three times lower conjugate concentration. Furthermore, the same result has been obtained for three different lectins, and there are no indications that patching or capping of cell surface materials can occur in the growing neurite. Furthermore, the freeze-fracture data reported below support our interpretation of the lectin binding studies. Thus, our observations suggest strongly that insertion of new membrane components occurs in the region of the growth cone, and that, during growth, apparently the full, appropriate carbohydrate complement is inserted into the growth cone plasmalemma.

The pulse-chase experiments just described are in accordance with *freeze-fracture observations* which have suggested earlier that the vesicles contained in the mounds may actually fuse with the plasmalemma and thus add new membrane to it (Pfenninger and Bunge, 1974; Pfenninger and Rees, 1976; Pfenninger, 1979). Interestingly, these vesicles are virtually free of intramembranous particles (IMP) as is the surface of the cytoplasmic protrusion. Furthermore, a density gradient of IMPs exists along the axis of the growing neurite, with very low particle counts at the level of the growth cone (approximately $120/\mu m^2$ for both leaflets) and an approximately 10-fold increase in IMP density at the level of the perikaryon. This IMP density gradient is readily explained by the proposed mechanism of plasmalemmal expansion, i.e., by the continuous insertion of particle-free membrane at the growing tip. Insertion into the membrane and/or appearance of IMPs seems to occur by a secondary, delayed process. These freeze-fracture observations also indicate that growth cone plasmalemma has at least one distinctive property, i.e., a very low density of IMPs, although this is not reflected in lectin labeling (cf. above).

It is not at all clear when integral membrane glycoproteins are structurally represented as IMPs (see, e.g., Pfenninger, 1978). Yet it seems rather unusual that the growth cone membrane which carries at least about $2000/\mu m^2$ lectin receptor sites should contain only about 1/20 that number IMPs. It would be interesting to know, therefore, whether plasmalemmal glycoconjugates of the growth cone are primarily *glycoprotein or glycolipid* or both. We do not have the answer to this problem; yet, pilot studies have shown that 70–80% of the receptors for both RCA I and RCA II (gal and galNAc, respectively) can be extracted from the growth cone membrane with chloroform-methanol, while resisting papain treatment. These preliminary results may suggest that a large proportion of glycoconjugates are glycolipid but they can be interpreted in other ways as well. More data and conclusive evidence will be needed to determine the nature of plasmalemmal glycoconjugates in the nerve growth cone.

SYNAPTOGENESIS

As pointed out earlier (Pfenninger and Rees, 1976; Pfenninger, 1979), the second step of the linkage event, recognition of a target cell by a nerve growth cone, triggers localized membrane differentiation in both the axonal and the target cell plasmalemma. This process leads to the formation of a synaptic junction. In other words, the growth cone membrane, whose specific properties are the basis for the recognition mechanism, gives way to a new type of membrane adapted to the special functional needs of the synapse. From the substantial cytochemical differences between synaptic axolemma and growth cone membrane (e.g., Pfenninger and Rees, 1976), it seems likely that synaptic membrane differentiation is the result of a change in the population of membrane glycoconjugates. We have therefore proceeded to investigate at what time and in which way axolemmal lectin receptors change right after contact with an appropriate target cell. The system under study consists of dissociated superior cervical ganglion neurons grown and synapsing with each other in vitro (Rees and Bunge, 1974). Although the synapses formed in this system do not seem to occur in the normal animal, this is a good and simple model system for studying synaptic membrane differentiation. This work is still in its earliest stages, and we have so far not been able to investigate lectin receptors within the (future) synaptic cleft region. However, it has become clear that, before synaptic maturity has been reached, the terminal axolemma of principal neurons of the superior cervical ganglion exhibits about twice as many RCA I binding sites as the growth cone plasmalemma prior to target contact (Simkowitz et al., 1978). This and other synapse-forming systems are currently being investigated in this laboratory with a series of different lectins in order to study nerve terminal membrane differentiation in greater detail.

CONCLUSIONS

Synaptogenesis may share with plasmalemmal expansion during neuritic growth the insertion of new membrane components. The mechanisms of synaptic membrane differentiation are not known, however, and modification of pre-existing membrane components is a possibility. In the case of plasmalemmal expansion during neuritic growth, evidence has been accumulated which suggests strongly that patches of pre-assembled membrane, with a full set of appropriate glycoconjugates, are inserted in a localized fashion by an exocytotic mechanism. Interestingly, this insertion of new glycoconjugates occurs primarily at the level of the growth cone, an area of the neurite that seems strategically important because it is the leading edge of the advancing cellular process. Thus, the neuron's genome and synthetic machinery can exert immediate influence on the surface carbohydrate composition of the growth cone membrane.

A further conclusion is concerned with the differentiation of neuroblasts into distinctive types of neurons. The comparative labeling studies of neurons during their process-forming phase as well as the labeling of developing neuroectoderm indicate that different types of neurons carry characteristic cell surface signatures in the form of differing amounts of certain carbohydrate residues. These plasmalemmal carbohydrate codes may be involved in the mechanisms governing morphogenetic events both at the grouping and at the linkage levels in nervous system development. However, we are far from being able to demonstrate a direct and causal relationship between the cell surface and cellular growth, differentiation and behavior. The finding of type-specific cell surface components does not necessarily imply that the interactions in which they may be involved are as selective as, e.g., antigen-antibody binding. Rather, cellular interactions and affinities seem to be of a graded nature; they may determine the broad rules for neuronal circuitry, whereas the finer details, such as point-to-point projection, could be controlled by other mechanisms.

As of today, we have not been able to investigate the full course of neuronal differentiation from neurulation and proliferation via migration, birth (i.e., cessation of mitosis), and process formation to synaptogenesis. However, the limited amount of data available suggests already that the composition in cell surface glycoconjugates changes dramatically as the neuron differentiates. In other words, the cell surface appears to indicate the differentiative course and state of a neuron and is likely to be involved in the signalling of this information to neighboring cells. Thus, the data presented here show that one kind of chemical specificity of the neuron resides on its plasmalemmal surface.

SUMMARY

On the basis of the hypothesis that the cell surface is an important element in cellular recognition and developmental control mechanisms, we have investigated distribution and changes of plasmalemmal glycoconjugates during neuronal differentiation. The data were obtained by cell surface labeling with ferritin-conjugated lectins that were then localized and quantified electron optically. The results indicate that both neural tube and crest cells and their derivatives acquire distinctive cell surface properties while still residing in the ectoderm. During the further differentiation of the neurons, surface glycoconjugate compositions change, but the difference between tube- and crest-derived neurons is maintained. In fact, within these two classes, each neuronal type expresses its own characteristic *surface carbohydrate signature* by the time it sends out axon and dendrites. During the neurite-forming phase of development, neurons increase their surface and maintain specific plasmalemmal properties by distal, *localized insertion of pre-assembled membrane.* Upon recognition of an appropriate target cell, axonal surface glycoconjugates are altered again during synaptogenesis, a process of localized membrane differentiation. Thus, we can conclude that neuronal specificity is expressed on the cell surface, in its glycoconjugates, indicating the neuron's type and differentiative state.

ACKNOWLEDGEMENTS

Expert technical and editorial assistance by Marian Johnson, Linda Siegel and Christine Wade is gratefully acknowledged.

This work is supported by USPHS Grant NS 13466, by Grant BNS 76-18513 from the National Science Foundation, and a Career Scientist Award from the I. T. Hirschl Trust Fund awarded to K.H.P.

REFERENCES

Abercrombie, M., Heaysman, J. E. M. and Pegrum, S. M. (1972) Locomotion of fibroblasts in culture. V. Surface marking with concanavalin A. *Exp. Cell Res.*, 73: 536–539.

Bray, D. (1970) Surface movements during the growth of single explanted neurons. *Proc. nat. Acad. Sci. (Wash.)*, 65: 905–910.

Bray, D. (1973) Model for membrane movements in the neural growth cone. *Nature (Lond.)*, 244: 93–96.

Brown, S. S. and Revel, J.-P. (1976) Reversibility of cell surface label rearrangement. *J. Cell Biol.*, 68: 629–641.

Currie, J. R., Pfenninger, K. H. and Maylié-Pfenninger, M.-F. (1978) Cell surface saccharides in developing neuroectoderm. *J. Cell Biol.*, 79: 56A.

Den, H., Malinzak, D. A. and Rosenberg, A. (1976) Lack of evidence for the involvement of β-D-galactosyl-specific lectin in the fusion of chick myoblasts. *Biochem. biophys. Res. Commun.*, 69: 621–627.

DeWaard, A., Hickman, S. and Kornfeld, S. (1976) Isolation and properties of β-galactoside binding lectins of calf heart and lung. *J. biol. Chem.*, 251: 7581–7587.

Edelman, G. M. (1976) Surface modulation in cell recognition and cell growth. *Science*, 192: 218–226.

Estridge, M. and Bunge, R. (1978) Compositional analysis of growing axons from rat sympathetic neurons. *J. Cell Biol.*, 79: 138–155.

Glaser, L., Santala, R., Gottlieb, D. I. and Merell, R. (1977) Cell-cell recognition in the embryonal nervous system. In *Cell and Tissue Interactions*, J. W. Lash and M. M. Burger (Eds.), Raven Press, New York, pp. 197–208.

Hatten, M. E. and Sidman, R. L. (1977) Plant lectins detect age- and region-specific differences in cell surface carbohydrates and cell reassociation behavior of embryonic mouse cerebellar cells. *J. supramol. Struct.*, 7: 267–275.

Hughes, A. F. (1953) The growth of embryonic neurites. A study on cultures of chick neural tissue. *J. Anat. (Lond.)*, 87: 150–162.

McLaughlin, B. J. and Wood, J. G. (1977) The localization of concanavalin A binding sites during photoreceptor synaptogenesis in the chick retina. *Brain Res.*, 119: 57–71.

Maylié-Pfenninger, M.-F. and Jamieson, J. D. (1979) Distribution of cell surface saccharides on pancreatic cells. I. General method for preparation and purification of lectins and lectin-ferritin conjugates. *J. Cell Biol.*, 80: 69–76.

Moscona, A. A. (Ed.) (1974) *The Cell Surface in Development*. Wiley and Sons, New York.

Moscona, A. A. and Hausman, R. E. (1977) Biological and biochemical studies on embryonic cell-cell recognition. In *Cell and Tissue Interactions*, J. W. Lash and M. M. Burger (Eds.), Raven Press, New York, pp. 173–185.

Nowak, T. P., Haywood, P. L. and Barondes, S. H. (1976) Developmentally regulated lectin in embryonic chick muscle and a myogenic cell line. *Biochem. biophys. Res. Commun.*, 68: 650–657.

O'Dell, D. S., Tencer, R., Monroy, A. and Brachet, J. (1974) The pattern of concanavalin A-binding sites during the early development of *Xenopus laevis*. *Cell Diff.*, 3: 193–198.

Pfenninger, K. H. (1978) Neuronal membrane organization. *Ann. Rev. Neurosci.*, 1: 445–471.

Pfenninger, K. H. (1979) Synaptic membrane differentiation. In *The Neurosciences; Fourth Study Program*, F. O. Schmitt (Ed.), MIT Press, Cambridge, Mass., pp. 779–795.

Pfenninger, K. H. and Bunge, R. P. (1974) Freeze-fracturing of nerve growth cones and young fibers. A study of developing plasma membrane. *J. Cell Biol.*, 63: 180–196.

Pfenninger, K. H. and Maylié-Pfenninger, M.-F. (1975) Distribution and fate of lectin binding sites on the surface of growing neuronal processes. *J. Cell Biol.*, 67: 322A.

Pfenninger, K. H. and Maylié-Pfenninger, M.-F. (1976) Differential lectin receptor content on the surface of nerve growth cones of different origin. *Neurosci. Abstr.*, 2: 224.

Pfenninger, K. H. and Maylié-Pfenninger, M.-F. (1977) Localized appearance of new lectin receptors on the surface of growing neurites. *J. Cell Biol.*, 75: 54A.

Pfenninger, K. H. and Maylié-Pfenninger, M.-F. (1978) Distribution and appearance of surface carbohydrates on growing neurites. In *Neuronal Information Transfer (Proceedings of the P&S Biomedical Science Symposia)*, H. J. Vogel, A. Karlin and V. M. Tennyson (Eds.), Academic Press, New York, pp. 373–386.

Pfenninger, K. H. and Rees, R. P. (1976) From the growth cone to the synapse: properties of membranes involved in synapse formation. In *Neuronal Recognition*, S. H. Barondes (Ed.), Plenum Press, New York, pp. 131–178, 357–358.

Rees, R. P. and Bunge, R. P. (1974) Morphological and cytochemical studies of synapses formed in culture between isolated rat superior cervical ganglion neurons. *J. comp. Neurol.*, 157: 1–12.

Roth, S., McGuire, E. J. and Roseman, S. (1971) Evidence for cell-surface glycosyltransferases: their potential role in cellular recognition. *J. Cell Biol.*, 51: 536–547.

Rutishauser, U., Thiéry, J.-P., Brackenbury, R. and Edelman, G. M. (1978) Adhesion among neural cells of the chick embryo. III. Relationship of the surface molecule CAM to cell adhesion and the development of histotypic patterns. *J. Cell Biol.*, 79: 371–381.

Sharon, N. and Lis, H. (1975) Use of lectins for the study of membranes. In *Methods in Membrane Biology*, E. D. Korn (Ed.), Plenum Press, New York, pp. 147–200.

Sieber-Blum, M. and Cohen, A. M. (1978) Lectin binding to neural crest cells. Changes of the cell surface during differentiation in vitro. *J. Cell Biol.*, 76: 628–638.

Simkowitz, P., Maylié-Pfenninger, M.-F. and Pfenninger, K. H. (1978) Early changes in cell surface glyco-conjugates during synaptogenesis. *J. Cell Biol.*, 79: 60A.

Mechanism of Action and Possible Sites of Synthesis of Nerve Growth Factor

H. THOENEN, Y.-A. BARDE, D. EDGAR, H. HATANAKA, U. OTTEN and M. SCHWAB

Department of Pharmacology, Biocenter of the University, Basel (Switzerland)

INTRODUCTION

The naming of nerve growth factor (NGF) dates back to the time when its most impressive effects were shown to be stimulation of an enormous volume increase of sensory and sympathetic ganglia, and a concomitant excessive neurite production (cf. Levi-Montalcini and Angeletti, 1968). Since that time, this factor has been identified as a protein, its sequence determined and its effects delineated in more detail, although we are still far from a complete understanding of its mechanism of action at the molecular level (cf. Mobley et al., 1977, Bradshaw, 1978).

We think that time has come to establish if the term "nerve growth factor" is appropriate and to delineate the categories into which its action can be divided. The term "growth" is justified only if it is used in the sense of neuronal volume increase without implying a mitogenic action on neuronal target cells. At least for the peripheral sympathetic nervous system it is now well established that the volume increase of the sympathetic ganglia effected by large doses of NGF in the early postnatal period results (a) from an augmented survival of sympathetic neurons, (b) from a very marked increase in the volume of the cell body of individual neurons, and (c) from an increase in the number of non-neuronal cells (cf. Hendry, 1977), which may be a consequence of the volume increase of the neurons. This increase in non-neuronal cell number is responsible for the elevated mitotic index induced by NGF in sympathetic ganglia in the early postnatal period.

During the early postnatal period NGF acts mainly as a survival factor as illustrated by the increased number of adrenergic neurons surviving under the influence of large doses of NGF, the necessity of NGF for the survival of dissociated sympathetic and sensory neurons in cultures free of non-neuronal cells and the drastic reduction of sympathetic neurons after administration of anti-NGF antibodies (cf. Levi-Montalcini and Angeletti, 1968; Herrup et al., 1974; Chun and Patterson, 1977; Hendry, 1977; Mobley et al., 1977). In addition, NGF exhibits hypertrophic effects – reflected by the volume increase of the neuronal perikarya – and enhances the differentiation of the adrenergic neurons reflected by an enhanced neuronal fiber outgrowth and a selective induction of tyrosine hydroxylase (TH) and dopamine-β-hydroxylase (DBH) (cf. Mobley et al., 1977; Thoenen et al., 1979).

In the following we will compare the effects of NGF on general growth with those on differentiation and then consider the possible role of NGF as a macromolecular messenger between effector cells and innervating neurons, reaching its site of action in the perikaryon by retrograde axonal transport. We then discuss diverse artifacts hindering the reliable determination of endogenous levels of NGF in blood and tissues. We end by briefly touching the possibility of another factor or factors representing alternatives to NGF.

COMPARISON OF GENERAL GROWTH EFFECTS OF NGF WITH THOSE ON DIFFERENTIATION

For any effects of NGF its interaction with high affinity receptors on the surface of the cell body or neuronal processes is necessary (cf. Herrup et al., 1974; Thoenen and Schwab, 1978). This interaction leads to the initiation of a cascade of events reflected by long- and short-term effects for which neither the detailed mechanism nor the possible inter-relationships are known.

As early effects of NGF, changes in neuronal phospholipid metabolism, transport of amino acids and RNA precursors have been described (cf. Varon, 1975; Lakshmanan, 1978). However, it is not known to what extent and by which mechanisms these relatively rapid effects are related to the long-term effects such as general growth (reflected by volume increase of the neuronal cell bodies) and differentiation (reflected by fiber outgrowth or selective induction of enzymes involved in specialized functions of the corresponding neurons).

In many biological systems events of rapid growth or regeneration are characterized by an early induction of ornithine decarboxylase (ODC), the rate-limiting enzyme in the synthesis of polyamines which are themselves involved in many regulatory processes of protein synthesis at the transcriptional and translational levels (cf. Tabor and Tabor, 1976).

In both organ cultures of sympathetic ganglia (MacDonnell et al., 1977; Otten et al., 1978) and in an NGF-responsive clonal cell line of a rat pheochromocytoma (Hatanaka et al., 1978), NGF initiates a marked induction of ODC by a cAMP-independent mechanism. In organ cultures of sympathetic ganglia the extent of ODC induction depends very much on

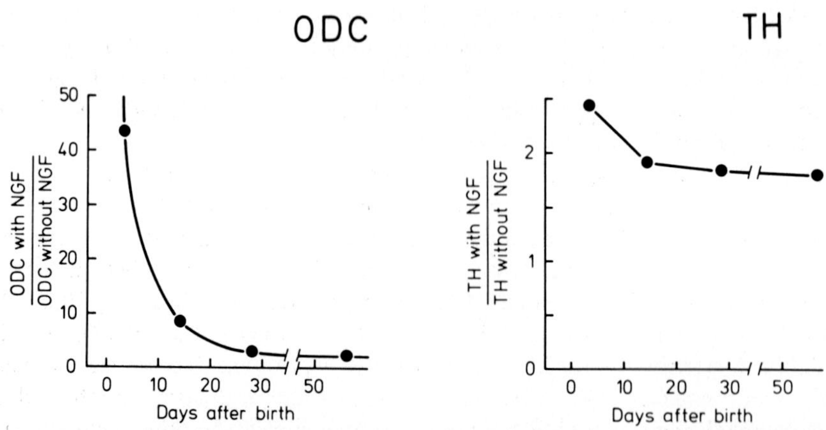

Fig. 1. Age dependency of NGF-mediated induction of ODC and TH. Superior cervical ganglia from rats of varying ages were cultured either in the absence or presence of 3 μg/ml of NGF for 7.5 hr. At this time the maximal effect on ODC was reached in both newborn and adult animals. ODC determinations were performed according to Russel and Snyder (1968). TH levels were determined according to Mueller et al. (1969) in animals of varying age 48 hr after the injection of 5 mg/kg of 2.5S NGF. At this time the maximal effect on TH was reached. The values presented represent the mean of 6 determinations.

the age of the animals from which the ganglia originate: in newborn animals NGF produces about a 50-fold increase in ODC activity, whereas with increasing age the maximal induction gradually decreases to a level 2–3-fold that of controls (Fig. 1). The age-dependent response of ODC induction strongly supports the assumption that its induction is related in this case, as in many other systems, to events of general growth which are prominent in the early postnatal period.

In contrast to the ODC induction, NGF-mediated TH induction – reflecting a differentiation-promoting action of NGF (cf. Thoenen et al., 1979) – remains virtually constant from birth to adulthood (Fig. 1). This indicates that NGF is essential for the regulation of the specialized function of transmitter production throughout life, an assumption which is supported by the observation that administration of a single dose of purified specific anti-NGF antibodies to adult animals results in a larger reduction of TH levels than of total proteins (Goedert et al., 1978).

There are additional differences between the regulation of ODC and TH by NGF. Beyond the time-requirement for the induction which is relatively short for ODC (maximal increase 6–8 hr after addition of NGF) and long for TH (maximal increase after 48 hr), the induction of ODC can be abolished both by cycloheximide and actinomycin D (Otten et al., 1978), whereas the induction of TH can only be abolished by cycloheximide but not by actinomycin D or α-amanitin (Rohrer et al., 1978). This indicates that the regulation of TH, in contrast to ODC, takes place at the post-transcriptional level. Such a selective regulation at the post-transcriptional level is remarkable as such, and particularly in connection with the acetylcholine-mediated transsynaptic enzyme induction which also results in a selective TH and DBH induction (cf. Thoenen et al., 1979): in contrast to the NGF-mediated TH and DBH induction, transsynaptic enzyme induction is abolished by α-amanitin and actinomycin D. Thus, one is confronted with the situation where a strikingly similar pattern of selective enzyme induction is not only effected by two differing agents, NGF versus acetylcholine, but also via two distinct mechanisms.

For both ODC and TH the mechanism of induction beyond the binding of NGF to its specific receptors is unknown. It is not clear whether very early events such as changes in the turnover of phosphatidylinositol (Lakshmanan, 1978) – an event frequently occurring in relation to ligand-receptor interaction (Michell, 1975) – or enhanced uptake of uridine or amino acids (cf. Varon, 1975) are causally related to later events such as induction of ODC and TH. The further analysis of such relationships urgently requires a simple model, i.e., a system of uniform cells available in sufficient quantities to allow detailed biochemical investigation. The PC12 pheochromocytoma clonal cell line (Greene and Tischler, 1976) may serve at least partially for such a purpose. As do sympathetic ganglia, PC12 cells respond to NGF with a fiber outgrowth (Greene and Tischler, 1976) and a marked ODC induction (Hatanaka et al., 1978). The latter effect on PC12 cells seems to be a cAMP-independent mechanism, as it is in sympathetic ganglia (Hatanaka et al., 1978; Otten et al., 1978). In other respects, however, there are marked differences between PC12 cells and sympathetic neurons. Even the initial effect, the interaction of NGF with the cell surface receptors seems to be different: the affinity of NGF for the PC12 receptors is an order of magnitude lower than for those of sympathetic and dorsal root ganglia (Herrup and Thoenen, 1979). Moreover, NGF does not induce TH in PC12 cells but produces an induction of choline acetyltransferase (Edgar and Thoenen, 1978), an enzyme not present in detectable quantities in normal adrenergic neurons.

Since information is lacking on the relationship between the initial binding step of NGF with its specific receptors and the subsequent intermediate and long-term effects, it is not known if NGF has to be internalized in order to exert its effects. At least it has clearly been demonstrated that NGF reaching the cell bodies of adrenergic neurons by retrograde axonal transport is able to induce TH (Paravicini et al., 1975). However, we do not know if an induction can also occur via the cell surface, implying that the retrograde transport represents nothing more than a transfer of peripheral receptors (including the possible complementary elements for the formation of second messenger(s)) to the perikaryon. The ultrastructural localization of NGF by quantitative electron microscopic autoradiography and histochemical procedures (using a coupling product of NGF with horseradish peroxidase) has shown that NGF is taken up by endocytosis and is transferred to the perikaryon enclosed in vesicles and smooth membrane cisternae (Schwab, 1977; Schwab and Thoenen, 1977). In the perikaryon these cisternae seem to fuse with other intracellular membranes and with lysosomal structures (dense and multivesicular bodies). No evidence for a release of intact NGF into the cytoplasm could be obtained, and similarly no evidence for any transfer to the cell nucleus. This is of particular interest with respect to recent reports that [^{125}I]NGF binds to the nuclear fraction of homogenates of sympathetic and dorsal root ganglia (Andres et al., 1977; Johnson et al., 1978). For the interpretation of these latter experiments contamination of the nuclear fraction by membrane fragments and redistribution of binding sites during the preparation of the nuclear fraction has to be considered. Such a redistribution of binding sites has been convincingly demonstrated for insulin (Bergeron et al., 1978).

Thus, in the light of direct morphological (autoradiographic and histochemical) evidence it seems to be unlikely that NGF exerts a direct effect on the regulation of the expression of specific genetic information either at the nuclear or at the ribosomal level; one has to assume a second messenger mechanism. Therefore, the question arises how the effects of NGF are mediated, and whether there are principal differences between the NGF effects mediated via surface receptors or after internalization and retrograde axonal transport. Unfortunately it has not yet been possible, under well controlled conditions in vitro, to block the internalization of NGF without severely impairing other general cell functions (unpublished observation).

There are 3 possible mechanisms by which NGF, in particular that moiety reaching the cell body by retrograde axonal transport, may exert its action (Fig. 2).

(a) The retrogradely transported NGF is transferred to the perikaryon associated with its receptors and additional membrane constituents necessary for the formation of second messenger(s). Consequently, the mechanism would be the same when NGF interacts with surface receptors of the cell body or when it reaches the perikaryon by retrograde axonal transport associated with the membrane of vesicles or cisternae (Fig. 2A).

(b) The fusion of intracellular cisternae or vesicles containing NGF with lysosomal structures is necessary for the initiation of the NGF action, e.g. the lysosomal proteases could form diffusible fragments of NGF which then act as "second" messenger(s). If such a mechanism should be involved, then the internalization either from the surface of the cell body, or from the nerve terminal with subsequent retrograde transport, would be necessary (Fig. 2B).

(c) During the internalization of NGF at the nerve terminals a sorting out of NGF receptors takes place, leaving behind the complementary elements necessary for the formation of second messenger(s). Thus, to become functional in the perikaryon, the vesicular or cisternal membranes carrying NGF must fuse with complementary membrane structures (Fig. 2C).

The localization of internalized NGF in vesicles and smooth membrane cisternae and the lack of evidence for NGF release into the cytoplasm must be considered in order to assess the physiological implications of the observation that high concentrations of NGF enhance

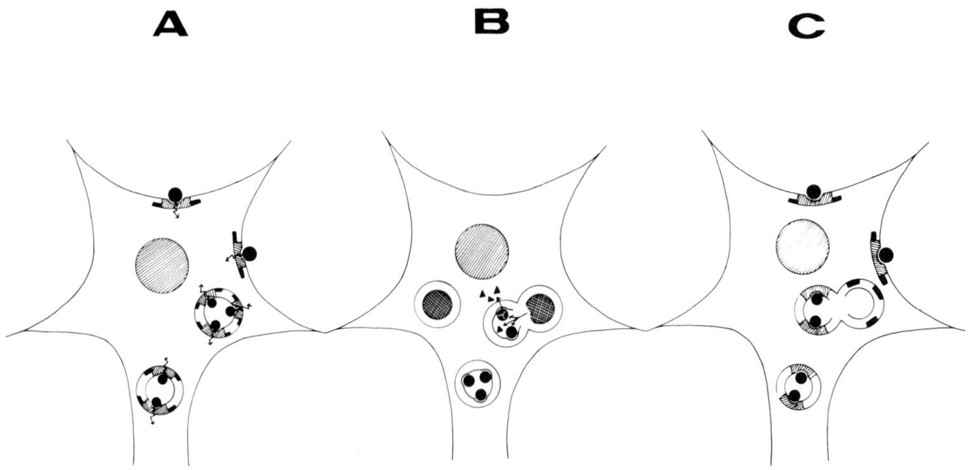

Fig. 2. Schematic presentation of the possible mechanisms of action of NGF reaching the perikaryon by retrograde axonal transport. A: transfer of NGF receptors from the periphery to the perikaryon including supplementary membrane constituents necessary for second messenger(s) formation. B: fusion of vesicles and cisternae containing NGF with lysosomes. The proteolytic cleavage products of NGF act as second messengers themselves. Internalization and fusion with lysosomes are necessary for the action of NGF. C: the retrograde axonal transport of NGF is linked with a sorting out of corresponding receptors. In order to become active (as the receptors on the surface of the cell body) a fusion with complementary membrane constituents is necessary.

the assembly of microtubules from tubulin in vitro (Calissano and Cozzari, 1974). In this case it would seem to be more plausible that the NGF-mediated enhanced assembly of microtubules observed in intact neurons (Levi-Montalcini et al., 1968) results from an indirect rather than from a direct effect of NGF.

RETROGRADE AXONAL TRANSPORT OF NGF; TRANSFER OF INFORMATION FROM EFFECTOR ORGANS TO INNERVATING ADRENERGIC NEURONS

In the preceding section evidence has been presented that the moiety of NGF taken up by adrenergic nerve terminals and transported retrogradely to the perikaryon is able to produce a selective induction of TH (Paravicini et al., 1975). There is good indirect evidence that the retrograde axonal transport of NGF is of physiological importance. The transection of adrenergic axons (Hendry, 1975a, b), the destruction of adrenergic nerve terminals by 6-hydroxydopamine (Levi-Montalcini et al., 1975) or the blockade of the axoplasmic transport with drugs leading to a disintegration of microtubules (Chen et al., 1977; Johnson, 1978) all have similar effects on the morphology and characteristic biochemical parameters of the cell bodies of adrenergic neurons. All these effects can be antagonized by the administration of exogenous NGF. Moreover, the effect of the functional or anatomical interruption of the connections between the periphery and the cell body is age dependent: in newborn animals the surgical or chemical interruption of these connections leads to irreversible damage, i.e., a degeneration of the cell bodies (Hendry, 1975a, b; Levi-Montalcini et al., 1975). With increasing age the effects become both smaller and reversible. Interestingly, the time-course of the effects of axotomy on the TH levels in rat superior cervical ganglia

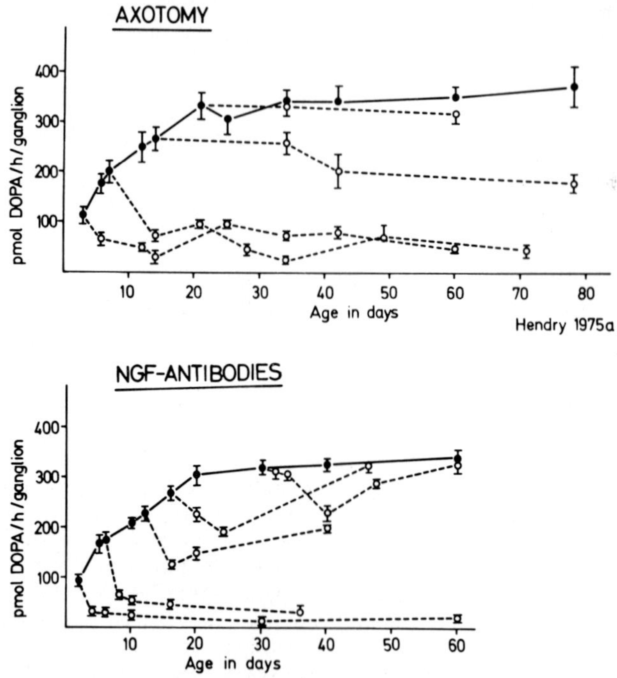

Fig. 3. Comparison between the effect of axotomy and administration of a single dose of purified NGF antibodies at different times after birth. Axotomy: transection of the postganglionic fibers of the rat superior cervical ganglia was performed from 3 to 21 days after birth. TH levels (representing a measure for the surviving adrenergic neurons) were determined up to 80 days (according to Hendry, 1975a). NGF antibodies: rats of different ages were injected with a single dose of 200 mg/kg of purified antibodies to NGF. TH levels were followed in a similar manner as after axotomy up to 60 days after birth (according to Goedert et al., 1978).

(Hendry, 1975a) and the administration of a single (large) dose of NGF antibodies (Goedert et al., 1978) are virtually identical (Fig. 3). This, together with the prevention by NGF administration of the above effects resulting from functional or anatomical interruption of the axons very much favor the interpretation that the effects of axotomy or blockade of axonal transport on adrenergic cell bodies result from an interruption of the supply of NGF or an NGF-like (immunologically cross-reacting) factor(s) to the cell body from the periphery. However, in order to directly demonstrate that this mechanism is of physiological importance, it must be shown that the corresponding effector organs possess the capability to accumulate or to produce NGF by either de novo synthesis or activation from a precursor. Unfortunately such an unambiguous demonstration has not been possible and the reasons for this failure are discussed in the following section.

PITFALLS IN THE IMMUNOLOGICAL AND BIOLOGICAL DETERMINATION OF NGF CONCENTRATIONS

The reliable and sensitive determination of NGF levels in both tissue samples and serum is necessary for the elucidation of the physiological role of NGF, in particular with respect to its function as a retrograde messenger between effector organs and innervating adrenergic neurons. To this end sensitive radioimmunoassays (RIA) have been developed, and with these assays high apparent NGF levels have been detected in virtually all the tissues and sera tested (cf. Suda et al., 1978). However, the range of the reported values, in particular those for serum of the same species, is embarrassingly large, ranging for instance in mouse serum from 2 to 1000 ng/ml (Johnson et al., 1971; Hendry and Iversen, 1973; Murphy et al., 1977). Most disturbing is the fact that the values obtained by RIA can generally not be confirmed by bioassays; the latter, although being semiquantitative, would be sensitive enough to detect the quantities of NGF predicted by RIA (Suda et al., 1978).

Below we illustrate the artifacts inherent to the determination of NGF in rat and mouse serum by a one-site RIA. We will also offer an explanation for these pitfalls and demonstrate how they can be avoided by the use of a two-site RIA.

In a competition assay (Fig. 4A), any decrease in radioactivity ([^{125}I]NGF) bound to the NGF receptors or NGF antibodies is interpreted as evidence for the presence of endogenous NGF. This interpretation applies to the various types of competition radioassays (the most commonly used in the case of NGF), such as receptor assays, solid-phase immunoglobulin RIA or immunoprecipitation RIA. Using a competition one-site RIA, we determined apparent values of 38 and 39 ng NGF/ml of serum for male and female rats, respectively (Suda et al., 1978). The corresponding values for mice were 12 and 9 ng/ml. These values are in agreement

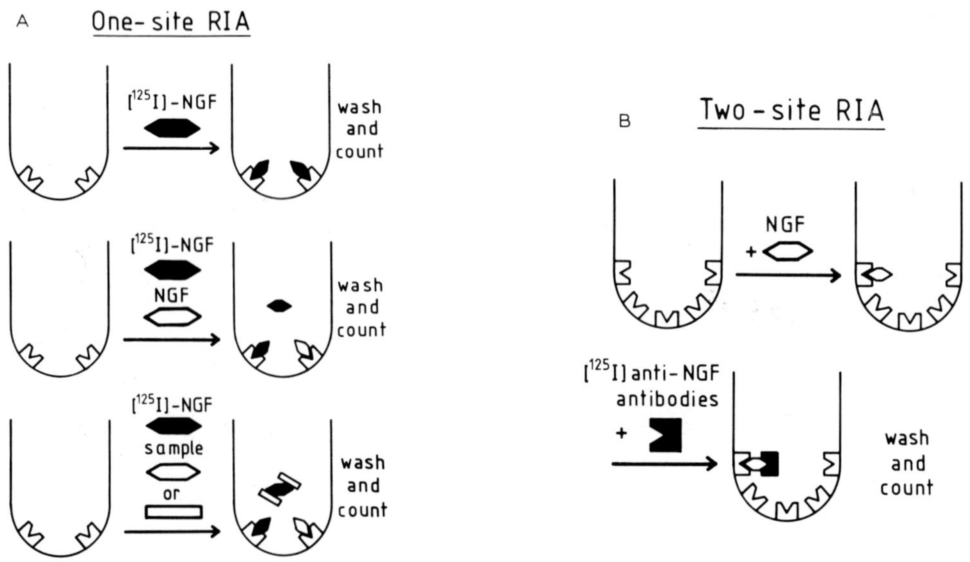

Fig. 4. Schematic comparison between one- and two-site radioimmunoassays (RIA). One-site RIA: a given concentration of labeled [^{125}I]NGF is competing with unknown concentrations of NGF for the limited number of solid-phase antibody binding sites. The binding of [^{125}I]NGF to high molecular soluble constituents mimics the presence of NGF. Two-site RIA: the bottom of the assay tube is covered with a large excess of specific NGF antibodies to which the NGF or NGF-like molecules are bound and subsequently quantified by the labeled [^{125}I]NGF antibodies. The large excess of solid-phase antibodies provides a more favorable situation for the competition with possible NGF-binding macromolecules in solution. Moreover, the interference by such binding components can be corrected for by determining the recovery of known amounts of added NGF.

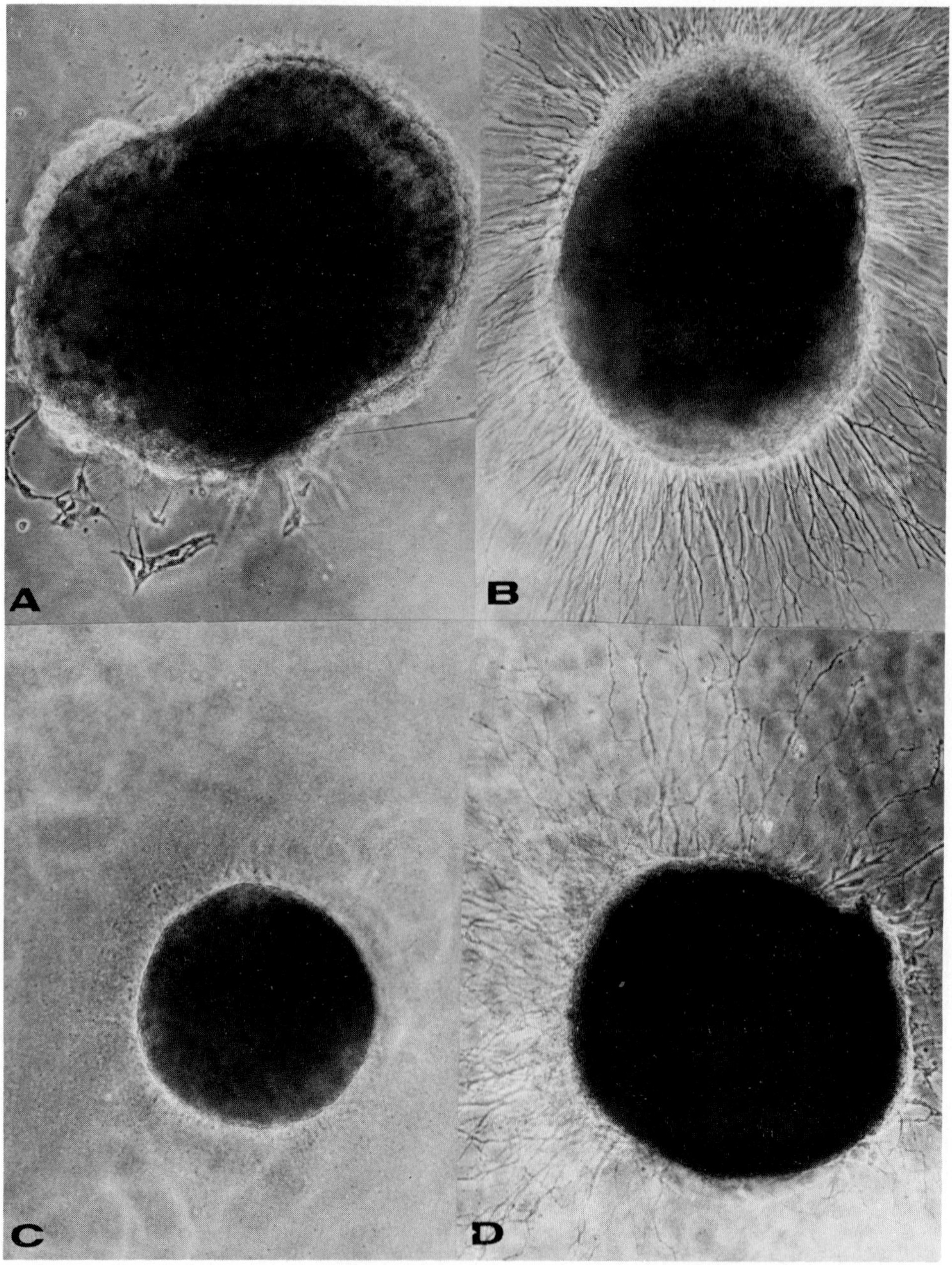

Fig. 5. Serum concentrations of NGF determined by bioassay. A: chick dorsal root ganglia were grown for 20 hr in control medium without NGF. B: addition of 2 ng/ml of NGF to control medium. C: ganglion incubated with rat serum (substituted for control medium). The NGF concentration predicted by one-site RIA was 30 ng/ml. D: rat serum supplemented with 2 ng/ml of NGF. In the two-site RIA no measurable amount of NGF could be detected, in agreement with the bioassay.

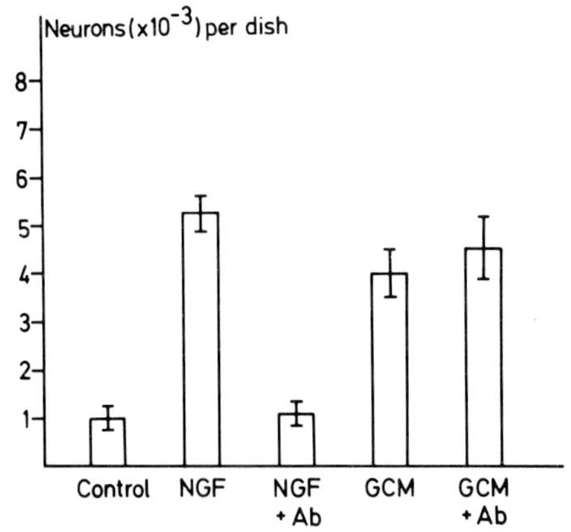

Fig. 6. Comparison between the effect of NGF and glial conditioned medium on the survival of chick dorsal root ganglia. Dorsal root ganglia of 10–12-day-old chick embryos were dissociated, plated and the survival of the neurons quantified 48 hr later (Barde et al., 1978). The concentration of NGF amounted to 1 ng/ml of 2.5S NGF and the purified specific NGF antibodies (Ab) to 100 ng/ml. The glial conditioned medium (GCM) was prepared from a rat glial tumor line (C6) according to a protocol described by Barde et al. (1978). The values given represent the total number (mean ± S.D.) of surviving neurons in a 35 mm culture dish.

with those reported by other investigators (Murphy et al., 1977), although in some cases considerably higher values have been determined (Johnson et al., 1971). However, if the same serum samples were tested in a biological assay, either no or only barely detectable amounts could be determined. This is illustrated in Fig. 5: it is shown (Fig. 5C) that a rat serum sample (with an apparent NGF concentration of 30 ng/ml, as determined by one-site RIA) did not exhibit the typical NGF response (see Fig. 5B). However, if only 2 ng/ml NGF were added to the same sample, a clear response could be seen (Fig. 5D). The effect of this concentration of NGF was somewhat smaller than that seen in the absence of rat serum, but it is still very clearly visible and in distinct contrast to the lack of effect of the same serum sample alone.

The discrepancy between the results of the bioassay (< 2 ng/ml) and the results of the one-site RIA (30 ng/ml) may be explained by the fact that serum components bind NGF. The affinity of these components is not very high ($K_d = 10^{-7}$ M) but their capacity is extremely large (up to 0.5 mg of NGF/ml of rat serum). The binding of [^{125}I]NGF to such components competes with its binding to the solid-phase antibodies ($K_d = 10^{-9}$ M) which must be present in limiting amounts for the one-site RIA. In order to overcome these difficulties, a two-site RIA has been developed (Suda et al., 1978), in which the amount of solid-phase antibody is not limiting (Fig. 4B), thus avoiding or at least markedly reducing problems of competition. Accordingly, an excess of purified anti-NGF immunoglobulins is bound to the solid phase. Using such a two-site RIA, correspondence between biological and immunological assays could be achieved (Suda et al., 1978), in that with these two assays of similar sensitivity, no NGF can be detected either in rat or mouse serum. So far we do not know if the binding of NGF by these serum components (proteins of MW $\sim$ 500,000 and $\sim$ 150,000) has a physiological role. Neither do we know if bound NGF is biologically active. In the bioassay, NGF is active in the presence of serum, even if sufficient time is allowed to achieve complete equilibration of NGF binding to the serum components by preincubating the two before the bioassay. It is thus possible that bound NGF is active, but it is equally possible that in the bioassay, the high affinity neuronal binding sites displace NGF from its serum binding sites, a situation very similar to that described for the two-site RIA.

In considering the correlation between NGF bioassays and RIA, it is also important to take into account the observation that antisera raised against 7S or β-NGF can contain immunoglobulins directed against unrelated mouse proteins such as mice γ-globulins (Tomita and Varon, 1971; Carstairs et al., 1977). It is very likely that in some cases, impurities in the antisera used can explain the erroneously high values obtained (see Discussion, Suda et al., 1978).

Problems in determining NGF levels are not confined to immunological assays but are also inherent to bioassays. Even if the most obvious pitfalls are avoided such as the misinterpretation of radial emigration of non-neuronal cells as neuronal fiber outgrowth, stringent criteria have to be considered in order to interpret correctly the results of the bioassay. There are a series of experimental conditions which lead to fiber outgrowth from explants of chicken dorsal root ganglia which are not caused by NGF (Roisen et al., 1972; Frazier et al., 1973; Hier et al., 1973; Saito et al., 1977). The specificity of the fiber outgrowth has to be verified by demonstrating that it can be suppressed by specific NGF antibodies. It has also to be shown that the amount of antibody used corresponds to the amount required to block a similar effect elicited by a known concentration of NGF.

The necessity to perform such controls has been illustrated recently. In two systems which are "par excellence" targets for NGF, namely the dissociated sensory ganglia of the chick embryo (Levi-Montalcini and Angeletti, 1963) and a pheochromocytoma clone, PC12 (Greene and Tischler, 1976), fiber outgrowth can be elicited by factor(s) obviously different from NGF. Indeed, medium conditioned by glial cells could be shown to have typical NGF effects in both systems (Barde et al., 1978; Edgar et al., 1979). However, neither in the case of sensory neurons nor in the case of PC12 cells could these effects be blocked by specific antibodies against NGF (Fig. 6), where the concentration of antibody used was enough to completely suppress the effects elicited by NGF in sister experiments. We can conclude, therefore, that NGF is not unique: molecules other than classical NGF have NGF-like properties. The isolation and chemical characterization of such factors together with the delineation of their relative specificity both with respect to individual species of neurons and their developmental stage are important and promising fields of future research.

SUMMARY

After an initial discussion of the justification of the term nerve "growth" factor (NGF), a brief survey is given on the role played by this protein in the ontogenesis and maintenance of function of sympathetic and sensory neurons.

The function of NGF as a trophic messenger between effector organs and innervating adrenergic neurons is then discussed more extensively: it is now established that NGF is taken up selectively by specific nerve terminals, is transported retrogradely to the perikaryon in smooth membrane compartments (vesicles and cisternae), some of which have been seen to fuse with lysosomal structures (dense bodies). Since there is no evidence that intact NGF leaves these membrane-limited compartments, it is improbable that the NGF-mediated regulation of microtubule and microfilament assembly or the regulation of the synthesis of specific proteins results from a direct interaction of NGF with the corresponding nuclear or cytoplasmic structures. The nature of the second messenger(s) and the relationship between short-term (enhanced uptake of protein and nucleic acid precursors) and long-term (general growth, selective enzyme induction) effects remain to be established.

The fact that the transection of axons, destruction of nerve terminals and blockade of axonal transport have the same effect on the cell body of adrenergic neurons as the neutralization of endogenous NGF or immunologically cross-reacting NGF-like factors by anti-NGF antibodies, provides strong but indirect evidence that NGF acts as a retrograde messenger from effector organs to innervating adrenergic neurons. However, an unambiguous direct quantitative determination of NGF in effector organs, and consequently a relationship between density of innervation and extent of de novo synthesis, accumulation or activation from a precursor has not yet been possible. Such investigations were hampered by pitfalls inherent to both radioimmuno- and bioassays. These pitfalls lead in many cases to erroneously high levels of NGF determined in serum and tissues: an explanation for these artifacts, in particular those found using competition radioimmunoassays, is given and their avoidance by use of an appropriate two-site radioimmunoassay is described. The discussion of possible pitfalls occurring in biological assays of NGF leads to a brief consideration of factors other than NGF but which have similar properties.

ACKNOWLEDGEMENTS

This work was supported by the Swiss National Foundation for Scientific Research (Grant No. 3.432.74), a grant from the Sandoz Foundation. David Edgar is a research fellow of EMBO and Hiroshi Hatanaka a visiting scientist of the Mitsubishi-Kasei Institute of Life Sciences, Tokyo, Japan.

We wish to thank Ms. Vreni Forster for preparing the figures and the manuscript.

REFERENCES

Andres, R. Y., Jeng, I. and Bradshaw, R. A. (1977) NGF receptors: identification of distinct classes in plasma membranes and nuclei of embryonic dorsal root neurons. *Proc. nat. Acad. Sci. (Wash.)*, 74: 2785–2789.

Barde, Y.-A., Lindsay, R. M., Monard, D. and Thoenen, H. (1978) New factor released by cultured glioma cells supporting survival and growth of sensory neurons. *Nature (Lond.)*, 274: 818.

Bergeron, J. J. M., Posner, B. I., Josefsberg, Z. and Sikstrom, R. (1978) Intracellular polypeptide hormone receptors. *J. biol. Chem.*, 253: 4058–4066.

Bradshaw, R. A. (1978) Nerve growth factor. *Ann. Rev. Biochem.*, 47: 191–216.

Calissano, P. and Cozzari, C. (1974) Interaction of NGF with the mouse-brain neurotubule protein(s). *Proc. nat. Acad. Sci. (Wash.)*, 71: 2131–2135.

Carstairs, J. R., Edwards, D. C., Pearce, F. L., Vernon, C. A. and Walter, S. J. (1977) Immunogenic contaminants in mouse NGF. *Europ. J. Biochem.*, 77: 311–317.

Chen, M. G. M., Chen, J. S., Calissano, P. and Levi-Montalcini, R. (1977) NGF prevents vinblastine destructive effects on sympathetic ganglia in newborn mice. *Proc. nat. Acad. Sci. (Wash.)*, 74: 5559–5563.

Chun, L. L. Y. and Patterson, P. H. (1977) Role of NGF in the development of rat sympathetic neurons in vitro. 1. Survival, growth and differentiation of catecholamine production. *J. Cell Biol.*, 75: 694–704.

Edgar, D. and Thoenen, H. (1978) Selective enzyme induction in a nerve growth factor-responsive pheochromocytoma cell line (PC12). *Brain Res.*, 154: 186–190.

Edgar, D., Barde, Y.-A. and Thoenen, H. (1979) Induction of fibre outgrowth and choline acetyltransferase in PC12 pheocromocytoma cells by conditioned media from glial cells and organ extracts. *Exp. Cell Res.*, in press.

Frazier, W. A., Ohlendorf, C. E., Body, L. F., Aloe, L., Johnson, E. M., Ferrendelli, J. A. and Bradshaw, R. A. (1973) Mechanism of action of nerve growth factor and cyclic AMP on neurite outgrowth in embryonic chick sensory ganglia: demonstration of independent pathways of stimulation. *Proc. nat. Acad. Sci. (Wash.)*, 70: 2448–2452.

Goedert, M., Otten, U. and Thoenen, H. (1978) Biochemical effects of antibodies against nerve growth factor on developing and differentiated sympathetic ganglia. *Brain Res.*, 148: 264–268.

Greene, L. A. and Tischler, A. S. (1976) Establishment of a noradrenergic clonal line of rat adrenal pheochromocytoma cells which respond to NGF. *Proc. nat. Acad. Sci. (Wash.)*, 73: 2424–2428.

Hatanaka, H., Otten, U. and Thoenen, H. (1978) NGF-mediated selective induction of ornithine decarboxylase in rat pheochromocytoma; a cyclic AMP-independent process. *FEBS Lett.*, 92: 313–315.

Hendry, I. A. (1975a) The effects of axotomy on the development of the rat superior cervical ganglion. *Brain Res.*, 90: 235–244.

Hendry, I. A. (1975b) The response of adrenergic neurones to axotomy and NGF. *Brain Res.*, 94: 87–97.

Hendry, I. A. (1977) Cell division in the developing sympathetic nervous system. *J. Neurocytol.*, 6: 299–309.

Hendry, I. A. and Iversen, L. L. (1973) Reduction in the concentrations of NGF in mice after sialectomy and castration. *Nature (Lond.)*, 243: 500–504.

Herrup, K. and Thoenen, H. (1979) Properties of the nerve growth factor receptor of a clonal line of rat pheocromocytoma (PC12) cells. *Exp. Cell Res.*, in press.

Herrup, K., Stickgold, R. and Shooter, E. M. (1974) The role of the NGF in the development of sensory and sympathetic ganglia. *Ann. N.Y. Acad. Sci.*, 228: 381–392.

Hier, D. B., Arnason, B. G. W. and Young, M. (1973) Nerve growth factor: relationship to the cyclic AMP system of sensory ganglia. *Science*, 182: 79–81.

Johnson, D. G., Gorden, P. and Kopin, I. J. (1971) A sensitive radioimmunoassay for 7S nerve growth factor antigens in serum and tissues. *J. Neurochem.*, 18: 2355–2362.

Johnson, Jr., E. M. (1978) Destruction of the sympathetic nervous system in neonatal rats and hamsters by vinblastine: prevention by concomitant administration of NGF. *Brain Res.*, 141: 105–118.

Johnson, E. M., Andres, R. Y. and Bradshaw, R. A. (1978) Characterization of the retrograde transport of NGF using high specific activity [^{125}I]NGF. *Brain Res.*, 150: 319–331.

Lakshmanan, J. (1978) Nerve growth factor induced turnover of phosphatidylinositol in rat superior cervical ganglia. *Biochem. biophys. Res. Commun.*, 82: 767–775.

Levi-Montalcini, R. and Angeletti, P. U. (1963) Essential role of the nerve growth factor in the survival and maintenance of dissociated sensory and sympathetic embryonic nerve cells in vitro. *Develop. Biol.*, 7: 653–659.

Levi-Montalcini, R. and Angeletti, P. U. (1968) Nerve growth factor. *Physiol. Rev.*, 48: 534–569.

Levi-Montalcini, R., Caramia, F., Luse, S. A. and Angeletti, P. U. (1968) In vitro effects of the nerve growth factor on the fine structure of the sensory nerve cells. *Brain Res.*, 8: 347–362.

Levi-Montalcini, R., Aloe, L., Mugnaini, E., Oesch, F. and Thoenen, H. (1975) NGF induces volume increase and enhances tyrosine hydroxylase synthesis in chemically axotomized sympathetic ganglia of newborn rats. *Proc. nat. Acad. Sci. (Wash.)*, 72: 595–599.

MacDonnell, P. C., Nagaiah, K., Lakshmanan, J. and Guroff, G. (1977) NGF increases activity of ornithine decarboxylase in superior cervical ganglia of young rats. *Proc. nat. Acad. Sci. (Wash.)*, 74: 4681–4684.

Michell, R. H. (1975) Inositol phospholipids and cell surface receptor function. *Biochim. biophys. Acta (Amst.)*, 415: 81–147.

Mobley, W. C., Server, A. C., Ishii, D. N., Riopelle, R. J. and Shooter, E. M. (1977) Nerve growth factor. *New Engl. J. Med.*, 297: 1096–1149, 1149–1158, 1211–1218.

Mueller, R. A., Thoenen, H. and Axelrod, J. (1969) Increase in tyrosine hydroxylase activity after reserpine administration. *J. Pharmacol. exp. Ther.*, 169: 74–79.

Murphy, R. A., Saide, J. D., Blanchard, M. H. and Young, M. (1977) NGF in mouse serum and saliva: role of the submandibular gland. *Proc. nat. Acad. Sci. (Wash.)*, 74: 2330–2333.

Otten, U., Hatanaka, H. and Thoenen, H. (1978) Effect of nerve growth factor on general growth and differentiation of sympathetic neurons: induction of ornithine decarboxylase and tyrosine hydroxylase as respective examples. In *4. Int. Catecholamine Symposium, Asilomar*, Pergamon Press, Oxford, in press.

Paravicini, U., Stoeckel, K. and Thoenen, H. (1975) Biological importance of retrograde axonal transport of nerve growth factor in adrenergic neurons. *Brain Res.,* 84: 279–291.

Rohrer, H., Otten, U. and Thoenen, H. (1978) On the role of RNA synthesis in the selective induction of tyrosine hydroxylase by nerve growth factor. *Brain Res.,* 159: 436–439.

Roisen, F. J., Murphy. R. A. and Braden, W. G. (1972) Neurite development in vitro. I. The effects of adenosine 3′,5′-cyclic monophosphate (cyclic AMP). *J. Neurobiol.,* 3: 347–368.

Russel, D. H. and Snyder, S. H. (1968) Amine synthesis in rapidly growing tissues: ornithine decarboxylase activity in regenerating rat liver, chick embryo and various tumors. *Proc. nat. Acad. Sci. (Wash.),* 60: 1420–1427.

Saito, H., Suda, K., Schwab, M. and Thoenen, H. (1977) Potentiation of the NGF-mediated nerve fiber outgrowth by ginsenoside RB_1 in organ cultures of chicken dorsal root ganglia. *Jap. J. Pharmacol.,* 27: 445–451.

Schwab, M. E. (1977) Ultrastructural localization of a NGF-horseradish peroxidase (NGF-HRP) coupling product after retrograde axonal transport in adrenergic neurons. *Brain Res.,* 130: 190–196.

Schwab, M. E. and Thoenen, H. (1977) Selective trans-synaptic migration of tetanus toxin after retrograde axonal transport in peripheral sympathetic nerves: a comparison with nerve growth factor. *Brain Res.,* 122: 455–474.

Suda, K., Barde, Y. A. and Thoenen, H. (1978) Nerve growth factor in mouse and rat serum: correlation between bioassay and radioimmunoassay determinations. *Proc. nat. Acad. Sci. (Wash.),* 75: 4042–4046.

Tabor, C. W. and Tabor, H. (1976) 1,4-Diaminobutane (Putrescine), spermidine, and spermine. *Ann. Rev. Biochem.,* 45: 285–306.

Thoenen, H. and Schwab, M. E. (1978) Physiological and pathophysiological implications of the retrograde axonal transport of macromolecules. In *Archives in Pharmacology and Therapeutics, Vol. 5, Neuropsychopharmacology (Proc. 7th int. Congr. Pharmacol., Paris),* C. Dumont (Ed.), Pergamon Press, Oxford, pp. 37–59.

Thoenen, H., Otten, U. and Schwab, M. (1979) Orthograde and retrograde signals for the regulation of neuronal gene expression; the peripheral sympathetic nervous system as a model. In *The Neurosciences, Fourth Study Program,* F. O. Schmitt and F. G. Worden (Eds.), MIT Press, Cambridge, Mass., pp. 911–928.

Tomita, J. T. and Varon, S. (1971) Preparation of antibodies to the three subunits of mouse 7S nerve growth factor. *Neurobiology,* 1: 176–190.

Varon, S. (1975) Nerve growth factor and its mode of action. *Exp. Neurol.,* 48: 75–92.

Effect of Prolonged Sodium Bromide Administration on the Fine Structure of Dendrites in the Superior Cervical Ganglion of Adult Rat

F. JOÓ*, W. DAMES and J. R. WOLFF

Max-Planck-Institute for Biophysical Chemistry, Department of Neurobiology/Neuroanatomy, Göttingen (G.F.R.)

INTRODUCTION

In a previous paper (Wolff et al., 1978b) we have described the effect of a long-lasting administration of γ-aminobutyric acid (GABA) on the dendrites of the principal ganglion cells in the superior cervical ganglion (SCG) of adult rats. These plastic changes consisted of the formation of non-innervated postsynaptic membrane thickenings (F-POST), changes in shape and the accumulation of microvesicles. As GABA was found to be present (Bertilsson et al., 1976) and controlled by neuronal activity in the SCG (Waniewski and Suria, 1977), the fine structural changes observed in our former study were tentatively interpreted as an amplification of normal GABA activity. It was also concluded that GABA might be involved in the physiological regulation of the number of synaptic contacts in the SCG. It is yet unknown how GABA produces these effects. Is it the interaction with extrasynaptic receptors changing the permeability for ions and thereby the electric properties of the neurons, or are these effects mediated by metabolic changes which might be specific for GABA?

The present study was undertaken to see if sodium bromide, a substance known to produce stable hyperpolarization in sympathetic ganglion of frogs (Riker and Montoya, 1978), was also capable of modifying the properties of receptive surfaces of neurons in the SCG of adult rat.

MATERIAL AND METHODS

Microinfusion of sodium bromide into the SCG

Adult rats (Sprague-Dawley) of both sexes were anesthetized with ether and the left SCG was exposed taking care to retain an intact blood and nerve supply. In 10 animals glass capillaries (outer diameter: 50 μm) connected to small glass bulbs containing sodium bromide (10 μl of 500 mM solution) and ethanol (0.2%) in distilled water were inserted into the

* On leave from: Laboratory of Molecular Neurobiology, Institute of Biophysics, Biological Research Center, Szeged, Hungary.

ganglia in aseptic conditions and then fixed with tissue glue (Histoacryl blau, Braun) at the m. longus colli (for further technical details see Dames et al., 1979). Glass bulbs filled with mock cerebrospinal fluid were inserted into the SCG of 5 control animals.

Electron microscopic processing

Ganglia were removed 1, 3, 7 and 31 days after the implantation of glass bulbs, fixed by immersion in 2.5% glutaraldehyde buffered with 0.1 M sodium cacodylate (pH 7.2) and processed by standard techniques for electron microscopy. After osmification (0.1% in 0.1 M sodium cacodylate) and dehydration in ascending series of ethanol, tissue blocks were embedded in Epon. Sections were cut on a Reichert OMU-2 microtome, mounted on copper grids with single hole, and double-stained with uranyl acetate and lead citrate. Sections were viewed and photographed in a JEOL 100B electron microscope.

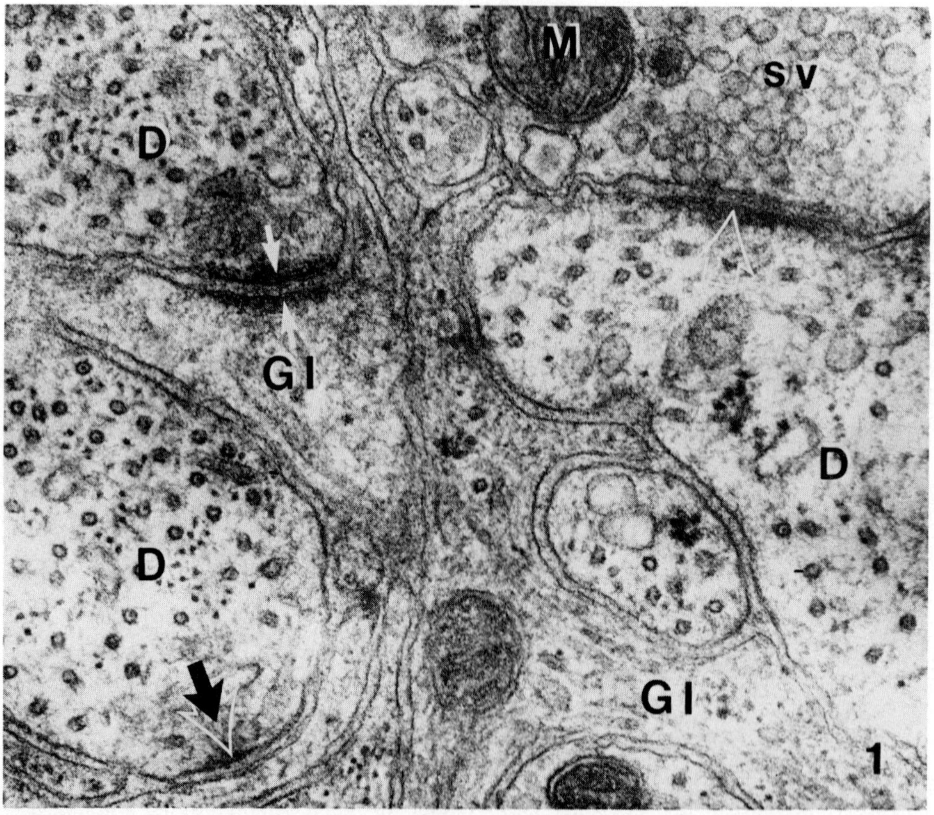

Fig. 1. Seven days after the beginning of sodium bromide microinfusion. Axon terminals with clear synaptic vesicles (sv) established Gray type I synapses (white empty arrow) at dendritic processes of the principal ganglion cells. M = mitochondrion, D = dendrites, Gl = glial processes. Black arrow points to a non-innervated postsynaptic membrane thickening (F-POST), while white solid arrows indicate symmetrical contacts. × 80,000.

Estimations of the amount of sodium bromide released from the implanted glass bulbs

As has been demonstrated for [^{3}H]GABA, substances contained in the glass bulbs are released continuously in a more or less linear manner (Dames et al., 1979). The actual amount of NaBr diffusing into the ganglia per unit of time can, however, not be directly determined. Several factors are influencing this value, such as the concentration in the glass bulb, the width of the capillary, the size of the ganglion, the vascular drainage, the distribution of the material within the ganglion, etc. All these may roughly be estimated to dilute the NaBr concentration within the glass bulb (500 mmol) by factors 10^{-3}–10^{-5}. According to this estimation the actual concentration which might be restricted to a region near to the tip of the glass pipet might vary between 5 and 500 μM of NaBr.

RESULTS

Fine structure of axons and axon terminals

A great number of myelinated, preterminal and synapsing axons were found in both control and experimental ganglia. Axon terminals contacted mainly with dendrites, but a few axosomatic synapses were also seen. Axonal endings establishing Gray type I synapses with dendritic branches of the principal ganglion cells were filled up with clear synaptic vesicles of 40–60 nm diameter and a few larger dense cored vesicles (Fig. 1). After the experimental intervention, no sign of axonal or terminal degeneration was observed.

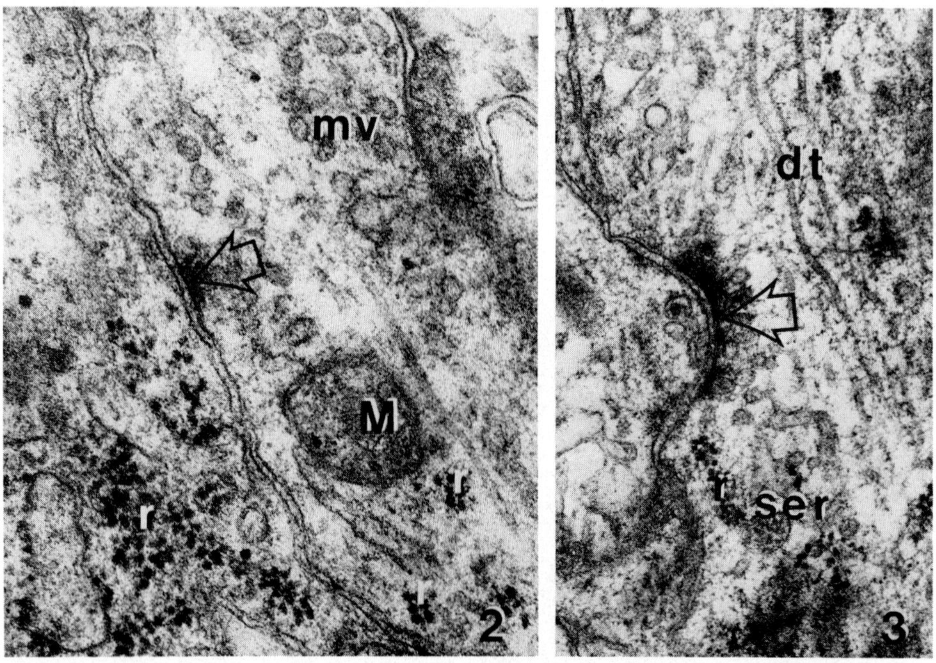

Figs. 2 and 3. Microvesicles (mv) were seen in great number in the dendrites both after 1 day (Fig. 2) and 31 days (Fig. 3) of sodium bromide treatment. Arrows indicate accumulated vesicles at specialized thickenings of dendrites. M = mitochondrion, r = ribosomes, ser = smooth endoplasmic reticulum, dt = dendritic tubules. Fig. 2, × 70,000; Fig. 3, × 45,000.

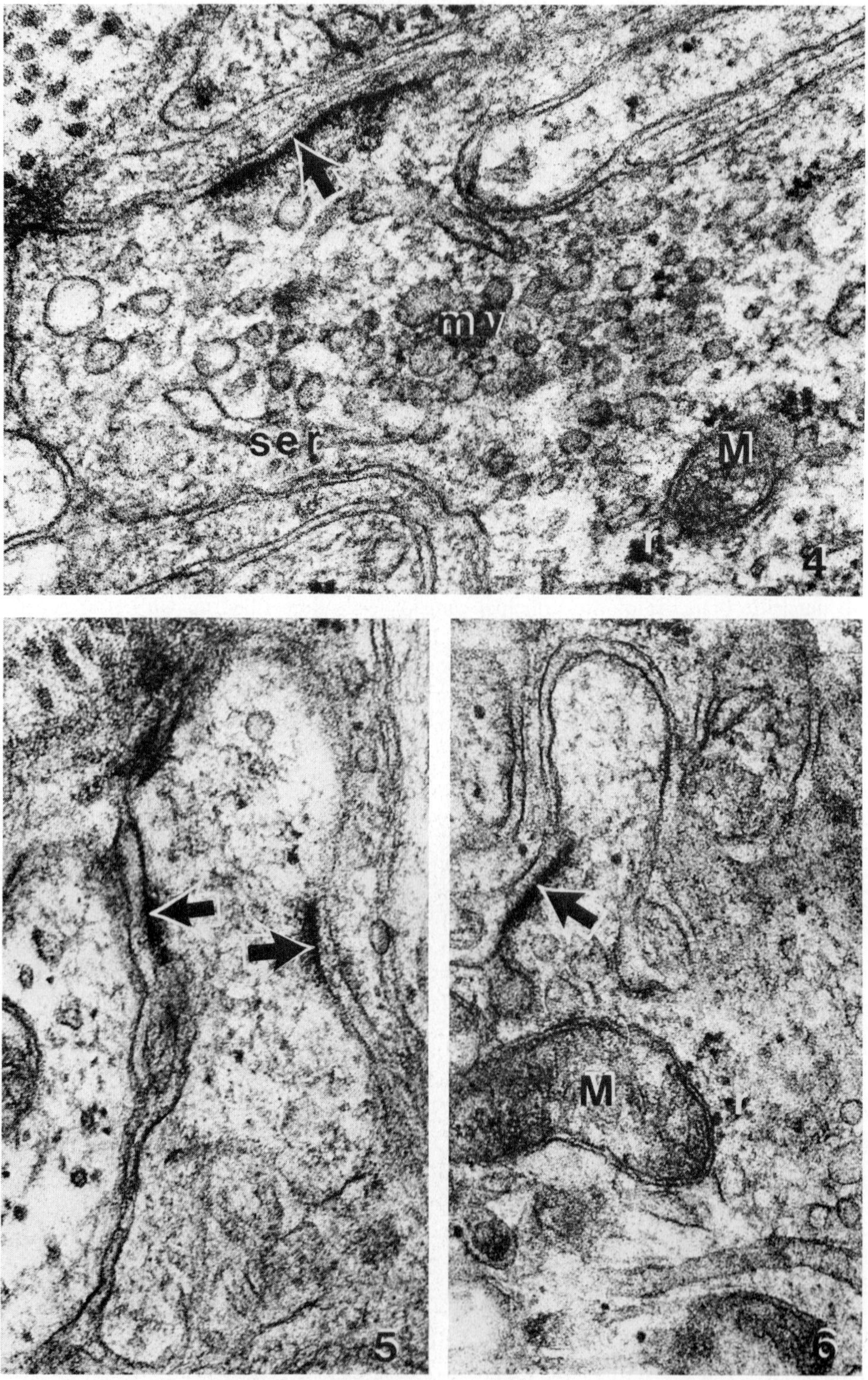

Figs. 4–6. Non-innervated, free postsynaptic membrane thickenings (arrows) on dendritic surfaces of the principal ganglion cells, 3 days (Fig. 4) and 7 days (Figs. 5 and 6) of sodium bromide treatment. mv = microvesicles, r = ribosomes, M = mitochondria, ser = smooth endoplasmic reticulum. Figs. 4 and 5, × 70,000; Fig. 6, × 80,000.

Formation of microvesicles in dendrites

Clear microvesicles of varying diameter had been formed in great number within the dendrites of principal ganglion cells already after one day of sodium bromide treatment. Some small clear vesicles contained a dense core (Fig. 2). Occasionally, a set of small microvesicles of 40–60 nm diameter appeared to aggregate at certain dendritic surfaces where membrane specializations resembling the presynaptic projections were also present (Fig. 3).

Production of F-POST on dendrites

In many cases, filamentous material aggregated to a varying extent along the inner aspect of plasma membrane and produced structural complexes similar in appearance to the postsynaptic membrane thickenings characteristic of Gray type I synapses (Figs. 4, 5 and 6). These structures were not in contact with intact axon terminals nor were axons and degenerating terminals found nearby. The majority of F-POST faced glial processes. Sometimes, those regions of the dendrites bearing F-POST had formed spiny branches.

In control ganglia, the dendrites contained microtubules and ribosomes in great number, but as a rule very few vesicles and spines were seen. The occurrence of F-POST was also negligible.

DISCUSSION

The electron microscopic findings described here after sodium bromide microinfusion appear to be similar in principle to that found in GABA-treated ganglia (Wolff et al., 1978b). In both experimental situations the fine structure of dendrites changed considerably including the appearance of F-POST, microvesicles and changes of shape. Regarding the possible molecular mechanism by means of which certain plasticity in dendrites can develop without interrupting the innervating axonal system, the following assumptions can be made. In addition to depressing the synaptic transmission in the SCG of cat (De Groat, 1970), rat (Adams and Brown, 1975) and dog (Kimura et al., 1977), GABA has been shown to increase the permeability of membranes to chloride ions in the SCG of rat (Adams and Brown, 1975). GABA depolarized ganglion cells (De Groat, 1970; Bowery and Brown, 1974; Adams and Brown, 1975), but induced hyperpolarization when ganglionic potential was less than –42 mV (Adams and Brown, 1975). On the other hand, sodium bromide has been reported to produce stable hyperpolarization in frog sympathetic ganglion (Riker and Montoya, 1978). It is conceivable that, similarly to GABA, sodium bromide microinfusion might have resulted in a long-lasting hyperpolarization of some ganglion cells as a result of displacing chloride. It cannot be excluded, however, that changes induced by GABA and/or sodium bromide were developed by altering directly the metabolism of nerve cells. The formation of microvesicles in dendrites after the experimental interventions might be indicative of a general cellular effect. On the other hand, it is accepted today that neurons in many regions of the central nervous system may have presynaptic properties at dendritic levels too (Sloper, 1971; Pasik et al., 1973; Szentágothai and Arbib, 1974). It may be pertinent to recall that, following X-ray irradiation, the perikarya and dendrites of the Golgi neurons in the cerebellum can be transformed to presynaptic structures which establish numerous synaptic contacts with spines and occasionally with shafts of Purkinje cell dendrites (Sotelo, 1977). Dendrites in the substantia nigra have been shown to contain clusters of small vesicles (Hajdu et al.,

1973) and release dopamine on depolarization (Geffen et al., 1976). In the light of the above mentioned data, one might interpret the formation of microvesicles in dendrites after continuous sodium bromide administration as morphological signs of dendritic transformation, but fully developed dendro-dendritic synapses have not been found in our material.

In our better understanding of the factors regulating different steps of the synaptogenesis, the question of formation and stabilization of postsynaptic membrane has always been of interest. Recently, fine structural investigations of the normal development of neurons have drawn attention to the transitory appearance of specialized postsynaptic membrane thickenings preceding the establishment of synaptic contacts by axon terminals in Gray type I synapses (Mugnaini, 1970; Stelzner et al., 1973; Westrum, 1975; Hinds and Hinds, 1976). In the occipital cortex these non-innervated free postsynaptic membrane thickenings (F-POST) occur more frequently in certain developmental stages and in certain laminae than in others (Wolff, 1978). Temporo-spatial aspects of the cortical development suggested that the maturation of GABA-accumulating cells including possible inhibitory neurons might have an impact on the formation of F-POST (Wolff et al., 1978a). Our previous results (Wolff et al., 1978b) have indicated that, after continuous GABA administration into the SCG of adult rat, plasticity in dendrites could be demonstrated. These plastic changes were independent of axonal degeneration, because neither axonal nor terminal degeneration were observed after the operation. Therefore, in contrast to the persisting or vacated postsynaptic sites seen after denervation (Sotelo, 1968, 1973; Raisman et al., 1974) F-POST observed in our study can be considered as newly formed membrane specializations (see also Wolff et al., 1979).

Whatever the exact molecular mechanism is, membrane thickenings resembling those found in Gray type I synapses can be produced without degeneration of normal preganglionic fibers by long-lasting continuous administration of GABA and/or sodium bromide in the SCG of adult rat. Whether or not these membrane thickenings (F-POST) have any functional significance, remains to be elucidated.

SUMMARY

Long-lasting sodium bromide microinfusion was provided into the superior cervical ganglion of adult rats. Ganglia from the experimental and control groups (infused with artificial cerebrospinal fluid) were processed for electron microscopy. Axons and synapsing terminals were frequently seen in the experimental as in control ganglia. After sodium bromide treatment, plastic changes were seen in dendrites which were similar in their main characteristics to those described earlier with GABA. These consisted mostly of the formation of non-innervated postsynaptic membrane thickenings, accumulation of microvesicles and changes in shape of dendrites.

The possible molecular mechanism of plastic change of dendrites is discussed.

ACKNOWLEDGEMENTS

The authors are grateful to Mrs. B. Pirouzmandi and Mrs. A. Wolff for skilful technical assistance and to Miss G. Kotte for typing the manuscript.

The study was supported by DFG, SFB 33, Proj. E3.

REFERENCES

Adams, P. R. and Brown, D. A. (1975) Action of γ-aminobutyric acid on the sympathetic ganglion cells. *J. Physiol. (Lond.)*, 250: 85–120.

Bertilsson, L., Suria, A. and Costa, E. (1976) γ-Aminobutyric acid in rat superior cervical ganglion. *Nature (Lond.)*, 260: 540–541.

Bowery, N. G. and Brown, D. A. (1974) Depolarizing actions of γ-aminobutyric acid and related compounds on rat superior cervical ganglia in vitro. *Brit. J. Pharmacol.*, 50: 205–218.

Dames, W., Joó, F. and Wolff, J. R. (1979) A method for localized and long-lasting microapplication of drugs into nervous tissue of freely moving rats. *Exp. Brain Res.*, in press.

De Groat, W. C. (1970) The actions of γ-aminobutyric acid and related amino acids on mammalian autonomic ganglia. *J. Pharmacol. exp. Ther.*, 172: 384–396.

Geffen, L. B., Jessell, T. M., Cuello, A. C. and Iversen, L. L. (1976) Release of dopamine from dendrites in rat substantia nigra. *Nature (Lond.)*, 260: 258–260.

Hajdu, F., Hassler, R. and Bak, I. J. (1973) Electron microscopic study of the substantia nigra and the strio-nigral projection in the rat. *Z. Zellforsch.*, 146: 207–221.

Hinds, J. W. and Hinds, P. L. (1976) Synapse formation in the mouse olfactory bulb. II. Morphogenesis. *J. comp. Neurol.*, 169: 41–62.

Kimura, T., Imamura, M. and Hashimoto, K. (1977) Facilitatory and inhibitory effects of γ-aminobutyric acid on ganglionic transmission in the sympathetic cardiac nerves of the dog. *J. Pharmacol. exp. Ther.*, 202: 397–403.

Mugnaini, E. (1970) The relation between cytogenesis and the formation of different types of synaptic contact. *Brain Res.*, 17: 169–179.

Pasik, P., Pasik, T., Hámori, J. and Szentágothai, J. (1973) Golgi type II interneurons in the neuronal circuit of the monkey lateral geniculate nucleus. *Exp. Brain Res.*, 17: 18–34.

Raisman, G., Field, P. M., Ostberg, A. J. C., Iversen, L. L. and Zigmond, R. E. (1974) A quantitative ultrastructural and biochemical analysis of the process of reinnervation of the superior cervical ganglion in the adult rat. *Brain Res.*, 71: 1–16.

Riker, W. K. and Montoya, G. (1978) Hyperpolarization and synaptic facilitation by sodium bromide in frog sympathetic ganglion. In *Proc. 7th Int. Congr. Pharmacol., Paris,* 1978.

Sloper, J. J. (1971) Dendro-dendritic synapses in the primate motor cortex. *Brain Res.*, 34: 186–192.

Sotelo, C. (1968) Permanence of postsynaptic specialization in the frog sympathetic ganglion cells after denervation. *Exp. Brain Res.*, 6: 294–305.

Sotelo, C. (1973) Permanence and fate of paramembranous synaptic specialization in "mutants" and experimental animals. *Brain Res.*, 62: 345–351.

Sotelo, C. (1977) Formation of presynaptic dendrites in the rat cerebellum following neonatal X-irradiation. *Neurosciences,* 2: 275–283.

Stelzner, D. J., Martin, A. H. and Scott, G. L. (1973) Early stages of synaptogenesis in the cervical spinal cord of the chick embryo. *Z. Zellforsch.*, 138: 475–488.

Szentágothai, J. and Arbib, M. A. (1974) Conceptual models of neural organization. *Neurosci. Res. Prog. Bull.*, 12: 399.

Waniewski, R. A. and Suria, A. (1977) Alterations in γ-aminobutyric acid content in the rat superior cervical ganglion and pineal gland. *Life Sci.*, 21: 1129–1142.

Westrum, L. E. (1975) Electron microscopy of synaptic structures in olfactory cortex of early postnatal rats. *J. Neurocytol.*, 4: 713–732.

Wolff, J. R. (1978) Ontogenetic aspects of cortical architecture: lamination. In *Architectonics of the Cerebral Cortex,* M. A. B. Brazier and H. Petsche (Eds.), Raven Press, New York, pp. 159–173.

Wolff, J. R., Chronwall, B. M. and Rickmann, M. (1978a) Morphogenetic relations between cell migration and synaptogenesis in the neocortex of rat. In *Proc. Europ. Soc. Neurochem., Vol. 1,* V. Neuhoff (Ed.), Verlag Chemie, Weinheim, pp. 158–173.

Wolff, J. R., Joó, F. and Dames, W. (1978b) Plasticity in dendrites shown by continuous GABA administration in superior cervical ganglion of adult rat. *Nature (Lond.)*, 274: 72–74.

Wolff, J. R., Joó, F., Dames, W. and Fehér, O. (1979) Induction and maintenance of free postsynaptic membrane thickenings in the adult superior cervical ganglion. *J. Neurocytol.*, in press.

Possible Mechanisms Underlying the Development of Central and Peripheral Cutaneous Afferent Connections (or, why I scratch my tummy when you tickle me on the back)

R. E. BAKER and M. A. CORNER

Netherlands Institute for Brain Research, IJdijk 28, Amsterdam (The Netherlands)

INTRODUCTION

Animals perceive their external environment through use of a variety of specialized sensory systems, each of which is designed to transduce a particular modality of stimuli into comprehensible interactions among neurons within the central nervous system (CNS). Since appropriate behavioral responses to environmental conditions are essential to survival, it is vital that the incoming sensory information reaches the proper brain centers for processing. Little is known, however, about the factors which assure the development of correct sensory projection pathways.

Most studies dealing with the ontogeny of sensory innervation have focused on submammalian vertebrates, where there is easy access to a variety of developmental stages and where excellent regeneration of cut nerves occurs in many species. (The assumption here is that regeneration adequately mimics the initial development of synaptic connections.) Anurans in particular appear to be suitable animals for analyzing the development of selective reflex connections. These animals characteristically give a variety of accurately aimed wiping responses to stimuli applied to the body surface. Such responses develop during and immediately after metamorphic climax, and thereafter remain constant throughout life. In addition, interchanging large pieces of dorsal and ventral skin during early or midlarval stages results in an irreversible change in the wiping movements, such that they become misdirected towards the original location of the transplanted skin rather than towards the point of stimulation (see Baker, 1976; Grinnell, 1977).

Broadly speaking, selective wiping reflexes could come about in one of two basic ways. There might exist either a *message specificity,* which involves distinctive timing sequences of action potentials generated in the afferent nerves, or a *channel specificity,* whereby selective anatomical connections occur between different peripheral end-organs and the CNS. The latter category can be broken down into 3 hypothetical ontogenetic mechanisms, one of which we have further subdivided into the 3 most plausible possibilities (Fig. 1). Any of these mechanisms could theoretically account for the development of both normal and misdirected reflexes in anurans.

IMPULSE PATTERNING MECHANISMS

Correct localization of tactile stimuli might come about through mechanisms other than anatomically specific pathways. For example, if belly and back skin receptors were able to reliably generate characteristic patterns of action potentials in the nerves connected to them, and if these differences could be recognized by the spinal cord and channelled to the appropriate motor centers, there would be no need to postulate the existence of highly localized cutaneous receptive fields (CRFs) to account for misdirected and normal wiping responses.

Recent experiments have therefore been conducted on the impulse traffic evoked in frog cutaneous nerve trunks by precisely controlled stimulation (Fig. 1; Corner and Baker, 1978). Single electrical shocks of varying intensity were applied to the skin in both normal and skin grafted *Discoglossus pictus* frogs. Such shocks elicited single action potentials in the nerve fibers activated by the stimulated skin, yet proved capable of evoking well organized behavioral responses from the animals. Reflexes elicited from normal skin were always correctly aimed at the site of stimulation and could not be distinguished from those elicited by tactile stimulation. Likewise, reflexes evoked from rotated skin grafts were misdirected, as had been the case for tactile stimuli. Repetitive electrical stimuli of high enough frequency to obliterate interspike interval fluctuations (500/sec) also elicited specific, accurately aimed, wiping reflexes according to the type of skin stimulated by the electrode. Such reflexes were not altered even when coupled with simultaneous subliminal mechanical stimuli applied to other areas of the body. In light of these observations, therefore, it seems inconceivable that temporal patterns of action potentials in single nerve fibers could provide the requisite information for correct localization of stimuli on the body surface.

It might be, however, that single impulses simultaneously evoked in a large number of nerve fibers could provide patterned information by arriving at the spinal reflex centers in characteristic temporal sequences due to their different conduction velocities (Fig. 1; Kornacker, 1963; Szèkely, 1974). Investigations to date have failed to indicate any differences in back and belly neuron responses which might bring about such differential signalling. Moreover, a large variation was noted in the conduction times of individual nerve fibers, depending upon where in a unit's CRF the stimulus was applied. These variations would introduce such a great uncertainty into the impulse spectrum generated in any given set of afferent nerve fibers that it is difficult to imagine how useful information could be transmitted about the location of receptors from which the action potentials originated.

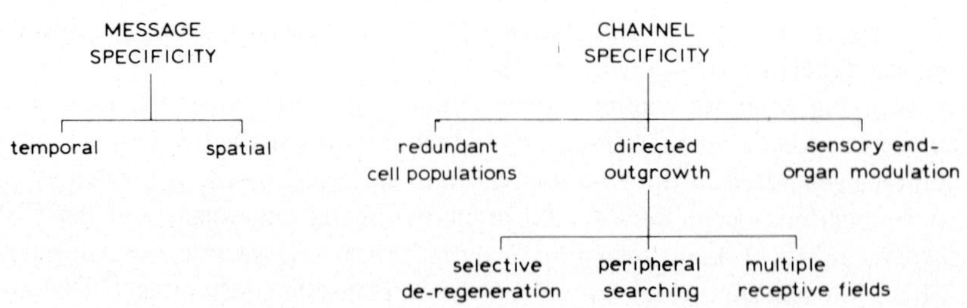

Fig. 1. Schema showing various mechanisms by which normal and misdirected reflex responses might come about in control and skin grafted frogs (see text for details).

SELECTIVE INNERVATION MECHANISMS

Appropriate connections between cutaneous mechanoreceptive neurons and the skin could be accomplished through selective (re)innervation of the proper skin types by neurons in the dorsal root ganglia (DRG). The most direct manner for selective (re)connections to be formed would be simply for the terminals of the neurites to continue growing until the appropriate skin type was encountered (*peripheral searching hypothesis;* Fig. 1). In skin grafted frogs, this means that the neurites would be able to recognize the presence of a wrong type of skin following rotation, and regrow over considerable distances until the correct skin type was located. Thus, the fibers would enter the skin at one point but in fact would be functionally connected with the proper skin type at a distance from the point of entry. Such a shift ought to be unmasked electrophysiologically, but no evidence in favor of this mechanism was found in any of the earlier studies conducted on skin grafted *Rana pipiens* (see Baker, 1976; Grinnell, 1977).

Since recent investigations have reopened the question of peripheral searching by sensory nerve fibers (Bloom and Tompkins, 1976; Heidemann, 1977), we have repeated the earlier experiments on *Rana pipiens* using the frog *Discoglossus pictus.* Skin grafting causes a general increase in the size of cutaneous receptive fields in this species (see Baker, 1978). Ventral nerve CRFs, which frequently extend onto the dorsum even in control animals, could account for some misdirected reflexes from the belly skin grafts on the dorsum in these animals. However, expanded ventral CRFs were occasionally seen to include considerable portions of grafted belly skin on the frog's mid-dorsal trunk, yet give rise to normally aimed dorsal wipes from most of these skin areas. Moreover, in other preparations, portions of the grafted belly skin from which misdirected wiping reflexes had been obtained were located well outside of the ventral nerve CRFs. We were able to demonstrate, by nerve crush experiments, that misdirected reflexes from these latter graft areas were indeed mediated via *dorsal* nerve trunks. Thus, although peripheral searching by DRG neurons could conceivably account for some of the misdirected reflexes observed in these animals, it cannot be the mechanism by which misdirected reflexes in general are elicited.

It is also conceivable that sensory neurons making contact with foreign skin withdraw their neurites and grow new ones directed to the original skin type, now in a different location on the animal's body (*selective degeneration-regeneration hypothesis;* Fig. 1). This hypothesis was tested by filling peripheral nerve trunks with cobalt, and then noting histologically where the stained cell bodies were located within the DRG (Baker et al., 1978). From 10 successfully filled dorsal nerve trunks, it was observed that the cell bodies both in control and 180° trunk skin grafted animals always predominate near the dorsal surface of the thoracic DRG. This topographical similarity suggests that selective de-regeneration could not have occurred in the skin grafted *D. pictus,* and thus cannot be the explanation for the occurrence of misdirected reflexes in these animals.

A third selective innervation mechanism, one which relies upon specificity between the neuron and its end-organ but not upon pathway specificity, involves *multiple branching* of individual ganglion cell neurites (Fig. 1). It is known, for example, that single cutaneous mechanoreceptive units in adult frogs occasionally possess split CRFs (see Baker, 1978), although such cells are not encountered frequently. However, multiple CRFs might be a more common phenomenon in embryonic stages, when the neurons are making their initial connections with the periphery. These multiple outgrowths would be free to travel through any established nerve trunk and, whenever the appropriate skin type was encountered, would establish functional connections. Those branches encountering a foreign skin type, on the other hand, would be withdrawn in the course of further development.

This alternative can be eliminated from consideration as the mechanism by which cutaneous reflexes are established on the basis of the following experiment. If the correct skin type normally stabilizes functional connections in only one of several widely separated neuritic outgrowths, then by increasing the amount of this skin type on the animal's trunk there ought to be an increase in the number of functional connections maintained by neurons which match that type of skin. Animals were therefore prepared which had essentially only one type of skin encircling the trunk (i.e., either belly skin or back skin on both the dorsum or ventrum) and were then investigated electrophysiologically for evidence of split, or abnormally large, receptive fields extending from the belly to the back. Only 3 out of 260 neurons examined possessed multiple or extended CRFs, which number is clearly insufficient to account for the misdirected reflexes which were seen in the animals' behavioral protocols (see Baker, 1978).

If it could be shown, finally, that the DRG cells providing innervation for belly skin were located in one area of the DRG, while neurons providing innervation for back skin were found predominantly in a different DRG location, then it should be possible to detect any shifts in their CRFs by recording unit responses from these areas of the ganglion. Such recordings would unmask changes in peripheral projections *regardless of what routes the nerve fibers might have taken to reach the correct skin types.* Electrophysiological experiments recently conducted on normal *Rana esculenta* and *D. pictus* frogs have demonstrated that a topographical segregation of cutaneous mechanoreceptive neurons does in fact exist within the thoracic DRG (see Baker, 1978). Cells providing innervation for dorsal skin areas are heavily predominant on the anterior dorsal surfaces, whereas cells innervating ventral skin areas predominate on the ventrocaudal surface. Animals with 180° skin rotation, despite their showing extensive misdirected reflexes, were found to have ganglionic topographies (back and belly skin neurons) which were no different from those in control animals. The failure to find any of the changes predicted by the selective (re)innervation hypothesis thus supports the negative results obtained in the previous 3 experiments described above.

CONCLUSIONS AND PERSPECTIVES

The elimination of the various mechanisms discussed above leaves us with only two hypotheses which might satisfactorily explain how cutaneous wiping reflexes arise during development. In the *sensory end-organ modulation hypothesis* (Fig. 1), cutaneous nerve fibers grow out *non-selectively* and innervate whatever skin type is encountered in the periphery. Information is supposed then to be transmitted from the skin to the DRG neurons, which subsequently form central reflex connections appropriate for the type of skin being innervated. Recent evidence from cutaneous nerve trunk cross-union in the axolotl appear to support this hypothesis (Johnston and Mark, 1977). In the frog, on the other hand, the existence of a clear-cut topographical organization in the thoracic spinal ganglia is difficult to reconcile with the idea of non-selective nerve outgrowth, and therefore suggests that mechanisms other than modulation are likely to be responsible for the development of reflex behavior. For example, flank and belly skin neurons are preferentially located in quite different areas of the ganglion, yet travel over considerable distances in a common nerve trunk before dividing to innervate their respective skin areas. Thus, while the ganglionic topography results do not definitively eliminate the possibility of sensory end-organ modulation, they cast doubt upon its validity since there is no longer any theoretical necessity to propose such a mechanism.

The last mechanism by which wiping reflexes might develop in anurans is that of *redundant cell populations* (Fig. 1). In this hypothesis, excessive numbers of neurons are produced throughout the ganglion, each specified for the type of skin which it must innervate peripherally. These neurons would send out fibers in a relatively non-directed fashion, with only those neurons surviving which make the correct peripheral connections. Electrophysiological recordings from the thoracic DRG have shown that, although there is a predominant population of cells from certain portions of the ganglion which innervate back or belly skin, there are always some neurons whose fibers project to the opposite body surface interspersed among these cells. Most neurites from belly skin neurons on the dorsal surface of the ganglion might normally travel towards the dorsum via the closest nerve trunk, only to die when confronted with back skin. The same thing would happen to the back skin neurons located near the ventral surface of the ganglion. In 180° trunk skin rotations, on the other hand, the reverse process would occur: e.g., the once doomed majority of belly skin neurons on the dorsal surface of the DRG would survive thanks to belly skin being located on the frog's dorsum, while cell death would now occur predominantly among *back* skin neurons (whose proper end-organs are located on the animal's ventrum).

Neither the electrophysiological nor anatomical mapping experiments so far reported would be able to identify different populations of cutaneous sensory neurons within a given topographical distribution pattern, and therefore are not suitable as a crucial test for these last two alternative hypotheses. What is required, therefore, is an experimental strategy which would allow us to distinguish between the redundant neuron hypothesis and the end-organ modulation hypothesis, an approach which still needs to be designed.

REFERENCES

Baker, R. E. (1976) Some comments on central and peripheral plastic changes in nerve connexions. In *Molecular and Functional Neurobiology*, W. H. Gispen (Ed.), Elsevier, Amsterdam, pp. 47–86.

Baker, R. E. (1978) Synapse selectivity in somatic afferent systems. *Progr. Brain Res.*, 48: 77–98.

Baker, R. E., Corner, M. A. and Veltman, W. A. M. (1978) Topography of cutaneous mechanoceptive neurones in dorsal root ganglia of skin grafted frogs. *J. Physiol. (Lond.)*, 284: 181–192.

Bloom, E. M. and Tompkins, R. (1976) Selective reinnervation in skin rotation grafts in *Rana pipiens*. *J. exp. Zool.*, 195: 237–246.

Corner, M. A. and Baker, R. E. (1978) Wiping reflexes and nerve impulse patterns evoked by electrical stimulation of the skin in frogs. *Physiol. Behav.*, 21: 789–792.

Grinnell, A. D. (1977) Specificity of neurons and their interconnections. In *Handbook of Physiology, Section I, The Nervous System*, E. R. Kandel (Ed.), American Physiological Society, Bethesda, Md., pp. 803–853.

Heidemann, M. K. (1977) Neurophysiological and behavioral evidence for selective reinnervation in skin-grafted *Rana pipiens*. *Proc. nat. Acad. Sci. (Wash.)*, 74: 5749–5753.

Johnston, B. T. and Mark, R. F. (1977) Plasticity of central actions of regenerated cutaneous nerves in axolotls. *Proc. int. Union Physiol. Sci.*, 13: 359.

Kornacker, K. (1963) Some properties of the afferent pathway in the frog corneal reflex. *Exp. Neurol.*, 7: 224–239.

Székely, G. (1974) Problems of neuronal specificity in the development of some behavioral patterns in amphibia. In *Aspects of Neurogenesis*, G. Gottlieb (Ed.), Academic Press, New York, pp. 115–150.

PART II

ORGANIZATION OF NEURAL ENSEMBLES

Chemically Coded Transmitter Systems

FLOYD E. BLOOM

Arthur Vining Davis Center for Behavioral Neurobiology, The Salk Institute, P. O. Box 1809, San Diego, Calif. 92112 (U.S.A.)

INTRODUCTION

Neuronal systems are most frequently classified with regard to 4 properties: (1) established or assumed functions, e.g., sensory or motor neurons; (2) cell shape or location, e.g., pyramidal, mitral or Purkinje neurons; (3) cell activity patterns, e.g., pacemakers, followers, bursting or silent cells; (4) neurochemical terms according to the transmitter the cell uses, e.g., cholinergic, GABAergic, or adrenergic. None of the classification systems necessarily includes or excludes the information described by the others. Participants in the present Symposium are focussing their attention on the chemical specificity of neurons as a key to the underlying development of basic principles of intercellular chemical interaction. My contribution to these considerations will attempt to employ the neurochemical classification of neurons as a mechanism by which to search for these principles of chemical intercellular communication. In this and related essays (Bloom, 1977, 1978, 1979; Bloom et al., 1978), I have attempted to develop some experimentally testable arguments by which such communicative events may be evaluated and compared.

WHAT IS BEING CODED?

When the term "chemically coded" is used with reference to neuronal systems, two levels of description are being employed. On the superficial level, the term means merely that the neuronal system has been neurochemically specified in terms of the transmitter substance or substances it secretes onto its target cells. A more complex level of consideration exists, however; namely, that the neurotransmitter molecule itself carries additional specific information which actually functions in the true sense of a code: a symbolic representation of a piece of instruction or information, or more simply a chemical representation of a functional signal. This latter level of discourse is the objective to be pursued here.

When there were few transmitters to be considered, many neuroscientists tacitly assumed that all transmitter molecules were functionally equivalent elements which differed only by producing either excitation or inhibition. Under that generalization, the transmitter for a given circuit did not really require identification so long as a qualitative sign could be defined. With the logic operations restricted to excitation and inhibition, theoretical constructs of neuronal ensembles to explain information processing appeared only to be matters of circuitry. Nevertheless, new candidate neurotransmitter substances are being discovered at a rapid rate, and the list of such candidates now numbers more than 2 dozen. This rapid rate of discovery has far outpaced the accurate determination of their probable sites and mechanisms of action. However, it seems illogical to assume that all these molecules are simply redundant carriers of the two simple commands, excitation and inhibition. What other types of information could the neurotransmitters be used to specify?

(1) Spatial signals

A transmitter could serve to identify the cell or cell population emitting the signal. If so, the number of transmitters in a given nervous system should bear a relationship to neuron number. However, if the response of a cell to a particular signal were to retain meaning as to the signal origin, and if there are multiple possible origins, additional features would be required. Each signalling molecule would also need an intracellular "symbolization" (Tomkins, 1975) in which each surface receptor system would be keyed to (for example) the production of a specific intracellular metabolite or ion. This symbolic perturbation would thus mediate the cell surface receptor's recognition of the agonist to which that receptor was on the alert. As currently conceived, all synaptic transmitters do change ion permeability or metabolite concentrations. The significance of such actions has been thought to lie only in the resultant change in membrane polarization or ion shunting, rather than in the specific molecular mechanism by which the change is effected. The number of ions (Na^+, K^+, Cl^-, Ca^{2+}) and intracellular metabolites (cyclic AMP, cyclic GMP) available to symbolize responses to individual transmitters is far smaller than the number of potential transmitters. Therefore, individual excitatory and inhibitory transmitters could not symbolize connectivity arrangements unless a given target cell received only one afferent system for each available intracellular symbol. A contrasting view is that cells accept signals blindly according to independent rules of connectivity and are regulated by the intracellular effects of these signals, oblivious of the origin or the molecular structure of the transmitter.

(2) Modality signals

The chemical output of a functional center (i.e., a nucleus, brain region, or any homotypic population of cells) might also be symbolized by a single transmitter. Thus, cells of the nucleus locus coeruleus are noradrenergic, the raphe nuclei cells are serotonergic, spinal motoneurons are cholinergic and cerebellar Purkinje cells are GABAergic. In this case, the number of transmitter species should be related to the number of cell classes but not necessarily to the number of cells. This hypothesis might also require the corollary that all neurons transmitting the same chemical message produce functionally equivalent effects. But nuclei that presumably employ the same transmitter do not share functional equality. For example, substance P and somatostatin are each found within some groups of primary sensory neurons in the dorsal root ganglia, and enkephalin, as well as neurotensin, are found in dorsal horn interneurons. However, these substances also occur within other groups of cells which have no known sensory function (Hökfelt et al., 1978).

Modality-derived codes could also be considered on the more common basis of excitation or inhibition. Each of these two general commands would appear to be generated by many of the transmitter substances, and further specification of the commands would seem warranted. At least 3 types of transmitter specific commands can now be documented: (1) changes in membrane potential associated with increased membrane conductance such as observed with amino acids and with nicotinic cholinergic receptors; (2) changes in membrane potential associated with no increased conductance or with decreased conductance, such as that seen with central beta-adrenergic receptors and peripheral muscarinic cholinergic receptors, and (3) changes in effectiveness through modulation of conductance changes due to other transmitters. While some peptide hormones act on their peripheral targets through activation of adenylate cyclase, there is as yet no compelling evidence now to ascribe this sort of "energy" transduction in mammals to centrally active peptides (see Nathanson, 1977).

Recently, the term "neuromodulator" has been used (Zieglgänsberger and Fry, 1976; Barker et al., 1978) to describe opioid and other peptides which alter "synaptic receptor-coupled conductances without direct activation of such conductances." Thus, enkephalins reduce the response of spinal cord neurons in vivo (Zieglgänsberger and Fry, 1976) or in vitro (Barker et al., 1978) to iontophoretic pulses of the excitant amino acid glutamate, but do not themselves appear to produce any change in membrane conductance. Similar "modulatory" effects have been reported for the effects of thyrotropin releasing hormone and substance P (Nicoll, 1978) on perfused frog spinal cords. This operational definition of neuromodulation provides precise grounds for future tests in which the choice of the test cell system will clearly be the critical issue. If the cells tested do not normally receive peptidic messages, the responses seen may have little physiologic relevance. Zieglgänsberger and Champagnat (1979) have recently demonstrated that the location of the glutamate receptor on distal dendrites of spinal motor neurons results in conductance changes which are not detectable in the perikaryon. Given this differential topography of receptors and receptor-coupled conductance changes, those remote synaptic receptors whose conductance change effects appear minimal may simply have escaped detection.

(3) Hierarchical position

Present concepts of the structural organization of the brain rely heavily on two principles of connectivity. In the primary sensory and motor pathways, the prevailing principle has been the classical concept of hierarchical relationships in which the transmission of information is highly sequential and specific. The key element of the hierarchical or "throughput" system is that destruction of one link incapacitates the chain. No transmitter molecule for any such throughput system, up or down, has as yet been identified, so it is not yet possible to determine whether specific chemicals are used to transmit between specific levels of such hierarchies.

The second widely applied principle of neuronal connectivity is that of the local circuit neuron (Rakic, 1975): typically a small, frequently unipolar, neuron whose efferent processes bear the morphology of dendrites. The basic feature of a local circuit neuron is that its connections are established exclusively within the local vicinity in which the cell body is found. Such small interneurons can exert significant control over information flowing through that locate, and may do so through "dendritic" release of their transmitter and without action potentials (Rakic, 1975). In some cases of inhibitory local circuits, the amino acids gamma-aminobutyric acid (GABA) or glycine (GLY) have been implicated as the transmitter (see Nicoll, 1978).

By comparison, monoaminergic neurons and presumptive peptidergic neurons operate over spatial domains which fit neither the concept of the local circuit neuron or the hierarchical throughput neuron exclusively. The dopamine-containing cell systems alone (Moore and Bloom, 1978) cover an extremely wide range from the ultra-short systems of the retina and olfactory bulbs to the longer, more highly arborized meso-cortical systems. On a spatial basis, the serotonergic systems seem to be as divergent and extensive as the noradrenergic systems. Cholinergic systems may also cover a broad spatial domain, but many aspects of specific circuits have yet to be determined (Krnjević, 1975).

Similarly, those neurons that contain biologically active peptides, as determined immunohistochemically (Uhl et al., 1977; Bloom et al., 1978; Hoffman et al., 1978; Hökfelt et al., 1978; Elde, this volume), do not appear as equivalent units of a single spatially predictable class: some presumptive peptidergic cells are small interneurons, such as the enkephalin- and neurotensin-containing cells (Hökfelt et al., 1978; Uhl et al., 1978), while others cover significantly broader spatial domains, such as those cells in the CNS and peripheral nervous system which are immunoreactive to antibodies against somatostatin, substance P, β-endorphin (Bloom et al., 1978) or luteinizing hormone releasing factor (Hoffman et al., 1978). Unfortunately, there are as yet no data with which to specify for any of these peptidergic systems the duration of the synaptic actions they may mediate.

(4) Macro-behavior coding

Finally, the use of the same transmitter could codify all those cells needed to execute individual steps leading to fundamental biobehavioral operations such as feeding, sleeping, mating, defending, or learning or even more detailed macro-functions such as body temperature or blood glucose regulation. Execution of this type of function might then require connections which coordinate the outputs of several chemically coded nuclei. Theoretical functional descriptions of specific transmitters (Barker and Smith, 1977; Brown et al., 1977) frequently employ this operational argument: the presence of the same peptides in multiple sites (e.g. brain, gut and endocrines) implies that the peptide integrates those tissues by evoking a concerted multicellular action. Despite the appeal of the "one transmitter–one behavioral function" concept, pharmacological approaches directed against neuronal cell populations containing the same monoamine transmitter have yet to provide compelling evidence that any complex behavioral function is so simply encoded. On the other hand, recent work on peptides related to drinking (Phillips et al., 1977) and pain perception (Hökfelt et al., 1978; Elde, this volume) may prove this philosophy to be more successful. However, what function could be subserved by somatostatin neurons in the cerebral cortex and somatostatin-secreting cells in pancreas (see Elde, this volume) to account for the spatial distribution of this peptide? The answer to this biological riddle may well lie in better understanding of the central representation of visceral-monitoring neurons and their ontogeny. In addition, more incisive operational definitions of the "purpose" of certain behaviors may also eventually provide general functional abstractions which will clarify the integral functions of widely separated cells sharing the same peptide or amine. Thus, cells secreting angiotensin (Phillips et al., 1977) or vasopressin (Swanson, 1977) could be seen not as signals for drinking or blood pressure elevation but rather as signals to control cell volume (MacKnight and Leaf, 1977) or extracellular fluid movement.

SPACE, TIME AND ENERGY OPERATIONS

These 4 possible bases for chemical codes among neurons should not be regarded as rigid categories of information content. Clearly other types of important information have not been considered here, for example, the importance of the phylogenetic origin of a class of neurons or type of intercellular command, and its manifestation within ontogenesis of the brain. Moreover, these same coding bases could easily be regrouped into information transfers on 3 standard physical domains: time, space and energy (Bloom, 1978; Bloom et al., 1978; Fig. 1).

To visualize how these 3 domains could be used to characterize the structure and function

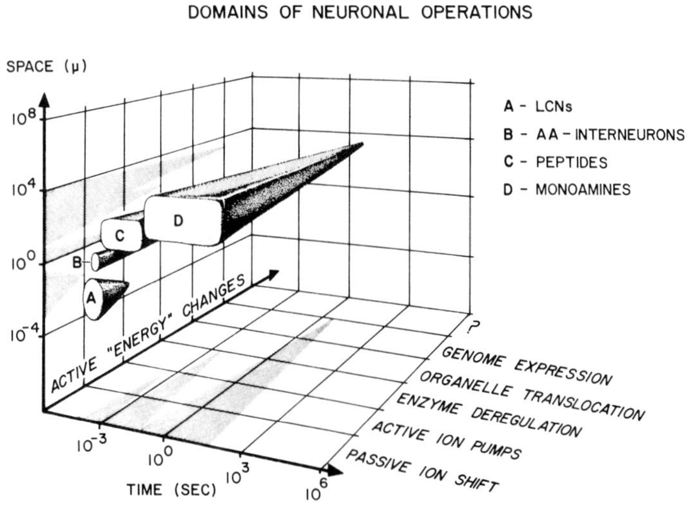

Fig. 1. Diagrammatic representation of the spatial, temporal and energy domains of neural circuits for which general chemical identification has been made. These multi-dimensional properties of nerve circuits are advanced as a meaningful basis on which to seek the informational content which transmitters may code (see Bloom, 1979).

of a specific chemically coded system, I conclude my essay with a consideration of the central noradrenergic neurons, reviewed in more detail elsewhere (Bloom, 1975; Bloom et al., 1978). Noradrenergic projections follow highly divergent trajectories in which a few norepinephrine-containing neurons reach out to target cells in many distant regions of the brain bearing no obvious direct functional relationship to each other. Spatially, in cerebral, cerebellar and hippocampal cortices, a major portion of the input seems to be directed towards the throughput output cells as targets. Temporally, noradrenergic projections operate on time domains with long latencies (30–50 msec or more) and long durations (300–600 msec or more) (Hoffer et al., 1973; Segal and Bloom, 1976a).

The effects of the coeruleo-cerebellar and coeruleo-hippocampal projections, and the iontophoretic simulations of the effects of coeruleo-cortical projections (Stone and Taylor, 1977) all fit closely into the interpretation that neurally released noradrenaline activates beta-adrenergic receptors coupled to adenylate cyclase and hence mediates according to the "second messenger" scheme of Sutherland (Siggins et al., 1971a, b; Bloom, 1975; Daly, 1977). The effects as judged by firing rates and transmembrane effects are overtly inhibitory, with hyperpolarizations accompanied by increased membrane resistance. However, when the effects are examined on other aspects of target cell functioning in different experimental contexts (Foote et al., 1975; Segal and Bloom, 1976a, b; Freedman et al., 1977) the effects of the locus coeruleus appear to fit better the designation of "biasing" or "enabling" (Hore et al., 1977) than simple "inhibition." The biasing or enabling function means only that in the epoch over which noradrenergic receptors are active, certain chemical messages received through other receptors can be enhanced or weighted (Moore and Bloom, 1978). Such enabling effects can be regarded as predictable outcomes of the observed changes in membrane properties (Weight, 1974).

As I have suggested elsewhere (Bloom, 1978, 1979; Bloom et al., 1978), the combination of electrophysiological and biochemical changes produced in target cells by the noradrenergic fibers may constitute a holistic set of responsive changes. The more easily observed electrophysiologic effects of this system (hyperpolarization, increased membrane impedance) are in this holistic view simply another index of the altered state of the target cells resulting from this form of neurotransmission. On one hand, these effects could be considered "modulatory" in the sense that adenylate cyclase-coupled noradrenergic receptors have altered information transmitted by other afferents for processing by the common target cell. However, the argument again returns to semantics. If the act of modulating is the physiologic function of locus coeruleus neurons, then surely their activity transmits that "modulate" or "enable" message.

CONCLUSIONS

Several aspects of emerging phenomena associated with chemically identified neurotransmitter systems in the brain suggest possible bases for seeking informational coding operations. Present evidence largely speaks against a tight and universal correlation of individual neurotransmitter codes with multi-celled complex behaviors. Nevertheless, experimental dissection of specific transmitter circuits and more precise definition of their operational goals may well provide some eventual primitive glimpses of the chemical and functional organization of brain cell systems.

SUMMARY

The chemical vocabulary of interneuronal communication resides in at least 3 specifiable variables: the transmitter molecules that neurons secrete, the temporal and spatial domains over which interconnected cells can regulate each other, and the resultant intracellular conditions imposed by these signals on their targets. Present data indicate that molecules acting as neurotransmitters fall into 3 chemical classes: amino acids, amino acid derivatives and peptides. Neuronal systems chemically coded by their transmitter substance exist within all structurally distinguishable classes of neuronal circuits. Characterization of chemical signals in the brain thus requires consideration of all 3 domains. The intracellular conditions imposed by the actions of transmitters on their target cells may provide the basis for a logic of intercellular operations which organizes individual neurons into responsive ensembles in order to produce phenomena recognizable as behavior. Furthermore, the ever-lengthening list of neuron-produced chemical signals allows ample possibilities for integrating time, space, and modality for rapid processing of biological information.

REFERENCES

Barker, J. L. and Smith, Jr., T. G. (1977) Peptides as neurohormones. *Neurosci. Symp.*, 2: 340.

Barker, J. L., Neale, J. H., Smith, Jr., T. G. and MacDonald, R. L. (1978) Opiate peptide modulation of amino acid responses suggest novel form of neuronal communication. *Science*, 199: 1451.

Bloom, F. E. (1975) The role of cyclic nucleotides in central synaptic function. *Rev. Physiol. Biochem. Pharmacol.*, 74: 1.

Bloom, F. E. (1977) Peptide transmitters: clues to the chemical cryptogram of interneuronal communication? *Biosystems*, 8: 179.

Bloom, F. E. (1978) Contrasting principles of synaptic physiology: peptidergic and non-peptidergic neurons. In *The 42nd Nobel Symposium on The Peptidergic Neuron*, K. Fuxe (Ed.), Plenum Press, New York, pp. 173–188.

Bloom, F. E. (1979) Chemical integrative processes in the central nervous system. In *The Neurosciences, 4th Intensive Study Program,* F. O. Schmitt and F. G. Worden (Eds.), MIT Press, Cambridge, Mass., in press.

Bloom, F. E., Battenberg, E. L. F., Rossier, J., Ling, N. and Guillemin, R. (1978) Neurons containing β-endorphin in rat brain exist separately from those containing enkephalin: immunocytochemical studies. *Proc. nat. Acad. Sci. (Wash.),* 75: 1591.

Brown, M., Rivier, J. and Vale, W. (1977) Neurotropic actions of central nervous system peptides. *Abstr. Int. Soc. Psychoneuroendocr.,* 177.

Daly, J. (1977) *Cyclic Nucleotides in the Nervous System.* Plenum Press, New York.

Foote, S., Freedman, R. and Oliver, A. P. (1975) Effects of putative neurotransmitters on neuronal activity in monkey auditory cortex. *Brain Res.,* 86: 229.

Freedman, R., Hoffer, B. J., Woodward, D. J. and Puro, D. (1977) Interaction of norepinephrine with cerebellar activity evoked by mossy and climbing fibers. *Exp. Neurol.,* 55: 269.

Hoffer, B. J., Siggins, G. R., Oliver, A. P. and Bloom, F. E. (1973) Activation of the pathway from locus coeruleus to rat cerebellar Purkinje neurons: pharmacological evidence of noradrenergic central inhibition. *J. Pharmacol. exp. Ther.,* 184: 553.

Hoffman, G. E., Knigge, K. M., Moynihan, J. A., Melnyk, V. and Arimura, A. (1978) Neuronal fields containing luteinizing hormone releasing hormone (LHRH) in mouse brain. *Neuroscience,* 3: 219.

Hökfelt, T., Elde, R., Johansson, O., Ljungdahl, Å., Schutzberg, A. and Fuxe, K. (1978) The distribution of peptide containing neurons in the nervous system. In *Psychopharmacology: a Generation of Progress,* M. A. Lipton, A. DiMascio and K. F. Killam (Eds.), Raven Press, New York, pp. 39–66.

Hore, J., Meyer-Lohmann, J. and Brooks, V. B. (1977) Basal ganglia coding disables learned arm movements of monkeys in the absence of visual guidance. *Science,* 195: 584.

Krnjević, K. (1975) Acetylcholine receptors in vertebrate CNS. *Handbook Psychopharmacol.,* 6: 190.

MacKnight, A. D. C. and Leaf, A. (1977) Regulation of cell volume. *Physiol. Rev.,* 57: 510.

Moore, R. Y. and Bloom, F. E. (1978) Central catecholamine neuron systems: anatomy and physiology of the dopamine systems. *Ann. Rev. Neurosci.,* 1: 129.

Moore, R. Y. and Bloom, F. E. (1979) Central catecholamine neuron systems: anatomy and physiology of the norepinephrine and epinephrine systems. *Ann. Rev. Neurosci.,* 2: 113.

Nathanson, J. (1977) Cyclic nucleotides and nervous system function. *Physiol. Rev.,* 57: 157.

Nicoll, R. A. (1978) Amino acids and peptides. In *Psychopharmacology: a Generation of Progress,* M. A. Lipton, A. DiMascio and K. F. Killam (Eds.), Raven Press, New York, p. 103.

Phillips, M. I., Felix, D., Hoffman, W. E. and Ganten, D. (1977) Angiotensin-sensitive sites in the brain ventricular system. *Neurosci. Symp.,* 2: 308.

Rakic, P. (1975) Local circuit neurons. *Neurosci. Res. Progr. Bull.,* 13: 293.

Segal, M. and Bloom, F. E. (1976a) The actions of norepinephrine in the rat hippocampus. III. Hippocampal cellular responses to locus coeruleus stimulation in the awake rat. *Brain Res.,* 107: 499.

Segal, M. and Bloom, F. E. (1976b) The action of norepinephrine in the rat hippocampus. IV. The effects of locus coeruleus stimulation on evoked hippocampal unit activity. *Brain Res.,* 107: 513.

Siggins, G. R., Hoffer, B. J. and Bloom, F. E. (1971a) Studies on norepinephrine-containing afferents to Purkinje cells of rat cerebellum. III. Evidence for mediation of norepinephrine effects by cyclic 3′5′-adenosine monophosphate. *Brain Res.,* 25: 535.

Siggins, G. R., Oliver, A. P., Hoffer, B. J. and Bloom, F. E. (1971b) Cyclic adenosine monophosphate and norepinephrine: effects on trans-membrane properties of cerebellar Purkinje cells. *Science,* 171: 192.

Stone, T. W. and Taylor, D. A. (1977) Microiontophoretic studies of the effects of cyclic nucleotides on excitability of neurone in the rat cerebral cortex. *J. Physiol. (Lond.),* 266: 523.

Swanson, L. (1977) Immunohistochemical evidence for a neurophysin-containing autonomic pathway arising in the paraventricular nucleus of the hypothalamus. *Brain Res.,* 128: 346.

Tomkins, G. (1975) The metabolic code. *Science,* 189: 760.

Uhl, G., Kuhar, M. and Snyder, S. (1977) Neurotensin: immunohistochemical localization in rat central nervous system. *Proc. nat. Acad. Sci. (Wash.),* 74: 4059.

Weight, F. F. (1974) Physiologic mechanisms of synaptic modulation. In *The Neurosciences – Third Study Program,* F. O. Schmitt (Ed.), M.I.T. Press, Cambridge, Mass., pp. 929–939.

Zieglgänsberger, W. and Champagnat, J. (1979) Cat spinal motoneurones exhibit topographic sensitivity to glutamate and glycine. *Brain Res.,* 160: 95.

Zieglgänsberger, W. and Fry, J. P. (1976) *Opiates and Endogenous Opioid Peptides.* Elsevier/North-Holland Biomedical Press, Amsterdam.

Hippocampal Plasticity

JOHN C. ECCLES

Max-Planck-Institut für biophysikalische Chemie, Abteilung für Neurobiologie, Göttingen (G.F.R.)

Memory is dependent on long enduring changes in the brain. There is general agreement that there are no gross structural changes, for example, in the growth of new pathways or of assemblages of nerve cells. All of these basic structures and connectivities are grown by genetic instructions prior to their usage. So in the learning process more subtle and prolonged changes in the synaptic communications (cf. Fig. 1B) between nerve cells have to be involved. Thus in the first place the study of memory resolves itself into an investigation of synaptic transmission in order to see if bursts of activity are followed by long lasting increases in synaptic potency that could be the elemental basis of memory. Such changes can be regarded as manifestations of synaptic plasticity.

In very recent investigations (Misgeld et al., 1977; Sarvey et al., 1979) advantage has been taken of the lamella organization (Andersen et al., 1971) by cutting strictly in the plane of the lamellae thin slices (about 0.4 mm thick) from the hippocampus of the guinea pig. These slices survive quite well for up to 12 hr in an appropriate oxygenated medium and are extremely well suited for the experimental investigation indicated in Fig. 2A. Recording is extracellular by a microelectrode in the zone of the CA3 pyramidal cell bodies. Stimulation

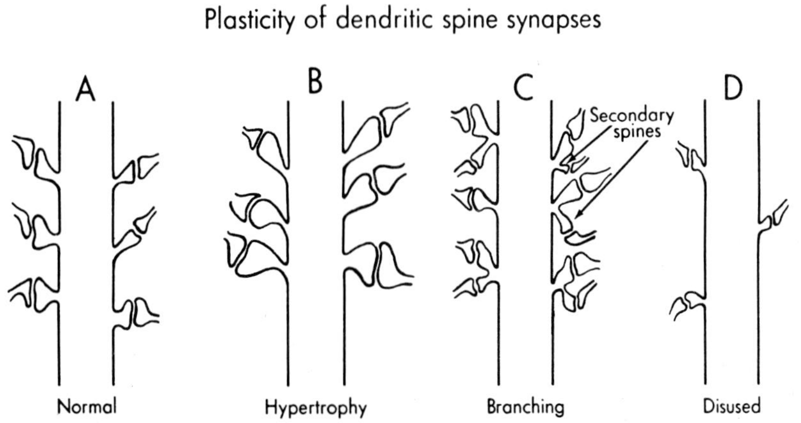

Fig. 1. Illustrations of proposed plasticity of dendritic spine synapses. The drawing are designed to convey the plastic changes in spine synapses that are postulated to occur with growth in B and C and with regression in D. Further description in text.

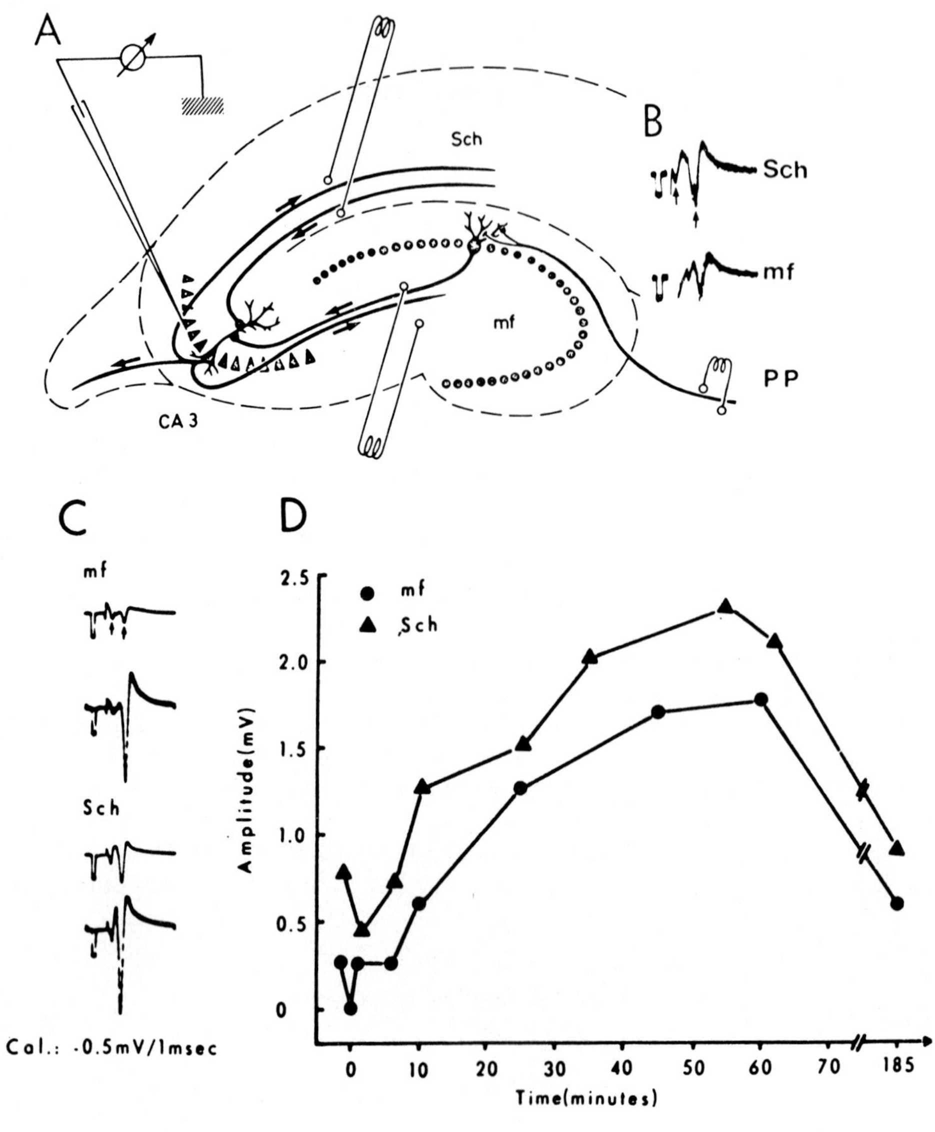

Fig. 2. A: drawing of a hippocampal slice in the plane of a lamella in order to indicate the electrode placements. The stimulating electrodes were located for stimulating selectively the Schaffer collaterals (Sch) and the mossy fibres (mf). The recording electrode was placed so as to record extracellularly from the somata of CA3 pyramidal cells. Also shown (pp) is the stimulating electrode in the entorhinal cortex for exciting the perforating pathway to the granule cells of the fascia dentata. B: the electrical responses with Sch and mf stimulation at a strength below twice threshold. Arrows on the Sch trace mark the double negative spike described in the text. C: the mf and Sch evoked responses in another experiment. The double negative spike is again marked by arrows. The lower responses in both the mf and Sch frames show the potentiation of the second spike 25 min after a conditioning tetanus to the mf input at 300/sec for 5 sec. The first spike was unaltered. D: the sizes of the second spike in mV were plotted against the times after the conditioning mf tetanus (Misgeld et al., 1977; Sarvey et al., 1979).

can be by 2 pairs of electrodes, one close to the mossy fibre (mf) input to the CA3 and the other close to the Schaffer collaterals (Sch). In Fig. 2B both the Sch and mf stimuli produced double negative spikes indicated by arrows, the smaller earlier one being due largely to the antidromic excitation of some of the pyramidal cells, the larger second to impulses set up by synaptic excitation of these same cells. This interpretation is based on carefully designed control experiments with intracellular recording. In C, after the control to the mf and Sch stimuli (upper traces), there was repetitive stimulation by the mf electrode, 300/sec for 5 sec. The lower traces show that there was a large potentiation of the second negative wave (the synaptic response) some 25 min after the tetanus with both the mf and the Sch responses. The testing stimulation was at the same strength as with the control, as is indicated by the unchanged size of the small initial negative spike potential. The similar time courses of the mf and Sch potentiations after an mf tetanus are shown in Fig. 2D. With much milder tetanic stimulation (200 stimuli at 2/sec to 18/sec) the potentiations were not as large as in Fig. 2, but had a similar prolonged time course.

A remarkable feature of Fig. 2C and D was that the synapses not stimulated (the Sch) participated in the potentiation almost as much as those stimulated (the mf). Very careful controls have been carried out with interaction of double stimulations at various short intervals, double by the same electrode or one stimulus through the mf and one through the Sch electrodes. These controls have shown facilitated responses to the second volley in the same afferent (mf or Sch) (Fig. 3A and D), but not when in different afferents (Fig. 3C and D).

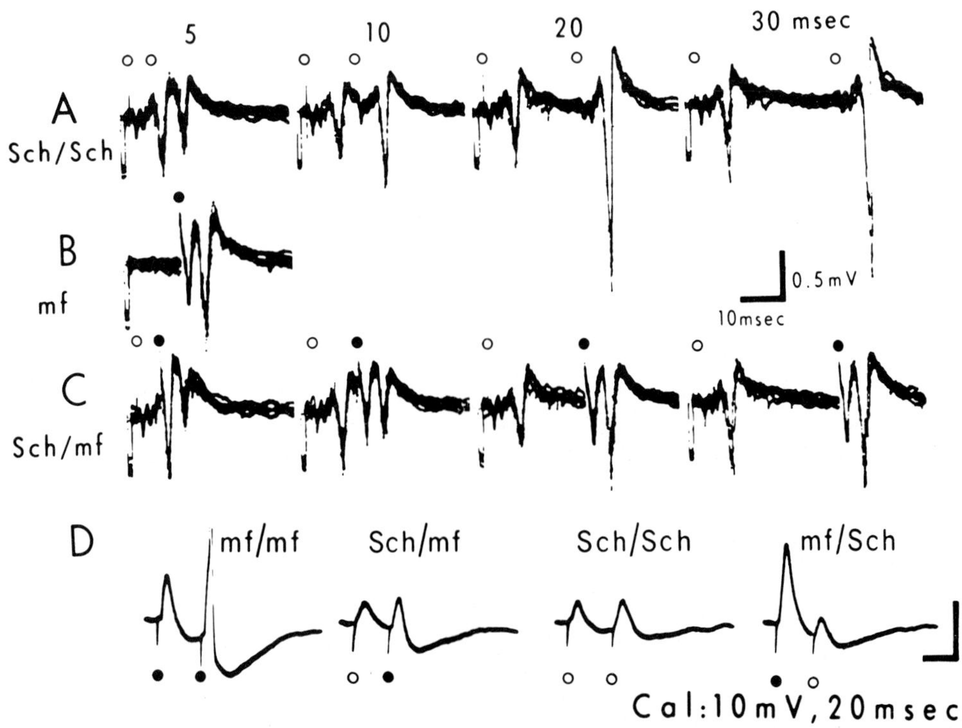

Fig. 3. Electrical responses evoked as in Fig. 2C by mf and Sch stimulation, mf responses being shown by filled circles and Sch by open circles. In A double Sch stimulation and in C Sch/mf stimulation as indicated, B showing control mf response. In D are intracellular double responses as indicated.

Thus it has been demonstrated that the mf and Sch electrodes were indeed exciting separate synaptic inputs to CA3 pyramidal cells, i.e. they were providing heterosynaptic inputs. Thus in the lower rows of Fig. 2C, there was heterosynaptic potentiation, and in the upper rows homosynaptic potentiation.

Prolonged homosynaptic potentiation was first demonstrated on the granule cells of the fascia dentata (Bliss and Lømo, 1973). The pathway from the entorhinal cortex via the perforating pathway (pp) is shown in Fig. 2A, the actual relationship of the fibres of the perforating pathway to the branching dendrites of the granule cells being illustrated in Fig. 4A. When recording extracellularly from the granule cells, there is a large negative potential (a population EPSP) when the electrode is at the level of the pp synapses (upper frame of Fig. 4A), and a large negative population spike, when at the level of the granule cell bodies (lower frame of Fig. 4A). In Fig. 4C entorhinal stimulation excited the pp pathway and the population spike of the granule cells was initially about 2 mV at a low control rate of stimulation (0.5/sec). The spike was potentiated over 4 times during an intercurrent higher frequency (15/sec for 15 sec) of stimulation. After the tetanus there was a brief initial depression, but soon this gave place to potentiation, which was almost double the initial size after 20 min. Fig. 4B shows a much longer potentiation of the population EPSP (upper frame of Fig. 4A) after 4 episodes of repetitive stimulation, as noted in the legend. The potentiation had diminished to about half at 10 hr after the last conditioning tetanus.

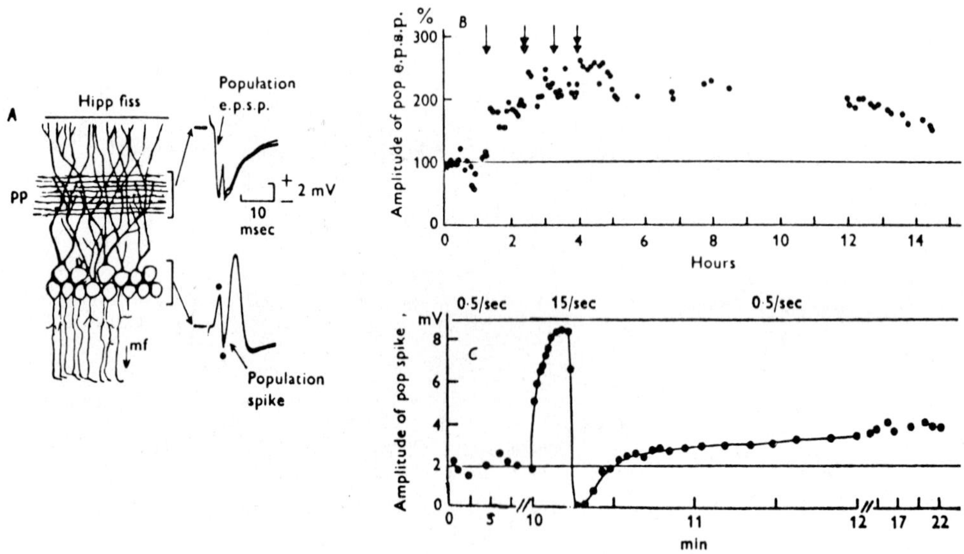

Fig. 4. Granule cells of the fascia dentata. A: drawing of granule cells with their bodies, dendrites and axons that form the mossy fibres (mf). The fibres of the perforating pathway (pp) are shown traversing the dendrites on which they make excitatory synapses. Recording the field potentials at the level of the pp synapses results in a large and prolonged negative potential, which is labelled population EPSP. When the recording electrode is advanced to the level of the cell bodies the sharp negative spike (population spike) signals the generation of impulses in the cell bodies. B: the relative amplitudes of the population EPSPS are plotted at up to 10 hr after 4 conditioning trains of stimulation indicated by the arrows. At single arrows there was stimulation at 15/sec for 15 sec, and at the double arrows 100/sec for 3 sec. The 100% line is drawn through the pre-stimulation responses at 0.5/sec and after the conditioning tetanus the same low rate was resumed. C: time course of post-stimulation potentiation as in B, but for the population spike. There was only a single conditioning tetanus of 15/sec for 15 sec (Bliss and Lømo, 1973).

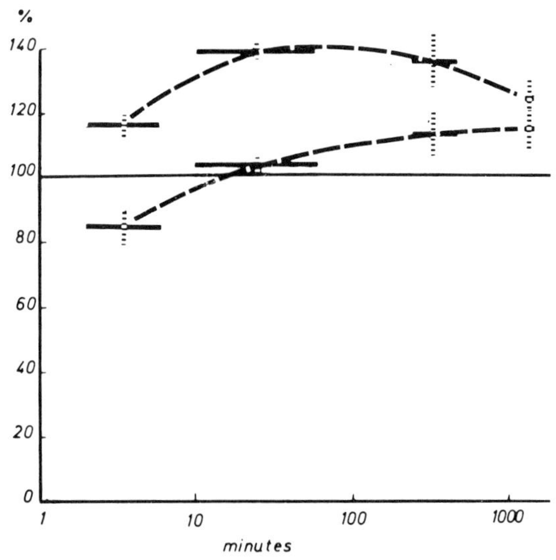

Fig. 5. Plotting of the effects of a conditioning tetanus of 15/sec for 15 sec on the sizes of the synaptic spines and the axon terminals, as measured in electron micrographs. The upper plotting is for the synaptic spines, the lower for the axon terminals. There has been pooling of post-stimulation intervals as indicated by the horizontal bars which are at the mean percentage levels relative to controls. The standard errors are shown for each pooled series by the vertical broken lines. Time scale as indicated is in minutes on a logarithmic scale. Ordinates are percentages relative to controls.

Of fundamental importance is the recent discovery by Fifková and Van Harreveld (1977) that a relatively mild repetitive stimulation (30/sec for 30 sec) of the entorhinal cortex by the electrode labelled pp in Fig. 2A resulted in a swelling of the stimulated spines of the granule cells, as observed in electron micrographs; and this was confirmed by most careful planimetric measurements on thousands of spines that have been identified by stringent criteria. The increase in area averaged about 35% and was highly significant relative to a similar series of planimetric measurements on the control synapses. It was also observed that the unstimulated commissural synapses on the proximal third of the dendrites did not participate in the enlargement, which was thus homosynaptic. In a total of 31 experiments the effects of stimulation were observed at times from 2 min to 23 hr afterwards. In Fig. 5 the course of the spine swelling is plotted on a logarithmic time scale with the standard errors indicated by vertical bars and with the ranges of the post-stimulation times for each statistical series shown by the horizontal bars. The swelling rose up to a maximum by about 100 min then slowly declined, though it was almost 25% at the longest test interval, 23 hr. When similarly plotted, the axon terminals (synaptic knobs) showed an initial shrinkage, and there seemed to be a later swelling to almost 15%, but for each set of data it was not statistically significant, though more significance would be obtained by pooling the data for the two longest testing periods.

There is a remarkable similarity in the time courses of the physiological potentiations illustrated in Fig. 4B and C and of the swellings in Fig. 5. In the growth theory of learning it has long been conjectured that excess activation of synapses resulted in their hypertrophy (Eccles, 1972), such postulated synapses being called *modifiable synapses.* Experiments such as those illustrated in Figs. 4 and 5 are a remarkable corroboration of this conjecture for the spine synapses from the perforating pathway onto the dendrites of hippocampal granule cells. An early diagrammatic representation of this conjecture in Fig. 1A and B corresponds very closely to the findings in Fig. 5.

If synaptic growth is required for learning, there must be an increase in brain metabolism of a special kind with the manufacture of proteins and other macromolecules required for the increases in membranes and in chemical transmission mechanisms. The specificities would be encoded in the structure, particularly in the synaptic connections of nerve cells, which are arranged in the unimaginably complex pattern that has already been formed in development. From then onward, all that seems to be required for the functional reorganization that is assumed to be the neuronal substrate of memory is merely the microgrowth of synaptic connections already in existence, as indicated in Fig. 1B and C, which can be regarded as models of the spine synapses on pyramidal cells.

Libet et al. (1975) described a conjunction operation in a sympathetic ganglion cell, where input by dopaminergic synapses results in a prolonged enhancement of the cholinergic synapses on the same cell. This potentiation by conjunction is mediated by an intracellular metabolic system utilizing cyclic adenosine monophosphate (AMP). This model proposed by Libet et al. is strictly heterosynaptic, as also is the instruction-selection theory of cognitive memory (Kornhuber, 1973; Eccles, 1978). The prolonged heterosynaptic potentiation illustrated in Fig. 2 is therefore of special interest as a model for learning processes in the cerebral cortex.

SUMMARY

Synaptic plasticity is manifested by long lasting changes in synaptic potency. Increased potency is of special importance in relation to the neural basis of memory. Even mild repetitive stimulation evokes large and prolonged potentiation of hippocampal synapses, as is revealed by electrical recording either in vivo or in vitro. More importantly there is a matching hypertrophy of the synaptic spines on the dendrites of hippocampal granule cells, as is shown by most convincing electromicrographs. There is brief reference to the metabolic processes that could be involved in this plastic response.

REFERENCES

Andersen, P., Bliss, T. V. P. and Skrede, K. K. (1971) Lamellar organization of hippocampal pathways. *Exp. Brain Res.*, 13: 222–238.

Bliss, T. V. P. and Lømo, T. (1973) Long-lasting potentiation of synaptic transmission in the dentate area of the anaesthetized rabbit following stimulation of the perforant path. *J. Physiol. (Lond.)*, 232: 331.

Eccles, J. C. (1972) Possible synaptic mechanism subserving learning. In *Brain and Human Behaviour*, A. Karczmar and J. C. Eccles (Eds.), Springer, Heidelberg, pp. 39–61.

Eccles, J. C. (1978) An instruction-selection hypothesis of cerebral learning. In *Cerebral Correlates of Conscious Experience*, P. Buser and A. Buser (Eds.), Elsevier, Amsterdam, pp. 155–175.

Fifková, E. and Van Harreveld, A. (1977) Long-lasting morphological changes in dendritic spines of dentate granule cells following stimulation of the entorhinal area. *J. Neurocytol.*, 6: 211.

Kornhuber, H. H. (1973) Neural control of memory into long term memory: limbic system and amnestic system in man. In *Memory and Transfer of Information*, H. P. Zippel (Ed.), Plenum Press, New York.

Libet, B., Kobayashi, H. and Tanaka, T. (1975) Synaptic coupling into the production and storage of a neuronal memory trace. *Nature (Lond.)*, 258: 155.

Misgeld, U., Sarvey, J. M. and Klee, M. R. (1977) Heterosynaptic post-tetanic potentiation in guinea pig hippocampal slice. *Electroenceph. clin. Neurophysiol.*, 43: 473.

Sarvey, J. M., Misgeld, U. and Klee, M. R. (1978) Long-lasting heterosynaptic post-activation potentiation (PAP) of CA3 neurons in guinea pig hippocampal slice. *Fed. Proc.*, 37: 251.

Factors Influencing Functional Connectivity during Hippocampal Development

PER ANDERSEN

Institute of Neurophysiology, University of Oslo, Oslo (Norway)

The hippocampal formation offers many advantages for the study of functional connectivity between identified cells. The main reasons are the well known structure and function of the participating cells, the lamellar and laminated arrangement of the connecting fibre systems and a large body of histochemical and pharmacological observations.

In the development of the hippocampus, as for other brain areas, there are 3 major developmental problems. (1) Which factors govern the migration of cells from the subependymal layer along the ventricles to their final position and organize the striking arrangement in nearly perfect register? (2) Which factors control the distribution of various axons to their proper target cells, and further to a specific part of the target cells? (3) Finally, how is the correct type of connection ensured? I should like to focus the interest upon the two last questions since certain histological and physiological observations may be pertinent for a discussion of the mechanisms that could be involved.

DISTRIBUTION OF AXONS TO THEIR CORRECT TARGET CELLS

Little seems to be known about the mechanisms that guide the growing axons to their correct receiving neurones. The granule cells migrate in part through clusters of CA3 neurones on their way from the subependymal zone to their final destination. Maybe the close contact when passing through allows the exchange of surface markers like glycoproteins which may guide the subsequent growth of the granule cell axons towards the CA3 neurones? If these mossy fibres grow towards some gradient the tip is probably more sensitive than the rest of the axon, since branching seldom occurs, and a given fibre produces a number of boutons en passage while proceeding towards the end of the CA3 region. The sudden stop at this position suggests a high degree of specificity of the postulated factor setting up the gradient. The giant mossy fibre/CA3 synapses may form even if a substantial fraction of other afferents destined for CA3 cells does not arrive. Thus, LaVail and Wolf (1973) found in tissue explants of neonatal hippocampi that mossy fibres made synapses showing normal morphology with CA3 cells. In this preparation, all commissural, septal and a considerable number of ipsilateral afferents must have been absent. Thus, the mossy fibres seem to find their correct position on correct cells and develop synapses of normal morphology whether or not other afferent systems are present.

DISTRIBUTION OF AXONS TO THE PROPER DENDRITIC AREA

Because most afferent fibres run parallel to each other and to the appropriate cell layer, the question of lamination of afferent axons and segregated synaptic territories is the same. One possible rule would be the temporal sequence of the arriving axons. In its simplest form, this theory seems to be contradicted by observations on the lamination pattern. The lateral and medial entorhinal areas develop simultaneously. However, their termination patterns on the dentate granule cells show definite stratification. If the sequence of arrival of the axons was the only determining factor, a mixture of the two terminal fields would be expected. Further, the CA1 and dentate commissural fibres end intermingled in the same zones as the ipsilateral fibres, although the ipsilateral fibres arrive before the commissural ones, a fact which should have given a stratified arrangement. Likewise, the late arriving mossy fibres acquire their position close to the CA3 soma although other afferent systems have had their axons present for a few days. For re-arrangement of synaptic systems in adult brain the modification of the sequential arrival idea proposed by Gottlieb and Cowan (1972) seems to have many merits. They propose that those axons that may reach a "vacant" synaptic territory first will occupy the area and prevent it from being taken over by other afferents. This theory adequately explains the lack of sprouting of perforant path fibres into the inner third of the granule cell dendritic tree following commissural degeneration. The presence of the ipsilateral fibres in this region will have an advantage being more closely located to the vacant sites than the perforant path fibres, so they prevent the latter from sprouting into this area. However, when the opposite experiment is done, causing degeneration of perforant path fibres, commissural and ipsilateral fibres do sprout into the vacant sites (Cotman et al., 1973; Zimmer, 1973). Both Nafstad (1967), Matthews et al. (1976) and our own studies (Sundberg and Andersen, unpublished observations) have shown that even the most extensive entorhinal lesion leaves at least 15% of the synapses in the dentate molecular layer unchanged. The source of these afferent fibres is unknown, but a subiculum or CA1 origin with fibres traversing the hippocampal fissure is a possibility. These fibres would be excellently suited to sprout and take over the vacant synapses. Why then are the ipsilateral and commissural fibres of the inner third able to sprout and grow into the former perforant path territory? One possibility is that there is a quantitative element in the competition. Maybe the parent fibres

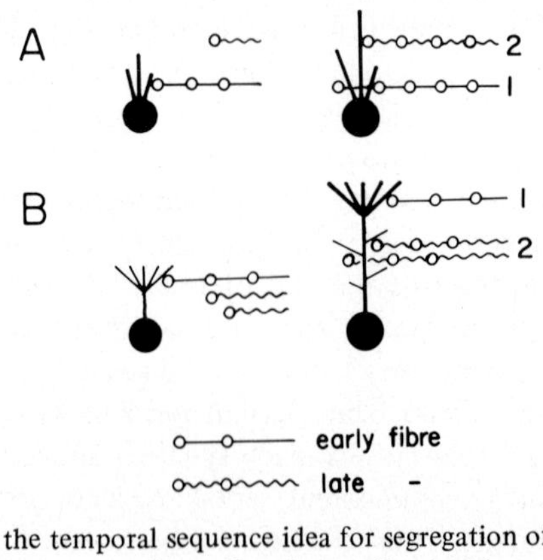

Fig. 1. A: diagram illustrating the temporal sequence idea for segregation of synapses. B: diagram over the modification of this idea. The late-coming fibres (2 and wavy lines) make contact with the rapidly growing apical dendrite and its thin side branches.

of the 15% remaining synapses after entorhinal lesions are too few to prevent sprouting of the commissural and ipsilateral axons. Another possibility is that the proximity factor may be outweighed by the speed of growth of particular fibres. For example, the sprouting is particularly efficient in young animals (Lynch et al., 1973a, b). Fibres from the inner third are able to sprout and fill the entire molecular layer. The proximity idea could still be applicable if the non-perforant path fibres to the molecular layer sprout relatively slowly.

Another interesting proposal to explain the lamination of hippocampal afferent systems was made by Stensaas (1967). The axons may contact postsynaptic sites as these become available within a critical "zone" of dendritic growth (Fig. 1). This would be compatible with the development of both the dentate granules and the stratum radiatum of CA1. In the latter, the molecular layer is relatively large early in maturation (Stensaas, 1967; Purpura and Pappas, 1968; Minkwitz and Holtz, 1975) while the lower part of the stem dendrites (stratum radiatum) develops relatively late. Thus, the temporal sequence of dendritic growth does not need to proceed gradually from the soma, but isolated growth of specific parts of the dendritic tree may attract afferent fibres arriving at that stage. The ability to find the correct dendritic area is not dependent on an arrangement of the target cell in register, and thereby a parallel position of the afferent fibres since both perforant path and commissural fibres make synaptic contact with the appropriate area also in Reeler mouse with their disorientated granule cells (Stanfield et al., 1975; Stirling and Bliss, 1978).

STABILITY OF AFFERENT LAMINATION SYSTEM

A remarkable topographical arrangement in the hippocampal formation is the parallel position of afferent fibres, much like the situation for the parallel fibres in the cerebellum. Not only are the fibres arranged in parallel lamellae nearly transverse to the longitudinal axis of the hippocampal formation (Blackstad et al., 1970; Andersen et al., 1971), but the fibres also run parallel in a plane containing the main dendritic extensions. This means that there is a remarkable tendency for the axons not to cross each others' path but to keep in register. However, many studies have shown that the central nervous system has a capability for rearrangement of fibres when certain parts of the cell are de-afferented (Raisman, 1969; Crain et al., 1973; Lynch et al., 1973a; Steward et al., 1973). The fact that the sharp borders between different termination fields are maintained under normal circumstances suggests that the tendency to sprouting into neighbouring areas is actively suppressed. Maybe the presynaptic axon or the synaptic contact area normally exerts a certain repressive action towards neighbouring fibres and synaptic contacts. This would be similar to the regressive action in muscle innervated by multiple afferent fibres in early development (Kuffler et al., 1977). It also would be compatible with the remarkable constancy of the number of synaptic complexes in the dentate area (Cotman, 1979). We have found the same situation for the synapses in both basal and apical dendritic layers of CA1. If this idea is extended so that the repressive action is stronger towards growing axons from a different source than towards axons from the same source, this could help in explaining the sharp lamination border found in the hippocampal formation both during development (Loy et al., 1977) and in the adult stage (Blackstad, 1956).

TYPES OF SYNAPTIC CONTACTS

Not only do hippocampal axons seek their correct target cell, but different afferent systems have distinct morphological features at their synaptic contacts (Hamlyn, 1963; Laatsch and Cowan, 1967). One possible explanation is that the presynaptic axon somehow programs the development of the postsynaptic structure. This would belong to the cyto-differentiation type of theories (Sperry, 1963). An alternative hypothesis to explain specificity has been proposed by Changeux and coworkers (Changeux and Danchin, 1976). This selective stabilization theory has many interesting features which may be used to explain the synaptic arrangement in the hippocampal formation. The theory implies several factors to control the stabilization of some synapses and the regression of others. These are an anterograde factor issued by the presynaptic fibre and an internal coupling factor produced inside the cell in response to afferent stimulation. Cooperation of these two factors may transform labile receptor proteins to a stable form and concentrate these at the synaptic contact site. Activity of the postsynaptic cell creates a "shut off" factor which stops the protein synthesis of the labile receptor protein. This activity-induced restriction of the postsynaptic structure could be used to restrict the number of synapses to a unit area as discussed above.

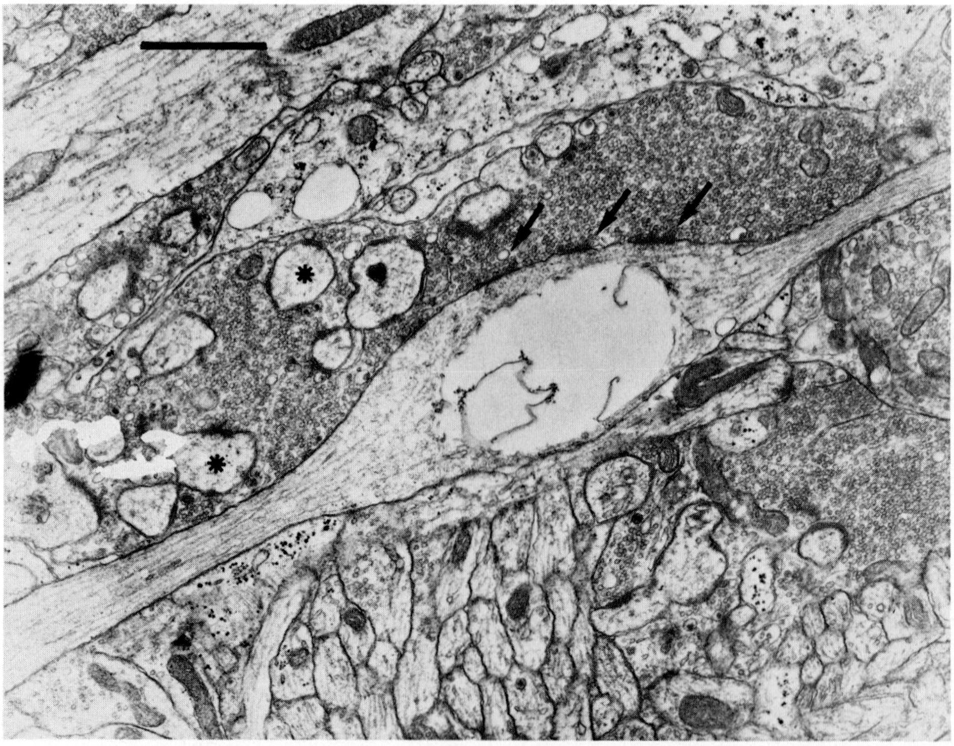

Fig. 2. Electron micrograph showing a mossy fibre making synaptic contacts both with the finger-like protrusions of dendritic spines of a CA3 pyramidal cell (asterisks) and with the beaded dendrite of an interneurone (arrows). The latter was identified by reconstruction from serial sections. Note many dense-core vesicles in the mossy fibre, some in close apposition to active sites. Bar, 1 μm.

If the selective stabilization theory should be used to explain the various morphological and functional forms of different synaptic structures in the hippocampal formation, it has to be expanded to incorporate a specific signal for the development of the postsynaptic site in parallel with the establishment of the synapse. In the developing mossy fibre/CA3 synapse, Bliss et al. (1974) found that the earliest form (2 days) contains few vesicles and very little specialization of the postsynaptic site. At 5 days of age, the structure had better developed synaptic vesicles and postsynaptic density. The synapse now showed signs of transmitter release in the form of extracellular field potentials. At 7 and 10 days of age the synapse approached the normal configuration with a large aggregation of synaptic vesicles and extensive growth of the synaptic site to a giant dendritic spine with finger-like processes invaginating the presynaptic bouton. This synaptic complex is unique for the mossy fibres. The arrangement requires considerably more than the aggregation of a set of correct receptor protein molecules in the membrane opposing the afferent fibre. The signal for the development may be issued by the presynaptic fibre or the program may reside postsynaptically and be triggered by the growing mossy fibre, or the process requires complementary reactions as proposed by Sperry (1963). Some of our own observations may be pertinent on this point. By reconstruction of elements from serial electron micrographs we have found that a single mossy fibre may make contact with both a CA3 giant dendritic spine and with the dendrites of interneurones (Fig. 2). The arrangement is probably serving forward inhibition. On the interneurone, the mossy fibre does not create a special type of ending, but a simple contact. Another feature is the extreme density with which the mossy and other afferent fibres end on the interneuronal dendrites. The surface of this dendrite is to a large extent covered with asymmetric synapses. Thus, the same growing afferent axon engages in widely different postsynaptic structures in functionally and morphologically different cells. Furthermore, the separation of spine-attached synapses, giving rise to a relatively fixed number of synapses per volume tissue, does not apply for the afferents to the interneurones. Here, the postulated repressive action clearly does not operate. The conclusion must be that the presynaptic axon cannot by itself or its anterograde factor prescribe the type or the density of its postsynaptic contacts. However, this discrepancy could be taken care of if different internal coupling factors are produced by the various postsynaptic cells. Furthermore, the type and concentration of the postsynaptic "shut off" factor could vary considerably from the cell. In this context, an adapted form of the specific stabilization theory could be compatible with the observed situation in the mossy fibre synaptic complex. When granule cells degenerate due to X-ray irradiation, normal lamination of the perforant path fibres are still found (Laurberg and Hjorth-Simonsen, 1977). In this case CA3 dendrites are elongated to make contact with these fibres, a connection which does not occur normally. Here, the presynaptic fibre seems essential for synaptic coupling.

Another instance which can teach us something about developmental principles is the distribution and action of interneurones in the hippocampal cortex. Somewhat surprising, interneurones are developed very early, even before the majority of pyramidal cells (Hine and Das, 1974; Minkwitz, 1976). Their migration has been studied both by [^{3}H]thymidine injections (Altman and Das, 1965; Angevine, 1965; Hine and Das, 1974) and by Golgi impregnation (Minkwitz, 1976). Thus, interneurones are present as targets for growing axons before the major dendritic development of the pyramidal cells takes place. Some of the interneurones are probably inhibitory. In neonatal kittens, Purpura et al. (1968) described a paucity of excitatory postsynaptic potentials but well developed hyperpolarizing inhibitory potentials. The afferent fibres could probably drive inhibitory interneurones which in turn produced IPSPs in the pyramidal cells. There is considerable evidence that some of these interneurones contain GABA synthesizing enzymes (Storm-Mathisen and Fonnum, 1971; Barber and Saito, 1976; Ribak et al., 1978), as glutamic acid decarboxylase (GAD).

The immunocytochemical localization of GAD supports the postulate of basket cell mediated inhibition on the pyramidal cell soma (Andersen et al., 1964). Iontophoretically applied GABA suppresses spontaneous and glutamate-induced spikes from hippocampal pyramids (Curtis et al., 1970). Intracellular recording has shown that locally applied GABA close to the soma of hippocampal pyramidal cells causes a large conductance mediated hyperpolarization (Langmoen et al., 1978) (Fig. 3A, B). The hyperpolarization is mediated by chloride ions and has the same equilibrium potential as that of recurrent IPSPs. The response is only found when the iontophoretic electrode is close to the soma of the impaled cell (15–30 μm). In the same cells iontophoretic application of GABA in dendritic territories gave an entirely different response (Fig. 3A, B). This dendritic induced GABA response consists of a depolarization with an intense conductance increase. The depolarization may lead to discharges (Fig. 3C) but at larger GABA doses the conductance increase was so intense that the spike mechanism decoupled and both excitatory and inhibitory synapses were inhibited by a conductance shunt mechanism. This effect of GABA may be mediated by interneurones located in stratum radiatum and moleculare. It would fit with the immunocytochemical distribution of GAD. Recently, Ribak et al. (1978) have shown GAD positive interneurones both in the oriens and in the stratum radiatum. The former could be the basket cells mediating the hyperpolarizing GABA response, while the latter could be the

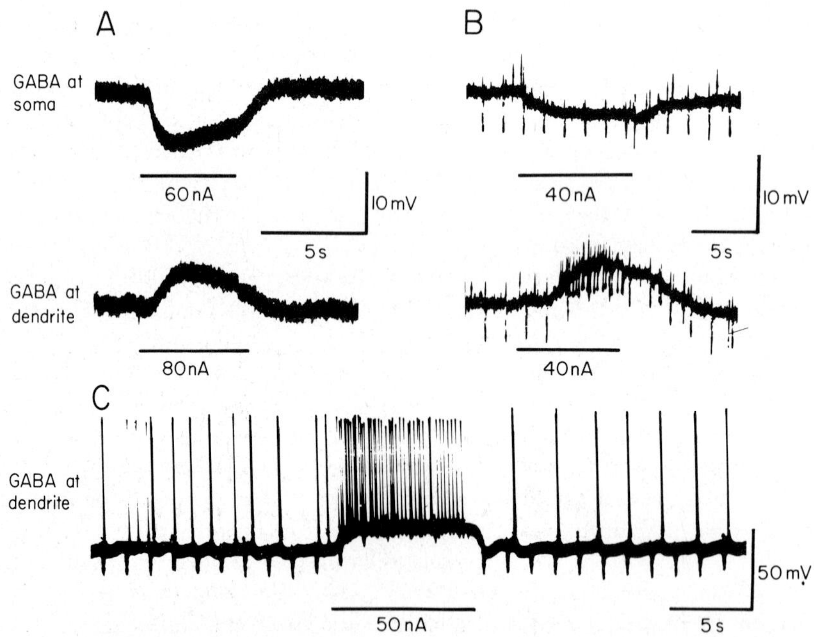

Fig. 3. Two effects of iontophoretically applied GABA to different parts of the surface of a CA1 pyramidal cell. A and B are from two different cells. Upper traces show hyperpolarization and lower traces show depolarizing response following application to soma, and to apical dendritic tree (100 μm somafugally), respectively. Downward strokes in B are hyperpolarizing constant current pulses. C: dendritic GABA application depolarizes CA1 pyramidal cell to give steady discharges.

interneurones responsible for dendritic effect mimicked by GABA application. Thus, cells using the same transmitter may cause widely different postsynaptic effects. The conclusion must be that the signal induced by the transmitter, according to Changeux and Danchin (1976) a good candidate for their anterograde factor, must be able to evoke different receptor proteins or at least receptor ionophore complexes. Again, it appears that the degree of specificity of the factors governing the development of the postsynaptic structure must be higher than that envisaged in theories relying upon activity as a major event in the establishment of a functionally polarized synapse.

A final example of the high degree of specificity required for establishing proper synaptic contacts in the hippocampus is given by experiments by Bjørklund et al. (1976). By removing the entorhinal area, perforant path degeneration was produced. In the trough left by the removal, small groups of amine-containing neurones were transplanted. In a number of cases, the transplants were accepted and sprouted fibres which by fluorescence histochemistry were shown to contain either dopamine, serotonin or norepinephrine. For the two first, the growing fibre copies the direction of the perforant path fibres. Swellings along the axons indicate en passage boutons. Although no proper functional studies have been made as yet, the appearance looks like other amine-containing contacts. The norepinephrine-containing fibres, however, take a different course. They penetrate the whole of the molecular layer to end around cells of the polymorph layer. The original norepinephrine fibres had been removed by chemical destruction. Thus, the vacancy of synaptic site is not a sufficient stimulus to guide growing fibres to the correct position. The norepinephrine fibres seek the same synaptic sites that norepinephrine fibres normally occupy. Thus, it appears that neither the presynaptic axons nor the postsynaptic structures are in themselves sufficient to establish the proper site for regenerating axons. Taken as a sum, although the selective stabilization theory can be used to explain many of the features in normal development of hippocampal connectivity and in regeneration studies, many observations seem to indicate that a complementary chemical specificity is needed of the type envisaged by Sperry in his chemo-affinity theory (1963).

REFERENCES

Altman, J. and Das, G. D. (1965) Autoradiographic and histological evidence of postnatal hippocampal neurogenesis in rats. *J. comp. Neurol.*, 124: 319–336.

Andersen, P., Eccles, J. C. and Løyning, Y. (1964) Location of postsynaptic inhibitory synapses of hippocampal pyramids. *J. Neurophysiol.*, 27: 592–607.

Andersen, P., Bliss, T. V. P. and Skrede, K. K. (1971) Lamellar organization of hippocampal excitatory pathways. *Exp. Brain Res.*, 13: 222–238.

Angevine, Jr., J. B. (1965) Time of neuron origin in the hippocampal region. An autoradiographic study in the mouse. *Exp. Neurol.*, 13 (Suppl. 2): 1–39.

Barber, R. and Saito, K. (1976) Light microscopic visualization of GAD and GABA-T in immunocytochemical preparations of rodent CNS. In *GABA in Nervous System Function, Vol. 5,* E. Roberts, T. N. Chase and D. B. Tower (Eds.), Raven Press, New York, pp. 113–132.

Bjørklund, A., Stenevi, U. and Svendgaard, N.-Aa. (1976) Growth of transplanted monoaminergic neurones into the adult hippocampus along the perforant path. *Nature (Lond.)*, 262: 787–790.

Blackstad, T. W. (1956) Commissural connections of the hippocampal region in the rat, with special reference to their mode of termination. *J. comp. Neurol.*, 105: 417–536.

Blackstad, T. W., Brink, K., Hem, J. and Jeune, B. (1970) Distribution of hippocampal mossy fibers in the rat. An experimental study with silver impregnation methods. *J. comp. Neurol.*, 138: 433–450.

Bliss, T. V. P., Chung, S. H. and Stirling, R. V. (1974) Structural and functional development of the mossy fibre system in the hippocampus of the post-natal rat. *J. Physiol. (Lond.)*, 239: 92P-94P.

Bliss, T. V. P., Chung, S. H. and Stirling, R. V. (1976) Electrophysiological and anatomical observations on the hippocampus of the Reeler mouse. *Exp. Brain Res.*, Suppl. 1: 235–236.

Changeux, J. P. and Danchin, A. (1976) Selective stabilisation of developing synapses as a mechanism for the specification of neuronal networks. *Nature (Lond.)*, 264: 705–712.

Cotman, C. W. (1979) Specificity of synaptic growth in brain: remodeling induced by kainic acid lesions. *This volume.*

Cotman, C., Taylor, D. and Lynch, G. (1973) Ultrastructural changes in synapses in the dentate gyrus of the rat during development. *Brain Res.*, 63: 205–213.

Crain, B., Cotman, C., Taylor, D. and Lynch, G. (1973) A quantitative electron microscopic study of synaptogenesis in the dentate gyrus of the rat. *Brain Res.*, 63: 195–204.

Curtis, D. R., Felix, D. and McLennan, H. (1970) GABA and hippocampal inhibition. *Brit. J. Pharmacol.*, 40: 881–883.

Das, G. D. (1971) Experimental studies on the postnatal development of the brain. I. Cytogenesis and morphogenesis of the accessory fascia dentata following hippocampal lesions. *Brain Res.*, 28: 263–282.

Fricke, R. and Cowan, W. M. (1977) An autoradiographic study of the development of the entorhinal and commissural afferents to the dentate gyrus of the rat. *J. comp. Neurol.*, 173: 231–250.

Gottlieb, D. I. and Cowan, W. M. (1972) Evidence for a temporal factor in the occupation of available synaptic sites during the development of the dentate gyrus. *Brain Res.*, 41: 452–456.

Hamlyn, L. H. (1963) An electron microscope study of pyramidal neurones in the Ammon's horn of the rabbit. *J. Anat. (Lond.)*, 97: 189–201.

Hámori, J. (1973) The inductive role of presynaptic axons in the development of postsynaptic spines. *Brain Res.*, 62: 337–344.

Hine, R. J. and Das, G. D. (1974) Neuroembryogenesis in the hippocampal formation of the rat. An autoradiographic study. *Z. Anat. Entwickl.-Gesch.*, 144: 173–186.

Kuffler, D., Thompson, W. and Jansen, J. K. S. (1977) The elimination of synapses in multiply-innervated skeletal muscle fibres of the rat: dependence on distance between end-plates. *Brain Res.*, 138: 353–358.

Laatsch, R. H. and Cowan, W. M. (1966) Electron microscopic studies of the dentate gyrus of the rat. I. Normal structure with special reference to synaptic organization. *J. comp. Neurol.*, 128: 359–396.

Laatsch, R. H. and Cowan, W. M. (1967) Electron microscopic studies of the dentate gyrus of the rat. II. Degeneration of commissural afferents. *J. comp. Neurol.*, 130: 241–262.

Langmoen, I. A., Andersen, P., Gjerstad, L., Mosfeldt Laursen, A. and Ganes, T. (1978) Two separate effects of GABA on hippocampal pyramidal cells in vitro. *Acta physiol. scand.*, 102: 28A-29A.

Laurberg, S. and Hjorth-Simonsen, A. (1977) Growing central axons deprived of normal target neurones by neonatal X-ray irradiation still terminate in a precisely laminated fashion. *Nature (Lond.)*, 269: 158–160.

LaVail, J. H. and Wolf, M. K. (1973) Postnatal development of the mouse dentate gyrus in organotypic cultures of the hippocampal formation. *Amer. J. Anat.*, 137: 47–66.

Loy, R., Lynch, G. and Cotman, C. W. (1977) Development of afferent lamination in the fascia dentate of the rat. *Brain Res.*, 121: 229–243.

Lynch, G. S., Mosko, S., Parks, T. and Cotman, C. W. (1973a) Relocation and hyperdevelopment of the dentate gyrus commissural system after entorhinal lesions in immature rats. *Brain Res.*, 50: 174–178.

Lynch, G. S., Stanfield, B. and Cotman, C. W. (1973b) Developmental differences in post-lesion axonal growth in the hippocampus. *Brain Res.*, 59: 155–168.

Matthews, D. A., Cotman, C. and Lynch, G. (1976) An electron microscopic study of lesion-induced synaptogenesis in the dentate gyrus of the adult rat. I. Magnitude and time course of degeneration. *Brain Res.*, 115: 1–21.

Minkwitz, H. G. (1976) Zur Entwicklung der Neuronenstruktur des Hippocampus während der prä- und postnatalen Ontogenese der Albinoratte. III. Mitteilung: Morphometrische Erfassung der ontogenetischen Veränderungen in Dendritenstruktur und Spinebesatz an Pyramidenneuronen (CA1) des Hippocampus. *J. Hirnforsch.*, 17: 255–275.

Minkwitz, H. G. und Holtz, L. (1975) Die ontogenetische Entwicklung von Pyramidenneuronen aus dem Hippocampus (CA1) der Ratte. *J. Hirnforsch.*, 16: 37–54.

Nafstad, P. H. J. (1967) An electron microscope study on the termination of the perforant path fibres in the hippocampus and the fascia dentata. *Z. Zellforsch.*, 76: 532–542.

Purpura, D. P. and Pappas, G. D. (1968) Structural characteristics of neurons in the feline hippocampus during postnatal ontogenesis. *Exp. Neurol.*, 22: 379–393.

Purpura, D. P., Prelevic, S. and Santini, M. (1968) Postsynaptic potentials and spike variations in the feline hippocampus during postnatal ontogenesis. *Exp. Neurol.*, 22: 408–422.

Raisman, G. (1969) Neuronal plasticity in the septal nuclei of the adult rat. *Brain Res.*, 14: 25–48.

Ribak, C. E., Vaughn, J. E. and Saito, K. (1978) Immunocytochemical localization of glutamic acid decarboxylase in neuronal somata following colchicine inhibition of axonal transport. *Brain Res.*, 140: 315–332.

Schwartz, I. R., Pappas, G. D. and Purpura, D. P. (1968) Fine structure of neurons and synapses in the feline hippocampus during postnatal ontogenesis. *Exp. Neurol.*, 22: 394–407.

Sperry, R. W. (1963) Chemoaffinity in the orderly growth of nerve fiber patterns and connections. *Proc. nat. Acad. Sci. (Wash.)*, 50: 703–710.

Stanfield, B. B., Caviness, Jr., V. S. and Cowan, W. M. (1975) The organisation of the afferents to the dentate gyrus of the hippocampal formation in the Reeler mutant mouse. *Neuroscience*, 1: 774.

Stensaas, L. J. (1967) The development of hippocampal and dorsolateral pallial regions of the cerebral hemisphere in fetal rabbits. III. Twenty-nine millimeter stage, marginal lamina. *J. comp. Neurol.*, 130: 149–162.

Steward, O., Cotman, C. W. and Lynch, G. S. (1974) Growth of a new fiber projection in the brain of adult rats. Reinnervation of the dentate gyrus by the contralateral entorhinal cortex following ipsilateral entorhinal lesions. *Exp. Brain Res.*, 20: 45–66.

Stirling, R. V. and Bliss, T. V. P. (1978) Observations on the commissural projection of the dentate gyrus in the Reeler mutant mouse. *Brain Res.*, 150: 447–465.

Storm-Mathisen, J. and Fonnum, F. (1971) Quantitative histochemistry of glutamate decarboxylase in the rat hippocampal region. *J. Neurochem.*, 18: 1105–1111.

Zimmer, J. (1973) Extended commissural and ipsilateral projections in postnatally de-entorhinated hippocampus and fascia dentata demonstrated in rats by silver impregnation. *Brain Res.*, 64: 293–311.

Zimmer, J. (1974) Proximity as a factor in the regulation of aberrant axonal growth in postnatally deafferented fascia dentata. *Brain Res.*, 72: 137–142.

On the Possible Role of Adenosine as a Modulatory Messenger in the Hippocampus and other Regions of the CNS

PETER SCHUBERT, MARTIN REDDINGTON and GEORG W. KREUTZBERG

Max-Planck-Institute for Psychiatry, Kraepelinstr. 2, 8000 Munich 40 (G.F.R.)

INTRODUCTION

Complex information processing in the brain can hardly be explained only in terms of nerve cell activation or inhibition mediated at the synapse by the transient and rigidly defined action of excitatory or inhibitory neurotransmitters. There is increasing evidence that the effect of such transmitter substances is also determined by other modulatory agents which interfere directly with transmitter action or which lead to a metabolically linked and longer lasting modification of cell responses. These agents might not only exert their effects on information transfer between neurons but also between neurons, glial cells and the vasculature.

One candidate for such a role as a neuronal signal having multiple targets is adenosine. This nucleoside might modulate the efficiency of synaptic input, could have a long term effect on cell function mediated via its stimulatory effect on the synthesis of cyclic AMP, and could participate in the regulation of local blood flow. In order to test whether such a role could be ascribed to adenosine, the following points were investigated: (1) the intraneuronal transport of adenosine derivatives and their release from neuronal processes; (2) the dependence of release on nerve cell activity; (3) factors determining the effective local extracellular concentration of adenosine; and (4) the action of adenosine on nerve cell function.

INTRANEURONAL TRANSPORT AND RELEASE

For studying the intraneuronal transport and release of adenosine derivatives we applied radioactive adenosine and analyzed its distribution by autoradiography. In fresh tissue more than 90% of applied [^{3}H]adenosine is recovered in a TCA-soluble form, predominantly as nucleotides. After processing for autoradiography, approximately 20% of this TCA-soluble material remains in the tissue and contributes to the autoradiographic labeling.

To study the transport of adenosine derivatives at the single cell level we applied [^{3}H]adenosine iontophoretically into the somas of individual cat spinal motor neurons. Adenosine derivatives were found to be transported into the dendrites by means of a fast transport system reaching the peripheral branches of the dendritic tree. Some of the transported material is released from the dendrites as indicated by the presence of labeled glial cells (Fig. 1; Schubert and Kreutzberg, 1975a). Released material also reaches blood vessels within the extension area of the dendritic tree (Schubert and Kreutzberg, 1976).

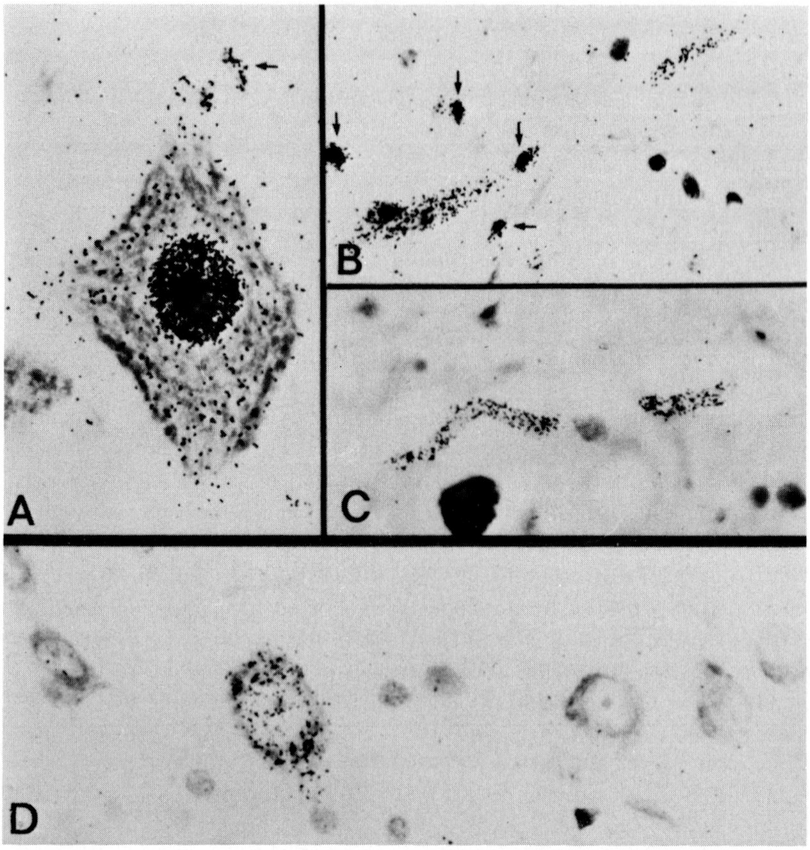

Fig. 1. A-C: transport of [^{3}H]adenosine derivatives in a cat spinal motoneuron after intracellular iontophoresis. A: incorporation in the soma, the site of injection. B: transport in a dendrite. Some of the transported radioactive adenosine derivatives are released as indicated by the presence of labeled glia cells (arrows). C: anterograde axonal transport. There is no obvious release along the axon demonstrable at the single cell level. D: retrograde axonal transport. Selective labeling of motoneurons in the nucleus ambiguus after injection of [^{3}H]adenosine into the cricothyroid muscle of squirrel monkey. Autoradiographs, stained with toluidine blue. Magnif.: A: × 850; B and C: × 550; D: × 400. (A–C: reprinted from Schubert and Kreutzberg, *Brain Res.*, 90 (1975); D: from Schubert and Jürgens, unpublished data.)

Adenosine derivatives are also transported down the axon (Austin et al., 1966; Casola et al., 1969; Rahman and Wolburg, 1971; Autilio-Gambetti et al., 1973; Ingoglia et al., 1973) as shown at the single cell level in Fig. 1C (Schubert and Kreutzberg, 1975a). The transport in axons occurs in both orthograde and retrograde directions (Hunt and Künzle, 1976; Wise and Jones, 1976; Kruger and Sapporta, 1977; Wise et al., 1978; see also Fig. 1D).

The release of adenosine derivatives from axon terminals in the CNS was studied in detail in various afferent projections to the hippocampus. The entorhinal-hippocampus system is particularly suitable for studying transneuronal transfer since the area of afferent fiber termination can be easily identified and distinguished from the cell body layer of the postsynaptic neurons. Axons originating in the entorhinal cortex terminate in well-defined layers on the dendrites of the hippocampal target neurons, i.e. the pyramidal cells and the granule

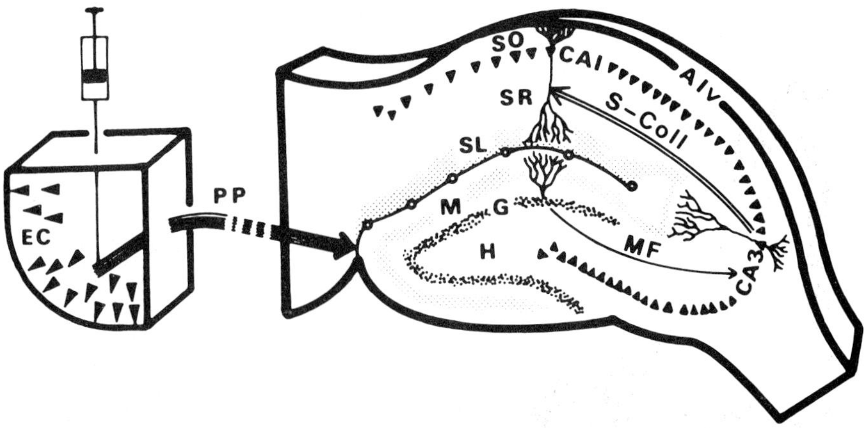

Fig. 2. The entorhino-hippocampal system. The neurons of the medial entorhinal cortex (EC, injection site) send their axons via the perforant pathway (PP) to the hippocampus. They terminate with the shaded area on the dendrites of their target neurons, i.e. in the middle molecular layer (M) on the granule cells (G), and in the stratum lacunosum moleculare (SL) on CA1 and CA3 pyramidal cells. The axons of the granule cells (MF) terminate exclusively on CA3 neurons which in turn are connected via the Schaffer collaterals (S-Coll) with the dendrites of CA1 neurons. H, hilus; SR, stratum radiatum; SO, stratum oriens; Alv, alveus.

cells of the dentate gyrus (Fig. 2). These are the areas found to be labeled when, as a control experiment, [^{3}H]leucine is injected into the entorhinal cortex (Fig. 3A). After injection of [^{3}H]adenosine, labeling is again found in the hippocampal terminal areas as a result of axonal transport but, in addition selective labeling appears in the somal layer of the postsynaptic neurons (Schubert et al., 1976, 1977; Fig. 3B). Since the axons of the granule cells terminate exclusively within the hippocampus on CA3 neurons and do not project back to the entorhinal cortex (the site of injection) their labeling cannot be the result of retrograde transport. The observed pattern of labeling strongly indicates that transported adenosine derivatives are released from the entorhinal axon terminals, taken up by the granule cell dendrites and accumulate in their somas. Labeling of different intensities, which appears to be proportional to the density of afferent termination, is also found in the somal layers of the other hippocampal target neurons, again indicating transfer (Fig. 3C).

Release of adenosine derivatives from axon terminals has been shown to occur in several systems in the CNS, i.e. the cortico-thalamic projection in the rabbit (Schubert and Kreutzberg, 1974, 1975b), the retino-tectal and tecto-thalamic fibers of the pigeon (Hunt and Künzle, 1976) and pathways originating in the somatosensory cortex as well as in thalamocortical pathways of the rat (Wise and Jones, 1976; Wise et al., 1978). This raises the question as to whether they are released together with the principal transmitters in the CNS, as has been shown to occur in peripheral monoaminergic and cholinergic nerves (e.g. Geffen and Livett, 1971; Silinsky and Hubbard, 1973; Burnstock, 1976). We therefore looked for the release of adenosine derivatives from septal fibers which project to the dentate gyrus (Raisman, 1966) and which have been convincingly shown to be cholinergic (Storm-Mathisen and Blackstad, 1964; Stumpf, 1965; Lynch et al., 1972; Bird and Aghajanian, 1975). Septal fibers are thought to terminate primarily, not on the granule cells themselves, but on interneurons (Mosko et al., 1973) originally described by Ramón y Cajal (1911). This suggestion is supported by our results. Following injection of adenosine into the septum an extremely

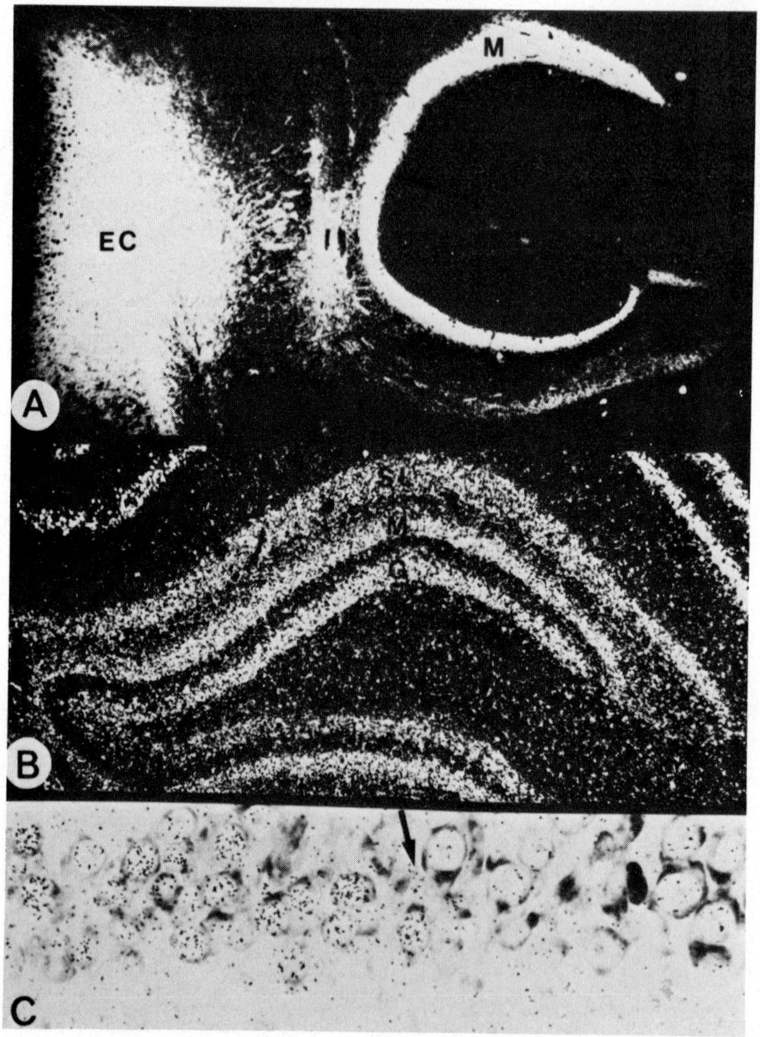

Fig. 3. Transfer of adenosine derivatives in the entorhino-hippocampal system (for orientation see Fig. 2). A: control experiment; 24 hr after [^{3}H]leucine injection into EC there is a transport of radioactive proteins into the axon terminals (M) in the dentate gyrus, but no label in the granule cells. Autoradiograph of a horizontal section, dark-field illumination, magnif.: × 30. B: 24 hr after [^{3}H]adenosine injection into EC, labeling is seen again in M, but in addition in G, indicating a release from the entorhinal axon terminals to granule cells. Also the terminal area (SL) of afferents to the CA1 and CA3 pyramidal cells are densely labeled. Autoradiograph of a cross-section, dark-field illumination, magnif.: × 70. C: in the pyramidal cell layer, CA1 neurons show a high grain density which decreases abruptly at the border to CA3 (arrow). This points to a selective transfer to CA1 neurons. For a possible explanation see Fig. 7. Autoradiograph, magnif.: × 500. (Reprinted from Schubert et al., *Brain Res.*, 147 (1977).)

high intensity of labeling is seen in individual neurons in the dentate gyrus which correspond in size and location to such interneurons (Rose and Schubert, 1977). This indicates that the release of adenosine derivatives from axon terminals can occur in addition to the principal transmitter and may be a general phenomenon at central synapses (Fig. 4).

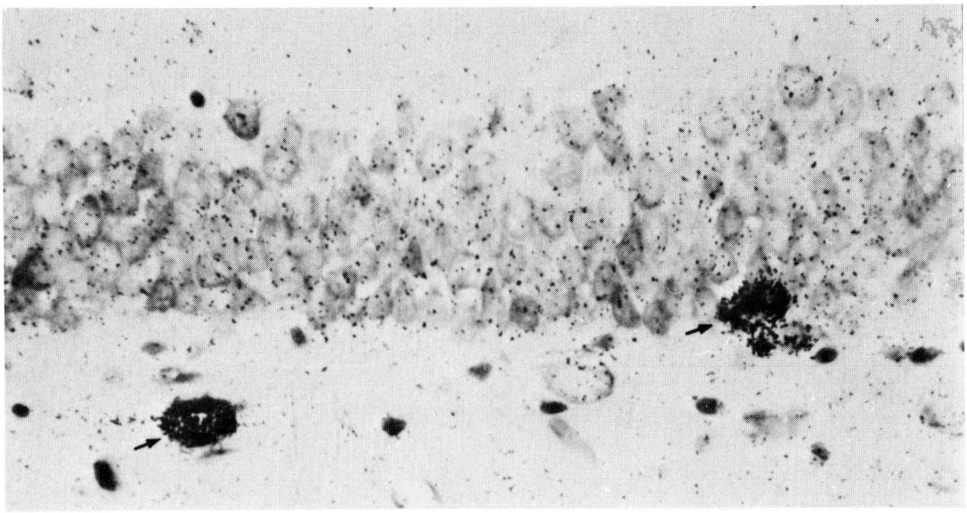

Fig. 4. Transfer of adenosine derivatives from septal afferents to single neurons in the dentate gyrus. These heavily labeled nerve cells (arrows), located in the hilus below the granule cell layer, are probably interneurons. Autoradiograph, stained with toluidine blue, magnif.: × 600. (Reprinted from Rose and Schubert, *Brain Res.*, 121 (1977).)

DEPENDENCE OF RELEASE FROM NERVE TERMINALS ON NERVE CELL ACTIVITY

An electrical stimulation-dependent release of adenosine derivatives was first demonstrated in vitro from brain slices by Pull and McIlwain (1972). In addition, following local application of [^{3}H]adenosine to brain cortex, release of labeled material could be demonstrated from that area on electrical field stimulation in vivo (Sulakhe and Phillis, 1975). In order to identify the axon terminals as structures from which release occurs during nerve cell activation we studied the effect of an electrophysiologically controlled synaptic stimulation on the release of adenosine derivatives after axonal transport. [^{3}H]Adenosine was injected in the entorhinal cortex of the rat. Using recordings of the extracellular field potentials as a guide, a stimulation electrode was inserted into a position in the injection site where it optimally activated the perforant pathway fibers (see Fig. 2). Mild stimulation (approx. 8 Hz) was applied for about 18 hr in the awake animal. Then the amount of radioactive TCA-soluble material recovered from the microdissected pre- and postsynaptic areas of the hippocampal dentate gyrus was measured by scintillation counting. Stimulation was found to increase the release and transfer from axon terminals to the postsynaptic granule cells by about 40% as compared to sham operated but unstimulated controls (Schubert et al., 1976). This demonstrates that the release of adenosine derivatives from axon terminals is related to nerve cell activity in vivo. Investigations with nerve ending preparations from brain in vitro, where field stimulation (100 pulses) of synaptosome beds led to a significant diminution of their adenine nucleotide content (Barberis and McIlwain, 1976), indicate that the axon terminals are a major site of release.

FACTORS DETERMINING THE EXTRACELLULAR CONCENTRATION OF ADENOSINE

The proposed function of adenosine as a molecular signal requires strict control of its effective concentration in the extracellular space. One controlling factor is obviously represented by the blood-brain barrier which is relatively impermeable to adenosine derivatives (Berne et al., 1974). This protects the nerve cell environment from fluctuations in levels of blood adenine nucleotides and makes the brain a virtually closed system in which the extracellular adenosine derivatives concentration is determined by intracerebral factors. One such factor is the activity-related release as described above. The question then arises as to the nature of the adenosine derivative released. Analysis of the material transported into the target area, e.g. from the entorhinal cortex to the hippocampus, shows that more than 94% was TCA-soluble. Nucleotides as well as nucleosides could be detected by thin-layer chromatography. However, the rapid interconversion of nucleosides and nucleotides and the rapid incorporation into RNA precludes identification of the actual substances released. Experiments designed to test specifically for the nature of the released material strongly indicate the release mainly of nucleotides. Thus, Barberis and McIlwain (1976) demonstrated 5′-AMP to be the most prominent adenosine derivative occurring in perfusates of cerebral synaptosomes and argued that it may be derived extracellularly from released ATP. The release of ATP has been directly shown from cerebral synaptosomes (White, 1978), from the electric organ of *Torpedo* (Zimmermann and Whittaker, 1974; Zimmermann, 1978) and from chromaffin granules (Douglas and Poisner, 1966; Smith and Winkler, 1972; Winkler, 1977). Further, it has been shown that extracellularly applied nucleotides are rapidly broken down to adenosine (Pull and McIlwain, 1977). A cascade of enzymatic degradations must therefore be present for the extracellular production of adenosine. This is a prerequisite for the formation of a membrane-permeable nucleoside which is necessary to explain the phenomenon of post-neuronal transfer.

The fine structural localization of the enzymes necessary for nucleotide degradation is currently under investigation. ATPase activity is found to be associated with both nerve and glial plasma membranes. 5′-Nucleotidase, the key enzyme catalyzing the final conversion of 5′-AMP to adenosine, is found, not on nerve cell membranes, but associated with glial plasma membranes. The presence of enzyme-bearing glial processes will therefore be an important factor in controlling the extracellular production of adenosine. High activity of 5′-nucleotidase can be found, for instance, on the plasma membranes of astrocytic processes engulfing synaptic complexes and on perivascular astrocytic footplates (Fig. 5; Kreutzberg et al., 1978). By changing the number or location of the glial carriers of 5′-nucleotidase, e.g. under pathological conditions, the site or extent of adenosine production could be modified according to functional demand (Kreutzberg and Barron, 1978).

The distribution of the adenosine-producing enzyme will also determine the sites where nucleotides can be converted into a membrane-permeable form for retrieval from the extracellular space. Uptake of adenosine occurs into pre- and postsynaptic neuronal elements as demonstrated by the retrograde transport and transneuronal transfer of adenosine derivatives

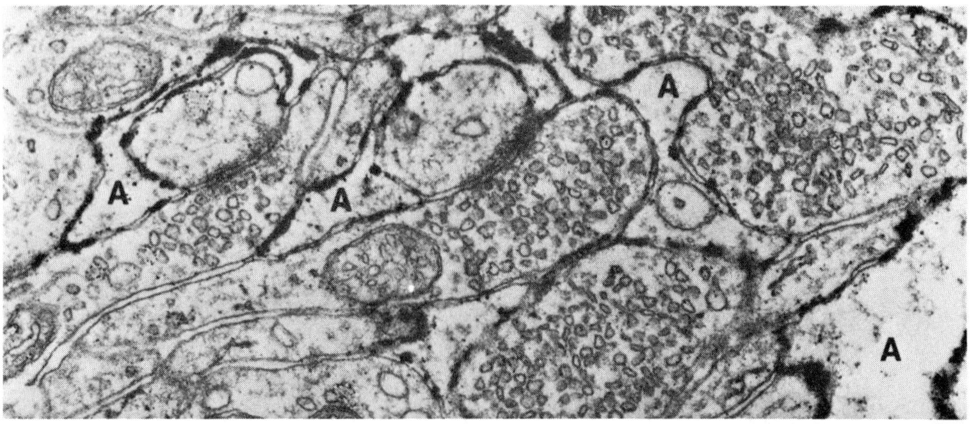

Fig. 5. 5′-Nucleotidase activity is demonstrated cytochemically by its hydrolysis of AMP. Black deposits of the reaction product are seen on the plasma membranes of astrocytic processes (A) as they cover axodendritic synapses. Rat, cerebellum, magnif.: × 4000. (Reprinted from Kreutzberg et al., *Brain Res.*, 158 (1978).)

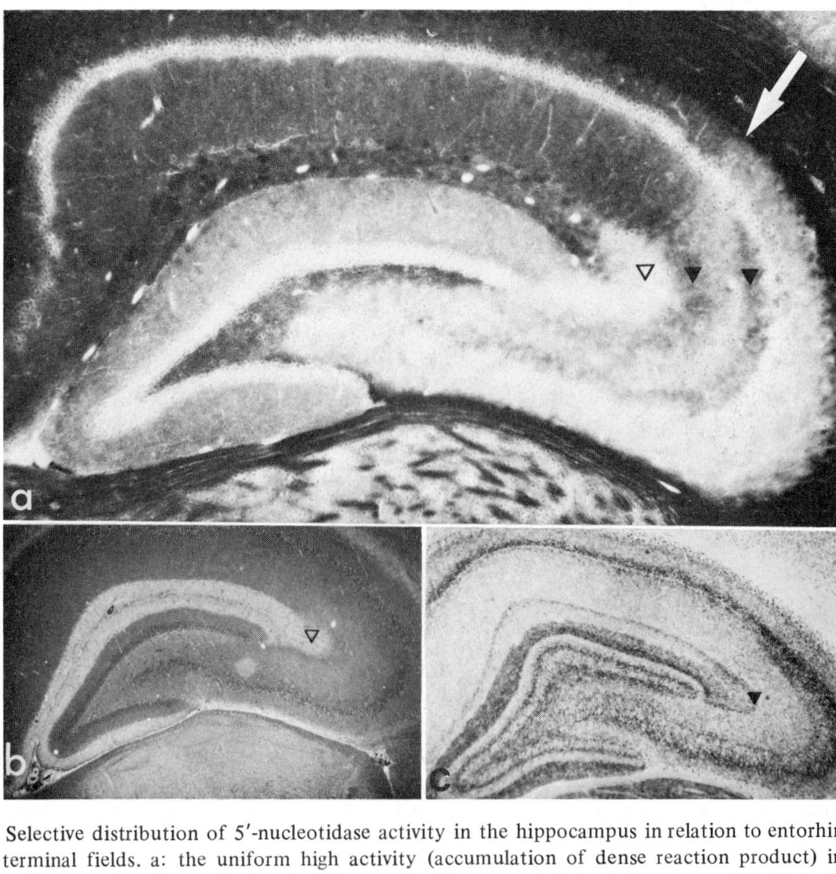

Fig. 6. Selective distribution of 5′-nucleotidase activity in the hippocampus in relation to entorhinal and septal terminal fields. a: the uniform high activity (accumulation of dense reaction product) in regio superior changes abruptly at the border (large arrow) to regio inferior. Here, a positive histochemical reaction is seen near the soma layer (▲) and in the U-shaped lamina where septal fibers terminate (▲, see also c). The entorhinal terminal field of CA3 (▽, see also b) shows no reaction product. Magnif., × 40. b: entorhinal terminal fields. 7 days after lesioning the medial and lateral entorhinal cortex, degenerating terminals were marked by silver impregnation. They appear light in the dark-field photography. Magnif., × 18. c: septal terminal fields are marked by the acetylcholine esterase activity (dark reaction product). Magnif., × 18. (Reprinted from Schubert et al., *Brain Res.* (1979).)

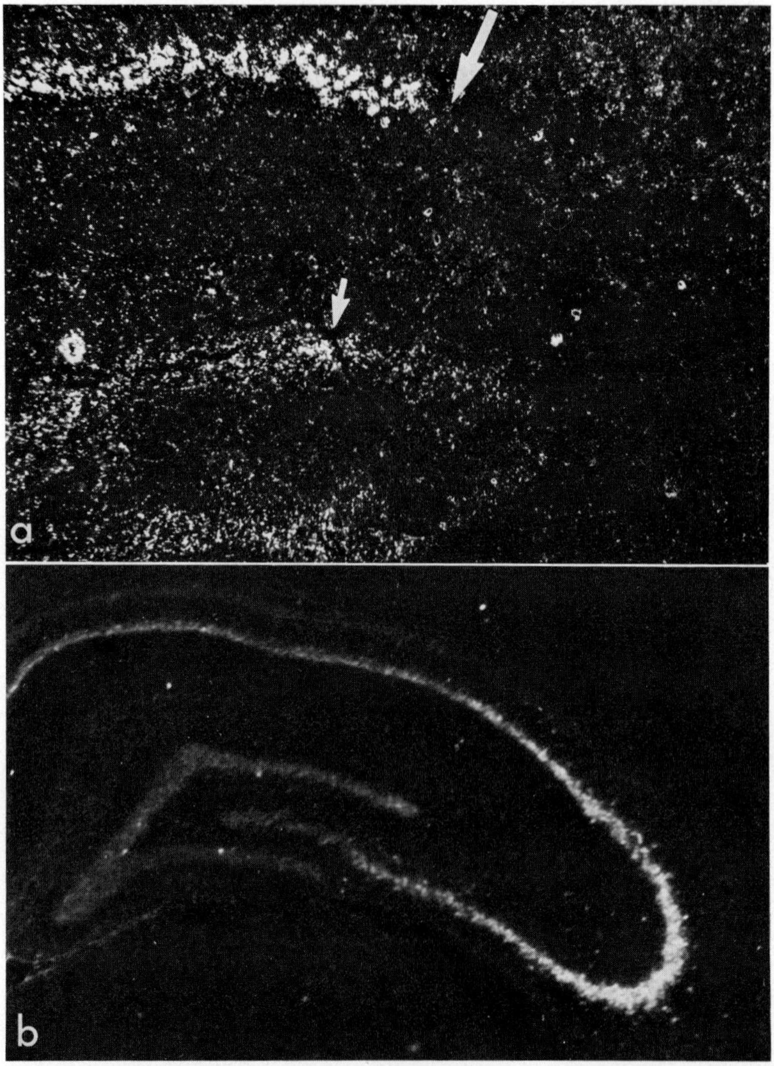

Fig. 7. a: 2 days after injection of [^{3}H]adenosine into the medial entorhinal cortex, silver grains are accumulated in the ring-like terminal field of the entorhinal afferents to CA3 neurons (small arrow). But in the somal layer of pyramidal neurons, dense labeling is only seen in the CA1 neurons breaking off abruptly at the border to regio inferior (large arrow). In the somal layer of CA3 neurons, grain density is even less than in the neighboring neuropil. Autoradiography, dark-field illumination. Magnif., × 120. b: 2 days after injection of [^{3}H]adenosine into the septum, the somal cell layer of CA3 neurons shows a dense labeling which is even more pronounced than in CA1 neurons and granule cells. Autoradiography, dark-field illumination. Magnif., × 30. (Reprinted from Schubert et al., *Brain Res.* (1979).)

(see above, Figs. 1, 3). It also occurs into glial cells as shown for material released from nerve terminals and dendrites (see Fig. 1B). Along the dendrites of a [^{3}H]adenosine-injected neuron, glial cells showed differences in labeling. It is likely that the labeled cells extend their processes to sites of nucleotide release and also carry the 5′-nucleotidase. Thus they are probably prominent elements in the retrieval of adenosine from the extracellular space. Such a recycling mechanism may be used for economic reasons to conserve substances requiring a complicated pathway of de novo synthesis. A retrieval process and/or enzymatic breakdown to a biologically inactive substance (adenosine deaminase action) must also be postulated to terminate the action of adenosine as a modulatory signal.

Of particular interest is the finding that the adenosine-producing enzyme, 5′-nucleotidase, shows striking differences in concentration in various brain regions, for example between closely neighboring areas in the hippocampus (Fig. 6). Here, transfer of adenosine derivatives was shown to be related to the topography of enzyme activity (Schubert et al., 1979). In regio superior, where the enzyme activity is high in all laminae, transfer to CA1 neurons occurs from both the entorhinal and septal afferents. In regio inferior, transneuronal labeling of CA3 neurons occurs only after septal but not entorhinal injection, most probably because 5′-nucleotidase is present in the septal terminal laminae but not in the entorhinal terminal laminae of CA3 (Fig. 7). Therefore, the specifically distributed 5′-nucleotidase seems to determine whether and where adenosine is produced as a consequence of an activity-related release of ATP from axon terminals. Thus, if ATP is released from nerve terminals in a region lacking 5′-nucleotidase it will have to diffuse in the extracellular space for some distance to meet enzyme-carrying structures at which adenosine can be produced. In this case adenosine formation will be extended both in time and space. On the other hand, if ATP can be broken down immediately near the site of release, adenosine could hit the target cells sooner, more precisely, and at a higher concentration.

POSSIBLE ACTIONS OF ADENOSINE

Adenosine has been described to have a vasodilatatory effect on cerebral blood vessels similar to its well-known action on the coronary vessels of the heart (Berne et al., 1974, 1976). Vasodilatation is thought to be mediated by Ca^{2+} affecting the contractile elements of the vascular cells (see Betz, 1976). By releasing nucleotides from neurons and the glia-controlled extracellular production of adenosine, vascular function and blood flow might thus be regulated in relation to local demand (Schubert and Kreutzberg, 1976). The regulation of local blood flow according to nerve cell function is indicated by a number of clinical and experimental observations (Ingvar, 1973; Kato et al., 1974).

One of the first effects of adenosine to be reported in the nervous system was its potent effect on cyclic AMP synthesis (Sattin and Rall, 1970). This has subsequently been shown to be due to a direct effect of adenosine on extracellular receptors coupled to adenyl cyclase, and not simply to an increase in the ATP pool available for cyclic AMP production. Thus, 2-chloroadenosine is also a powerful stimulator of cyclic AMP accumulation in brain slices although it is unable to serve as a precursor in cyclic AMP synthesis (Sturgill et al., 1975). Further, stimulation of cyclic AMP accumulation by adenosine is potentiated when the uptake of adenosine into the intracellular compartment is blocked (Huang and Daly, 1974). More recently, adenosine or 2-chloroadenosine have been shown to stimulate adenyl cyclase directly in homogenates of various brain regions (Fredholm, 1977; Prémont et al., 1977). In these studies, as well as in earlier investigations using brain slices (Huang et al., 1972), theophylline was shown to antagonize adenosine-stimulated cyclic AMP synthesis.

An interesting property of the adenosine-stimulated production of cyclic AMP in brain slices is its synergistic interaction with biogenic amine-stimulated adenyl cyclase systems (Sattin and Rall, 1970; Schultz and Daly, 1973; Mah and Daly, 1976). This observation could have important implications when considering possible functional effects of adenosine. Thus, a specific metabolic effect which is dependent on a particularly high level of cyclic AMP could be achieved only if both adenosine and biogenic amines act together. Cyclic AMP produced in response to adenosine could mediate a number of events, particularly the long term and metabolically linked modulation of cell function. Such effects are well known to be exerted by neurons and are commonly referred to as trophic effects.

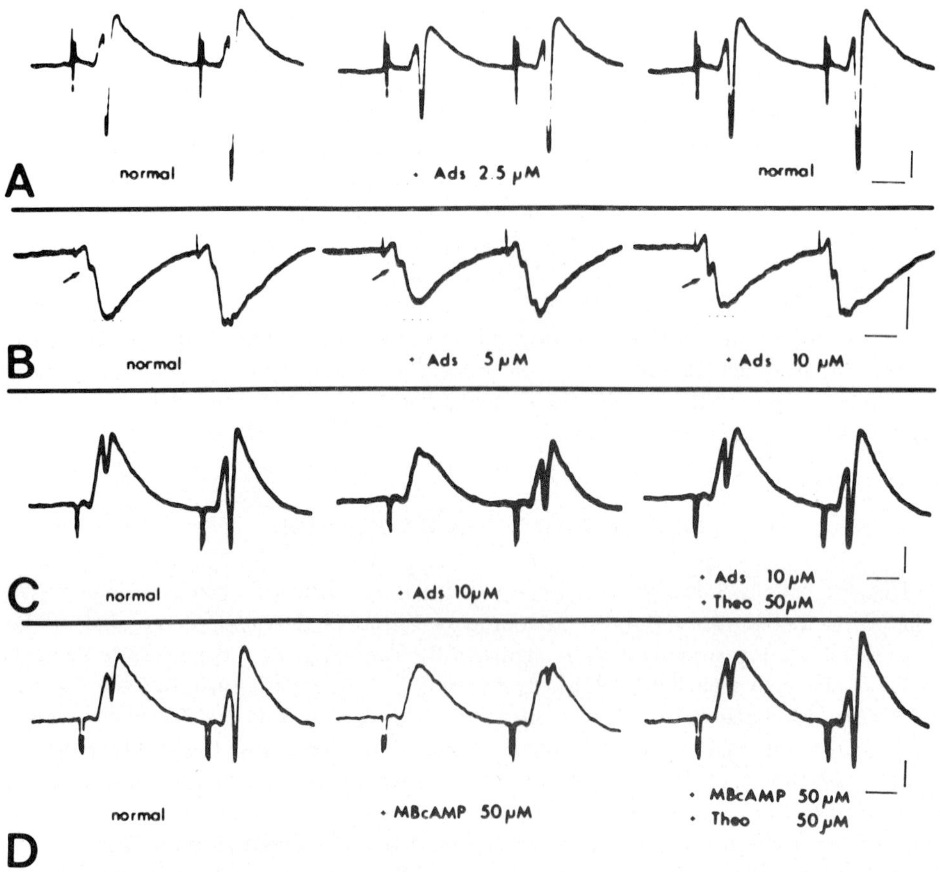

Fig. 8. Effect of micromolar concentrations of adenosine on evoked potentials recorded extracellularly from hippocampal CA1 neurons. Each trace gives the responses to two stimuli which were applied with a short interval to the afferent radiatum fibers and resulted in frequency potentiation. Horizontal scale: 5 msec, vertical scale: 1 mV. Recordings were taken 15 min after starting superfusion of the indicated medium. A: concentration-dependent depression of the population spikes. B: depression of the dendritic potentials (extracellular EPSPs) by 15–20% is seen in the presence of 5 μM adenosine under constant input conditions (unchanged fiber potentials, arrows). The depressive effect of 10 μM adenosine is not completely overcome when considerably increasing the strength of the afferent input (60% increased fiber potential). C and D: the depressive effect of both adenosine and monobutyryl-cAMP (MBcAMP) is antagonized by theophylline.

The most prominent action of adenosine on nerve cell function which is accessible to electrophysiological investigation is its depressive effect on nerve cell activity. Thus, iontophoretically applied adenosine has been shown to depress spontaneous nerve cell activity in various areas of the brain including the hippocampus (Phillis, 1977). Adenosine was also reported to depress evoked potentials elicited in slice preparations of olfactory cortex (Okada and Kuroda, 1975; Kuroda et al., 1976). The critical question when evaluating such effects is whether they can be elicited at concentrations expected to be in the physiological range. Although direct measurements of extracellular adenosine concentrations are lacking, the amount of adenosine in cerebral tissue is reported to be 0.6% of the total adenine nucleotide content (Pull and McIlwain, 1972), i.e. an overall concentration of adenosine of around 10 μM can be expected. We therefore investigated the effects of micromolar concentrations of adenosine on evoked responses in a hippocampal slice preparation (Schubert and Mitzdorf, 1979).

On stimulation of the afferent fibers in the stratum radiatum (see also Fig. 2), the responses evoked in the CA1 target neurons were recorded extracellularly via two recording electrodes, one located in the soma and the other in the dendritic region where the stimulated afferent fibers terminate. The nature of the recorded extracellular responses has been analyzed and described by Andersen's group (see Andersen, 1975). The negative deflexion recorded from the dendritic region (referred to as "dendritic potential") is thought to represent the evoked postsynaptic potential (extracellular EPSP). The "population spike" recorded from the soma layer gives information about how many neurons reach the threshold required to produce an action potential as a result of afferent stimulation. The sizes of the "dendritic potential" and the population spike can be used as a measure of the efficiency of afferent stimulation. Both were found to be depressed in a concentration-dependent manner by 2.5–10 μM adenosine added to the medium with which the slices were constantly superfused (Fig. 8). By controlling for the size of the fiber potential which precedes the dendritic potential and which can be taken as a measure for the strength of afferent input (see Andersen et al., 1977), input-output curves were constructed. They showed that at a given afferent input the dendritic potential (extracellular EPSP) was significantly reduced in the presence of adenosine, suggesting a direct effect of the nucleoside on synaptic transmission (Fig. 8B).

Further information about the site of adenosine action was sought from a current source density analysis (Schubert and Mitzdorf, 1979). This technique gives rather precise information about the size and local distribution of current fluxes which flow into and out of the neuron during activation. The inward currents generated by the transmitter-mediated ion fluxes in the synaptic region, i.e. the synaptic currents, can be clearly identified and were found to be depressed in the presence of adenosine. They reappeared during subsequent superfusion with medium lacking adenosine (Fig. 9). These results also suggest that adenosine reduces the efficiency of a given synaptic input by interfering with the mechanism of synaptic transmission.

The depressive effect of adenosine is abolished if it is superfused together with adenosine deaminase, which converts adenosine to the obviously biologically inactive inosine. Moreover, the depressive action of 5′-AMP on spontaneous nerve cell activity as described by Phillis (1977) seems to depend on prior breakdown to adenosine since the response is abolished by adenosine deaminase and since non-hydrolyzable methyl-substituted AMP is without effect. This indicates that depression of the efficiency of synaptic input is a result of the direct action of adenosine.

Theophilline antagonizes the depressive effect of adenosine on hippocampal neurons (Fig. 8C) as well as blocking the stimulation of cyclic AMP synthesis by adenosine. This

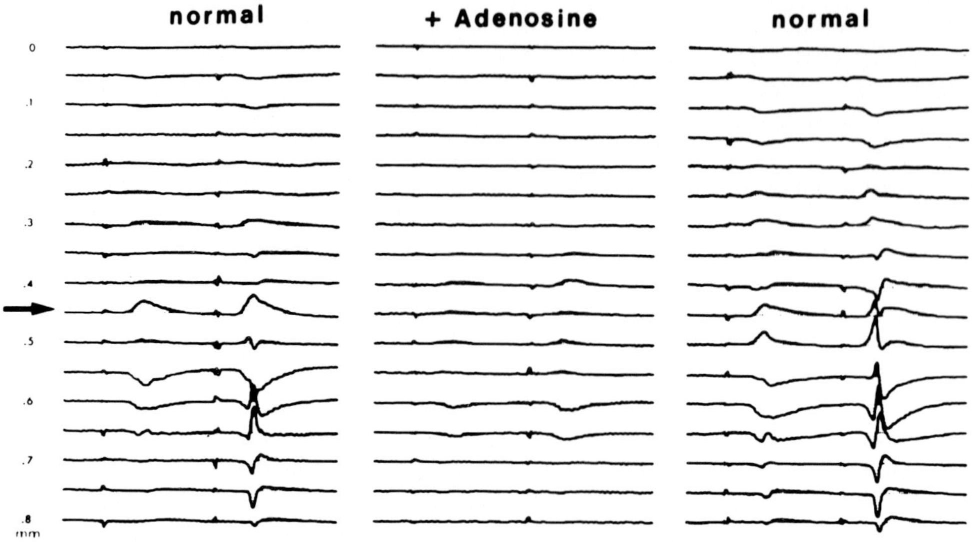

Fig. 9. Current density analysis during synaptic activation of CA1 neurons via paired-pulse stimulation of radiatum afferents. The currents were computed at different levels along the extension of CA1 neurons in steps of 50 μm, from the peripheral apical dendrites (at 0 mm) to the soma region (at 0.6 mm) and further to the peripheral basal dendrites (at 0.8 mm). The area where the stimulated afferent radiatum fibers terminate on the CA1 dendrites is marked by an arrow. Here, a synaptic inward current is generated as indicated by an upward deflection (downward deflection represents outward current). In the presence of 10 μM adenosine these synaptic currents are markedly depressed. They reappear during superfusion of normal medium.

might be taken to indicate a similarity between the adenosine receptors mediating these biochemical and electrophysiological responses. Monobutyryl cyclic AMP, a stable cyclic nucleotide derivative which directly activates protein kinase activity, also depresses evoked potentials (Fig. 8D). This is consistent with a cyclic AMP-mediated mechanism of adenosine action. Surprisingly, however, theophylline also abolished the effect of monobutyryl cyclic AMP, indicating an action of theophylline at a site other than interfering with the adenosine-mediated cyclic AMP increase (Fig. 8D; Reddington and Schubert, 1979). Therefore, the parallelism between the effects of theophylline on the biochemical and electrophysiological parameters cannot be used as an argument for a cyclic AMP-mediated mechanism. Nevertheless, if this were indeed the case, it would be expected that the adenosine receptors mediating the increase in cyclic AMP content and the physiological response would exhibit identical properties with respect to the relative affinities towards adenosine receptor agonists. However, this proved not to be the case. Half maximal inhibition of the population spike was obtained with approximately 5 μM adenosine or 0.1 μM 2-chloroadenosine, i.e. with an EC_{50} ratio of 50:1. On the other hand, a ratio of only 2:1 was obtained for the concentrations of adenosine and 2-chloroadenosine required to half-maximally stimulate cyclic AMP accumulation under identical conditions. In this case the EC_{50} values were 28 μM and 12 μM for adenosine and 2-chloroadenosine respectively (Reddington and Schubert, 1979). These results raise the possibility of multiple receptor sites having different relative affinities for these two ligands and cast doubt on the existence of a direct relationship between cyclic AMP production and the depression of synaptic activity in hippocampus slices.

Although it would be premature to rule out the participation of a cyclic AMP-mediated mechanism in evoked potential suppression, alternative explanations must clearly be considered. Thus, monobutyryl cyclic AMP might in this case exert its inhibitory effect by a secondary action such as changing intracellular free calcium concentration; this possibility has been discussed in some detail by Phillis (1977). A modulatory effect on transmembrane Ca^{2+} fluxes would appear therefore to be an attractive mechanism also for the electrophysiologically observed effects of adenosine. The feasibility of such a mechanism is shown by the results of Schrader et al. (1975) who demonstrated that adenosine suppresses calcium-mediated slow action potentials in heart muscle cells. In nerve tissue, by using Ca^{2+}-sensitive electrodes, Ten Bruggencate et al. (1977) found that the stimulation-induced drop in extracellular Ca^{2+} concentration is decreased in the presence of adenosine. These data suggest that adenosine suppresses Ca^{2+} influx into intracellular compartments. Such a depression of Ca^{2+} flux, if occurring presynaptically, could result in a reduction in transmitter release. This is indeed shown from studies in peripheral monoaminergic (Hedqvist and Fredholm, 1976; Clanachan et al., 1977) and cholinergic (Sawynok and Jhamandas, 1976; Vizi and Knoll, 1976; Israel and Meunier, 1977) nerves which demonstrate a reduction of transmitter release in the presence of adenosine or ATP.

SUMMARY AND CONCLUSION

A schematic summary of the reported data and the suggested row of events concerning the action of adenosine as a modulatory signal is given in Fig. 10. Adenosine derivatives,

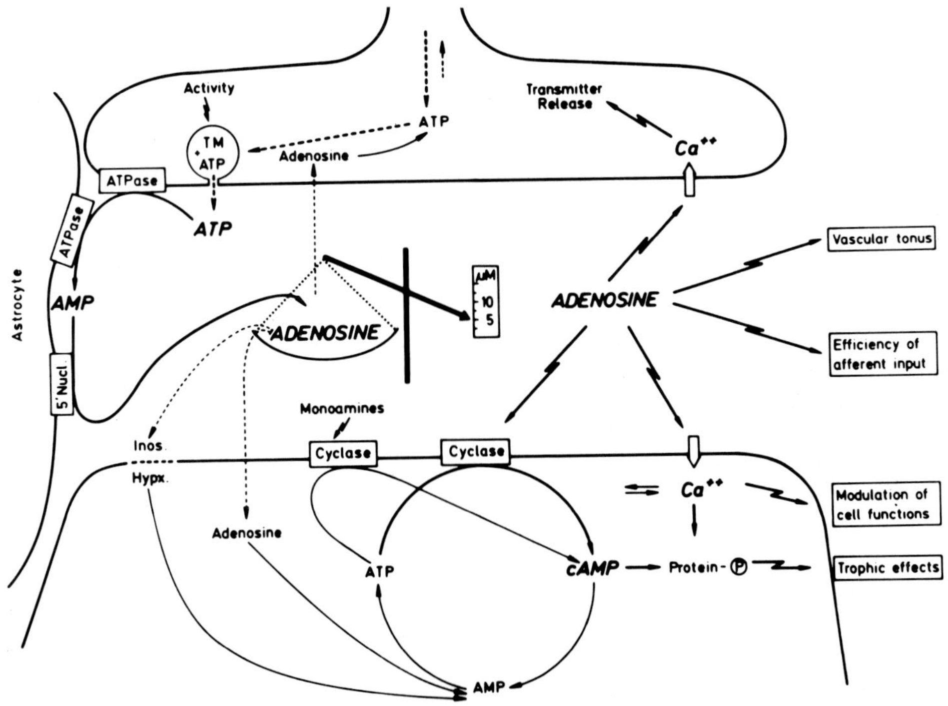

Fig. 10. Row of events involved in the suggested modulatory actions of adenosine in the CNS (see Summary and Conclusions).

probably in the form of nucleotides, are transported in axons and dendrites and are released from both nerve cell processes. The release from axon terminals appears to be a general phenomenon. It is related to nerve cell activity and probably occurs in the form of ATP together with the principle transmitter from synaptic vesicles. ATP is broken down in the extracellular space by a cascade of enzyme reactions resulting in adenosine. The key enzyme in adenosine production is 5′-nucleotidase which is associated with glia plasma membranes and shows striking differences in activity in various brain regions.

Thus, the local extracellular level of adenosine is obviously controlled by the interaction of two factors, i.e. the activity-related neuronal release of ATP and its subsequent enzymatic breakdown. The latter prescribes in a topographically specific manner the range within which the local adenosine concentration can be varied according to nerve cell activity.

This represents a novel principle concerning how a neuronal messenger is brought into action. In contrast to a classical transmitter, adenosine is probably a neuronal messenger, common to all nerve cells, but which is released in an inactive form. The translation of its message into a modulatory effect on target cell function is encoded in the environment and may thus be related to the particular local demands.

Adenosine could exert a number of effects in various target cells. It depresses evoked potentials at the expected average physiological concentration. Variations of its extracellular level lead to an enhancement or attenuation of its depressive action. Therefore, controlling the local extracellular adenosine concentration as described above, might be a mechanism of determining and modulating the efficiency of synaptic input in that region.

The powerful effect of adenosine on cyclic AMP synthesis suggests that adenosine could also influence cell metabolism and thus have a long term modulatory effect on cell function such as mediating trophic effects of neurons. Further, it may be involved in the regulation of local blood flow and vascular function.

REFERENCES

Andersen, P. (1975) Organization of hippocampal neurons and their interconnections. In *The Hippocampus, Vol. I,* R. L. Isaacson and K. H. Pribram (Eds.), Plenum Press, New York, pp. 155–175.

Andersen, P., Sundberg, S. H., Sveen, D. and Wigström, H. (1977) Specific long-lasting potentiation of synaptic transmission in hippocampal slices. *Nature (Lond.),* 266: 736–737.

Austin, L., Bray, J. J. and Young, R. J. (1966) Transport of proteins and ribonucleic acid along nerve axons. *J. Neurochem.,* 13: 1267–1269.

Autilio-Gambetti, L., Gambetti, P. and Shafer, B. (1973) RNA and axonal flow. Biochemical and autoradiographic study in the rabbit optic system. *Brain Res.,* 53: 387–399.

Barberis, C. and McIlwain, H. (1976) 5-Adenine mononucleotides in synaptosomal preparations from guinea pig neocortex: their change on incubation, superfusion and stimulation. *J. Neurochem.,* 26: 1015–1021.

Berne, R. M., Rubio, R. and Curnish, R. R. (1974) Release of adenosine from ischaemic brain. *Circulat. Res.,* 35: 262–272.

Berne, R. M., Herlihy, J. T., Schrader, J. and Rubio, R. (1976) Effect of adenosine on contraction of vascular smooth muscle. In *Ionic Actions on Vascular Smooth Muscle,* E. Betz (Ed.), Springer Verlag, Heidelberg, pp. 137–140.

Betz, E. (1976) (Ed.) *Ionic Actions on Vascular Smooth Muscle.* Springer Verlag, Heidelberg.

Bird, S. J. and Aghajanian, G. K. (1975) Denervation supersensitivity in the cholinergic septohippocampal pathway: a microiontophoretic study. *Brain Res.,* 100: 355–370.

Burnstock, G. (1976) Do some nerve cells release more than one transmitter? *Neuroscience,* 1: 239–248.

Casola, L., Davis, G. A. and Davis, R. E. (1969) Evidence for RNA transport in rat optic nerve. *J. Neurochem.,* 16: 1037–1041.

Clanachan, A. S., Johns, A. and Paton, D. M. (1977) Presynaptic inhibitory actions of adenine nucleotides and adenosine on neurotransmission in the rat vas deferens. *Neuroscience,* 2: 597–602.

Douglas, W. W. and Poisner, A. M. (1966) On relation between ATP splitting and secretion in the adrenal chromaffin cell. Extrusion of ATP (unhydrolysed) during release of catecholamines. *J. Physiol. (Lond.),* 183: 249–256.

Fredholm, B. B. (1977) Activation of adenylate cyclase from rat striatum and tuberculum olfactorium by adenosine. *Med. Biol.,* 55: 262–267.

Geffen, L. B. and Livett, B. G. (1971) Synaptic vesicles in sympathetic neurons. *Physiol. Rev.,* 51: 98–157.

Hedqvist, P. and Fredholm, B. B. (1976) Effects of adenosine on adrenergic transmission; prejunctional inhibition and postjunctional enhancement. *Naunyn-Schmiedeberg's Arch. exp. Path. Pharmak.,* 293: 217–223.

Huang, M. and Daly, J. W. (1974) Adenosine-elicited accumulation of cyclic AMP in brain slices: potentiation by agents which inhibit uptake of adenosine. *Life Sci.,* 14: 489–503.

Huang, M., Shimizu, H. and Daly, J. W. (1972) Accumulation of cyclic adenosine monophosphate in incubated slices of brain tissue. 2. Effects of depolarizing agents, membrane stabilizers, phosphodiesterase inhibitors, and adenosine analogues. *J. med. Chem.,* 15: 462–466.

Hunt, S. P. and Künzle, H. (1976) Bidirectional movement of label and transneuronal transport phenomena after injection of [^{3}H]adenosine in the central nervous system. *Brain Res.,* 112: 127–132.

Ingoglia, N. A., Grafstein, B., McEwen, B. S. and McQuarrie, I. G. (1973) Axonal transport of radioactivity in the goldfish optic system following intraocular injection of labeled RNA precursors. *J. Neurochem.,* 20: 1605–1616.

Ingvar, D. H. (1973) Cerebral blood flow metabolism in complete apallic syndroms, in states of severe dementia, and in akinetic mutism. *Acta neurol. scand.,* 49: 233–244.

Israel, M. and Meunier, F. (1977) Postsynaptic release of adenosine triphosphate induced by acetylcholine, a retroaction able to inhibit transmitter release. *Proc. int. Soc. Neurochem.,* 6: 33.

Kato, M., Ueno, H. and Black, P. (1974) Regional cerebral blood flow of the main visual pathways during photic stimulation of the retina in intact and split-brain monkeys. *Exp. Neurol.,* 42: 65–77.

Kreutzberg, G. W. and Barron, K. D. (1978) 5′-Nucleotidase of microglial cells in the facial nucleus during axonal reaction. *J. Neurocytol.,* 7: 601–610.

Kreutzberg, G. W., Barron, K. D. and Schubert, P. (1978) Cytochemical localisation of 5′-nucleotidase in glial plasma membranes. *Brain Res.,* 158: 247–257.

Kruger, L. and Sapporta, S. (1977) Axonal transport of [^{3}H]adenosine in visual somatosensory pathways. *Brain Res.,* 122: 132–136.

Kuroda, Y., Saito, M. and Kobayashi, K. (1976) Concomitant changes in cyclic AMP level and postsynaptic potentials of olfactory cortex slices induced by adenosine derivatives. *Brain Res.,* 109: 196–201.

Lynch, G., Matthews, D. A., Mosko, S., Parks, T. and Cotman, C. W. (1972) Induced AChE-rich layer in rat dentate gyrus following entorhinal lesions. *Brain Res.,* 42: 311–318.

Mah, H. D. and Daly, J. W. (1976) Adenosine-dependent formation of cyclic AMP in brain slices. *Pharmacol. Res. Commun.,* 8: 65–79.

Mosko, S., Lynch, G. and Cotman, C. W. (1973) The distribution of septal projections to the hippocampus of the rat. *J. comp. Neurol.,* 152: 163–174.

Okada, Y. and Kuroda, Y. (1975) Inhibitory action of adenosine and adenine nucleotides on the postsynaptic potential of olfactory cortex slices of guinea pig. *Proc. Jap. Acad.,* 51: 491–494.

Phillis, J. W. (1977) The role of cyclic nucleotides in the CNS. *Canad. J. neurol. Sci.,* 4: 151–189.

Prémont, J., Perez, M. and Bockaert, J. (1977) Adenosine-sensitive adenylate cyclase in rat striatal homogenates and its relationship to dopamine- and Ca^{2+}-sensitive adenylate cyclases. *Mol. Pharmacol.,* 13: 662–670.

Pull, I. and McIlwain, H. (1972) Adenine derivatives as neurohumoral agents in the brain. *Biochem. J.,* 130: 975–981.

Pull, I. and McIlwain, H. (1977) Adenine mononucleotides and their metabolites liberated from and applied to isolated tissues of the mammalian brain. *Neurochem. Res.,* 2: 203–216.

Rahman, H. und Wolburg, H. (1971) Intra-axonaler Transport von ^{3}H-Uridin Verbindungen im Tractus opticus von Teleosteern. *Experientia (Basel),* 27 (Suppl. V): 903–904.

Raisman, G. (1966) The connexions of the septum. *Brain Res.,* 89: 317–348.

Ramón y Cajal, S. (1911) *Histologie du Système Nerveux de l'Homme et des Vertébrés, Vol. II.* Maloine, Paris.

Reddington, M. and Schubert, P. (1979) Parallel investigations of the effects of adenosine on evoked potentials and cyclic AMP accumulation in hippocampus slices. Submitted for publication.

Rose, G. and Schubert, P. (1977) Release and transfer of [^{3}H]adenosine derivatives in the cholinergic septal system. *Brain Res.*, 121: 353–357.

Sattin, A. and Rall, T. W. (1970) Cyclic AMP content of guinea pig cerebral cortex slices. *Mol. Pharmacol.*, 6: 13–23.

Sawynok, J. and Jhamandas, K. H. (1976) Inhibition of acetylcholine release from cholinergic nerves by adenosine, adenine nucleotides and morphine: antagonism by theophylline. *J. Pharmacol. exp. Ther.*, 197: 379–390.

Schrader, J., Rubio, R. and Berne, R. M. (1975) Inhibition of slow action potentials of guinea pig atrial muscle by adenosine: a possible effect on Ca^{++} influx. *J. mol. cell. Cardiol.*, 7: 427–433.

Schubert, P. and Kreutzberg, G. W. (1974) Axonal transport of adenosine and uridine derivatives and transfer to postsynaptic neurons. *Brain Res.*, 76: 526–530.

Schubert, P. and Kreutzberg, G. W. (1975a) Dendritic and axonal transport of nucleoside derivatives in single motoneurons and release from dendrites. *Brain Res.*, 90: 319–323.

Schubert, P. and Kreutzberg, G. W. (1975b) [^{3}H]Adenosine, a tracer for neuronal connectivity. *Brain Res.*, 85: 317–319.

Schubert, P. and Kreutzberg, G. W. (1976) Communication between the neuron and the vessels. In *The Cerebral Vessel Wall*, J. Cervós-Navarro et al. (Eds.), Raven Press, New York, pp. 207–213.

Schubert, P. and Mitzdorf, U. (1979) Electrophysiological evaluation of the depressive effect of adenosine on evoked potentials in hippocampus slices. *Brain Res.*, in press.

Schubert, P., Lee, K., West, M., Deadwyler, S. and Lynch, G. (1976) Stimulation-dependent release of ^{3}H-adenosine derivatives from central axon terminals to target neurones. *Nature (Lond.)*, 260: 541–542.

Schubert, P., Rose, G., Lee, K., Lynch, G. and Kreutzberg, G. W. (1977) Axonal release and transfer of nucleoside derivatives in the entorhinal-hippocampal system: an autoradiographic study. *Brain Res.*, 134: 347–352.

Schubert, P., Komp, W. and Kreutzberg, G. W. (1979) Correlation of 5′-nucleotidase activity and selective transneuronal transfer of adenosine in the hippocampus. *Brain Res.*, in press.

Schultz, J. and Daly, J. W. (1973) Adenosine 3′,5′-monophosphate in guinea pig cerebral cortical slices: effects of β-adrenergic agents, histamine, serotonin and adenosine. *J. Neurochem.*, 21: 573–579.

Silinsky, E. M. and Hubbard, I. I. (1973) Released ATP from rat motor nerve terminals. *Nature (Lond.)*, 243: 404–405.

Smith, A. D. and Winckler, H. (1972) Fundamental mechanisms in the release of catecholamines. In *Handbuch der experimentellen Pharmakologie, Vol. XXXIII*, H. Blaschko and E. Muscholl (Eds.), Springer Verlag, Berlin, pp. 538–617.

Storm-Mathisen, J. and Blackstad, T. W. (1964). Cholinesterase in the hippocampal region. Distribution and relation to architechtonics and afferent systems. *Acta anat. (Basel)*, 56: 216–253.

Stumpf, C. (1965) Drug action on the electrical activity of the hippocampus. *Int. Rev. Neurobiol.*, 8: 77–137.

Sturgill, T. W., Schrier, B. K. and Gilman, A. G. (1975) Stimulation of cyclic AMP accumulation by 2-chloroadenosine: lack of incorporation of nucleoside into cyclic nucleotides. *J. Cyclic Nucl. Res.*, 1: 21–30.

Sulakhe, P. V. and Phillis, J. W. (1975) The release of ^{3}H-adenosine and its derivatives from the cat sensory motor cortex. *Life Sci.*, 17: 551–556.

Ten Bruggencate, G., Steinberg, R., Stöckle, H. and Nicholson, C. (1977) Modulation of extracellular Ca^{++} and K^+ levels in the mammalian cerebellar cortex. In *Iontophoresis and Transmitter Mechanisms in the Mammalian Central Nervous System*, J. S. Kelly (Ed.), Elsevier, Amsterdam, pp. 412–415.

Vizi, E. S. and Knoll, J. (1976) The inhibitory effect of adenosine and related nucleotides on the release of acetylcholine. *Neuroscience*, 1: 391–398.

White, T. D. (1978) Release of ATP from a synaptosomal preparation by elevated extracellular K^+ and by veratridine. *J. Neurochem.*, 30: 329–336.

Winkler, H. (1977) The biogenesis of adrenal chromaffin granules. *Neuroscience*, 2: 657–683.

Wise, S. P. and Jones, E. G. (1976) Transneuronal or retrograde transport of [^{3}H]adenosine in the rat somatic sensory system. *Brain Res.*, 107: 127–131.

Wise, S. P., Jones, E. G. and Berman, N. (1978) Direction and specificity of the axonal and transcellular transport of nucleosides. *Brain Res.*, 139: 197–217.

Zimmermann, H. (1978) Turnover of adenine nucleotides in cholinergic synaptic vesicles of the *Torpedo* electric organ. *Neuroscience,* 3: 827–836.

Zimmermann, H. and Whittaker, V. P. (1974) Effect of electrical stimulation of the yield and composition of synaptic vesicles from the cholinergic synapses of the electric organ of *Torpedo. J. Neurochem.,* 22: 435–450.

Localization of Neurotransmitters, Particularly Glutamate, in Hippocampus, Septum, Nucleus Accumbens and Superior Colliculus

FRODE FONNUM, RAGNAR LUND KARLSEN, DIDRIK MALTHE-SØRENSSEN, KNUT K. SKREDE and IVAR WALAAS

Norwegian Defence Research Establishment, Division for Toxicology, N-2007 Kjeller (Norway)

INTRODUCTION

In the present survey we will try to identify the neurotransmitter in certain well defined fibres in the hippocampal-septal system including the nucleus accumbens septi. The latter structure will also be discussed as a ventral part of striatum, and its efferent projection as a ventral striato-pallidal pathway. Superior colliculus is, like the hippocampus, a laminar structure where many of the afferent fibres are well known. It is therefore included in this survey.

The techniques employed in our laboratory in an attempt to identify a neurotransmitter are the estimation of proper neurotransmitter marker in microdissected samples of the region under investigation. The transmitters present in the neurones are identified by correlating the distribution of the transmitter marker to the distribution of axon terminals as defined by previous anatomical investigation; by studying the changes in the marker after interruption of specific afferent fibres and after destruction of intrinsic neurones by local injection of kainic acid; and also by studying the release of transmitter marker after stimulating specific nerve fibre bundles. The use of kainic acid has been shown to be an excellent tool when carefully used (Olney et al., 1974; Hattori and McGeer, 1977; Schwarcz and Coyle, 1977; Fonnum and Walaas, 1978a; Walaas and Fonnum, 1979b).

It is well established that the enzymes choline acetyltransferase (ChAT) and glutamate decarboxylase (GAD) are the most specific markers for neurones using acetylcholine and γ-aminobutyric acid (GABA) as transmitters respectively. The enzymes are easy to measure, are highly concentrated in presynaptic structures and do not diffuse on preparation of the tissue. (For more detailed discussion, see Fonnum, 1972, 1973; Fonnum and Storm-Mathisen, 1978.) The localization of catecholaminergic and serotonergic fibres are well described through histofluorescence (Dahlström and Fuxe, 1965; Lindvall and Björklund, 1978), immunohistochemical studies (Hökfelt et al., 1977) and combined neurotoxic and radio-autographic methods (Azmitia and Segal, 1978).

MARKERS FOR LOCALIZATION OF ASPARTATE AND GLUTAMATE AS NEUROTRANSMITTERS

The acidic amino acids aspartate (ASP) and glutamate (GLU) are thought to be important candidates for excitatory neurotransmitters in the brain. The two amino acids produce powerful excitation with rapid on- and offset when applied to neurones in the brain by microiontophoresis with an apparent change in ionic conductance (Curtis and Johnston, 1974; Krnjević, 1974; Tebēcis, 1974).

The two acidic amino acids occupy a central position in the general metabolism and it is difficult to separate the metabolic GLU from the transmitter GLU. In addition it has not been possible to find an enzyme which is rate-limiting for the supply of transmitter GLU. According to current views on the metabolic compartmentation of amino acids in brain, glucose, pyruvate and citrate are the major precursors for glutamate in a large glutamate compartment which comprises nerve terminals, whereas acetate is the major precursor for the small glutamate compartment which comprises glial cells (Balázs et al., 1973; Van den Berg et al., 1975; Berl and Clarke, 1978). Glutamine, which is synthesized in the glial cell by the enzyme glutamine synthetase (Martinez-Hernandez et al., 1977), diffuses freely into the nerve terminals and is a major precursor for the neuronal pools of glutamate, aspartate and GABA (Bradford et al., 1978; Cotman and Hamberger, 1978). Inhibition of glutaminase by NH_4^+ ions decreases the potassium evoked release of endogenous GLU. Glutaminase therefore plays an important part in the synthesis of these amino acids. Studies have revealed that this enzyme is distributed in subcellular fractions in the same way as the general mitochondrial marker fumarase (Blokhuis and Veldstra, 1970). This infers that the enzyme may synthesize glutamate for other purposes than neurotransmission. Other enzymes involved in glutamate or aspartate metabolism are glutamate dehydrogenase and aspartate aminotransferase. Glutamate dehydrogenase is mainly localized to mitochondria outside nerve terminals (Reijnierse et al., 1975) and cannot therefore be heavily involved in the supply of transmitter GLU. There are also some histochemical evidences for this enzyme in rat astrocytes (Norenberg, 1976). Aspartate aminotransferase in brain is present as two different isoenzymes, one of them is a general cytoplasmic marker and the other is a general mitochondrial marker (Fonnum, 1968). It is therefore unlikely that this enzyme specifically supplies the transmitter pool of GLU or ASP. The contribution of these enzymes for amino acid transmitters may be studied from the loss of enzyme activities following degeneration of glutamergic, aspartergic and GABAergic nerve terminals.

During the last 3 years, work in our own and other laboratories has led to the establishment of several parameters which we believe indicate the presence of glutamergic and aspartergic nerve terminals or neurones. These parameters comprise the sodium-dependent high affinity uptake (HA uptake) of the amino acids, the calcium-dependent release of the amino acids and changes in the endogenous levels of the amino acids.

It is generally accepted that brain mini-slices and synaptosomes have the ability to accumulate several putative neurotransmitters, such as catecholamines, serotonin, glycine and GABA (see Snyder et al., 1973).

The K_m of these uptake mechanisms is of the order of 1–20 μM ("high affinity"), and the uptake is dependent on Na^+ ions. Several amino acids may be taken up by HA mechanism, but only those regarded as neurotransmitters have Na^+-dependent uptake (Bennett et al., 1973). Kinetic evidence shows that L-glutamate (GLU) and D- and L-aspartate (ASP) all seem to be taken up by the same HA uptake system (Balcar and Johnston, 1972; Davies and Johnston, 1976). The maximal velocity of D-ASP is equal to that of L-GLU and higher than that of L-ASP (Takagaki, 1978). This makes D-ASP, which is not metabolized in brain, an acceptable tool for uptake studies (Lund Karlsen and Fonnum, 1978; Storm-Mathisen and Woxen Opsahl, 1978; Walaas and Fonnum, 1979b) and release studies (this chapter).

The HA uptake of GLU shows a distinct regional distribution with the highest uptake in thalamus and almost negligible uptake in globus pallidus (Walaas and Fonnum, 1979b). There are also several studies which have shown a significant decrease in the HA uptake of D-ASP and/or L-GLU after destruction of nerve terminals which may use ASP or GLU as neurotransmitter. Thus, viral infections of hamsters leading to a disappearance of granular cells of the cerebellum, led to a 70% loss of both L-GLU and L-ASP HA uptakes in homogenates from cerebellum, but no decrease in the uptake of other amino acids (Young et al., 1974). Destruction of the corticostriatal input was accompanied by a 50–70% decrease of both D-ASP and L-GLU HA uptake in striatal homogenate, but no change in the corresponding uptake of GABA (Divac et al., 1977; Fonnum, 1978). In contrast there were no changes in the HA GLU uptake after destruction of thalamic nuclei projecting to the striatum. In rat there was a 70% decrease in both D-ASP and L-GLU HA uptake in homogenate prepared from the lateral geniculate body following destruction of the visual cortex, but no changes after retinal ablation (Lund Karlsen and Fonnum, 1978). In these studies the main part of the uptake in unoperated animals and the changes in the lesioned animals were found to be localized to the synaptosome fraction. Several examples quoted below will show a specific loss of HA uptake of GLU after degeneration of excitatory fibres in hippocampus, septum, n. accumbens and superior colliculus.

There are other results indicating that also glial cells show HA uptake of L-GLU and such an uptake may interfere with HA uptake as a marker for glutamergic nerve terminals. Thus, HA uptake of both GLU, ASP and GABA occurs in bulk prepared glial cells although the tissue/medium ratio is much lower than for synaptosomes (Hamberger et al., 1976, 1978). Glial cells grown in tissue culture also show HA GLU uptake (Henn et al., 1974). Glial cells prepared in this way may, however, have changed their membrane properties. Bulk isolated glial cells do not conform to the suggested specificity (Iversen and Schon, 1973) for glial and nerve terminal uptake of GABA-like compounds (Sellström and Hamberger, 1975; Sieghart et al., 1977). Intact dorsal root ganglion also possesses a slow HA GLU uptake which is probably of glial origin (Roberts, 1976).

Autoradiography after intracerebral injection of L-[^{3}H]GLU previously indicated a predominant glial localization of radioactivity (Hökfelt and Ljungdahl, 1972; Schon and Kelly, 1974), but more recent studies have clearly shown that a predominance of label is in nerve terminals (Beart, 1976; Iversen and Storm-Mathisen, 1976). When labelled L-GLU or GABA is taken up into whole rat retina, the main proportion of the label is localized to the glial cells of the retina (the Müller cells) (Neal, 1976). However, the changes in the HA GLU uptake in retinal homogenates or in the whole retina after local injection of α-aminoadipic acid, which destroys the Müller cells, and after glutamate treatment, which destroys the neurones, are consistent with the view that glial uptake dominates in the intact retinae whereas nerve terminal uptake dominates in the retinal homogenate (Lund Karlsen, 1978). In addition almost complete lack of HA uptake of D-ASP in a homogenate from globus pallidus or the almost total loss of HA uptake of L-GLU or D-ASP, but not of other transmitter markers, in combined surgical and chemical lesions of n. accumbens (Walaas and Fonnum, 1979b) or of superior colliculus (Lund Karlsen, to be published), makes us believe that glial uptake in a brain homogenate is not very substantial. The same conclusion can be reached after the many examples of substantial decrease in HA uptake of GLU and/or ASP after surgical or chemical lesions which promote gliosis.

In conclusion, although glial uptake of these amino acids may be important in vivo and even in slices where the glial structures are well preserved, we believe that HA uptake in homogenates is a reliable parameter for localization of glutamergic or aspartergic nerve terminals.

Since HA uptake cannot differentiate between L-GLU or L-ASP as a transmitter, this can only be determined by amino acid analysis. Thus, both in the cerebellum deprived of granule cells (Young et al., 1974), in striatum after removal of the corticostriatal terminals (Fonnum, Storm-Mathisen and Divac, see Fonnum, 1978) and in the lateral geniculate body after removal of the corticothalamic fibres (Lund Karlsen and Fonnum, 1978), there was a specific loss of endogenous glutamate but not of aspartate, alanine, glycine or GABA. The loss in the endogenous amino acid was much less pronounced than the corresponding loss in HA uptake. Even so the loss of endogenous glutamate must be much larger than the loss of tissue in striatum and lateral geniculate body, since the concentration of other amino acids or transmitter parameters did not change. The concentration of glutamate in the glutamergic nerve terminals must therefore be substantial.

Another useful parameter for localization of nerve terminals using acidic amino acids as their neurotransmitter is chemical or electrical stimulus evoked release. Ca^{2+} dependency or antagonism by Mg^{2+} is usually taken as absolute requirements to distinguish between nerve terminal release and release from other compartments. The experiments can either be carried out by studying the release of exogenously added labelled L-GLU or D-ASP in response to a depolarizing concentration of K^+ or veratridin or by analyzing the release of endogenous amino acids.

In the case of preloading of slices one is again confronted with the problem of glial uptake and release. The strict dependency of the release on Ca^{2+} is additional indirect evidence that the uptake is also confined to nerve terminals in slices. Exogenously labelled D-[^{3}H]ASP or L-GLU have been chemically released from cortical slices (Mulder and Snyder, 1974), striatal synaptosomes (Fonnum, unpublished), cerebellar synaptosomes (Sandoval and Cotman, 1978) or hippocampal slices (Nadler et al., 1977), and release of endogenous amino acids has also been studied after chemical depolarization of cortical synaptosomes, hypothalamic synaptosomes (Bradford et al., 1978), hippocampal slices (Nadler et al., 1976), cerebellar synaptosomes (Sandoval and Cotman, 1978) and slices from visual cortex (Clark and Collins, 1976). Such studies only tell us that aspartergic or glutamergic nerve terminals are present in the slice. Changes in the release after surgical lesions give indications of the identity of the nerve terminals. Thus, destruction of parallel fibres by neonatal X-irradiation of the cerebellum was accompanied by a decrease of L-[^{3}H]GLU release from cerebellar synaptosomes, indicating that the release originated from the parallel fibre endings (Sandoval and Cotman, 1978).

Release of preloaded exogenous amino acids after electrical stimulation of specific nerve fibres represents a much higher degree of specificity than chemical release. The method cannot differentiate between GLU or ASP, but many of the problems of unspecific release or glial interaction are abolished with this technique. Below are shown such examples using the transverse hippocampal slice. Another example is the release of [^{3}H]GLU from olfactory cortex slice after stimulation of lateral olfactory tract (Yamamoto and Matsui, 1976).

Release of endogenous amino acids after stimulation of specific nerve fibres is one of the most important criteria for transmitter identification. Re-uptake of neurotransmitter during perfusion represents a major technical problem which may obscure release. Uptake inhibitors may be used but they often exchange with the endogenous substance or depolarize the terminals. An example of such studies is the specific release of endogenous GLU, but not

ASP, glycine or glutamine from olfactory cortex after stimulation of the lateral olfactory tract (Bradford and Richards, 1976).

HIPPOCAMPUS

Hippocampus is a laminated structure where the pyramidal and granular cells are distributed in single layers that extend throughout the hippocampus proper and area dentata respectively. In subiculum the cell bodies are more heterogenously organized. The hippocampal neurones are excited by a series of known fibres such as commissural, perforant path, mossy fibres and Schaffer collaterals, and inhibited by e.g. basket cells. The fibres are organized in a layered manner parallel to the cell bodies. In addition, all major neuronal excitatory members as well as the arteries to the hippocampal formation are arranged in lamellae parallel to each other in a plane nearly transverse to the longitudinal axis of the hippocampus (details in Ramón y Cajal, 1911; Lorente de Nó, 1934; Blackstad, 1967; Andersen, 1975; Storm-Mathisen, 1977). The laminar structure of hippocampus lends itself readily to topographical and histochemical studies of neurotransmitters or neurotransmitter markers. Such studies combined with surgical lesions of efferent and afferent projections have led to an accurate description of the neurotransmitter content of the different fibre projections (see reviews of Fonnum, 1977; Storm-Mathisen, 1977). The recent introduction of the glutamate analogue kainic acid, that destroys local neurones but not traversing axons or nerve terminals, has been of considerable help in elucidating the neurotransmitter of local fibres (Fonnum and Walaas, 1978a, b).

GLUTAMATE AND ASPARTATE AS TRANSMITTERS IN HIPPOCAMPUS

The pyramidal cells are extremely sensitive to intrahippocampal kainic acid injection (Fonnum and Walaas, 1978a). Injection of 1 μg kainic acid into dorsal hippocampus was accompanied by a loss of the pyramidal cells and by a loss in both HA uptake of GLU and in endogenous content of GLU and ASP in that part of hippocampus (Table I). Depolarization

TABLE I

THE EFFECT OF INTRAHIPPOCAMPAL INJECTION OF KAINIC ACID ON NEUROTRANSMITTER MARKERS IN HIPPOCAMPUS

	Unoperated	*Injected*
	(μmol/hr/g protein)	*(% unoperated)*
GLU uptake	2.67 ± 0.18	37 ± 4
GAD	192 ± 14	26 ± 4
ChAT	62 ± 6	90 ± 7
AAD	3.7 ± 0.2	97 ± 3
	(μmol/g protein)	
GLU	92 ± 10	63 ± 7
ASP	14 ± 2	59 ± 8
GABA	25 ± 3	51 ± 9

of hippocampal slices by potassium was also accompanied by release of exogenously added L-GLU and L-ASP and in endogenous release of L-GLU and L-ASP (Nadler et al., 1977, 1978). These experiments strongly suggest the presence of intrinsic glutamergic or aspartergic nerve terminals in the hippocampus.

CA3 AXON COLLATERALS

An important intrahippocampal fibre connection is the excitatory Schaffer collaterals originating from the CA3 pyramidal cells and terminating in the stratum radiatum of CA1 with characteristic en passage synapses on the pyramidal cell apical dendrites (Andersen et al., 1971, 1978; Andersen, 1975, 1976). In addition to the Schaffer collateral the CA3 axons dichotomize, sending a second main branch to the lateral septal nucleus through fimbria/fornix (Andersen et al., 1973b, c; Andersen, 1976; Swanson and Cowan, 1977).

Surgical lesions aimed to degenerate the pyramidal cells of CA3/4 plus the commissural fibres led to a substantial fall in HA uptake of GLU (Storm-Mathisen, 1977b) in CA1. The lesion also led to a specific loss of endogenous GLU, and to a lesser extent, of ASP in stratum oriens/radiatum of CA1 (Fonnum and Storm-Mathisen, unpublished). Both findings indicate that GLU and/or ASP may be the transmitters of the Schaffer collaterals or CA1 afferent commissural fibres.

Previous investigations have shown that electrical stimulation (by small current pulses) of fibres, located in the stratum radiatum of CA1 in the transverse hippocampal slice, excites CA1 pyramidal neurones and only to a small, or no, extent neurones in the dentate gyrus (Skrede and Westgaard, 1971; Andersen et al., 1978; Schwartzkroin and Prince, 1978).

Thus, transverse hippocampal slices were preloaded with D-[^{3}H]ASP under HA uptake conditions. The slices were washed for 30 min with normal Krebs-Ringer solution. When the slices were selectively stimulated in stratum radiatum (Fig. 1A), a maximum stimulated release of 200–300% (definition: Potashner, 1978) was regularly obtained. The release was Ca^{2+} dependent (Fig. 1B) and did not occur when D-[^{3}H]ASP was exchanged with [^{3}H]leucine. The mean maximum stimulated release was 155% ± 10 (mean ± S.E.M., 23 observations); the highest value was found to be 350%.

Since the transverse hippocampal slice contains other fibre systems such as perforant path, mossy fibres and fibres from pyramidal cells of CA1 to subiculum which may be glutamergic or aspartergic, we dissected out the CA3/CA1 region, avoiding area dentata subiculum and the CA1 molecular layer (Fig. 2A). Stimulation of the isolated CA3/CA1 preparation evoked an increased release of D-[^{3}H]ASP in a similar manner to the intact slice (Fig. 2B). Mean maximum stimulated release of the dissected slice was 196 ± 25% (mean ± S.E.M., N = 10), and therefore higher than in the intact slice. The difference is significant ($P < 0.005$, Wilcoxon's two-sample rank test) and is most probably due to the lack of contribution of spontaneous release of D-[^{3}H]ASP from the regions removed by dissection. The electrically evoked release could be completely abolished by a lesion carefully placed to section all afferents coursing caudally through the stratum radiatum and to avoid cutting the pyramidal layer and the stratum oriens/alveus (Fig. 2A). In this case the slices were only stimulated at position 1. This procedure has previously been used to abolish the evoked population and unit discharges in CA1 after stimulation in CA3 (Andersen et al., 1978; Schwartzkroin and Prince, 1978).

The evoked release of D-[^{3}H]ASP is therefore most likely due to the activation of the Schaffer collaterals (Skrede and Teyler, unpublished). The CA3 cells could selectively be

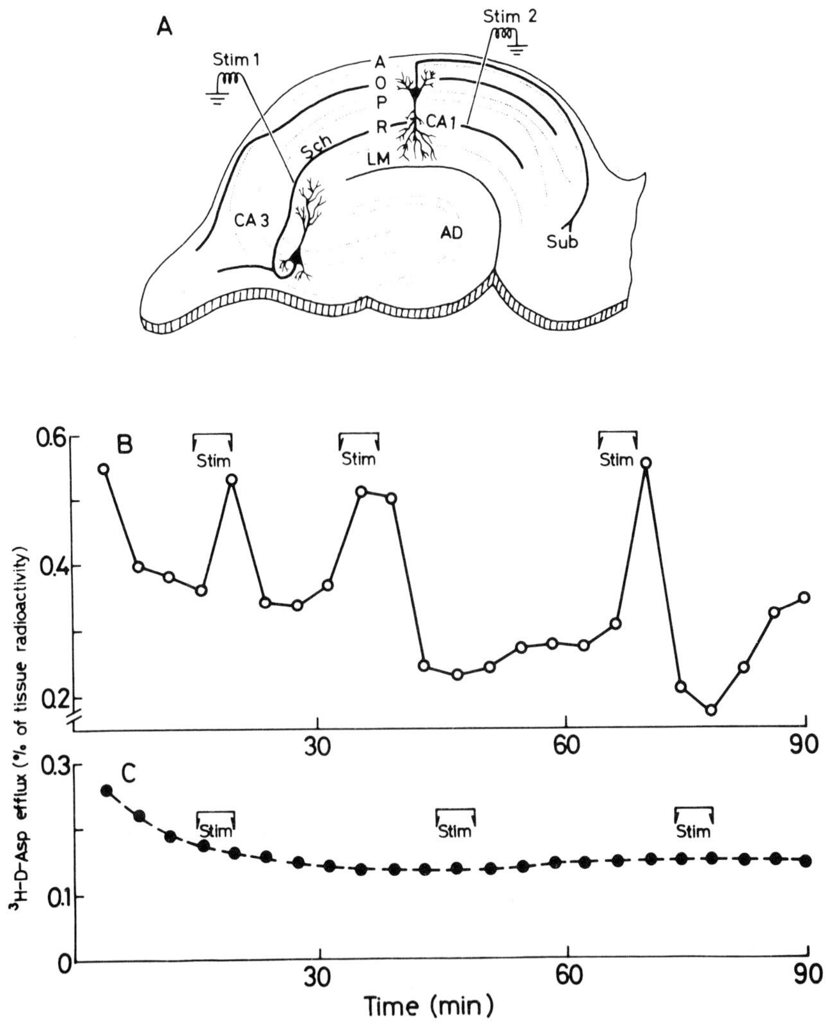

Fig. 1. A: diagram of a transverse hippocampal slice. Abbreviations mark the histological layers and subfields: AD, dentate area; CA3, hippocampus regio inferior; CA1, hippocampus regio superior; Sub, subiculum; A, O, P, R, LM, alveus, stratum oriens, pyramidale, radiatum and lacunosum moleculare respectively of hippocampus CA1; nomenclature according to Lorente de Nó (1934). Positions of the stimulation sites (Stim 1, Stim 2) are indicated near the employed fibres in stratum radiatum. For clarity, only one heavily outlined Schaffer collateral (Sch) is drawn, leaving out, e.g., the commissural fibres and other CA1 excitatory afferent fibre systems which possibly may be activated by stimulation in the stratum radiatum. Afferents to the pyramidal cell basal dendrites are indicated by a heavy line in stratum oriens. B: spontaneous and stimulus evoked release of D-[^{3}H]aspartate from intact slices in the presence of 1.5 mM calcium. Each point represents the radioactivity of 1 ml Krebs-Ringer perfusion solution collected each 4 min from perfusion cell. The perfusion flow rate was 0.25 ml/min. The values are expressed as percentage of the D-[^{3}H]aspartate remaining in tissue at the time of fraction collection. C: the spontaneous and stimulated release of D-[^{3}H]aspartate in the absence of calcium but in the presence of 1.5 mM EGTA in the perfusion solution. Otherwise as in B. In all experiments the stimulation frequency was 25 Hz. Each stimulation period (Stim) represents 4 slices stimulated twice for 15 sec with an interval of 15 sec. The monopolar stimulation was carried out with microcathodes of isolated tungsten wire with a naked tip of 20–40 μm. Stimuli (0.2 msec, 100–150 μA) were delivered to the fibres in the slices. Field potential or unit discharges were regularly recorded to test the viability of the slices and to secure that the spread of current was negligible.

destroyed by local injection of a low concentration (0.1–0.2 μg) of kainic acid into the dorsal hippocampus. This will selectively destroy the Schaffer collaterals. Such chemical lesions were accompanied by a 40% loss in HA uptake of GLU in the homogenate of a transverse hippocampal slice. When such a CA3/CA1 slice was subjected to Ca^{2+}-dependent potassium evoked release of D-[^{3}H]ASP, the fractional release (in per cent of slice content) was reduced by 30–40% compared to a control slice. The total amount of D-[^{3}H]ASP released was reduced by 70–80% of that in a control slice.

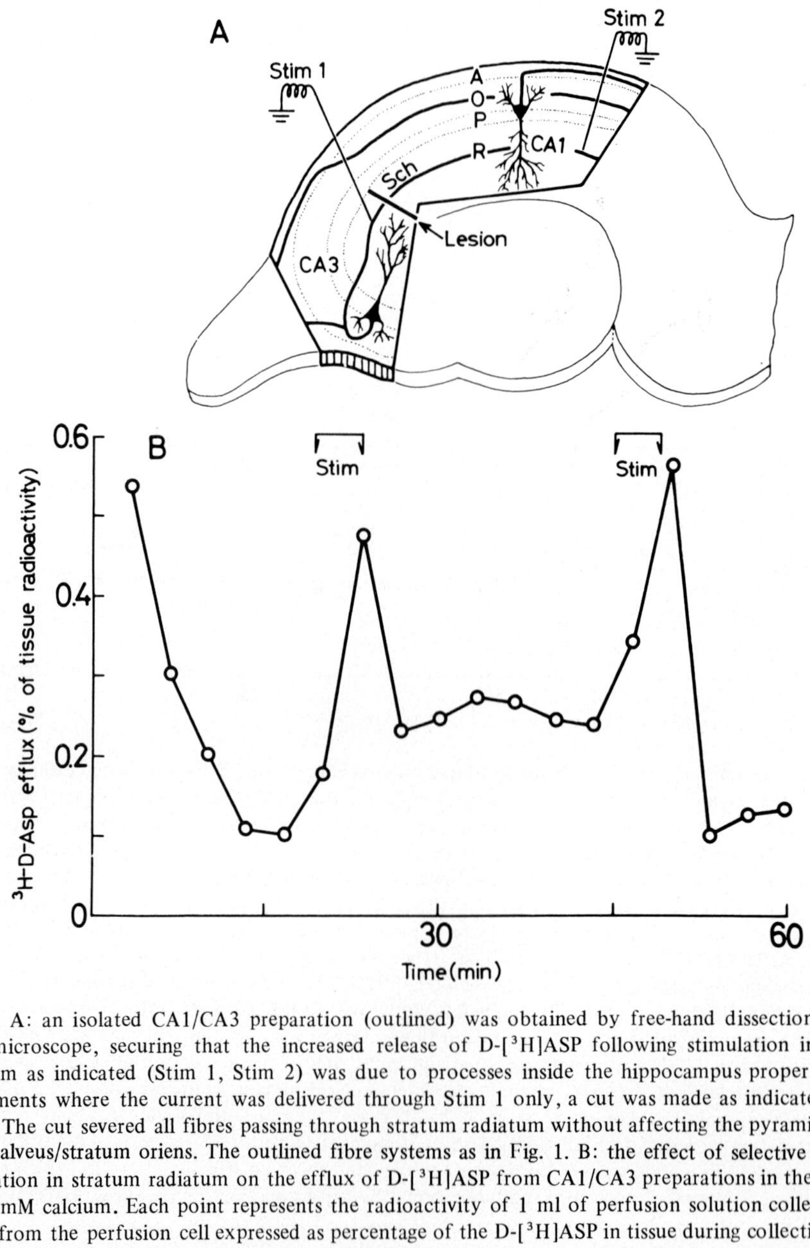

Fig. 2. A: an isolated CA1/CA3 preparation (outlined) was obtained by free-hand dissection under a stereomicroscope, securing that the increased release of D-[^{3}H]ASP following stimulation in stratum radiatum as indicated (Stim 1, Stim 2) was due to processes inside the hippocampus proper. In some experiments where the current was delivered through Stim 1 only, a cut was made as indicated by the arrow. The cut severed all fibres passing through stratum radiatum without affecting the pyramidal layer, or the alveus/stratum oriens. The outlined fibre systems as in Fig. 1. B: the effect of selective electrical stimulation in stratum radiatum on the efflux of D-[^{3}H]ASP from CA1/CA3 preparations in the presence of 1.5 mM calcium. Each point represents the radioactivity of 1 ml of perfusion solution collected each 4 min from the perfusion cell expressed as percentage of the D-[^{3}H]ASP in tissue during collection of the effluent. Stimulation parameters as in Fig. 1. Two stimulation periods (Stim) are indicated.

TABLE II

NEUROTRANSMITTERS IN LATERAL AND MEDIAL SEPTUM

Treatment	*Parameter*	*Lateral*	*Medial*
		μmol/hr/g protein	
Untreated	GLU uptake	2.66 ± 0.13	0.95 ± 0.14
	GAD	262 ± 15	93 ± 8
	ChAT	45 ± 2	120 ± 16
	AAD	7.3 ± 0.9	7.4 ± 0.4
		per cent untreated	
Kainic acid Dorsal hippocampus	GLU uptake	65 ± 6	86 ± 10
Unilateral fimbria	GLU uptake	59 ± 5	88 ± 11
Bilateral fimbria	GLU uptake	30 ± 5	91 ± 9
Bilateral fimbria	GLU	67 ± 3	–
	ASP	91 ± 8	–
	GLN	116 ± 17	–

In conclusion, the changes in HA uptake of GLU or D-ASP and in the endogenous content of GLU after surgical and chemical lesions together with studies of electrically evoked and potassium evoked release strongly suggest that the Schaffer collaterals use GLU as their neurotransmitter.

In addition to the Schaffer collaterals the CA3 cells send axons through fimbria/fornix to the lateral, but not the medial septum on both sides. In agreement, unilateral transection of these fibres was accompanied by 40% reduction in HA uptake of GLU in the lateral septum of both sides. Bilateral transection increased the reduction to 70% as expected (Table II; Fonnum and Walaas, 1978a). No changes were detected in medial septum or of other transmitter markers in the lateral septum. Similar findings were obtained by Storm-Mathisen and Woxen Opsahl (1978). Intrahippocampal injection of various concentrations of kainic acid (1–0.1 μg), which destroyed either all the pyramidal cells or cells in CA3 only, led to a specific reduction in HA uptake in the dorsal part of lateral septum (Fonnum and Walaas, 1978a). In addition, bilateral transection of fimbria was accompanied by a reduction in 30% of endogenous GLU. No changes in the content of other amino acids, e.g., ASP and GABA, were found (Table II).

The CA3/CA4 fibres to septum were also amenable to electrically induced release studies. Sagittal slices of the lateral septum which adhered to the fimbria were dissected out and preloaded with D-[^{3}H]ASP as described in detail for the transverse hippocampal slice. Electrically evoked stimulation of the fimbria was then accompanied by an increase in release of D-ASP which was 2–4 times higher than the resting release. Also in this case was the release found to be Ca^{2+}-dependent.

In conclusion, surgical lesions of the CA3/CA4 pyramidal cell axons or chemically induced lesions of the pyramidal cell itself were accompanied by a decrease in HA uptake of GLU and D-ASP and in the endogenous content of GLU in samples taken from the terminal area of these axons. Electrical stimulation of the axons, either to CA1 or to lateral septum, was also consistent with the concept that these axons use GLU as their transmitter. It is in accordance with Dale's principle that the two axon branches use the same transmitter.

PERFORANT PATH

Appreciable amount of work has been carried out on the identification of the transmitter of the perforant path. The perforant path arises from cells in the entorhinal cortex and ends in the molecular layer of area dentata (Nafstad, 1967; Lømo, 1971). Destruction of the perforant path leads to a complex pattern of sprouting of other inputs to this region (for discussion, see Cotman, this volume). Slices of area dentata show a potassium evoked release both of exogenously added [^{3}H]GLU and endogenous GLU. A lesion in entorhinal cortex destroying the perforant path terminals was followed by a significant decrease in potassium evoked release of endogenous GLU but not ASP (Nadler et al., 1976). Autoradiographic studies in hippocampal slices submitted to HA uptake of GLU have previously been studied in our laboratory (Storm-Mathisen, 1977b; Taxt et al., 1977). Deafferentation of perforant path was accompanied by a loss of grains in the outer two-thirds of the molecular layer, in agreement with a loss of 52% in HA uptake of GLU in homogenates containing perforant path synaptosomes (Storm-Mathisen, 1977b). In agreement, Nadler et al. (1976, 1978) found changes both in HA uptake of GLU and chemically stimulated Ca^{2+}-dependent release of [^{3}H]GLU as well as endogenous GLU from slices of the lower blade of the dentata area. Interestingly, they did not detect a significant change in the endogenous content of GLU and ASP in the slices after lesion (Nadler et al., 1978). Possibly their slices contain too much material which does not belong to the terminal region of perforant path. Evidence is therefore still favouring GLU as a transmitter of the perforant path fibres.

COMMISSURAL FIBRES

The commissural fibres are derived from the pyramidal cells of the contralateral hippocampus and enter hippocampus through fimbria and the ventral psalterium (Blackstad, 1956; Andersen, 1959). According to Storm-Mathisen (1978), intersection of contralateral axons resulted in only 20% loss of D-[^{3}H]ASP uptake in oriens/radiatum of CA1. After commissurotomy Nadler et al. (1978) observed a significant decrease in the Ca^{2+}-dependent release of endogenous GLU and ASP from slices of regio superior and endogenous ASP from the area dentata slices. They did not find any changes in the total content of the amino acids in these slices. In contrast, Nitsch et al. (this volume) found a decrease in endogenous GLU in CA1 stratum oriens after commissurotomy. In conclusion therefore, the situation is unclear with regard to neurotransmitters of the commissural fibre. At present both ASP and GLU are possible candidates.

MOSSY FIBRES

The mossy fibres are derived from the dentate granule cells and they end in a narrow layer on the apical dendrites of CA3 pyramids (Blackstad and Kjærheim, 1961; Blackstad et al., 1970). Autoradiography after HA uptake of L-[^{3}H]GLU into slices revealed that a few of these terminals possessed a high density of grains (Iversen and Storm-Mathisen, 1976), and could possibly use GLU or ASP as their transmitter.

However, neonatal X-irradiation, which destroyed 80% of the granule cells and therefore inhibited the development of the mossy fibres, was not accompanied by a reduced release of GLU or ASP in CA3 slices (Nadler et al., 1978). This discrepancy may be explained if only a few of the mossy fibres contain ASP/GLU or if the release from mossy fibre only accounts for a small part of the total release of endogenous GLU and ASP from CA3. An additional complication is the possible fragile nature of hippocampal mossy fibres (cf. cerebellar mossy fibres; Israël and Whittaker, 1965).

CHOLINERGIC FIBRES

Choline acetyltransferase in hippocampus has by subcellular fractionation been shown to be present in synaptosomes (Fonnum, 1970). The highest enzyme activity was by micro-dissection found in two narrow infra- and suprapyramidal zones in hippocampus proper. In area dentata the highest activities are localized around the granular cell layers (Fonnum, 1970). In the hippocampal region there is a good correlation between acetylcholine esterase (AChE) and ChAT activities (Fonnum, 1970).

The cholinergic input to hippocampus is derived from medial septum or from the nucleus of the diagonal band (Shute and Lewis, 1961; Oderfeld-Nowak et al., 1974) and enters hippocampus through fimbria (Storm-Mathisen, 1972).

Kainic acid injections into the nucleus of the diagonal band were more effective than injection into septum to destroy the cholinergic activity in the hippocampus and seem to be the main site of origin of these fibres (Table III). There is a small proportion of cells with strong AChE staining in area 31 of CA1 (Srebro and Mellgren, 1974) even after fimbrial transection and these cells may be intrinsic cholinergic cells. These cells could account for the small loss of ChAT (5–10%) after intrahippocampal kainic acid injection (Table I).

TABLE III

THE EFFECT OF LOCAL KAINIC ACID INJECTION INTO SEPTUM OR INTO NUCLEUS OF DIAGONAL BAND

Kainic acid, 2 or 3 μg in 0.5 μl, was injected over 4 min and the animals killed after 7 days. When injection site was lateral septum, the kainic acid diffused over most of septum. When injection site was nucleus of diagonal band a part also diffused into the ventral septal parts.

Injection site	*Marker*	*Septum*	*Diagonal band*	*Hippocampus*
			Per cent of untreated	
Septum	ChAT	80 ± 12	–	90 ± 4
	GAD	33 ± 3	–	102 ± 9
Nucleus of diagonal band	ChAT	28 ± 6	37 ± 4	20 ± 4
	GAD	42 ± 5	55 ± 5	102 ± 7
	HA GLU	90 ± 5	75 ± 8	–

TABLE IV

MANIPULATION OF CHOLINERGIC ACTIVITY IN HIPPOCAMPUS

Treatment	*ACh level (nmol/g protein)*	*ACh turnover (nmol/g protein/hr)*
Control	270	3400
Acute fimbrial transection	390	720
Chronic fimbrial transection	44	200
Septal stimulation	270	8380

Following an acute septal lesion, i.e. 1 hr after transection of fimbria, a transient rise in the content of ACh (Sethy et al., 1973) and a dramatic decrease in the ACh turnover are observed (Table IV; Malthe-Sørenssen et al., 1978b). The increase in the ACh level may be explained as a continued ACh synthesis in the absence of ACh release and indicates a poor regulation mechanism for ACh level in the nerve terminal. After chronic fimbrial lesion (1 week) when the cholinergic terminals have degenerated, there is a simultaneous decrease in both ACh content and turnover in hippocampus. Stimulation in septum and thereby activation of cholinergic fibres to hippocampus is followed by an increase in ACh release in hippocampus (Smith, 1974; Dudar, 1975). Such stimulation does not lead to any change in ACh level, but a clear increase in its turnover. These simple experiments clearly show that ACh turnover, but not the level, is the important parameter when studying modulation of cholinergic activity. Intraventricular injection of several peptides did therefore, as expected, not change the ACh content in hippocampus (Table V). Somatostatin and α-melanocyte stimulating hormone (α-MSH), however, increased, whereas substance P reduced ACh turnover in hippocampus (Malthe-Sørenssen et al., 1978a, b; Wood et al., 1978). The effect of substance P, but not of the two other peptides, could be mimicked by intraseptal injection. This makes us believe that α-MSH and somatostatin interfere with the cholinergic terminals in hippocampus, whereas substance P in some way acts by modifying the cholinergic cell

TABLE V

THE EFFECT OF INTRAVENTRICULAR INJECTION OF PEPTIDES ON CHOLINERGIC ACTIVITY IN HIPPOCAMPUS

Treatment	*nmol*	*ACh level (nmol/g protein)*	*ACh turnover (nmol/g protein/hr)*
Saline	–	280	3500 ± 900
TRH	28	220	4400 ± 800
Somatostatin	48	230	6800 ± 300*
Substance P	10	280	1700 ± 300*
α-MSH	5	340	6800 ± 500*
Neurotensin	6	220	2900 ± 400
Angiotensin II	2	300	3600

* $P < 0.05$.

bodies in the nucleus of the diagonal band. It is in this connection interesting to recall that a high density of nerve terminals is shown to contain somatostatin-like material in CA1/2 of the dorsal hippocampus (Petrusz et al., 1977) and that somatostatin excites the pyramidal cells when applied to the cell bodies in this region (Dodd and Kelly, 1978).

OTHER TRANSMITTERS

Topographical studies of GAD activity in the hippocampal region have demonstrated that the enzyme activity is bimodally distributed with peaks in the neuronal cell body layers and in the molecular layers (Fonnum and Storm-Mathisen, 1969; Storm-Mathisen and Fonnum, 1971). The bimodal localization has been confined both by autoradiography after HA uptake of GABA (Hökfelt and Ljungdahl, 1972; Iversen and Schon, 1973; Taxt et al., 1977) and after immunohistochemical demonstration of GAD (Ribak et al., 1977). Intrahippocampal injection of kainic acid was also accompanied with a major loss of GAD and GABA concomitant with the loss of hippocampal neurones (Table I; Fonnum and Walaas, 1978a). Taken together with the previously reported resistance of GAD to hippocampal deafferentation (Storm-Mathisen, 1972), these results indicate that all GAD activity is localized to intrinsic neurones in hippocampus.

The serotonergic fibres in hippocampus are mainly derived from median raphe nucleus (Lorens and Guldberg, 1974; Azmitia and Segal, 1978), but a small part may also come from the dorsal raphe (Azmitia, 1978). The fibres enter the hippocampus mainly through a dorsal route consisting of fimbria, fornix superior and cingulum and a small part ventrally passing through amygdala (Storm-Mathisen and Guldberg, 1974). Inhibition seems to be the dominant effect of serotonin in hippocampus (Stefanis, 1964, 1968). The noradrenergic projection is derived from cells in locus coeruleus (Lindvall and Björklund, 1974; Ross and Reis, 1974) and also this projection is mainly inhibitory (Stefanis, 1964; Segal and Bloom, 1974a, b). The noradrenergic fibres enter the hippocampus along 3 routes: rostrally through the septal area, along the cingulum bundle and through the piriform and entorhinal cortex (Lindvall and Björklund, 1974; Storm-Mathisen and Guldberg, 1974; for review see Lindvall and Björklund, 1978). The level of dopamine in the hippocampus is extremely low, about 1% of the noradrenaline level (Malthe-Sørenssen, personal communication) and rejects any possibility of a dopaminergic input to the hippocampus (see, however, Bischoff et al., 1979).

GLUTAMATE AS A TRANSMITTER OF OTHER HIPPOCAMPAL EFFERENTS

Recent work indicates that most fibres in the descending fornix originate in the pyramidal cells of the subiculum (Meibach and Siegel, 1977; Swanson and Cowan, 1977). These fibres have a widespread distribution with major terminal fields in the bed nucleus of stria terminalis, nucleus accumbens and the mammillary body (Swanson and Cowan, 1977). A bilateral transection of the descending fornix was therefore made. This led to a decrease in the HA GLU uptake in all these nuclei by approx. 50%, and a decrease in the level of endogenous GLU but not in ASP, glutamine or other amino acids (Table VI; Walaas and Fonnum, 1979b). These fibres therefore probably use GLU as transmitter. Thus, GLU seems to be the most important transmitter candidate of the pyramidal cells in the hippocampal formation (Fig. 3).

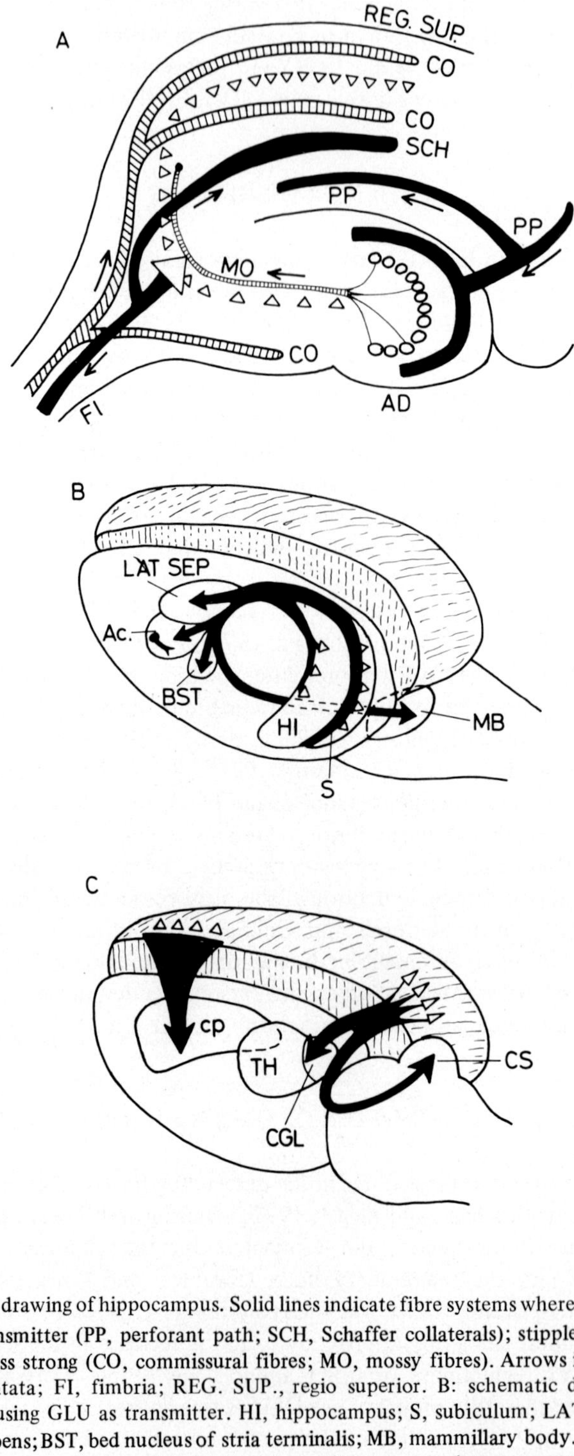

Fig. 3. A: schematic drawing of hippocampus. Solid lines indicate fibre systems where experimental evidence favours GLU as transmitter (PP, perforant path; SCH, Schaffer collaterals); stippled lines indicate fibres where evidence is less strong (CO, commissural fibres; MO, mossy fibres). Arrows indicate impulse direction. AD, area dentata; FI, fimbria; REG. SUP., regio superior. B: schematic drawing of allocortical efferents probably using GLU as transmitter. HI, hippocampus; S, subiculum; LAT SEP, lateral septum; Ac., nucleus accumbens; BST, bed nucleus of stria terminalis; MB, mammillary body. C: schematic drawing of neocortical efferents probably using GLU as transmitter. cp, caudate putamen; TH, thalamus; CGL, corpus geniculatum laterale; CS, colliculus superior.

TABLE VI

THE EFFECT OF FORNIX TRANSECTION ON HA UPTAKE OF GLU AND AMINO ACID CONTENT IN N. ACCUMBENS, BED NUCLEUS OF STRIA TERMINALIS AND CORPUS MAMMILLARE

	N. accumbens		*Bed nucleus of stria terminalis*		*Corpus mammillare*	
	N (*μmol/hr/g prot.*)	*L* (*% of N*)	*N* (*μmol/hr/g prot.*)	*L* (*% of N*)	*N* (*μmol/hr/g prot.*)	*L* (*% of N*)
HA GLU uptake	2.67 ± 0.16	48 ± 4*	1.39 ± 0.16	57 ± 8*	1.68 ± 0.08	45 ± 11*
Amino acids	(*μmol/g prot.*)	(*% of N*)	(*μmol/g dry wt.*)	(*% of N*)	(*μmol/g dry wt.*)	(*% of N*)
GLU	103	67 ± 6*	57	67 ± 7*	45	68 ± 9*
GLN	95	87	28	150	32	97
ASP	26	78	19	111	17	115
TAU	–	–	18	120	16	95
GABA	45	91	–	–	–	–

* $P < 0.02$.

TRANSMITTERS IN SEPTUM

We have already discussed the possibility that GLU may be the transmitter of CA3 axons to the lateral septal nucleus. In addition, the medial septum and especially the diagonal band nucleus display considerable HA GLU uptake. The uptake in these nuclei is resistant to local kainic acid injection (Table III), as also is the GLU uptake in the lateral septum. Thus, except for the fibres from hippocampus to the lateral septum, the origin of the putative GLU fibres in these regions is unknown. The transmitters in other afferents are incompletely known. ChAT is concentrated in the nucleus of the diagonal band and in the medial septum, while GAD is concentrated in the lateral septum (Palkovits et al., 1974; Tappaz et al., 1976; Fonnum and Walaas, 1978a). Catecholamine and serotonin fibres arrive mostly through the medial forebrain bundle (Lindvall and Björklund, 1974; Azmitia and Segal, 1978), but a transection of this bundle has no effect on ChAT or GAD activities (Fonnum et al., 1977). We have, therefore, tested whether these enzymes could be present in local neurones. Kainic acid injection into the septum decreased GAD activity, but was without effect on ChAT. When the kainate injection was into the diagonal band nucleus, however, ChAT decreased in both septum, the diagonal band nucleus and in hippocampus (Table III). It is therefore likely that most of the cholinergic fibres in the septum originate in the diagonal band nucleus. The GABA neurones in septum are probably mostly short-axon local cells.

This finding is coherent with electrophysiological work which suggests that the septal area contains inhibitory interneurones which are activated locally by recurrent collaterals (DeFrance et al., 1971, 1972; McLennan and Miller, 1974a, b).

NUCLEUS ACCUMBENS SEPTI

The nucleus accumbens has previously been considered to be a septal nucleus, mostly connected with the "limbic" system (Powell and Leman, 1976). Recent anatomical evidence, however, has indicated that the nucleus could be involved in the interaction between the limbic system and the basal ganglia (reviews Heimer and Wilson, 1975; Graybiel and Ragsdale, this volume). Nucleus accumbens may therefore have an important intermediate position as a link between limbic structures and basal ganglia, and it has been regarded by some authors as "ventral striatum". We have therefore studied the localization of neurotransmitters in n. accumbens and its efferent and afferent connections and compared the results with the transmitters of the basal ganglia (Fonnum and Walaas, 1978b; McGeer et al., this volume).

The major afferent projections to neostriatum and nucleus accumbens originate in the cortex. In the rat, nucleus accumbens receives excitatory fibres (DeFrance and Yoshihara, 1975) from the allocortex, mainly the subiculum (Swanson and Cowan, 1977), while the neostriatum receives excitatory fibres mainly from the motor cortex. Destruction of the subicular fibres leads to a 50% decrease in the HA uptake of GLU and a less pronounced, but still significant, decrease in the endogenous GLU concentration in nucleus accumbens (Table VI; Walaas and Fonnum, 1979a), whereas the fall in these parameters in neostriatum after frontal cortical lesions is even more pronounced (Table VII; Divac et al., 1977; Fonnum, 1978). No change in AAD, GAD, HA uptake of GABA or ChAT is found after these lesions, indicating that a selective population of glutamatergic fibres has been destroyed by the lesion. Light microscopic studies indicate that the neurones in the nucleus accumbens display the same sensitivity to kainic acid as those in neostriatum (Coyle et al., 1978; Walaas and Fonnum, 1979b). Stereotactic kainate injections into the nucleus accumbens have therefore been used in order to selectively destroy local neurones and were found to induce dramatic decreases in GAD and ChAT (Table VII) without affecting AAD activity (Walaas and Fonnum, 1979b). In addition, the GLU uptake decreased by 45%. The nerve terminals responsible for this GLU uptake do not belong to the fibres from subiculum, as the decrease in uptake following a combined kainate/fornix lesion is additive and results in almost 90% decrease. Thus, the major part of cholinergic and GABAergic terminals in both nucleus accumbens and neostriatum belongs to local neurones. Nucleus accumbens, unlike neostriatum, also seems to contain a considerable part of intrinsic glutamergic neurones.

The monoaminergic fibres to both neostriatum and nucleus accumbens are known to originate in the mesencephalon. The dopaminergic fibres derive from the A9 and A10 cell

TABLE VII

LESIONS INDUCING DECREASE IN TRANSMITTER MARKERS IN NEOSTRIATUM AND NUCLEUS ACCUMBENS OF RAT BRAIN

Data summarized from Fonnum et al. (1977), Schwarcz and Coyle (1977), Fonnum (1978), and Walaas and Fonnum (1979a, b)

	Neostriatum		*N. accumbens*	
Transmitter marker	*Lesions*	*% change*	*Lesions*	*% change*
AAD	hemitransection	– 85	MFB transection	– 85
ChAT	kainic acid	– 70	kainic acid	– 76
GAD	kainic acid	– 68	kainic acid	– 70
GLU uptake	frontal decortication	– 80	fornix lesion kainic acid	– 50 – 45
GLU concentration	frontal decortication	– 50	fornix lesion	– 30

groups in substantia nigra and the adjacent ventral tegmental area, respectively (Ungerstedt, 1971). The serotonergic fibres derive from the dorsal raphe (Azmitia and Segal, 1978). In agreement with this, both a hemitransection through the hypothalamus and a medial forebrain bundle (MFB) transection decrease AAD in neostriatum and nucleus accumbens respectively by 85% (Table VII; Fonnum et al., 1977; Walaas and Fonnum, 1979b).

The transmitter composition of the efferent projections of the neostriatum has been intensively investigated and important GABAergic (Fonnum et al., 1978) and peptidergic (review by McGeer et al., this volume) fibres have been found. Recently we (Walaas and Fonnum, 1979a) have obtained evidence that nucleus accumbens also has significant GABAergic fibre projections. The dominating efferent accumbens projection, the "ventral striatopallidal fibres", terminates in the rostral part of the substantia innominata, which both morphologically and histochemically seems to be a ventral extension of the globus pallidus (Heimer and Wilson, 1975; Williams et al., 1977; Walaas and Fonnum, 1979a). This region displays very high GAD activity, even higher than the activity in substantia nigra pars reticulata (Fonnum et al., 1977; Walaas and Fonnum, 1979a). Following electrocoagulation of nucleus accumbens, a consistent fall in GAD occurs both in this part and, to a slightly lesser extent, in a restricted rostroventral part of the supracommissural globus pallidus (Table VIII). In contrast, GAD in the central part of globus pallidus and other adjacent regions is unchanged, and no change in ChAT in any of these regions is found. Thus, an important GABAergic projection originates in nucleus accumbens and terminates in the rostral substantia innominata and a ventral part of the globus pallidus, in striking parallel to the GABA fibres from neostriatum to the supracommissural globus pallidus (Fonnum et al., 1978a). This gives neurochemical support to the suggestion that the accumbens fibres represent ventral striatopallidal fibres, and indicates that this part of the basal forebrain may be regarded as a "ventral pallidum" (Heimer, 1978).

In conclusion, the nucleus accumbens reveals striking similarities with neostriatum regarding the transmitter composition of afferent, local and efferent neurones. However, it should also be mentioned that there are neurochemical differences between the accumbens and neostriatum, especially regarding the concentration of peptide transmitter candidates present (Kanazawa and Jessell, 1976; Hong et al., 1977; Kobayashi et al., 1977). It is therefore for the moment probably best to regard the nucleus accumbens as a distinct entity comparable to – but not identical with – the neostriatum.

TABLE VIII

GAD IN GLOBUS PALLIDUS AND "VENTRAL PALLIDUM" AFTER ACCUMBENS LESIONS

Results given as range, summarized from Walaas and Fonnum (1979a)

Extent of lesion	*Ventral pallidum*	*Rostroventral pallidum* *per cent of control*	*Central pallidum*
Large	29 – 49*	52 – 62**	85 – 94
Intermediate	56 – 73***	65 – 87***	82 – 99
Small	96 – 99	100	108

* $P < 0.01$.
** $P < 0.02$.
*** $P < 0.05$.

SUPERIOR COLLICULUS

The superior colliculus is a layered structure which both on a functional and on an anatomical basis can be divided into a superficial visual part and a deeper non-visual part (Harting et al., 1973; Ingle and Sprague, 1975; Grofová et al., 1978). It is rather surprising, however, that so little is known about neurotransmitters in this functionally important part of the CNS when compared to other laminar structures such as hippocampus. It has previously been demonstrated in our laboratory, based on decrease in HA uptake of GLU and decrease in endogenous GLU, that glutamate is a strong candidate as neurotransmitter in the projection from the visual cortex to the superior colliculus in the rat (Lund Karlsen and Fonnum, 1978). In this species, however, in contrast to the pigeon (Henke et al., 1976), there are no indications for glutamate being a neurotransmitter in the optic nerve (Lund Karlsen, 1978). Local injection of kainic acid (0.5 μg in 0.5 μl) reduced the HA uptake of L-glutamate in the SC by 50% (Table IX), which suggests that a considerable proportion of intrinsic glutamate neurones is located in the superior colliculus. As visual cortex ablation reduced the HA uptake of glutamate to the same extent as kainic acid injection (both 50%), the glutamate uptake systems can be fully accounted for by these two lesions in the SC. This suggestion is further supported by several surgical lesions aimed to deafferentate the SC, all failing to affect glutamate transport mechanisms in the structure (commissurotomy of the SC, destruction of the connections from the inferior colliculus and destruction of the connections from the tegmental region and from the preoptic region). The GAD activity, GABA concentration and HA uptake of GABA are all very high in the superior colliculus (Okada, 1976; Lund Karlsen and Fonnum, 1978).

From previous work it has been thought that the GABA neurones, at least in the superficial layers, are purely interneurones (Okada, 1974). However, recent work has demonstrated that GABA is a putative transmitter in the nigrotectal projection (Vincent et al., 1978). Anatomically, however, this projection is described to terminate in the deeper, non-visual layers of the SC (Grofová et al., 1978). In the present work (Table IX), disruption of the nigrotectal projection reduced GAD activity to the same extent (30%) both in visual and non-visual parts of the SC. However, the surgical approach used to interrupt the nigrotectal projection (lateral knife lesion) might also have destroyed the parabigeminal projection. By kainic acid injection into the SC there was a 50% reduction in GAD activity, indicating that about 50% of GAD activity is located to interneurones. Other surgical lesions, as described previously, failed to reduce GAD activity in the SC, which is in agreement with previous work (Okada, 1974).

By histochemical staining for AChE a laminated pattern is easily demonstrated. Recent work has also shown that the deep lamina stained for AChE is organized in a columnar way (Graybiel, 1978). It has previously been described in the literature that the mesencephalic reticular nucleus projects cholinergic fibres to the third layer of the SC and that this layer further supplies the most superficial layer with cholinergic fibres (Shute and Lewis, 1967). In disagreement with this assumption, however, injection of kainic acid into the SC (even at a very high dose; 1.5 μg) failed to reduce ChAT activity in the structure (Table IX). This observation strongly suggests that the cell bodies of the cholinergic fibres supplying the most superficial layer are neither localized to layer 3, nor to intrinsic neurones of the SC. Anatomically, however, the parabigeminal nucleus is demonstrated to project to this layer (Grofová et al., 1978). In agreement with this observation, surgical interruption of the fibres from the parabigeminal nucleus to the SC reduced ChAT activity by 40% (Table IX). Complete undercutting of the SC with a tungsten wire knife intended to destroy both the con-

TABLE IX

EFFECTS OF SURGICAL AND CHEMICAL LESIONS ON CHOLINE ACETYLTRANSFERASE ACTIVITY (ChAT), GLUTAMATE DECARBOXYLASE ACTIVITY (GAD) AND HIGH AFFINITY UPTAKE OF L-GLUTAMATE (HA GLU) IN THE SUPERIOR COLLICULUS OF THE RAT

The results represent mean ± S.D. from 6 separate experiments expressed as: enzyme activity nmole/hr/mg protein; uptake activity pmole/3 min/mg protein. Enzyme activities and uptake activity after lesion are expressed in per cent of normal activities.

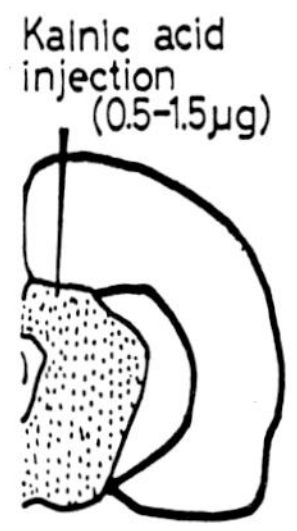

Fig. 1.

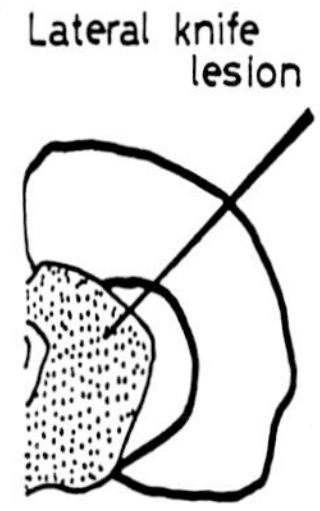

Fig. 2.

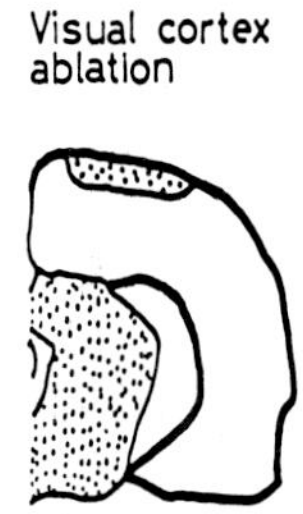

Fig. 3.

	Control values	*Kainic acid lesion*	*Lateral knife lesion*	*Visual cortex ablation*
ChAT	60.8 ± 10.2	105	55*	100
GAD	635.0 ± 23.9	41*	72*	102
HA GLU	90.5 ± 16.2	54*	93	48*

* $P < 0.05$. Wilcoxon Signed Rank Distribution Test.

nections from the mesencephalic reticular nucleus and from the parabigeminal nucleus and abolished completely the staining for AChE both in layer 1 and 3, thus supporting the neurochemical work. As previously mentioned for glutamate uptake, the other surgical lesions failed to reduce ChAT activity in the structure.

REFERENCES

Andersen, P. (1959) Interhippocampal impulses. I. Origin, course and distribution in cat, rabbit and rat. *Acta physiol. scand.*, 47: 63–90.

Andersen, P. (1975) Organization of hippocampal neurons and their interconnections. In *The Hippocampus., Vol. I,* R. L. Isaacson and K. H. Pribram (Eds.), Plenum Press, New York, pp. 155–175.

Andersen, P. (1976) Some properties of synapses near to and far from the soma of hippocampal pyramids. In *Afferent and Intrinsic Organization of Laminated Structures in the Brain,* O. Creutzfeldt (Ed.). *Exp. Brain Res.,* Suppl. I: 202–206.

Andersen, P., Bliss, T. V. P. and Skrede, K. K. (1971) Lamellar organization of hippocampal excitatory pathways. *Exp. Brain Res.,* 13: 222–238.

Andersen, P., Teyler, T. and Wester, K. (1973a) Long-lasting change of synaptic transmission in a specialized cortical pathway. *Acta physiol. scand.,* Suppl. 396: 34.

Andersen, P., Bland, B. H. and Dudar, J. (1973b) Lamellar hippocampal input to the septal nuclei. Abstract from the Meeting of the Scandinavian Physiological Society in Uppsala, 24–25th November, 1972. *Acta physiol. scand.,* 9A–10A.

Andersen, P., Bland, B. H. and Dudar, J. D. (1973c) Organization of the hippocampal output. *Exp. Brain Res.*, 17: 152–168.

Andersen, P., Silfvenius, H., Sundberg, S. H., Sveen, O. and Wigström, H. (1978) Functional characteristics of unmyelinated fibres in the hippocampal cortex. *Brain Res.*, 144: 11–18.

Azmitia, E. C. (1978) The serotonin-producing neurons of the midbrain median and dorsal raphe nuclei. In *Handbook of Psychopharmacology, Vol. 9,* L. L. Iversen, S. D. Iversen and S. H. Snyder (Eds.), Plenum Press, New York, pp. 233–314.

Azmitia, E. C. and Segal, M. (1978) An autoradiographic analysis of the differential ascending projections of the dorsal and median raphe nuclei in the rat. *J. comp. Neurol.*, 179: 641–667.

Balázs, R., Machiyama, Y. and Patel, A. I. (1973) Compartmentation and the metabolism of γ-amino-butyrate. In *Metabolic Compartmentation in the Brain,* R. Bálazs and J. E. Cremer (Eds.), Plenum Press, New York, pp. 57–70.

Balcar, V. J. and Johnston, G. A. R. (1972) The structural specificity of the high affinity uptake of L-glutamate and L-aspartate by rat brain slices. *J. Neurochem.*, 19: 2657–2666.

Beart, P. M. (1976) The autoradiographic localization of L-[^{3}H]glutamate in synaptosomal preparations. *Brain Res.*, 103: 350–355.

Bennett, J. P., Logan, W. J. and Snyder, S. M. (1973) Amino acids as central nervous transmitters: the influence of ions, amino acid analogues and ontogeny on transport systems for L-glutamic and L-aspartic acids and glycine into central nervous synaptosomes of the rat. *J. Neurochem.*, 21: 1533–1550.

Berl, S. and Clarke, D. D. (1978) Metabolic compartmentation of the glutamate-glutamine system: glial contribution. In *Amino Acids as Chemical Transmitters,* F. Fonnum (Ed.), Plenum Press, New York, pp. 691–708.

Bischoff, S., Scatton, B. and Korf, J. (1979) Biochemical evidence for a transmitter role of dopamine in the rat hippocampus. *Brain Res.*, 165: 161–165.

Blackstad, T. W. (1956) Commissural connections of the hippocampal region in the rat, with special reference to their mode of termination. *J. comp. Neurol.*, 205: 417–537.

Blackstad, T. W. (1967) Cortical gray matter. A correlation of light and electron microscopic data. In *The Neuron,* H. Hydén (Ed.), Elsevier, Amsterdam, pp. 49–118.

Blackstad, T. W. and Kjærheim, A. (1961) Special axodendritic synapses in the hippocampal cortex: electron and light microscopic studies on the layer of mossy fibres. *J. comp. Neurol.*, 117: 133–160.

Blackstad, T. W., Brink, K., Hem, J. and Jume, B. (1970) Distribution of the mossy fibres in the rat. An experimental study with silver impregnation methods. *J. comp. Neurol.*, 138: 433–450.

Blokhuis, G. G. D. and Veldstra, H. (1970) Heterogeneity of mitochondria in rat brain. *FEBS Lett.*, 2: 197–199.

Bradford, H. F. and Richards, C. D. (1976) Specific release of endogenous glutamate from piriform cortex stimulated in vitro. *Brain Res.*, 105: 168–172.

Bradford, H. F., de Belleroche, J. and Ward, H. K. (1978) On the metabolic and intrasynaptic origin of amino acid transmitters. In *Amino Acids as Chemical Transmitters,* F. Fonnum (Ed.), Plenum Press, New York, pp. 367–378.

Clark, R. M. and Collins, G. G. S. (1976) The release of endogenous amino acids from the rat visual cortex. *J. Physiol. (Lond.)*, 262: 383–400.

Cotman, C. W. and Hamberger, A. (1978) Glutamate as a CNS neurotransmitter: properties of release, inactivation and biosynthesis. In *Amino Acids as Chemical Transmitters,* F. Fonnum (Ed.), Plenum Press, New York, pp. 379–412.

Coyle, J. T., Molliver, M. E. and Kuhar, M. J. (1978) In situ injection of kainic acid: a new method for selectively lesioning neuronal cell bodies while sparing axons of passage. *J. comp. Neurol.*, 180: 301–324.

Crawford, I. L. and Connor, J. D. (1973) Localization and release of glutamic acid in relation to the hippocampal mossy fibre pathway. *Nature (Lond.)*, 244: 442–443.

Curtis, D. R. and Johnston, G. A. R. (1974) Amino acid transmitters in the mammalian central nervous system. *Ergebn. Physiol.*, 69: 98–188.

Dahlström, A. and Fuxe, K. (1965) Evidence for the existence of monoamine containing neurons in the central nervous system. I. Demonstration of monoamines in the cell bodies of brain stem neurons. *Acta physiol. scand.*, 62 (Suppl. 232): 1–55.

Davies, L. P. and Johnston, G. A. R. (1976) Uptake and release of D- and L-aspartate by rat brain slices. *J. Neurochem.*, 26: 1007–1014.

DeFrance, J. F. and Yoshihara, H. (1975) Fimbria input to the nucleus accumbens septi. *Brain Res.*, 90: 159–163.

DeFrance, J. F., Shimono, T. and Kitai, S. T. (1971) Anatomical distribution of the hippocampal fibres afferent to the lateral septal nucleus. *Brain Res.*, 34: 176–180.

DeFrance, J. F., Shimono, T. and Kitai, S. T. (1972) Hippocampal inputs to the lateral septal nucleus: patterns of facilitation and inhibition. *Brain Res.*, 37: 333–339.

DeFrance, J. F., Kitai, S. T. and Shimono, T. (1973) Electrophysiological analysis of the hippocampo-septal projections. Vol. II. Functional characteristics. *Exp. Brain Res.*, 17: 463–476.

Divac, I., Fonnum, F. and Storm-Mathisen, J. (1977) High affinity uptake of glutamate in terminals of corticostriatal axons. *Nature (Lond.)*, 266: 377–378.

Dodd, J. and Kelly, J. S. (1978) Is somatostatin an excitatory transmitter in the hippocampus? *Nature (Lond.)*, 273: 674–675.

Dudar, J. D. (1975) The effect of septal nuclei stimulation on the release of acetylcholine from the rabbit hippocampus. *Brain Res.*, 83: 123–133.

Fonnum, F. (1968) The distribution of glutamate decarboxylase and aspartate transaminase in subcellular fractions of rat and guinea-pig brain. *Biochem. J.*, 106: 291–298.

Fonnum, F. (1970) Topographical and subcellular localization of choline acetyltransferase in rat hippocampal region. *J. Neurochem.*, 17: 1029–1037.

Fonnum, F. (1972) Application of microchemical analysis and subcellular fractionation techniques to the study of neurotransmitters in discrete areas of mammalian brain. In *Advances in Biochemistry and Psychopharmacology, Vol. 6*, E. Costa, L. L. Iversen and R. Paoletti (Eds.), Raven Press, New York, pp. 75–88.

Fonnum, F. (1973) Recent developments in biochemical investigations of cholinergic transmission. *Brain Res.*, 62: 497–507.

Fonnum, F. (1977) Acetylcholine and amino acids: transmitter candidates in rhinencephalon. In *Bel-Air Symposium, V*, George and Co., Geneva, pp. 61–78.

Fonnum, F. (1978) Comments on the localization of neurotransmitters in the basal ganglia. In *Amino Acids as Chemical Transmitters*, F. Fonnum (Ed.), Plenum Press, New York, pp. 143–154.

Fonnum, F. and Storm-Mathisen, J. (1969) GABA synthesis in rat hippocampus correlated to the distribution of inhibitory neurons. *Acta physiol. scand.*, 76: 35A-37A.

Fonnum, F. and Storm-Mathisen, J. (1978) Localization of GABAergic neurons in the CNS. In *Handbook of Psychopharmacology, Vol. 9*, S. Snyder, S. D. Iversen and L. L. Iversen (Eds.), Plenum Press, New York, pp. 357–401.

Fonnum, F. and Walaas, I. (1978a) The effect of intrahippocampal kainic acid injections and surgical lesions on neurotransmitters in hippocampus and septum. *J. Neurochem.*, 31: 1173–1181.

Fonnum, F. and Walaas, I. (1978b) Neurotransmitters in neostriatum. In *Workshop on Neostriatum*, I. Divac (Ed.), in press.

Fonnum, F., Walaas, I. and Iversen, L. (1977) Localization of GABAergic, cholinergic and aminergic structures in the mesolimbic system. *J. Neurochem.*, 29: 221–230.

Fonnum, F., Gottesfeld, Z. and Grofová, I. (1978) Distribution of glutamate decarboxylase, choline acetyltransferase and aromatic amino acid decarboxylase in the basal ganglia of normal and operated rats. Evidence for striatopallidal, striatoentopeduncular and striatonigral GABAergic fibres. *Brain Res.*, 143: 125–138.

Graybiel, A. M. (1978) A stereometric pattern of distribution of acetylthiocholinesterase in the deep layers of the superior colliculus. *Nature (Lond.)*, 272: 539–541.

Grofová, I., Ottersen, O. P. and Rinvik, E. (1978) Mesencephalic and diencephalic afferents to the superior colliculus and periaqueductal gray substance demonstrated by retrograde axonal transport of horseradish peroxidase in the cat. *Brain Res.*, 146: 205–220.

Hamberger, A., Nyström, B., Sellström, A. and Woiler, C. T. (1976) Amino acid transport in isolated neurons and glia. In *Advances in Experimental Medicine and Biology, Vol. 69*, G. Levi, L. Battistin, and A. Lajtha (Eds.), Plenum Press, New York, pp. 221–237.

Hamberger, A., Sellström, Å and Woiler, C. T. (1978) Glial cells and amino acid transmitters. In *Amino Acids as Chemical Transmitters*, F. Fonnum (Ed.), Plenum Press, New York, pp. 653–662.

Harting, J. K., Hall, W. C., Diamond, I. T. and Martin, G. F. (1973) Anterograde degeneration study of the superior colliculus in *Tupaia glis:* evidence for a subdivision between superficial and deep layers. *J. comp. Neurol.*, 148: 361–386.

Hattori, T. and McGeer, E. G. (1977) Fine structural changes in the rat striatum after local injections of kainic acid. *Brain Res.*, 129: 174–180.

Heimer, L. (1978) The olfactory cortex and the ventral striatum. In *The Continuing Evaluation of the Limbic System Concept*, K. Livingston and O. Hornykiewicz (Eds.), Plenum Press, New York, pp. 95–187.

Heimer, L. and Wilson, R. (1975) The subcortical projections of the allocortex: similarities in the neural associations of the hippocampus, the piriform cortex and the neocortex. In *Perspectives in Neurobiology, Golgi Centennial Symposium,* M. Santini (Ed.), Raven Press, New York, pp. 177–193.

Henke, H., Schenker, T. M. and Cuénod, M. (1976) Effects of retinal ablation on uptake of glutamate, glycine, GABA, proline and choline in pigeon tectum. *J. Neurochem.,* 26: 131–137.

Henn, F. A., Goldstein, M. N. and Hamberger, A. (1974) Uptake of the neurotransmitter candidate glutamate by glia. *Nature (Lond.),* 249: 663–664.

Henn, F. A., Venema, R. and Sellström, Å. (1978) Interaction between neurotransmitters and astroglial cells. In *Amino Acids as Chemical Transmitters,* F. Fonnum (Ed.), Plenum Press, New York, pp. 663–668.

Hong, J. S., Yang, H.-Y. T., Fratta, W. and Costa, E. (1977) Determination of methionine enkephalin in discrete regions of rat brain. *Brain Res.,* 134: 383–386.

Hökfelt, T. and Ljungdahl, Å. (1972) Autoradiographic identification of cerebellar and cerebral cortical neurons accumulating labelled gamma-aminobutyric acid (^{3}H-GABA). *Exp. Brain Res.,* 14: 354–362.

Hökfelt, T., Johansson, O., Fuxe, K., Goldstein, M. and Park, D. (1977) Immunohistochemical studies on the localization and distribution of monoamine neuron systems in the rat brain. II. Tyrosine hydroxylase in the telencephalon. *Med. Biol.,* 55: 21–40.

Ingle, D. and Sprague, J. M. (1975) Sensorimotor function of the midbrain tectum. *Neurosci. Res. Progr. Bull.,* 13: 169–288.

Israël, M. and Whittaker, V. P. (1965) The isolation of mossy fibre endings from the granular layer of the cerebellar cortex. *Experientia (Basel),* 21: 325–326.

Iversen, L. L. and Schon, F. F. (1973) The use of autoradiographic techniques for the identification and mapping of transmitter specific neurones in CNS. In *New Concepts in Neurotransmitter Regulation,* A. J. Mandell (Ed.), Plenum Press, New York, pp. 153–193.

Iversen, L. L. and Storm-Mathisen, J. (1976) Uptake of [^{3}H]glutamic acid in excitatory nerve endings in the hippocampal formation of the rat. *Acta physiol. scand.,* 96: 22A-23A.

Jasper, H. H., Khan, R. T. and Elliott, K. A. C. (1965) Amino acid released from the cerebral cortex in relation to its state of activation. *Science,* 147a: 1448–1449.

Kanazawa, I. and Jessell, T. (1976) Post mortem changes and regional distribution of substance P in the rat and mouse nervous system. *Brain Res.,* 117: 362–367.

Kobayashi, R. M., Brown, M. and Vale, W. (1977) Regional distribution of neurotensin and somatostatin in rat brain. *Brain Res.,* 126: 584–588.

Krnjević, C. (1974) Chemical nature of synaptic transmission in vertebrates. *Physiol. Rev.,* 54: 418–540.

Lindvall, O. and Björklund, A. (1974) The organization of the ascending catecholamine neuron system in the rat brain. *Acta physiol. scand.,* Suppl. 412: 1–48.

Lindvall, O. and Björklund, A. (1978) Organization of the catecholamine neurons in the rat CNS. In *Handbook of Psychopharmacology, Vol. 9,* L. L. Iversen, S. D. Iversen and S. H. Snyder (Eds.), Plenum Press, New York, pp. 192–194.

Lorens, S. A. and Guldberg, H. C. (1974) Regional 5-hydroxytryptamine following selective midbrain raphe lesions in the rat. *Brain Res.,* 78: 45–56.

Lorente de Nó, R. (1934) Studies on the structure of the cerebral cortex. II. Continuation of the study of the ammonic system. *J. Psychol. Neurol. (Lpz.),* 46: 113–177.

Lømo, T. (1971) Patterns of activation in a monosynaptic cortical pathway: the perforant path input to the dentate area of the hippocampal formation. *Exp. Brain Res.,* 12: 18–45.

Lund Karlsen, R. (1978) Neurotransmitters in the mammalian visual system. In *Amino Acids as Chemical Transmitters,* F. Fonnum (Ed.), Plenum Press, New York, pp. 241–256.

Lund Karlsen, R. and Fonnum, F. (1978) Evidence for glutamate as a neurotransmitter in the corticofugal fibres to the dorsal lateral geniculate body and the superior colliculus in rats. *Brain Res.,* 151: 457–467.

Malthe-Sørenssen, D., Cheney, D. L. and Costa, E. (1978a) Modulation of acetylcholine metabolism in the hippocampal cholinergic pathway by intraseptally injected substance P. *J. Pharmacol. exp. Ther.,* 206: 21–28.

Malthe-Sørenssen, D., Wood, P. L., Cheney, D. L. and Costa, E. (1978b) Modulation of the turnover rate of acetylcholine in rat brain by intraventricular injections of thyrotropin-releasing hormone, somatostatin, neurotensin and angiotensin II. *J. Neurochem.,* 31: 685–691.

Martinez-Hernandez, A., Bell, K. P. and Norenberg, M. D. (1977) Glutamine synthetase glial localization in brain. *Science*, 195: 1356–1358.

McLennan, H. and Miller, J. J. (1974a) The hippocampal control of neuronal discharges on the septum of the rat. *J. Physiol. (Lond.)*, 237: 607–624.

McLennan, H. and Miller, J. J. (1974b) γ-Aminobutyric acid and inhibition in the septal nuclei of the rat. *J. Physiol. (Lond.)*, 237: 625–633.

Meibach, R. C. and Siegel, A. (1977) Efferent connections of the hippocampal formation in the rat. *Brain Res.*, 124: 197–224.

Moroni, F., Malthe-Sørenssen, D., Cheney, D. L. and Costa, E. (1978) Modulation of ACh turnover in the septal-hippocampal pathway by electrical stimulation and lesioning. *Brain Res.*, 150: 333-341.

Mulder, A. H. and Snyder, S. H. (1974) Potassium-induced release of amino acids from cerebral cortex and spinal cord slices of the rat. *Brain Res.*, 76: 297–308.

Nadler, J. V., Vaca, K. W., White, W. F., Lynch, G. S. and Cotman, C. W. (1976) Aspartate and glutamate as possible transmitters of excitatory hippocampal afferents. *Nature (Lond.)*, 260: 538–540.

Nadler, J. V., White, W. F., Vaca, K. W., Redburn, D. A. and Cotman, C. W. (1977) Characterization of putative amino acid transmitter release from slices of rat dentate gyrus. *J. Neurochem.*, 2: 279–290.

Nadler, J. V., White, W. F., Vaca, K. W., Perry, B. W. and Cotman, C. W. (1978) Biochemical correlates of transmission mediated by glutamate and aspartate. *J. Neurochem.*, 31: 147–155.

Nafstad, P. H. J. (1967) An electron microscope study on the termination of the perforant path fibres in the hippocampus and the fascia dentata. *Z. Zellforsch.*, 76: 532–542.

Neal, M. J. (1976) Amino acid transmitter substances in the vertebrate retina. *Gen. Pharmacol.*, 7: 321–332.

Norenberg, M. D. (1976) Histochemical studies in experimental portosystemic encephalopathy. *Arch. Neurol. (Chic.)*, 33: 265–269.

Oderfeld-Nowak, B., Narkiewicz, O., Bialowas, J., Dabrowska, J., Wieraszko, A. and Gradkowska, M. (1974) The influence of septal nuclei lesions on the activity of acetylcholinesterase and choline acetyltransferase in the hippocampus of the rat. *Acta Neurobiol. exp. (Warszawa)*, 34: 583–601.

Okada, Y. (1974) Distribution of γ-aminobutyric acid (GABA) in the layers of superior colliculus of rabbit. *Brain Res.*, 75: 363–365.

Okada, Y. (1976) Role of GABA in the substantia nigra. In *GABA in Nervous System Function, Kroc Foundation Series, Vol. 5*, E. Roberts, T. N. Chase and D. B. Tower (Eds.), Raven Press, New York, pp. 235–243.

Olney, J., Rhee, V. and Ho, O. L. (1974) Kainic acid: a powerful neurotoxic analogue of glutamate. *Brain Res.*, 77: 507–512.

Palkovits, M., Saavedra, M., Kobayashi, R. M. and Brownstein, M. (1974) Choline acetyltransferase content of the limbic nuclei of the rat. *Brain Res.*, 79: 443–450.

Petrusz, P., Sar, M., Crossman, G. H. and Kizer, J. S. (1977) Synaptic terminals with somatostatin-like immunoreactivity in the rat brain. *Brain Res.*, 137: 181–187.

Potashner, S. J. (1978) The spontaneous and electrically evoked release, from slices of guinea-pig cerebral cortex, of endogenous amino acids labelled via metabolism of D-[U-^{14}C]glucose. *J. Neurochem.*, 31: 177–186.

Powell, E. W. and Leman, R. B. (1976) Connections of the nucleus accumbens. *Brain Res.*, 105: 389–406.

Ramón y Cajal, S. (1911) *Histologie du Système Nerveux de l'Homme et des Vertébrés, Vol. 2*, Maloine Paris, 993 pp.

Reijnierse, G. L. A., Veldstra, H. and Van den Berg, C. J. (1975) Short-chain fatty acid synthesis in brain. *Biochem. J.*, 152: 477–484.

Ribak, C. E., Vaughn, J. E. and Saito, K. (1977) Immunocytochemical localization of glutamic acid decarboxylase in neuronal somata following colchicine inhibition of axonal transport. *Brain Res.*, 140: 315–332.

Roberts, P. J. (1976) Amino acid transport in spinal and sympathetic ganglia. In *Advances in Experimental Medicine and Biology, Vol. 69*, G. Levi, L. Battistin and A. Lajtha (Eds.), Plenum Press, New York, pp. 165–178.

Ross, R. A. and Reis, D. J. (1974) Effects of lesions of locus coeruleus on regional distribution of dopamine-β-hydroxylase activity in rat brain. *Brain Res.*, 73: 161–166.

Sandoval, M. E. and Cotman, C. W. (1978) Evaluation of glutamate as a neurotransmitter of cerebellar parallel fibres. *Neuroscience*, 3: 199–206.

Schon, F. and Kelly, J. S. (1974) Autoradiographic localization of [^{3}H]GABA and [^{3}H]glutamate over satellite glial cells. *Brain Res.,* 66: 275–288.

Schwarcz, R. and Coyle, J. T. (1977) Striatal lesions with kainic acid: neurochemical characteristics. *Brain Res.,* 127: 235–249.

Schwartzkroin, P. A. and Andersen, P. (1975) Glutamic acid sensitivity of dendrites in hippocampal slices in vitro. In *Properties of Dendrites. Advances in Neurology, Vol. 12,* G. Kreutzberg (Ed.), Raven Press, New York, pp. 45–51.

Schwartzkroin, P. A. and Prince, D. A. (1978) Cellular and field potential properties of epileptogenic hippocampal slices. *Brain Res.,* 147: 117–130.

Segal, M. and Bloom, F. E. (1974a) The action of norepinephrine in the rat hippocampus. I. Iontophoretic studies. *Brain Res.,* 72: 79–97.

Segal, M. and Bloom, F. E. (1974b) The action of norepinephrine in the rat hippocampus. II. Activation of the input pathway. *Brain Res.,* 72: 99–114.

Sellström, Å. and Hamberger, A. (1975) Neuronal and glial cell systems for γ-aminobutyric acid transport. *J. Neurochem.,* 24: 847–852.

Sethy, V. H., Kuhar, M. J., Root, R. A., Van Woert, M. A. and Aghajanian, G. K. (1973) Cholinergic neurons: Effect of acute septal lesion on acetylcholine and choline content of rat hippocampus. *Brain Res.,* 55: 481–484.

Shute, C. C. D. and Lewis, P. R. (1961) The use of cholinesterase techniques combined with operative studies to follow nervous pathways in the brain. Histochemistry of cholinesterase. *Bibl. anat. (Basel),* 2: 34–47.

Shute, C. C. D. and Lewis, P. R. (1967) The ascending cholinergic reticular system: neocortical, olfactory and subcortical projections. *Brain,* 90: 497–520.

Sieghart, W., Sellström, Å. and Henn, F. A. (1977) γ-Aminobutyric acid transport in bulk-isolated glial, C-6 glioma and ganglional glial cells. A comparison. In press.

Skrede, K. K. and Westgaard, R. H. (1971) The transverse hippocampal slice: a well-defined cortical structure maintained in vitro. *Brain Res.,* 35: 589–593.

Smith, C. M. (1974) Acetylcholine release from the cholinergic septo-hippocampal pathway. *Life Sci.,* 14: 2159–2166.

Snyder, S. H., Young, A. B., Bennett, J. P. and Mulder, A. H. (1973) Synaptic biochemistry of amino acids. *Fed. Proc.,* 32: 2039–2047.

Srebro, B. and Mellgren, S. I. (1974) Changes in postnatal development of acetylcholinesterase in the hippocampal region after early septal lesions in the rat. *Brain Res.,* 79: 119–131.

Stefanis, C. (1964) Hippocampal neurons: their responsiveness to microelectrophoretically administered endogenous amines. *Pharmacologist,* 6: 171.

Stefanis, C. (1968) Discussion of serotonin effects on central neurons. *Advanc. Pharmacol.,* 6A: 414–418.

Storm-Mathisen, J. (1972) Glutamate decarboxylase in the rat hippocampal region after lesions of the afferent fibre systems: evidence that the enzyme is localized in intrinsic neurons. *Brain Res.,* 40: 215–225.

Storm-Mathisen, J. (1977a) Localization of transmitter candidates in the brain: the hippocampal formation as a model. *Progr. Neurobiol.,* 8: 119–181.

Storm-Mathisen, J. (1977b) Glutamic acid and excitatory nerve endings: reduction of glutamic acid uptake after axotomy. *Brain Res.,* 120: 379–386.

Storm-Mathisen, J. (1978) Localization of putative transmitters in the hippocampal formation. With a note on the connections to septum and hypothalamus. In *Functions of the Septo-Hippocampal System, Ciba Found. Symp. 58,* K. Elliott and J. Whelan (Eds.), Excerpta Medica, Amsterdam, pp. 47–79.

Storm-Mathisen, J. and Fonnum, F. (1971) Quantitative histochemistry of glutamate decarboxylase in the rat hippocampal region. *J. Neurochem.,* 18: 1105–1111.

Storm-Mathisen, J. and Guldberg, H. C. (1974) 5-Hydroxytryptamine and noradrenaline in the hippocampal region: effect of transection of afferent pathways on endogenous levels, high affinity uptake and some transmitter-related enzymes. *J. Neurochem.,* 22: 793–803.

Storm-Mathisen, J. and Woxen Opsahl, M. (1978) Aspartate and/or glutamate may be transmitters in hippocampal efferents to septum and hypothalamus. *Neurosci. Lett.,* 9: 65–70.

Swanson, L. W. and Cowan, W. M. (1977) An autoradiographic study of the organization of the efferent connections of the hippocampal formation in the rat. *J. comp. Neurol.,* 172: 49–84.

Takagaki, G. (1978) Properties of the accumulation of D-[^{14}C]aspartate into rat cerebral crude synaptosomal fraction. In *Amino Acids as Chemical Transmitters,* F. Fonnum (Ed.), Plenum Press, New York, pp. 357–362.

Tappaz, M. L., Brownstein, M. J. and Palkovits, M. (1976) Distribution of glutamate decarboxylase in discrete brain nuclei. *Brain Res.*, 108: 371–379.

Taxt, T., Storm-Mathisen, J., Fonnum, F. and Iversen, L. L. (1977) Glutamate (GLU)/aspartate (ASP) in three defined systems of excitatory nerve endings in the hippocampal formation. *Proc. int. Soc. Neurochem.*, 6: 647.

Tebēcis, A. K. (1974) *Transmitters and Identified Neurons in the Mammalian Central Nervous System.* Scientechnica, Bristol, 340 pp.

Ungerstedt, U. (1971) Stereotaxic mapping of the monoamine pathways in the rat brain. *Acta physiol. scand.*, Suppl. 367: 1–48.

Van den Berg, C. J., Matheson, D. F., Ronda, G., Reijnierse, G. L. A., Blokhuis, G. G. D., Kroon, M. C., Clarke, D. D. and Garfinkel, D. (1975) A model of glutamate metabolism in brain: a biochemical analysis of a heterogeneous structure. In *Metabolic Compartmentation and Neurotransmission,* S. Berl, D. D. Clarke and D. Schneider (Eds.), Plenum Press, New York, pp. 515–558.

Vincent, S. R., Hattori, T. and McGeer, E. G. (1978) The nigrotectal projection: a biochemical and ultrastructural characterization. *Brain Res.*, 151: 159–164.

Walaas, I. and Fonnum, F. (1979a) The distribution and origin of glutamate decarboxylase and choline acetyltransferase in ventral pallidum and other basal forebrain regions. *Brain Res.*, In press.

Walaas, I. and Fonnum, F. (1979b) The effects of surgical and chemical lesions on neurotransmitter candidates in nucleus accumbens. *Neuroscience,* 4: 209–216.

Williams, D. J., Crossman, A. R. and Slater, P. (1977) The efferent projections of the nucleus accumbens in the rat. *Brain Res.*, 130: 217–227.

Wood, P. L., Malthe-Sørenssen, D., Cheney, D. L. and Costa, E. (1978) Increase of hippocampal acetylcholine turnover rate and the stretching-yawning syndrome elicited by alpha-MSH and ACTH. *Life Sci.*, 22: 673–678.

Yamamoto, C. and Matsui, S. (1976) Effect of stimulation of an excitatory nerve tract on release of glutamic acid from olfactory cortex slices in vitro. *J. Neurochem.*, 26: 487–491.

Young, A. B., Oster-Granite, M. L., Herndon, R. M. and Snyder, S. H. (1974) Glutamic acid: selective depletion by viral-induced granule cell less in hamster cerebellum. *Brain Res.*, 73: 1–13.

The Commissural Fibers in Rabbit Hippocampus: Synapses and their Transmitter

CORDULA NITSCH, JONG-KYU KIM* and CHICACO SHIMADA**

Department of Neurobiology, Max-Planck-Institut für Hirnforschung, Deutschordenstr. 46, Frankfurt/M. (G.F.R.)

INTRODUCTION

In the last years, evidence has grown indicating that the highly excitatory amino acid L-glutamic acid (Glu), is a major neurotransmitter in hippocampus. In particular, it has been proposed that Glu is the transmitter in the intrahippocampal mossy fiber system (Crawford and Connor, 1973), of the hippocampo-subicular efferents (Nitsch et al., 1978; Storm-Mathisen and Woxen Opsahl, 1978) and of the entorhinal perforant path fibers (Nadler et al., 1976; Storm-Mathisen, 1977; White et al., 1977). Controversy still exists as to whether Glu (Storm-Mathisen, 1977) or the other neuroexcitatory amino acid, L-aspartic acid (Asp) (Nadler et al., 1976, 1978), is the specific neurotransmitter of the interhippocampal commissural system.

Most of the present data have been obtained by studying high affinity membrane transport or Ca^{2+}-evoked release. Since Glu is a major metabolite (Balázs et al., 1973), identification as a neurotransmitter based on its decrease in the target area of a lesioned pathway has been questioned (Nadler et al., 1978). Nevertheless, Kim et al. (1977) observed a significant decrease in striatal Glu content – which is absent for other neurotransmitter candidates – 4 weeks after ablation of the frontal motor cortex in rats. These findings not only parallel the observations of Divac et al. (1977) and McGeer et al. (1977) on reduced Glu uptake in striatum after this kind of lesion, suggesting that Glu is the neurotransmitter of the cortico-striatal projections, but also indicate that it is well possible to observe decreases in Glu concentration in the target regions of Glu-ergic pathways. The hippocampus as a layered structure offers itself for a more detailed analysis of Glu content by studying its concentration in well defined, functionally and morphologically rather uniform layers. Thus, using a highly sensitive assay system for Glu, we studied the distribution of this amino acid in single layers of the rabbit hippocampus after complete removal of its commissural input.

---

* On leave of absence from: Department of Physiology, Catholic Medical College, Seoul 110, Korea.

** Permanent address: Department of Neurochemistry, Tokyo Metropolitan Institute for Neurosciences, Fuchu-shi, Tokyo, Japan.

METHODS

In male rabbits, anesthetized with phenobarbital, the entire hippocampal-subicular formation was removed by suction through a small hole in the parietal bone (Fig. 1). Rabbits with a lesion of the parietal cortex served as sham-operated controls. The animals were allowed to survive for 20 days, since directly after removal of large brain regions, the level of several amino acids may be altered, but will have returned to normal 3–4 weeks after operation, whereas only the specific transmitter will remain decreased in the target area of the removed brain structure (Kim et al., 1977).

Freeze-dried, 16 μm thick perpendicular sections of the hippocampus contralateral to the lesion were prepared as already described (Nitsch and Okada, 1979). From the sections, single layers were dissected out under the stereomicroscope as shown in Fig. 2. The samples were weighed using a fishpole quartz-fiber balance weighing in the range of 0.1–0.4 μg, and then introduced into the oil well (Lowry and Passonneau, 1972). The principle of the assay is the determination of Glu via the enzymatic production of NADH. The NADH present is amplified, using the NAD-cycling procedure described by Kato et al. (1973). The product of the cycling reaction, malate, is determined fluorometrically after formation of NADH with malate dehydrogenase. For details of the procedure see Nitsch and Okada (1979).

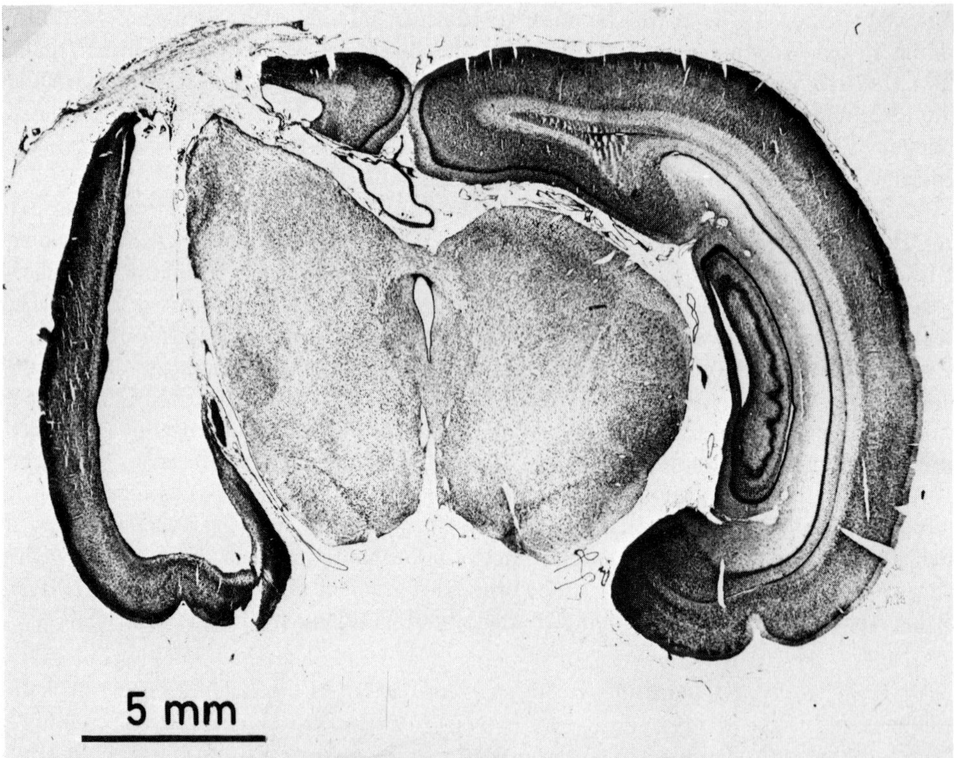

Fig. 1. Rabbit, formalin perfusion 20 days after unilateral hippocampus extirpation. Cresyl violet-stained coronal paraffin section.

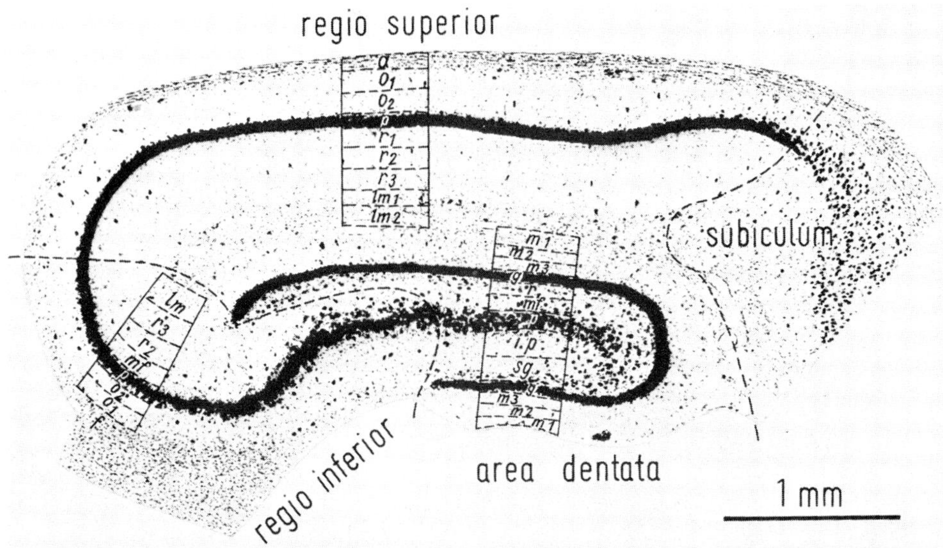

Fig. 2. Cresyl violet-stained perpendicular section of rabbit hippocampus. The subdivision of the hippocampal fields, regio superior, regio inferior and area dentata, in individual layers is indicated as cut under the stereomicroscope from freeze-dried sections. Abbreviations: a, alveus; f, fimbria; g, stratum granulare; ip, infrapyramidal layer; lm, stratum lacunosum moleculare; m, stratum moleculare; mf, mossy fiber layer or stratum lucidum; o, stratum oriens; p, stratum pyramidale; r, stratum radiatum; sg, subgranular layer. The indices indicate the splitting of a stratum in several layers.

To control on a substructural level the extent of the commissural deafferentation after this type of lesion, rabbits were perfused transaortically with an aldehyde fixative, 2, 4 and 6 days after unilateral hippocampus extirpation. Samples of regional brain areas were processed for electron microscopy.

RESULTS AND DISCUSSION

Two to 6 days after unilateral hippocampus extirpation, numerous axon terminals in the target layers of the commissural pathways exhibited typical signs of degeneration such as shrinkage of the bouton, darkening of its matrix, clumping of the vesicles, and engulfment of the boutons by astroglial processes (Figs. 3 and 4). Numerous axon terminals degenerated along the whole extent of the stratum oriens, in the regio superior (Fig. 3a), in the regio inferior (Fig. 4a), and in the infrapyramidal zone of the hilus area dentata. Thus, also with the present preparation, we could confirm that a major part of the commissural pathway ends in the stratum oriens (Stephan, 1975; Hjorth-Simonsen, 1977).

Twenty days after the lesion, the Glu concentration after hippocampus extirpation, as compared with the sham-operated controls, was significantly decreased in stratum oriens of the hippocampus proper and in the infrapyramidal and subgranular layers of the area dentata (Fig. 5). The overall largest decrease with 35% was present in o_1 of the regio superior. This result indicates that Glu is located in the commissural nerve endings in stratum oriens. In view of the evidence from other systems (Kim et al., 1977; Lund Karlsen and Fonnum,

1978) and other neurotransmitters (Pepeu et al., 1973; Sethy et al., 1973; Storm-Mathisen and Guldberg, 1974), it may be speculated that the commissural system is using Glu as its transmitter. The role of the other possible neurotransmitter in this system, Asp, and its behavior after commissural deafferentation remain to be established.

Extensive degeneration of terminal and en passant boutons was also observed in the center of the stratum radiatum, in the regio superior (Fig. 3b), and in the regio inferior directly adjacent to the stratum lucidum and sometimes even intruding into this layer

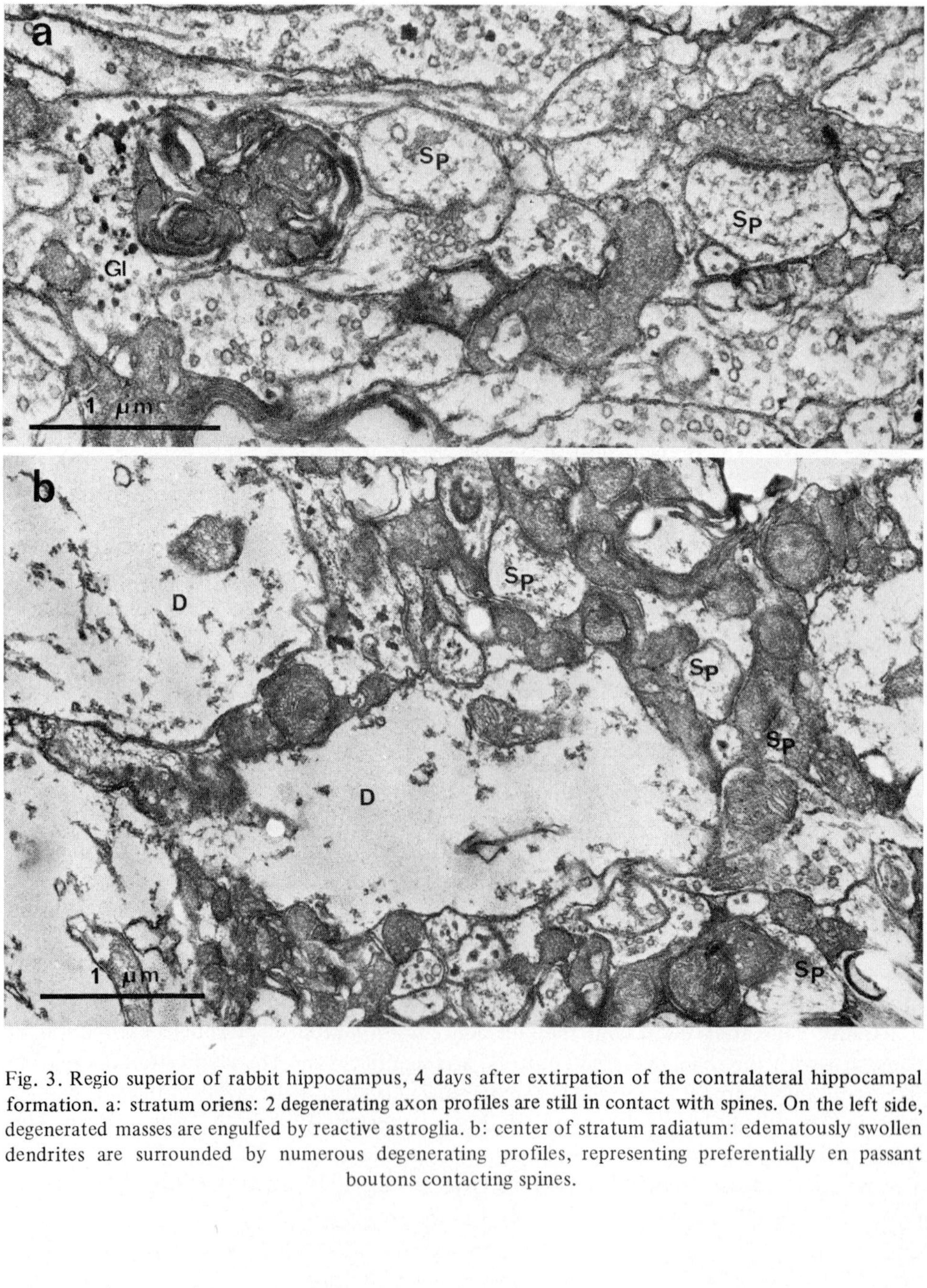

Fig. 3. Regio superior of rabbit hippocampus, 4 days after extirpation of the contralateral hippocampal formation. a: stratum oriens: 2 degenerating axon profiles are still in contact with spines. On the left side, degenerated masses are engulfed by reactive astroglia. b: center of stratum radiatum: edematously swollen dendrites are surrounded by numerous degenerating profiles, representing preferentially en passant boutons contacting spines.

(Fig. 4b). The same is true for the juxtagranular third of the stratum moleculare, in confirmation with the earlier reports of Hjorth-Simonsen (1977) and Stephan (1975). In these layers, the Glu content 20 days after hippocampus extirpation was either unchanged (in r_2 of regio superior and m_3 of area dentata) or even increased (in r_1 and r_3 of regio superior and r_2 of regio inferior, Fig. 5). In addition, significant increases in the Glu level took place after hippocampus extirpation in some layers in which no degenerated boutons were found, and which were situated adjacent to those denervated zones in which no Glu decrease occurred (in r_3 and lm_{1-2} of regio superior, in mf of regio inferior and in m_2 of the dentate stratum moleculare, Fig. 5).

These increases in Glu level could be caused by a deranged metabolism resulting from extensive degeneration and reactive gliosis, indicated by the insignificantly increased Glu levels in the cell layers. Nevertheless, this hypothesis does not explain why Glu decreases significantly in stratum oriens, but not in the other layers receiving commissural afferents.

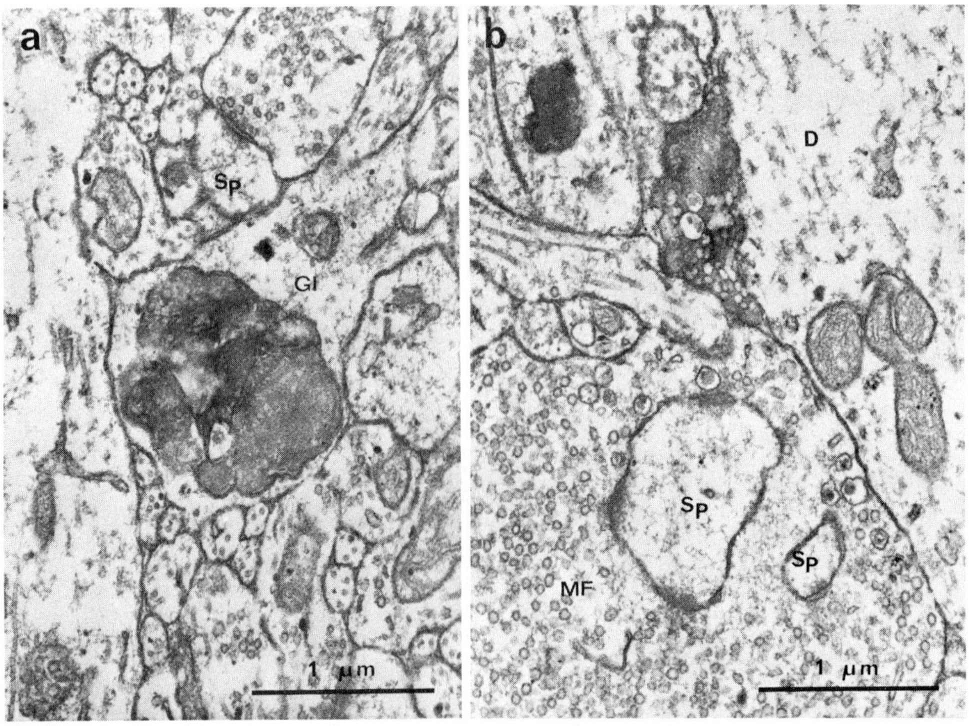

Fig. 4. Regio inferior of rabbit hippocampus, 4 days after extirpation of the contralateral hippocampal formation. a: stratum oriens: a degenerated profile, in which still vesicular and mitochondrial structures can be recognized, is completely engulfed by reactive astroglia. b: border between stratum lucidum and stratum radiatum: directly adjacent to a giant mossy fiber bouton, a degenerating axon terminal with numerous vesicles is contacting the apical dendrite of a pyramidal cell.

Most of the layers exhibiting increased Glu levels after disruption of the commissural input do contain either endings of the Schaffer's collaterals or receive entorhinal perforant path fibers (Stephan, 1975). The entorhinal afferents probably use Glu as a neurotransmitter (Nadler et al., 1976; Storm-Mathisen, 1977; White et al., 1977). Glu may also be located in the Schaffer's collaterals, since these are collaterals of the hippocampo-septal fibers, which probably use this amino acid as neurotransmitter (Nitsch et al., 1979; Storm-Mathisen and Woxen Opsahl, 1978). In contrast, in the stratum oriens, the only major input besides the commissural one is the cholinergic septo-hippocampal pathway (Lewis et al., 1967).

Sprouting of nerve fibers into denervated zones has been shown to occur as early as 5 days after denervation, as for example the proliferation of septal fibers into layers normally possessed by the terminals of the entorhinal perforant path (Nadler et al., 1977). Since in the present experiments the survival time after deafferentation was 20 days, such a sprouting of neighboring axons may have taken place. In the case of the stratum radiatum and the

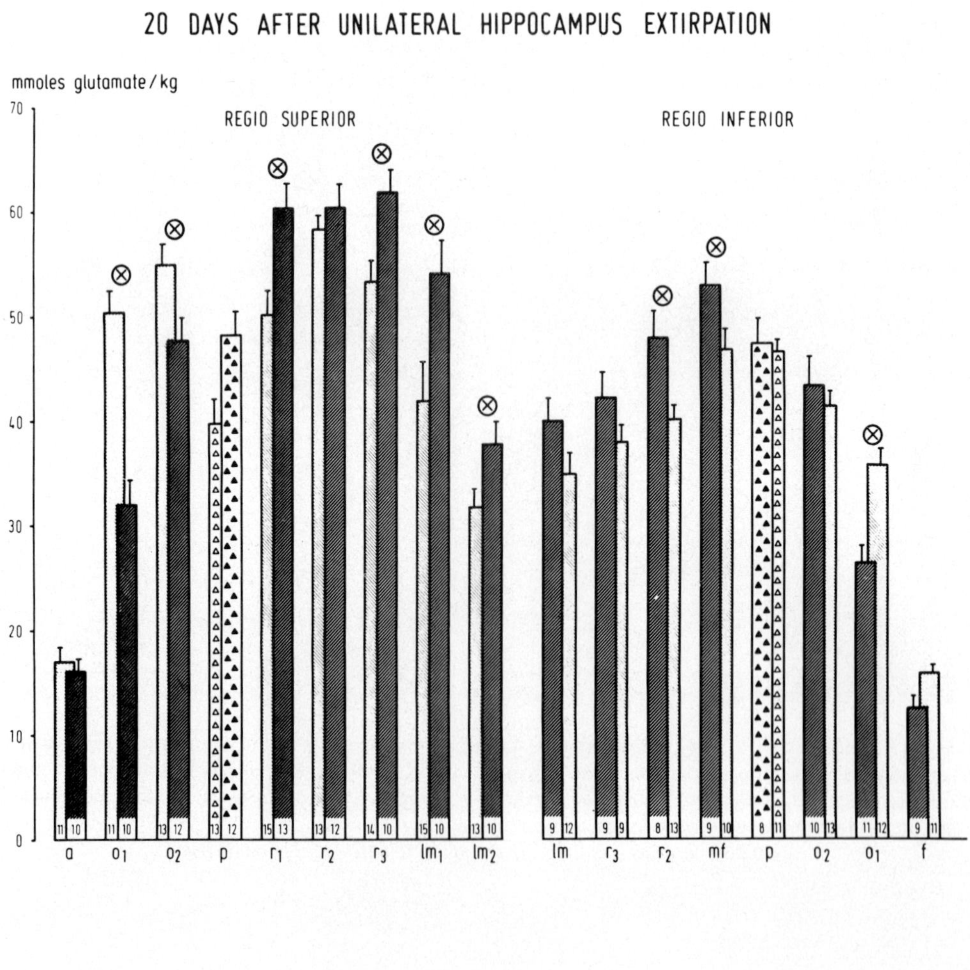

stratum moleculare, the proliferation of adjacent Glu-ergic fibers may have resulted in the normalization of Glu levels, whereas in the stratum oriens sprouting of cholinergic endings will not have this effect. The increased Glu content in those layers where the sprouting originates may be taken as a reflection of the proliferation of these afferents into the denervated zones.

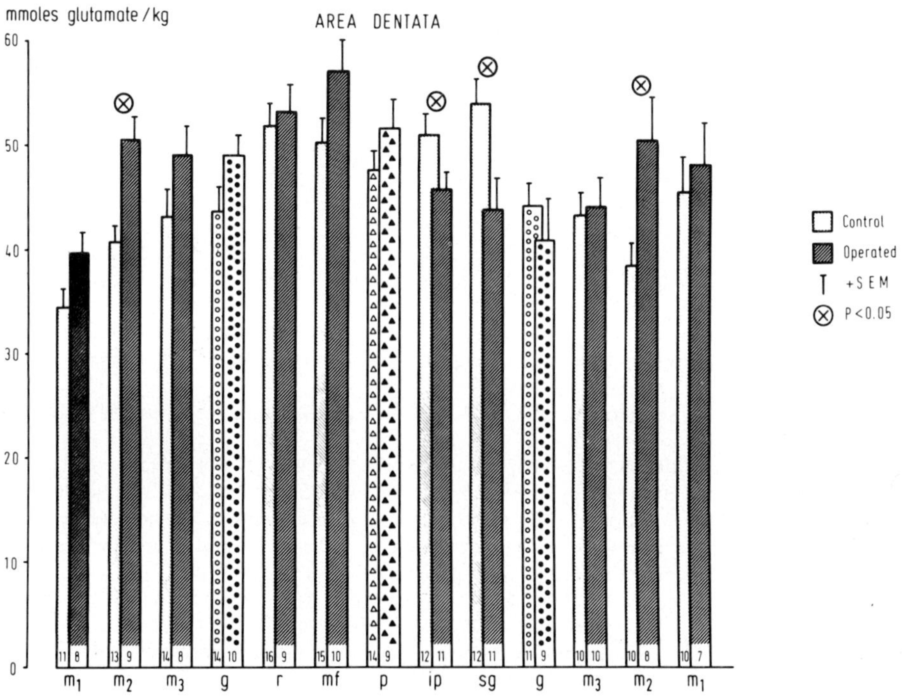

Fig. 5. Histogram of the Glu content in the individual layers of the rabbit hippocampus, in sham-operated controls and 20 days after hippocampus extirpation. Values are given in mmoles/kg dry tissue ± S.E.M. (vertical bars). The number of assays per layer is indicated at the bottom of the column. The abbreviations are the same as in Fig. 2.

SUMMARY

In rabbits, a complete unilateral hippocampus extirpation was performed. The degree of commissural deafferentation in the contralateral hippocampus was investigated electron microscopically. Glutamate (Glu) levels were determined in single layers of the hippocampal fields, regio superior, regio inferior and area dentata, 20 days after the operation and compared to those found in sham-operated controls. After commissural deafferentation, Glu content decreased significantly in stratum oriens, but no decreases were observed in the other layers receiving commissural endings. Additionally, Glu level increased in layers containing the supposed Glu-ergic terminals of the entorhinal perforant path fibers and the Schaffer's collaterals. To explain these findings, it is proposed that Glu is located in the commissural nerve endings, but that as a result of the sprouting of neighboring Glu-ergic terminals of other origin, Glu content may normalize in some of the denervated zones.

REFERENCES

Balázs, R., Patel, A. J. and Richter, D. (1973) Metabolic compartments in the brain: their properties and relation to morphological structures. In *Metabolic Compartmentation in the Brain*, R. Balázs and J. E. Cremer (Eds.), MacMillan, London, pp. 167–184.

Crawford, I. L. and Connor, J. D. (1973) Localization and release of glutamic acid in relation to hippocampal mossy fiber pathway. *Nature (Lond.)*, 244: 442–443.

Divac, I., Fonnum, F. and Storm-Mathisen, J. (1977) High affinity uptake of glutamate in terminals of corticostriatal axons. *Nature (Lond.)*, 266: 377–378.

Hjorth-Simonsen, A. (1977) Distribution of commissural afferents to the hippocampus of the rabbit. *J. comp. Neurol.*, 176: 495–514.

Kato, T., Berger, S. J., Carter, J. A. and Lowry, O. H. (1973) An enzymatic cycling method for nicotinamide-adenine dinucleotide with malic and alcohol dehydrogenases. *Anal. Biochem.*, 35: 86–97.

Kim, J. S., Hassler, R., Haug, P. and Paik, K.-S. (1977) Effect of frontal cortex ablation on striatal glutamic acid level in rat. *Brain Res.*, 132: 370–374.

Lewis, P. R., Shute, C. C. D. and Silver, A. (1967) Confirmation from choline acetylase analysis of a massive cholinergic innervation to the rat hippocampus. *J. Physiol. (Lond.)*, 191: 215–224.

Lowry, O. H. and Passonneau, J. V. (1972) *A Flexible System of Enzymatic Analysis.* Academic Press, New York.

Lund Karlsen, R. and Fonnum, F. (1978) Evidence for glutamate as a neurotransmitter in corticofugal fibers to the dorsal lateral geniculate body and the superior colliculus in rats. *Brain Res.*, 151: 457–467.

McGeer, P. L., McGeer, E. G., Scherer, U. and Singh, K. (1977) A glutamatergic corticostriatal path? *Brain Res.*, 128: 369–373.

Nadler, J. V., Vaca, K. W., White, W. F., Lynch, G. S. and Cotman, C. W. (1976) Aspartate and glutamate as possible transmitters of excitatory hippocampal afferents. *Nature (Lond.)*, 260: 538–540.

Nadler, J. V., Cotman, C. W. and Lynch, G. S. (1977) Histochemical evidence of altered development of cholinergic fibers in the rat dentate gyrus following lesions. I. Time course after complete unilateral entorhinal lesion at various ages. *J. comp. Neurol.*, 171: 561–588.

Nadler, J. V., White, W. F., Vaca, K. W., Perry, B. W. and Cotman, C. W. (1978) Biochemical correlates of transmission mediated by glutamate and aspartate. *J. Neurochem.*, 31: 147–155.

Nitsch, C. and Okada, Y. (1979) Distribution of glutamate in layers of the rabbit hippocampal fields CA1, CA3, and dentate area. *J. Neurosci. Res.*, in press.

Nitsch, C., Kim, J.-K., Shimada, C. and Okada, Y. (1979) Effect of hippocampus extirpation in the rat on glutamate level in target structures of hippocampal efferents. *Neurosci. Lett.*, 11: 295–299.

Pepeu, G., Mulas, A. and Mulas, M. L. (1973) Changes in the acetylcholine content in the rat brain after lesions of the septum, fimbria, and hippocampus. *Brain Res.*, 57: 153–164.

Sethy, V. H., Roth, R. H., Kuhar, M. J. and Van Woert, M. H. (1973) Choline and acetylcholine: regional distribution and effect of degeneration of cholinergic nerve terminals in the rat hippocampus. *Neuropharmacology,* 12: 819–823.

Stephan, H. (1975) *Allocortex. Handbuch der mikroskopischen Anatomie des Menschen, 4. Band, Nervensystem, 9. Teil.* Springer, Berlin, pp. 494–602.

Storm-Mathisen, J. (1977) Glutamic acid and excitatory nerve endings: reduction of glutamic acid uptake after axotomy. *Brain Res.,* 120: 379–386.

Storm-Mathisen, J. and Guldberg, H. C. (1974) 5-Hydroxytryptamine and noradrenaline in the hippocampal region: effect of transection of afferent pathways on endogenous levels, high affinity uptake and some transmitter-related enzymes. *J. Neurochem.,* 22: 793–803.

Storm-Mathisen, J. and Woxen Opsahl, M. (1978) Aspartate and/or glutamate may be transmitters in hippocampal efferents to septum and hypothalamus. *Neurosci. Lett.,* 9: 65–70.

White, W. F., Nadler, J. V., Hamberger, A., Cotman, C. W. and Cummins, J. T. (1977) Glutamate as transmitter of hippocampal perforant path. *Nature (Lond.),* 270: 356–357.

Specificity of Synaptic Growth in Brain: Remodeling Induced by Kainic Acid Lesions

CARL W. COTMAN

Department of Psychobiology, University of California, Irvine, Calif. 92717 (U.S.A)

INTRODUCTION

The basic circuitry of the brain is formed during development. However, brain circuitry is not fixed once it is formed. Even in the adult it is plastic, mutable, so that many perturbations, from environmental to experimental, can initiate new functional connections. Data providing the strongest support for this concept arise from studies of the responses elicited by partial denervation. Destruction of a portion of the input to a target often allows the remaining undamaged inputs to grow and create new functional synapses. This phenomenon is commonly referred to as axon sprouting or reactive synaptogenesis.

The initial suggestion that partial denervation can induce new synapse formation originated from studies of the neuromuscular junction. In 1885, Exner suggested that the rapid recovery of neuromuscular contraction following partial transection of a motor nerve, but prior to regeneration, might be the result of fiber sprouting and the growth of new connections by the residual fibers. In the late forties and early fifties Edds (1950), Hoffmann (1950) and others showed by anatomical and histochemical methods that this was in fact the case. Studies of reactive fiber growth in response to denervation were extended to nerve-nerve connections in the sympathetic ganglion by Murray and Thompson in 1957, to the spinal cord in 1958 by Liu and Chambers and to the brain in 1969 by Raisman.

The basic paradigm in all such studies involves removing a portion of the input by various experimental means, and examining, over time, the response of the remaining afferents using anatomical, chemical or electrophysiological methods. It is now clear that new connections will form in response to denervation in a number of areas throughout the brain (see Cotman, 1978). At present, studies in the hippocampus provide the most thorough documentation of the nature of these events in the brain and their underlying mechanisms.

GENERAL PRINCIPLES

As a result of studies in the hippocampus and a variety of other brain systems, it is possible to derive the following general conclusions (Cotman and Lynch, 1976; Cotman and Nadler, 1978).

(1) Partial denervation stimulates some fibers to grow and form new synapses. These synapses usually are similar in overall appearance to the original ones. In the cases where the synapses have been tested they are functional.

(2) In mature animals synapses first form at approximately 5–9 days after a lesion; synaptogenesis may continue for 1–2 months.

(3) The rate of reactive fiber growth can be changed. It can be accelerated if a small lesion precedes, by a few days, a larger one; it can be slowed down by the administration of glucocorticoids.

(4) The capacity to form new synapses in response to a lesion persists throughout the life of an animal. It occurs in aged animals as well as mature adults although in aged animals the rate is slower and the extent of growth is reduced.

(5) Synapse formation is selective in that only particular afferents respond in particular places to particular lesions. An afferent reactive to one type of lesion may not respond to another.

(6) In the adult nervous system, an efferent cannot reinnervate a new cell type. Existing inputs to a cell are increased and/or reorganized. Synapses may grow into areas of a dendritic field not previously innervated, i.e. grow outside their normal lamina. In all cases studied so far reactive afferents are adjacent to a denervated zone.

CURRENT MAJOR ISSUES

The most critical issue at present is to understand the basis of selectivity. Why do only particular afferents grow to particular places? The answer to this question would give considerable insight into reactive synaptogenesis. It has often been suggested that reactive synaptogenesis may not simply be a repair process, but that it may reflect an underlying mechanism the brain has at its disposal to remodel its circuitry throughout life. Studies on the specificity of synapse formation induced by lesions may provide clues on the hierarchy of changes normally permissible and their underlying mechanisms. More directly, knowledge of which fibers will reconnect should provide a basis to predict the usefulness of circuitry rearrangements for the recovery of function after brain damage. Will the new connections aid or hinder recovery? It might be possible to encourage beneficial changes and discourage nonbeneficial ones.

In this paper I shall describe the basic changes which take place in the hippocampus following select lesions and I will examine some of the basic mechanisms insofar as they are understood. Through the use of kainic acid we have recently been able to gain new insights into the nature of reactive synaptogenesis.

Kainic acid was isolated in 1953 by Murakami and coworkers as the active ingredient in a crude extract of the red marine alga *Digenea simplex* used in the treatment of ascariasis. Subsequently it has been found that kainic acid is a cytotoxic agent structurally related to glutamate which destroys cell bodies while sparing those afferents impinging on these cells (see McGeer et al., 1978; Nadler, 1978). The use of kainic acid in the hippocampus has enabled us to selectively destroy cell groups previously inaccessible to experimental manipulation. This has made it possible to examine a number of questions on selectivity which previously could not be studied in detail. Is selectivity in reactive synaptogenesis related at all to the nature of the transmitter? To the nearest fibers? To the most abundant afferent? To the extent of denervation? To selective initiation of growth only in particular fibers?

Besides serving as an experimental approach for understanding selectivity, the use of kainic acid provides, for the first time, a means to experimentally imitate the cell loss that occurs in the hippocampus as a result of stroke, epilepsy and senile dementia. The hippocampus is well known to be a primary target of these dibilitating diseases (Minckler, 1971; Blackwood and Corsellius, 1976). What, if any, is the nature of synaptic growth and recovery following the loss of intrinsic cell populations?

BASIC ORGANIZATION OF THE HIPPOCAMPUS

The hippocampal formation consists of the dentate gyrus and the hippocampus proper which is divided into subfields CA1, CA2, CA3 and CA4 (see Fig. 1). The hippocampal formation offers a number of important advantages for studies on reactive growth. It contains predominately two cell types, pyramidal cells in the hippocampal fields and granule cells in the dentate gyrus. These neurons and their axonal and dendritic processes are well separated by a large scale regional architecture. The circuitry within the hippocampus is relatively simple and well defined. Extrinsic inputs arise primarily from the septum, entorhinal cortex and various brain stem nuclei. Intrinsic inputs include several intrahippocampal projections as well as reciprocal connections between the two hippocampi. These, plus a few interneurons, appear to account for the vast majority of all connections. The connections are organized in discrete lamina, as we shall discuss (see Cotman and Nadler (1978) for a recent comprehensive review of hippocampal circuitry).

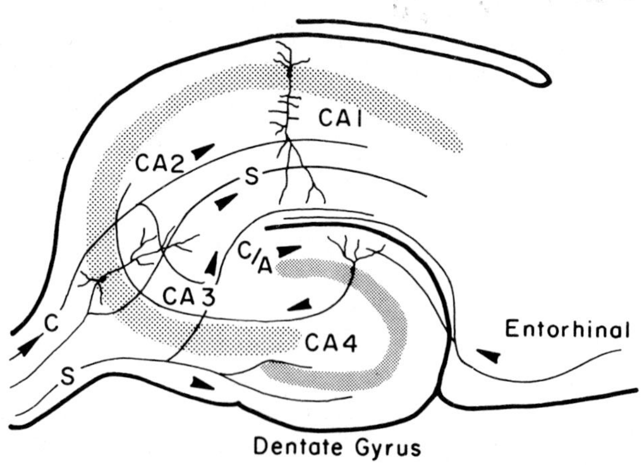

Fig. 1. Schematic of the hippocampus showing the major subfields and connections.

INTRAVENTRICULAR KAINIC ACID

We have studied the effects of intraventricularly administered kainic acid as a means of selectively eliminating hippocampal neurons. We have found that the type of response obtained depends markedly on the dose administered (Nadler et al., 1978a, c). Low doses (0.1–0.3 μg) act quite selectively on CA3 pyramidal neurons. By 3 days after kainic acid administration, sections stained with cresyl violet show an extensive reduction in CA3 neurons (see Fig. 2). Most pyramidal cells are lost from areas CA3a and CA3b and a few are absent

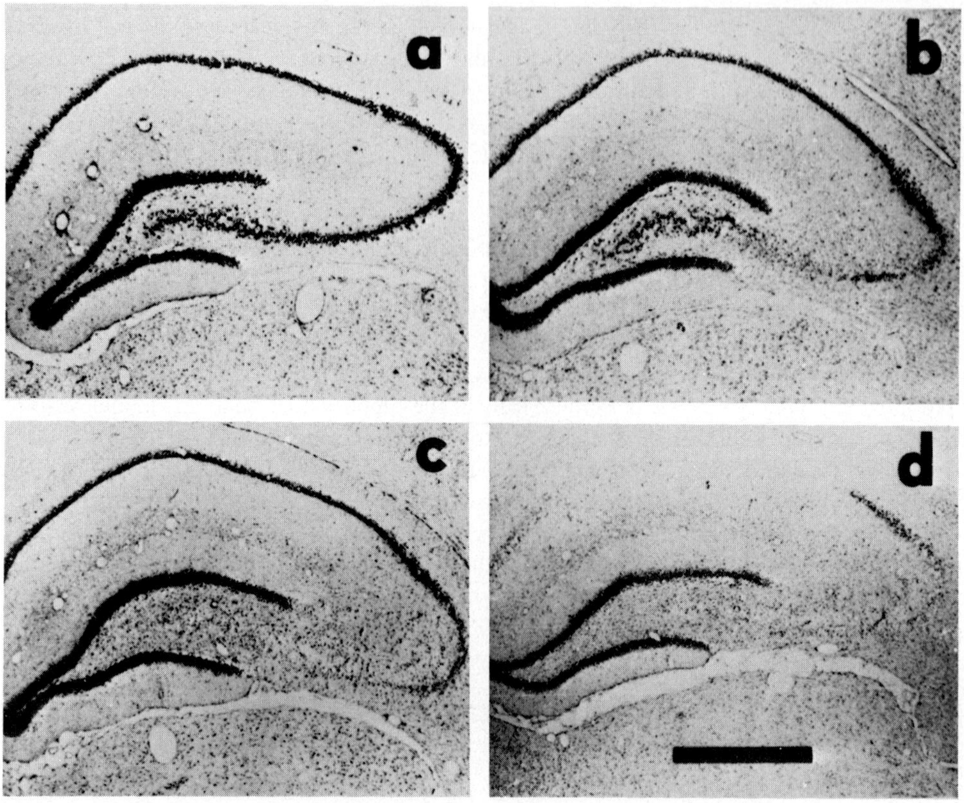

Fig. 2. Effect of intraventricular kainic acid on hippocampal neurons. a: vehicle injected; b: 0.3 μg; c: 0.8 μg; d: 1.1 μg. All pictures are from animals 3 days after the injection.

from area CA3c. Cell loss is greatest in the septal portion of the hippocampus. Granule cells, CA2, and CA1 neurons are not killed at this dose.

At higher concentrations (approximately 1.1 μg), kainic acid has a remarkable effect. In addition to the loss of the CA3 neurons, subfields CA4 and CA1 are destroyed. Dentate granule cells are resistant to kainic acid as are CA2 cells.

Intermediate doses (0.8 μg) produce a relatively selective lesion of CA3 and CA4 pyramidal cells. More than 90% of CA3 cells are lost as well as most CA4 cells except those at the apex of the dentate. CA1 is unaffected as are CA2 pyramidal cells and dentate granule cells. Some subicular neurons are lost. Doses above about 3 μg are usually fatal, and in the few animals which survive, hippocampal destruction is massive.

Thus, kainic acid appears to destroy specific intrinsic hippocampal neurons as a function of the applied dose. From our studies, we have identified the order of sensitivity to kainic acid as CA3a pyramids $>$ CA3b pyramids, CA3c pyramids $>$ CA4 pyramids = subicular pyramids $>$ CA1 pyramids $>$ CA2 pyramids $\gg$ dentate granule cells. Kainic acid does not appear to damage extrinsic afferents or intrinsic connections other than those emanating from the cells which are destroyed. The septal projection, for example, remains intact. The presence of acetylcholinesterase (AChE) in the cholinergic septohippocampal fibers provides a simple, convenient means of studying this projection. Following kainic acid there is no demonstrable loss in AChE staining in the hippocampus indicating that the septal afferents remain intact, despite the loss of intrinsic hippocampal neurons.

Before turning to a discussion of reactive growth, it is appropriate to comment on the selectivity of kainic acid. It is clear that kainic acid at low concentrations acts selectively on the hippocampus. Intraventricular kainic acid also affects structures outside the hippocampus when used at high concentrations. For example, at low doses (approximately 0.5 μg) there is occasional damage in the lateral septum adjacent to the site of injection but little damage elsewhere. Thus, at these or lower doses, kainic acid produces a fairly pure hippocampal lesion. With increasing doses, degenerating neurons appear in some of the thalamic nuclei, amygdala and deep layers of the cerebral cortex. No degenerating cells are seen in areas known to project to the hippocampal formation, except in nucleus reuniens of the thalamus and layer III of the entorhinal cortex. The striatum and hypothalamus are invariably spared, except for the lateral nucleus and premammillary area at high doses.

The basis of selectivity in the hippocampus is not known, but it is not due to selective diffusion since, within the hippocampus, the CA2 field and granule cells are spared even when CA1 or CA4 neurons are destroyed. Also, areas directly adjacent to the injection site, such as the medial septum, are unaffected. Kainic acid appears to exert its effect directly on the hippocampus and not through an action elsewhere in the brain since low doses injected directly into the hippocampus produce a similar hierarchy of destruction.

In order to obtain selective destruction of hippocampal neurons by intraventricular administration, we have found it necessary to carefully regulate the dose and the time over which the drug is administered. We inject kainic acid over a 30 min period at a fairly constant rate in order to minimize local concentration gradients and non-selective destruction. Rapid administration of high concentrations directly into brain tissue destroys most cells, illustrating that kainic acid can be non-selective when not precisely controlled.

We have found that the effects of kainic acid are not confined to adults but can be used as an effective cytotoxic agent in developing animals. Intraventricular kainic acid, as in adults, generally spares granule cells and acts preferentially on the hippocampal subfields. The main difference appears to be that the effective doses required are approximately 10-fold higher.

REORGANIZATION WITHIN THE HIPPOCAMPUS AFTER KAINIC ACID LESIONS

As mentioned above, one of our goals in pursuing studies with kainic acid is to examine the response to a clinically relevant form of hippocampal damage. Kainic acid lesions in rats closely mimic the selective destruction of hippocampal neurons seen in man following various neural pathologies. The CA3 field in the rat is homologous to the end folium in man, a subfield of hippocampus particularly susceptible to disease. The CA1 area plus subiculum of the rat is homologous to the Somner sector in man, an area also susceptible to disease. CA2 pyramidal cells, homologous to h_2 cells in man, and dentate granule cells are nearly always spared. Thus, the lesion produced by 1.1 μg of kainic acid appears very similar to that which results from various human pathologies. In view of this finding, and the potential for mechanistic analyses not possible with other lesions, we performed a variety of histological and ultrastructural studies to determine whether the connections destroyed by kainic acid are replaced.

Rats were injected bilaterally with an intermediate dose of kainic acid and the extent of reinnervation was studied. As noted above, intermediate doses of kainic acid (0.8 μg) destroy nearly every CA3 and CA4 pyramidal cell. In normal or vehicle-injected rats, the synaptic density in stratum radiatum of CA1 is about 35 synapses/100·μm^2. In animals sacrificed

1–7 days after kainic acid injection, there is extensive presynaptic degeneration in this zone and the synaptic density falls to about 6 synapses/100 μm^2. This reflects the loss of the dense innervation by the Schaffer collateral and commissural fibers. Many of the residual synapses feature boutons with flattened vesicles in symmetric contact, characteristics thought to signify inhibitory connections. A few asymmetric excitatory contacts are also preserved. Do the synapses return over time and, if so, what are their sources?

When stratum radiatum is examined at 41 or 55 days after kainic acid administration, the synaptic density is normal (35 synapses/100 μm^2), and the newly formed synapses resemble those normally present. In fact, in the electron microscope there is little, if any, difference between the recovered neuropil and that seen in normal animals. The dimensions of stratum radiatum are not affected by the drug treatment. Thus, it must be that extensive new growth has occurred. The total number of intact synapses increases at least 6-fold, illustrating one of the most extensive examples of reactive synaptogenesis yet reported.

Which afferents contributed to this recovery? Few of the afferents adjacent to stratum radiatum appear to grow. It might be expected that the mossy fibers which are left without their target cells might extend into CA1. Normally, the mossy fibers terminate sharply at the CA3–CA2 border. After kainic acid lesions, we never saw a case where the mossy fibers invaded the CA2 or the CA1 subfields. Thus, afferents without their target do not always mobilize and take the nearest target.

Similarly, septal fibers retain their usual boundaries. AChE histochemistry shows that the septo-hippocampal fibers do not change their innervation in stratum radiatum. Finally, autoradiographic studies of the temporo-ammonic tract show that this afferent does not grow into the denervated zone from its normal termination in an adjacent lamina, stratum lacunosum moleculare. Thus, translaminar growth by adjacent fibers innervating the CA1 field does not appear responsible for reconstituting the population of synapses. At present, we have not identified the source of the new synapses. It appears likely that they arise from interneuronal proliferation, CA1 collaterals or extensive growth of fibers from the few residual CA3 pyramidal cells. These data indicate a strong selectivity in the systems responsible for reinnervation.

It is interesting to note that kainic acid, administered to developing animals in doses which destroy the CA3 field, promotes the growth of mossy fibers into the CA1 field (Fig. 3). Thus, it is clear that some of the constraints present in mature animals are not active in developing animals.

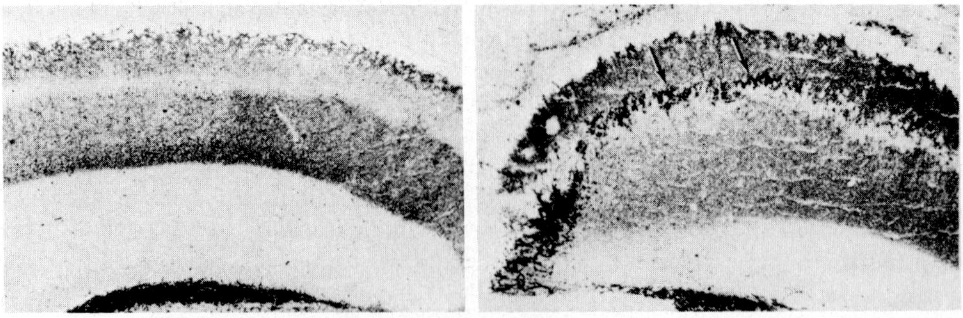

Fig. 3. Growth of the mossy fiber projection into the CA1 field when the CA3 field is destroyed in immature rats by kainic acid. No such changes occur following kainic acid destruction in mature animals. The figure on the left shows the pattern in normal animals, that on the right from kainic acid treated animals. The arrow shows part of the new innervation by the mossy fibers.

Kainic acid at intermediate doses selectively denervates the dentate gyrus. The normal organization of inputs on the granule cell dendrites is illustrated in Fig. 4. The outer three-fourths of the dendritic field consist primarily of a dense innervation from the ipsilateral entorhinal cortex and a sparse innervation from the septum and contralateral entorhinal cortex. The inner one-fourth of the dendritic field contains primarily the commissural and associational fibers originating from the contralateral and ipsilateral pyramidal cells of CA4, respectively. It contains, in addition, a very few septal fibers and mossy fibers (collaterals of the granule cells).

In previous work, it has been shown that residual afferents extensively rewire their circuitry following an entorhinal lesion (Cotman and Lynch, 1976; Cotman and Nadler, 1978). Septal fibers and temporo-ammonic fibers proliferate within the denervated zone;

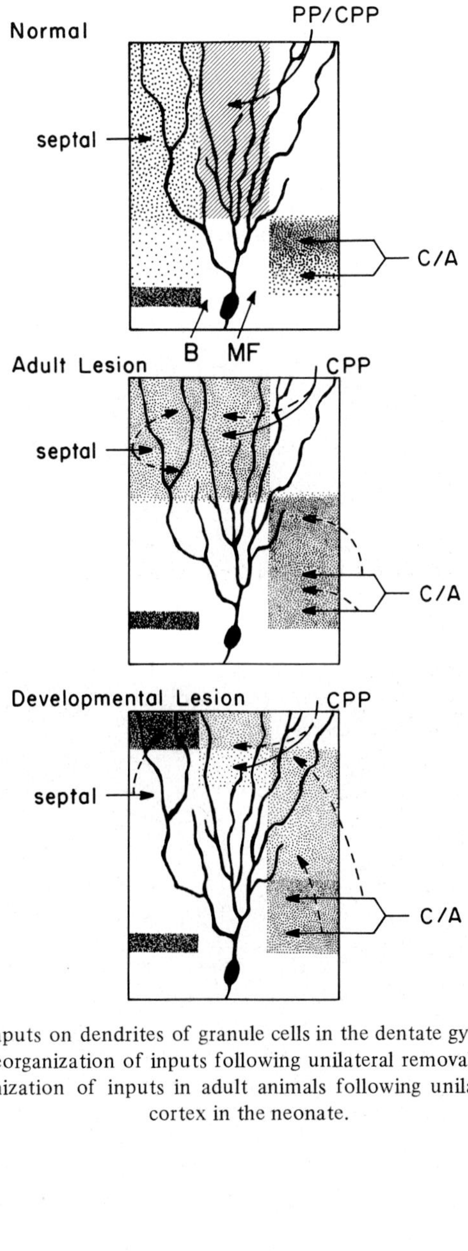

Fig. 4. Organization of inputs on dendrites of granule cells in the dentate gyrus. Upper: normal organization of inputs. Middle: reorganization of inputs following unilateral removal of the entorhinal cortex in adult rats. Lower: organization of inputs in adult animals following unilateral removal of entorhinal cortex in the neonate.

commissural and associational fibers grow and form a new boundary pathway into the denervated zone.

Bilateral injections destroy both the commissural and associational projections which terminate in the inner one-fourth of the granule cell dendritic field. This type of lesion provides a particularly unique opportunity to examine selectivity of growth within a defined and highly plastic population of neurons. Kainic acid lesions provide a way of examining the nature of the reinnervation response on a single cell type to different forms of denervation and allow the extent of denervation to be varied. What is the nature of the reinnervation process?

Destruction of the contralateral hippocampal CA4 neurons results in the loss of approximately 20% of the synaptic input, which is restored over time (McWilliams et al., 1975; McWilliams and Lynch, 1978). The new synapses appear to originate from the associational system. Septal fibers and mossy fibers do not appear to change. What happens when approximately 50% of the input to the commissural-associational zone is lost? Kainic acid injected bilaterally at intermediate doses (about 0.8 μg) increases the extent of denervation because it partially destroys the associational system. Again, electron microscopic analysis illustrates that the synaptic population returns to normal within 50 days (Nadler and Cotman, in preparation). Septal fibers do not appear to change as indicated by a normal AChE staining pattern. However, mossy fibers grow extensive collaterals and proliferate specifically within the denervated zone (see Fig. 5A). It is surprising that the septal system does not react; the

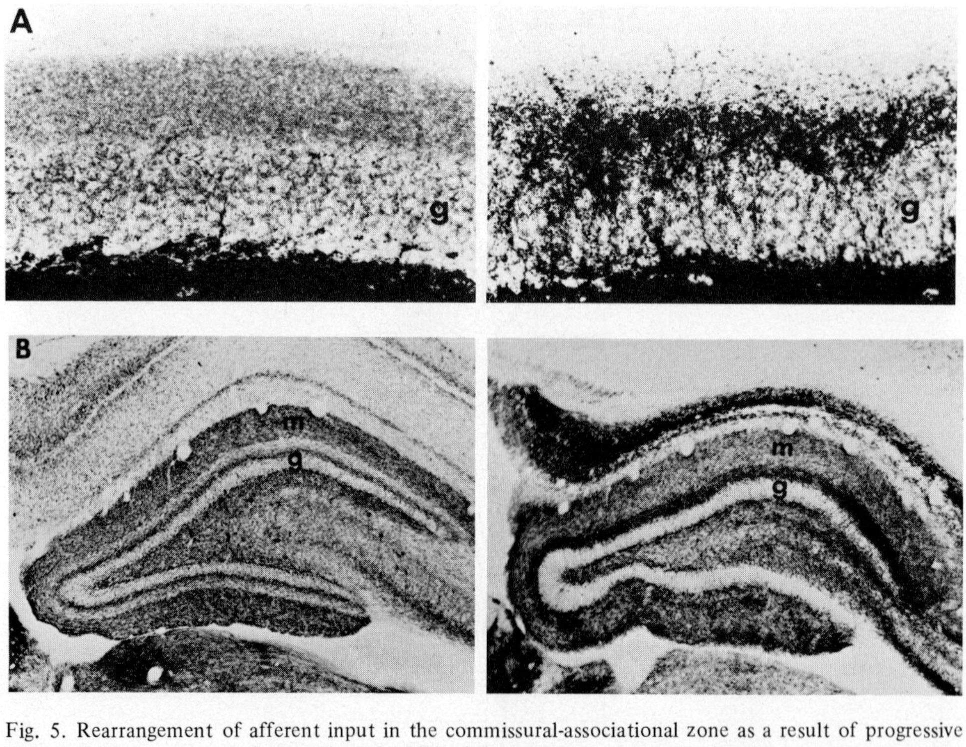

Fig. 5. Rearrangement of afferent input in the commissural-associational zone as a result of progressive denervation. A: removal of approximately 50% of the synapses releases the growth of mossy fibers but not septal fibers, 105 days after injection; left normal, right denervated. B: removal of approximately 80% of the synapses releases the growth of septal fibers; left normal, right denervated. g = granule cells, m = molecular layer of dentate gyrus.

response of this system appears directly related to the extent of denervation. If higher doses of kainic acid are used so that nearly all the synapses in the commissural-associational zone are removed, the entire dendritic layer above the supragranular band stains uniformly for AChE (Fig. 5B). Entorhinal projections remain unchanged after all 3 lesions. These results are summarized in Fig. 6.

Clearly, the nature of the response in the hippocampus depends markedly on the nature of the lesion. There is a progressive hierarchy of reorganization depending precisely on the extent of denervation. In addition, the response depends on the nature of the particular afferent removed. Growth may be specific with no translaminar rearrangements as described for the CA1 field or dentate commissural-associational zone. Alternately, extensive translaminar growth may be displayed as shown by the expansion of commissural-associational fibers after an entorhinal lesion. What mechanisms appear to account for this remarkably specific growth?

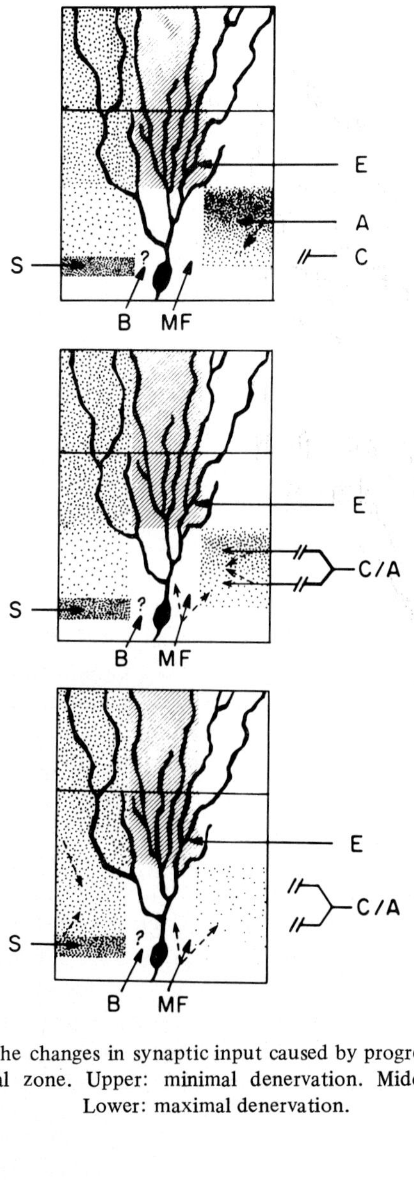

Fig. 6. Diagram illustrating the changes in synaptic input caused by progressive removal of synapses from the commissural-associational zone. Upper: minimal denervation. Middle: intermediate denervation. Lower: maximal denervation.

Transmitter identity clearly does not account for the specificity. The septal system, for example, is cholinergic (see Storm-Mathisen, 1977) and grows in place of systems which clearly do not use acetylcholine as their transmitter. The entorhinal projections and the commissural and associational projections appear to use glutamate and/or aspartate as their neurotransmitters (Nadler et al., 1977, 1978b; Sandoval et al., 1978; White et al., 1978, 1979). Similarly, the distance between the cells of origin of the reactive fibers and the denervated terminal field does not account for selectivity. For example, septal neurons are further from the zone of denervation than entorhinal neurons. Yet septal fibers react to extensive commissural-associational denervation whereas entorhinal fibers never do. Competition based on the abundance of particular afferent systems also does not appear to account for selectivity. The mossy fibers and the septal input are present, it appears, in similar abundance and, as we have discussed, mossy fibers grow under conditions in which the septal fibers do not. It should be noted that it may be that the mossy fiber and supragranular septal inputs are innervating interneurons rather than granule cells. Nonetheless, one system reacts before the other so that the differential response cannot be related to selective denervation in either case. A differential innervation pattern would need to exist and there is no evidence at present for this. Other examples also tend to rule out competition based strictly on afferent abundance (see Cotman and Nadler, 1978).

Selectivity might lie, at least in part, in the initiation process so that only certain fibers will grow under certain circumstances. Or, it might lie in some mechanism beyond initiation such as a specific affinity between afferents and target cells. Finally, there may be a selective suppression of growth.

A simple experiment can be performed which provides a way to determine if selective initiation accounts for the differential responses. As noted above, septal fibers will proliferate in response to a complete or partial entorhinal lesion or an, e.g., extensive commissural-associational lesion. If initiation underlies the selective response in the commissural-associational zone, it should be possible to initiate growth with minor commissural-associational denervation by simultaneously performing an entorhinal and a partial commissural-associational lesion. That is, once the septal system is reactive, it should react generally. Alternatively, if processes other than initiation are involved, there should be no change. We found that the AChE pattern is the same in response to an entorhinal lesion or a combination entorhinal and partial commissural-associational lesion (Cotman and Nadler, 1978, and in preparation).

It does appear, however, that with complete commissural-associational lesions the characteristic expansion of the clear zone in the inner molecular layer does not occur. This zone expands in response to an entorhinal lesion alone.

Geometry is clearly an essential factor in establishing the pattern of reinnervation and, at one level of analysis, it accounts for some of the selectivity. Afferents must be adjacent to a denervated zone in order to react, indicating that the presence of a normal field is prohibitive to growth. Proximity, however, while necessary is an insufficient growth condition in itself. As we have discussed, fibers adjacent to a denervated zone may not react, e.g., entorhinal fibers after a complete commissural-associational lesion. It appears that specific membrane properties and factors that inhibit growth are the most acceptable explanation for the selectivity at present.

The presence of growth suppression factors was postulated by Cajal in order to account for the termination of growth during development. Evidence favoring such factors in axon sprouting has been rallied recently by Diamond et al. (1976) based on studies on the salamander hind limb. Reducing axoplasmic flow (via colchicine treatment) without actually destroying fibers triggers sprouting by adjacent untreated fibers. We have performed similar experiments in the CNS (Goldowitz and Cotman, 1978). We found that colchicine treatment which does not cause a net loss of synapses can promote synapse formation. These data are consistent with a regulation of synaptic growth by so-called negative trophic factors. Thus, as in the peripheral nervous system, it may be that growth suppression factors supplied to the terminal by axoplasmic flow are responsible for maintaining the brain in a suppressed state of growth. There may be an interactive effect between the presence of existing fibers and the growth of new fibers.

Growth, it appears, may need to be constantly held back. In the course of development and reinnervation, neurons accept a finite and fixed number of synapses. Denervation, whether through the actual loss of synapses or a disturbance of their metabolic impact on their target, releases synaptic growth. Progressive denervation may allow a progressive release of growth in residual afferents.

CRITICAL AFFERENT MODEL OF LAMINATION

The notion that certain afferents can suppress the growth of others appears to explain a number of our observations. Specifically it is proposed that the commissural-associational system can suppress or repel the growth of the septal system. The septal fibers do not react in the commissural-associational zone until all, or nearly all, of these fibers are depleted. In contrast, septal fibers respond to a partial, as well as complete, entorhinal lesion. Moreover, septal fibers in the inner molecular layer appear to be displaced from part of their field by reactive commissural-associational fibers as evidenced by an expanded clear zone. This clear zone exactly corresponds to that of expanded commissural-associational fibers which sprout partway into the denervated entorhinal area. It may be that these expanded commissural-associational fibers have forced the septal fibers out of their normal zone. If this is the case, removal of commissural-assocational fibers would prevent the clearing of septal fibers. Rats were treated with kainic acid in order to destroy commissural-associational fibers, given a unilateral entorhinal lesion 30 days later and stained for AChE 15 days post-lesion. The pattern of AChE staining showed that the AChE clear zone failed to develop. Thus, it appears that commissural-associational fibers can repel reactive septal fibers. Commissural-associational fibers appear to serve as a critical afferent which can establish the pattern of septal reactivity and reorganization.

SUMMARY

The data discussed in this chapter illustrate that highly selective synaptic growth can occur in the adult brain. In order to trigger synaptic growth we have used kainic acid. Kainic acid kills certain neurons in the hippocampus when injected at low concentrations into the lateral ventricle. The CA3 subfield is most sensitive to the cytotoxic action followed by CA4, CA1 and subiculum. The CA2 field and dentate gyrus are particularly resistant to kainic acid.

The lesions produced by kainic acid in rats resemble, in many respects, the types of lesions produced in man as a result of epilepsy, senile dementia and stroke. In man, the Somner sector (homologous to CA1 and subiculum in rat) and the end folium (homologous to CA3 field in rat) are particularly vulnerable to cell loss.

Over time, we find that the residual connections reorganize and a new circuitry emerges. Denervated cells become repopulated with new synaptic connections. The circuits which recover after intrinsic hippocampal cell loss depend not only on the cell group lost but on the extent of their loss. Particular fibers grow only in particular areas. In the commissural-associational zone of the dentate gyrus fibers react sequentially as a function of the extent of denervation. It appears as if, in some cases, those fibers most related to the lost input react. When a particular extent of denervation is achieved, the reaction becomes less specific. Growth is always selective and hierarchical.

The mechanisms which underlie selectivity are complex indeed. At present, it does not seem that transmitter identity, afferent competition, or proximity to the denervated zone can account for the findings. Moreover, selective initiation of growth to particular fibers can be ruled out in some cases.

It is argued that the reactivity of septal fibers is selectively restrained by the commissural-associational fibers and further, that reactive commissural-associational fibers can actually displace reactive septal fibers. Thus, growth suppression may play a critical role in reactive synaptogenesis. It may be that growth is normally retarded but can be released when such factors are reduced either by destruction of inputs or by reducing the axoplasmic flow of substances along afferent fibers. Thus, it may be that synapses are always trying to form in the mature brain and that there is a constant struggle between maintaining and changing synaptic connections.

REFERENCES

Blackwood, W. and Corsellius, J.A.N. (Eds.) (1976) *Greenfield's Neuropathology*. Edward Arnold, London.

Cotman, C.W. (Ed.) (1978) *Neuronal Plasticity*. Raven Press, New York.

Cotman, C.W. and Lynch, G.S. (1976) Reactive synaptogenesis in the adult nervous system. In *Neuronal Recognition*, S. Barondes (Ed.), Raven Press, New York, pp. 69–108.

Cotman, C.W. and Nadler, J.V. (1978) Reactive synaptogenesis in the hippocampus. In *Neuronal Plasticity*, C.W. Cotman (Ed.), Raven Press, New York, pp. 227–271.

Diamond, J., Cooper, E., Turner, C. and MacIntyre, L. (1976) Trophic regulation of nerve sprouting. *Science*, 193: 371–377.

Edds, Jr., M.V. (1950) Collateral regeneration of residual motor axons in partially denervated muscles. *J. exp. Zool.*, 113: 517.

Exner, S. (1885) Notiz zur der Frage von der Fuservertheilung mehrerer Nerven in einem Muskel. *Arch. gen. Physiol.*, 36: 572.

Goldowitz, D. and Cotman, C.W. (1978) Evidence that neurotrophic interactions control synapse formation in the adult rat brain. *Brain Res.*, Submitted.

Hoffmann, H. (1950) Local reinnervation in partially denervated muscle: a histophysiological study. *Aust. J. exp. Biol med. Sci.*, 28: 383–397.

Liu, C.N. and Chambers, W.W. (1958) Intraspinal sprouting of dorsal root axons: development of new collaterals and preterminals following partial denervation of the spinal cord in the cat. *Arch. Neurol. Psychiat. (Chic.)*, 79: 46.

McGeer, E.G., Olney, J.W. and McGeer, P.L. (Eds.) (1978) *Kainic Acid as a Tool in Neurobiology*. Raven Press, New York.

McWilliams, J.R. and Lynch, G.S. (1978) Terminal proliferation and synaptogenesis following partial deafferentation. *J. comp. Neurol.*, 180: 581–615.

McWilliams, J.R., Lynch, G.S. and Cotman, C.W. (1975) Synaptic reinnervation in the inner molecular layer of the dentate gyrus following partial deafferentation: an electron microscopic study in the rat. *Neurosci. Abstr.*, 1: 517.

Minckler, J. (Ed.) (1971) *Pathology of the Nervous System, Vol 2.* McGraw-Hill, New York.

Murakami, S., Takemoto, T., Shimizu, Z. and Daigo, K. (1953) Effective principle of *Digenea*. *Jap. J. Pharm. Chem.*, 25: 571–574.

Murray, J.G. and Thompson, J.W. (1957) The occurrence and function of collateral sprouting in the sympathetic nervous system of the cat. *J. Physiol. (Lond.)*, 135: 133.

Nadler, J.V. (1978) Kainic acid: neurophysiological and neurotoxic action. *Life Sci.*, in press.

Nadler, J.V., White, W.F., Vaca, K.W., Redburn, D.A. and Cotman, C.W. (1977) Characterization of putative amino acid transmitter release from slices of rat dentate gyrus. *J. Neurochem.*, 29: 279–290.

Nadler, J.V., Perry, B.W. and Cotman, C.W. (1978a) Preferential vulnerability to intraventricular kainic acid. In *Kainic Acid as a Tool in Neurobiology*, E.G. McGeer, J.W. Olney and P.L. McGeer (Eds.), Raven Press, New York, pp. 591–596.

Nadler, J.V., White, W.F., Vaca, K.W., Perry, P.W. and Cotman, C.W. (1978b) Biochemical correlates of transmission mediated by glutamate and aspartate. *J. Neurochem.*, 31: 147–155.

Nadler, J.V., Perry, B. and Cotman, C.W. (1978c) Intraventricular kainic acid in hippocampal pyramidal cells. *Nature (Lond.)*, 271: 676–677.

Raisman, G. (1969) Neuronal plasticity in the septal nuclei of the adult rat. *Brain Res.*, 14: 25.

Sandoval, M.E., Horch, P. and Cotman, C.W. (1978) Evaluation of glutamate as a hippocampal neurotransmitter: glutamate uptake and release from synaptosomes. *Brain Res.*, 142: 285–299.

Storm-Mathisen, J. (1977) Localization of transmitter candidates in the brain: the hippocampal formation as a model. *Progr. Neurobiol.*, 8: 119–181.

White, W.F., Nadler, J.V., Hamberger, A., Cotman, C.W. and Cummins, J.T. (1978) Glutamate as transmitter of hippocampal perforant path. *Nature (Lond.)*, 270: 356–357.

White, W.F., Nadler, J.V. and Cotman, C.W. (1979) The effect of acidic amino acid antagonists on synaptic transmission in the hippocampal formation in vitro. *Brain Res.*, 164: 177–194.

Bursting Neurons in Cultures of Rat Hypothalamus

B. H. GÄHWILER and J. J. DREIFUSS

Biological and Medical Research Division, Sandoz Ltd., Basle and Department of Physiology, University of Geneva Medical School, Geneva (Switzerland)

The hormones oxytocin and vasopressin are synthesized by neurosecretory cells of the paraventricular and supraoptic nuclei and released from their axonal endings in the posterior pituitary (Cross et al., 1975). Electrophysiologically, supraoptic and paraventricular neurons display two main patterns of spontaneous neuronal firing: a majority show random (more or less continuous) firing, the remainder display a phasic discharge pattern, characterized by bursts of activity alternating with silent periods (Dreifuss et al., 1976a). It has been proposed that phasic activity may be confined to the vasopressinergic neurons. The nature of this bursting pattern is still obscure, but it has been speculated that it may be due to an inherent property of neurosecretory cells rather than to an exogenous synaptic drive (Dreifuss et al., 1976b; Poulain et al., 1977). Direct evidence for this hypothesis is, however, still lacking, since cells cannot be synaptically isolated in the intact preparation, and intracellular recordings from these neuroendocrine cells proved to be extremely difficult to carry out. To partially circumvent these problems, we have cultured hypothalamic explants of the supraoptic nucleus area from young rats (Gähwiler et al., 1978).

The cultures are prepared from 1–7-day-old rats by means of the roller-tube technique (Gähwiler et al., 1973). After 3–10 weeks of culture, electrophysiological recordings were carried out from large nerve cells, 20–30 μm in diameter. Electron microscopic studies revealed the existence within the cultures of neurons containing neurosecretory granules in axons and perikarya (Gähwiler et al., 1978).

Spontaneous activity was recorded intracellularly from a total of 60 cells, the majority of which fired randomly. The activity of approximately 30% of the cells could be termed phasic (Fig. 1), based on the existence of bursts of activity alternating with silent periods. Mean cycle time (i.e. interval between the onset of bursts) (35.8 ± 11.1 sec, n = 21, ± S.E.M.) and mean burst duration (8.8 ± 3.5 sec, n = 21, ± S.E.M.) varied considerably from culture to culture. Computation of the instantaneous frequency during bursts (Fig. 1B) revealed that the frequency was highest at the onset of the bursts and then decreased gradually until the cell suddenly became silent. In a proportion of these cells, the bursts were composed of even shorter phasic units riding on an oscillatory membrane potential (Fig. 2).

In an attempt to determine whether the phasic activity was an endogenous property of these cells, they were exposed to solutions known to block synaptic transmission. In most cells, addition of 0.4 mM Co^{2+} or 4 mM Mg^{2+} reversibly abolished all activity. Moreover, the phasic activity was not a function of membrane potential. Intracellular current injections through the recording electrode altered neither cycle time nor burst duration. Prominent EPSPs appeared during strong hyperpolarization of the membrane (Fig. 3).

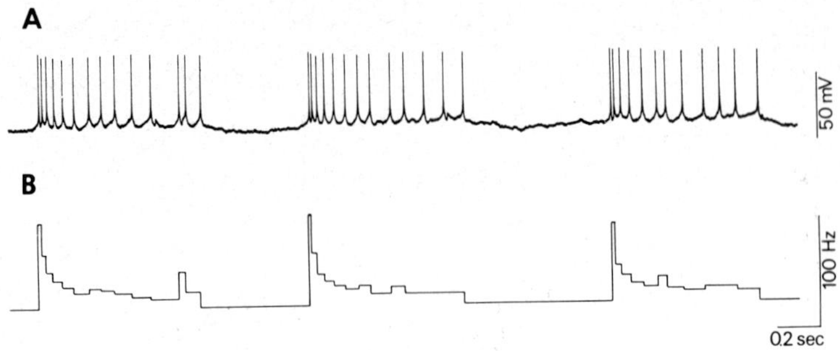

Fig. 1. Intracellular record of phasic activity from a hypothalamic neuron in culture. B: display of the instantaneous frequency. Age of culture, 23 days.

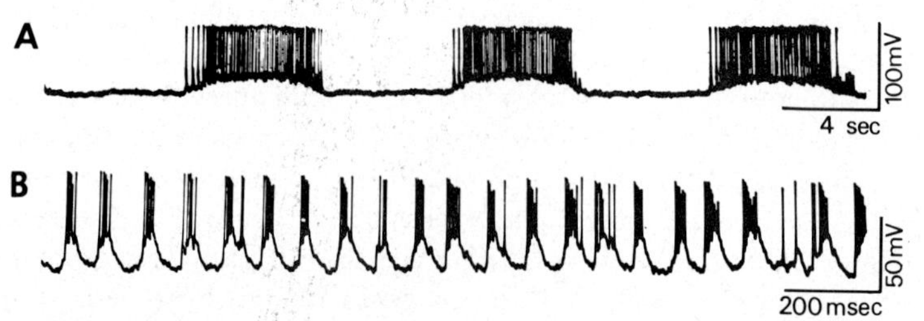

Fig. 2. Spontaneous bursts of activity in a 44-day-old culture. B shows the recording on a faster time scale during one of the bursts illustrated in A. Note the occurrence of phasic units within the bursts. Resting membrane potential, –62 mV.

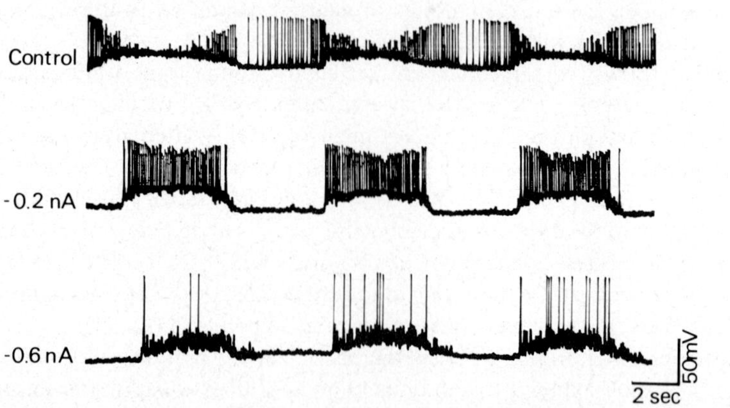

Fig. 3. Hyperpolarization abolished the spikes during the interburst intervals, but it had no effect on cycle time and burst duration. In A, the spike generating mechanism was partly inactivated during the bursts. Strong hyperpolarization resulted in the phasic appearance of prominent EPSPs (C). Resting membrane potential, –65 mV. 44-day-old culture.

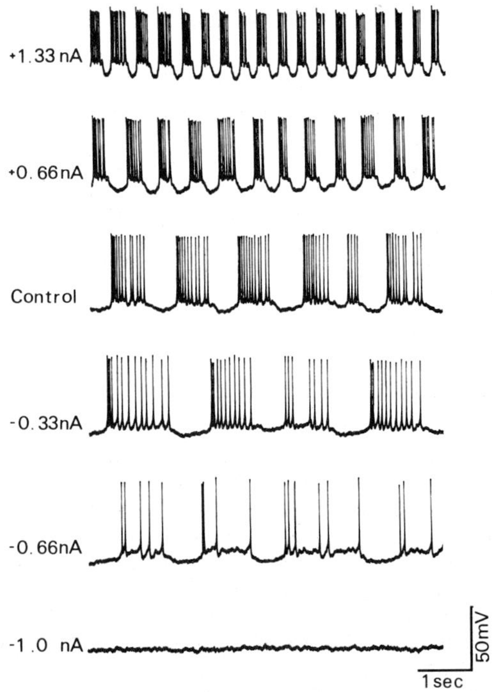

Fig. 4. Spontaneous activity recorded in pacemaker neuron during application of 2 mM Co^{2+}. Depolarization decreased, hyperpolarization increased mean cycle time, burst duration and intraburst spike interval. Note the complete absence of EPSPs during strong hyperpolarization of the membrane (–1 nA).

Although the majority of cells turned out to be follower cells, activity was also recorded from neurons which met all the criteria for pacemaker cells. The activity of the cell illustrated in Fig. 4 persisted in a solution containing 2 mM Co^{2+}, a concentration which is 5-fold that needed to block discharges in follower cells. Furthermore, in this cell, cycle time and burst duration were found to be markedly dependent upon the amplitude of the membrane potential. Depolarization accelerated, hyperpolarization slowed the phases. No EPSPs became apparent as a result of strong membrane hyperpolarization.

The data presented demonstrate that a proportion of hypothalamic neurons of the supraoptic nucleus area displayed phasic activity in vitro. Cycle time and burst duration were comparable to those recorded from rat vasopressinergic neurons in situ (Dreifuss et al., 1976a).

The activity of the majority of phasically active cells exhibited the typical features of follower cells, since the phases were independent of membrane polarization but were abolished by addition of Co^{2+} and Mg^{2+} ions. Spontaneous activity must originate within the confines of the culture, and it is therefore not suprising that cells were found which could be identified as pacemaker neurons. These pacemaker cells probably contribute to the synchronization of discharges which is observed in the cultures (Gähwiler et al., 1978). Although similar bursting discharges had been reported to occur in invertebrate neurosecretory cells (Yagi et al., 1971; Gainer, 1972), they had never before been unequivocally identified in the mammalian brain.

SUMMARY

A proportion of cultured hypothalamic neurons of the supraoptic nucleus area displayed spontaneous phasic activity characterized by high frequency bursts alternating with silent periods. The phasic activity of the majority of cells was shown to be synaptic in origin. Hyperpolarization of the membrane by current injection through the recording electrode did not alter the duration of their interburst periods, and their activity was abolished by addition of Co^{2+} or high concentrations of Mg^{2+}. In contrast, endogenous pacemaker activity was demonstrated to be a function of membrane potential and it persisted during application of Co^{2+}.

REFERENCES

Cross, B. A., Dyball, R. E. J., Dyer, R. G., Jones, C. W., Lincoln, D. W., Morris, J. F. and Pickering, B. T. (1975) Endocrine neurones. *Recent Progr. Hormone Res.*, 31: 243–294.

Dreifuss, J. J., Harris, M. C. and Tribollet, E. (1976a) Excitation of phasically firing hypothalamic supraoptic neurones by carotid occlusion in rats. *J. Physiol. (Lond.)*, 257: 337–354.

Dreifuss, J. J., Tribollet, E., Bärtschi, A. J. and Lincoln, D. W. (1976b) Mammalian endocrine neurones: control of phasic activity by antidromic action potentials. *Neurosci. Lett.*, 3: 281–286.

Gähwiler, B. H., Mamoon, A. M. and Tobias, C. A. (1973) Spontaneous bioelectric activity of cultured Purkinje cells during exposure to agents which prevent synaptic transmission. *Brain Res.*, 53: 71–79.

Gähwiler, B. H., Sandoz, P. and Dreifuss, J. J. (1978) Neurones with synchronous bursting discharges in organ cultures of the hypothalamic supraoptic nucleus area. *Brain Res.*, 151: 245–253.

Gainer, H. (1972) Electrophysiological behaviour of an endogenously active neurosecretory cell. *Brain Res.*, 39: 403–418.

Poulain, D. A., Wakerley, J. B. and Dyball, R. E. J. (1977) Electrophysiological differentiation of oxytocin and vasopressin-secreting neurones. *Proc. roy. Soc. B*, 196: 367–384.

Yagi, K., Iwasaki, S., Sawaki, Y. and Satow, Y. (1971) Electrophysiological studies on the neuroendocrine neuron. *Med. J. Osaka Univ.*, 21: 75–90.

Immunohistochemical Studies of Central and Peripheral Peptidergic Neurons

ROBERT ELDE*, TOMAS HÖKFELT, RAYMOND HO**, VIRGINIA SEYBOLD, H. DAVID COULTER, PAUL MICEVYCH and NIHAL DE LANEROLLE***

(R.E., R.H., V.S., H.D.C. and P.M.) Departments of Anatomy and (N. de L.) Pharmacology, University of Minnesota, Minneapolis, Minn. (U.S.A.) and (T.H.) Department of Histology, Karolinska Institute, Stockholm (Sweden)

INTRODUCTION

Immunohistochemical analysis of molecular constituents of the nervous system has been in widespread use for less than a decade. The techniques used have enabled localization of a variety of macromolecules, including glia-specific proteins, neurotransmitter synthesizing enzymes, classical neurotransmitters (see Steinbusch et al., 1978), and biologically active neuropeptides. Investigations of the latter have rapidly burgeoned, due to the increasing number and variety of peptides isolated from the nervous system (see Otsuka and Takahashi, 1977; Guillemin, 1978b).

Prior to the advent of immunohistochemical analysis of the nervous system, few techniques were available that would allow combined molecular and cellular mapping. One of these exceptions was the elegant formaldehyde-induced fluorescence method of Falck and Hillarp (Falck et al., 1962) which enabled mapping of monoaminergic neurons and their pathways (see Dählstrom and Fuxe, 1964; Fuxe, 1965). The present depth of understanding of monoaminergic mechanisms has been greatly aided by the detailed knowledge of the transmitter-specific circuitry of the monoamines.

Advances in isolation and synthesis of molecules of the nervous system, as well as advances in producing antibodies to these substances, now permit immunohistochemical identification of a wide variety of nervous system constituents (see also Raff et al., this volume). In the present chapter, we will briefly review aspects of the distribution of presently characterized neuropeptides revealed by immunohistochemical techniques. The distribution of some of these peptides as determined by radioimmunoassay techniques has recently been reviewed (Brownstein, 1977).

---

* Address correspondence to: Dr. Robert Elde, Department of Anatomy, 262 Jackson Hall, 321 Church St. S.E., University of Minnesota, Minneapolis, Minn. 55455, U.S.A.

** Present address: Department of Anatomy, Ohio State University, Columbus, Ohio 43210, U.S.A.

*** Present address: Department of Psychiatry, Yale University, New Haven, Conn. 06510, U.S.A.

METHODOLOGICAL CONSIDERATIONS

Much of the immunohistochemical analysis of neuropeptides to date has been accomplished with the indirect immunofluorescence technique as described by Coons (1958). Localization of potentially diffusable substances, such as the neuropeptides or cytoplasmic enzymes, is facilitated by fixation of the tissues with 4% paraformaldehyde (Pease, 1962; Hökfelt et al., 1975b). Such fixation diminishes the quantity of immunoreactive peptides to approximately 75% of the value found in fresh tissue as determined by radioimmunoassay (Coulter and Elde, 1979). In spite of this decrement in immunoreactive peptide, the tissues and peptide antigens are stabilized to an extent that permits incubations of immunochemical reagents on tissue sections with no further loss of immunoreactivity or tissue integrity. For the routine immunofluorescence procedure, we obtain sections of frozen tissue from a microtome-cryostat. In our hands, sections of paraffin or epoxy embedded tissues are not optimal since chemical dehydration through increasing concentrations of ethanol (as used to render the tissue miscible with molten paraffin and its solvents, or epoxy resins and their solvents) is extremely deleterious to preservation of neuropeptide immunoreactivity. After ethanol dehydration less than 15% of the original immunoreactivity is retained in either fixed or unfixed tissue (Coulter and Elde, 1979).

Antisera to the various peptides in our studies have been raised in rabbits or guinea pigs after immunization with covalent complexes of synthetic peptides and larger carrier proteins such as hemocyanin, thyroglobulin or serum albumin. Several of our antisera to peptides have been characterized in competitive peptide binding studies in order to examine specificity and possible cross-reactions with other, presently identified peptides (e.g., Arimura et al., 1978). Specificity of immunohistochemical localization is also established by treating a working dilution of an antiserum with an excess of its antigen prior to its use on tissue sections. Immunohistochemical specificity is inferred if such pretreated antiserum does not stain tissue elements that are stained in an adjacent section after exposure to untreated antiserum.

More refined characterization of immunohistochemical staining has recently been obtained by Schultzberg et al. (1979). For example, staining resultant to a leu-enkephalin antibody could be abolished in a dose-dependent fashion by pretreatment of antiserum with incremental additions of leu-enkephalin. Staining was also abolished in a dose-dependent manner with addition of met-enkephalin to the leu-enkephalin antibody, although 100 times more met-enkephalin than leu-enkephalin was required to produce an equivalent inhibition of staining.

From these studies, it would appear that localizations with this leu-enkephalin antiserum would be restricted to leu-enkephalin in the tissue section. However, in spite of such exhaustive controls, it remains possible that the antiserum may localize a biosynthetic precursor or intermediate in addition to the characterized peptide. Therefore, immunohistochemical analysis can only reveal the location of immunoreactivity *similar* to the peptide in question.

Although we have primarily used immunofluorescence to study the cellular distribution of neuropeptides, the labeled (Nakane, 1971) and unlabeled antibody peroxidase variants (Sternberger, 1974) have also been demonstrated to be effective immunohistochemical approaches. They are uniquely useful in localization studies at the electron microscopic level. Several investigators have reported the ultrastructural localization of neuropeptides in the pre-embedding modification of the technique. However, morphological aspects of tissue processed by such means are compromised, making detailed analysis of synaptology difficult. Furthermore, because of the thickness of tissues used during the immunohistochemical procedure, it is not feasible to localize other neuropeptides in neighboring terminals, thereby preventing the study of relationships between different peptidergic systems.

Theoretically, this can be overcome by the use of the postembedding staining techniques. In this case, the immunochemical staining reaction is conducted on the ultrathin section of epoxy-embedded tissue. Such an approach has been useful in the hypothalamic median eminence where the concentration of hypophysiotropic peptides is very high. However, outside this area, little success has been reported. This is most likely due to the extraction of most of the peptide immunoreactivity during dehydration in ethanol as discussed above. We have recently been successful in preserving peptide immunoreactivity in ultrathin, epoxy-embedded sections of frozen dried neural tissue (Coulter and Elde, 1979). Dehydration is accomplished without exposure to ethanol, thereby leaving the peptide stores intact. This tissue has good morphological characteristics at the ultrastructural level (Coulter and Terracio, 1977). The extent of the preservation of immunoreactivity is best demonstrated at the light microscopic level in ultrathin sections (Fig. 1). Further characterization of immunoreactivity at the ultrastructual level is presently being investigated. This approach promises to be a useful method to the study of neuropeptide-containing structures at the synaptic level.

DISTRIBUTION OF NEUROPEPTIDES

The large number of presently characterized neuropeptides, as well as the complexity of neuronal circuits containing neuropeptide immunoreactivity, precludes a comprehensive review of their distribution. Furthermore, our knowledge of the distribution of these peptides is, in many cases, rather fragmentary. Of the neuropeptides, definitive mapping is presently available only for substance P (Cuello and Kanazawa, 1978; Ljungdahl et al., 1978). In this review the focus will be on peptides that are especially prominent in certain regions of the central nervous system (CNS) and peripheral nervous system (PNS) or where their appearance is noteworthy because of the implications to broader areas of neurobiological investigation.

In general terms, neuropeptides are prominent in areas of the CNS that are involved in (1) central regulation of autonomic function (viz., nucleus tractus solitarius, dorsal motor nucleus of cranial nerve X, nucleus parabrachialis, several hypothalamic nuclei, (2) neuroendocrine phenomenon (viz., various hypothalamic nuclei, external layer of the median eminence, posterior pituitary, (3) "extrapyramidal" structures (viz. globus pallidus, caudate-putamen, substantia nigra), (4) limbic system structures (amygdaloid nuclei, septal nuclei, various hypothalamic nuclei), and (5) pain pathways. Immunoreactivity of only a few neuropeptides (somatostatin, vasoactive intestinal polypeptide, and the carboxy-terminal octapeptide of cholecystokinin) has been reported in the cerebral cortex. Little or no immunoreactivity to presently characterized neuropeptides has been described in the cerebellum. Within the PNS, some neuropeptides are found in primary afferent neurons and in numerous structures of the peripheral autonomic nervous system.

Most of the data presently available reflect the distribution of neuropeptides in a single species – the laboratory rat. Some data are available on the occurrence of peptides in the guinea pig nervous system, and only scattered reports describe immunohistochemical localization of neuropeptides in other mammals and in non-mammalian vertebrates*. As discussed below in more detail, preliminary phylogenetic studies on neuropeptides have revealed striking differences in neuropeptide content in what are assumed to be homologous neuronal

* An exception is LHRH, the distribution of which has been described in numerous species (see review by Sternberger and Hoffman, 1978).

circuits. However, unless otherwise noted, the following descriptions of neuropeptide immunoreactivity are derived from immunohistochemical localizations performed on rat tissue.

Central nervous system

Neuroendocrine peptides

The posterior pituitary hormones vasopressin and oxytocin were the first peptides to be isolated from the CNS, sequenced and characterized for their hormonal activity upon target organs (Du Vigneaud, 1954). They arise biosynthetically in association with larger peptides termed neurophysins (Sachs and Takabatake, 1964; Gainer et al., 1977). The major neuronal circuits containing vasopressin, oxytocin and neurophysin immunoreactivity arise from magnocellular perikarya in the hypothalamic supraoptic and paraventricular nuclei (see Defendini and Zimmerman, 1978). Most of the axons from these nuclei project as the hypothalamo-neurohypophyseal tract and terminate adjacent to capillaries in the posterior pituitary. Nerve terminals originating from paraventricular perikarya with vasopressin immunoreactivity are also found in the external layer of the median eminence (Antunes et al., 1977; Elde and Hökfelt, 1978). The vasopressin immunoreactivity contained within these terminals is suspected of acting as a corticotropin releasing factor (Stillman et al., 1977). Further support for a releasing factor role for external layer vasopressin is derived from our recent studies of this system after reserpine administration (Elde et al., 1978; Seybold et al., 1978). Briefly, dose- and time-response data on the disappearance of vasopressin and neurophysin immunoreactivity from the external layer of the median eminence parallel the disappearance of bioassayable corticotropin releasing activity (Bhattacharya and Marks, 1969). Thus, it is possible that vasopressin is one of several hypothalamic factors responsible for control of corticotropin release from the pituitary.

A minor group of perikarya with vasopressin immunoreactivity is found in the suprachiasmatic nucleus and is thought to project to the thalamus, septum and some other extrahypothalamic areas (Sofroniew and Weindl, 1978). Rather sparse pathways containing vasopressin and oxytocin immunoreactivity project to certain brain stem nuclei (Swanson, 1978) and the intermediate and dorsal horns of the spinal cord (Swanson, 1977; Elde and Hökfelt, 1978) and are thought to arise from perikarya in the paraventricular nucleus.

Thyrotropin releasing hormone (TRH) was the first of the neuropeptides characterized as a hypophysiotropic hormone or releasing factor (Burgus et al., 1970; Nair et al., 1970). Radioimmunoassay data first suggested the widespread distribution of immunoreactivity similar to TRH outside of the hypothalamus (Brownstein et al., 1974; Jackson and Reichlin, 1974; Oliver et al., 1974; Winokur and Utiger, 1974). Thus, in addition to a neuroendocrine system with immunohistochemically demonstrable terminals in the external layer of the median eminence (Hökfelt et al., 1975c; Choy and Watkins, 1977), terminals containing TRH immunoreactivity are found in nucleus accumbens, nucleus interstitialis stria terminalis, the lateral septal nucleus, several brain stem nuclei and the intermediolateral and ventral horns of the spinal cord (Hökfelt et al., 1975c). Neuronal perikarya containing TRH immunoreactivity have thus far been described only in the hypothalamic dorsomedial nucleus and perifornical area (Hökfelt et al., 1977a).

Luteinizing hormone releasing hormone (LHRH) is a decapeptide which stimulates release of luteinizing and follicle stimulating hormones from the pituitary (Amoss et al., 1971; Schally et al., 1971). Immunohistochemical localizations of this peptide have shown it in densely packed terminals in the lateral aspect of the external layer of the median eminence (Barry et al., 1973; Leonardelli et al., 1973). Considerable controversy has arisen regarding the distribution of neuronal perikarya containing LHRH immunoreactivity. These perikarya are found in several hypothalamic nuclei and are discussed in detail elsewhere (Hoffman et al., 1978; Silverman and Krey, 1978; Sternberger and Hoffman, 1978).

Somatostatin (SOM) is a tetradecapeptide that was isolated in crude form by Krulich et al. (1968) and completely characterized and synthesized by Brazeau et al. (1973). It was named for its ability to inhibit the release of growth hormone from the pituitary. However, its widespread distribution outside of the hypothalamic neuroendocrine system and its manifold capacity to inhibit the function of cells in numerous organs make it clear that the designation somatostatin is a misnomer (see Guillemin, 1978a).

Immunoreactive SOM is found in perikarya in the hypothalamic periventricular nucleus (Elde and Parsons, 1975; Alpert et al., 1976). Their axons seem to project exclusively to the external layer of the median eminence where they terminate in a broad zone and extend into the pituitary stalk (Elde and Hökfelt, 1978; see also Brownstein et al., 1977; Epelbaum et al., 1977).

In addition, immunoreactive nerve terminals from unknown sources innervate portions of the hypothalamic ventromedial, arcuate and suprachiasmatic nuclei (Hökfelt et al., 1975a; Elde and Hökfelt, 1978). Lesion studies have shown that these nerve terminals are not collaterals from the SOM-containing neuroendocrine system that has cell bodies in the periventricular nucleus.

Approximately 75% of the total CNS SOM immunoreactivity occurs outside of the hypothalamus (Brownstein, 1978). Prominent areas of SOM immunoreactive nerve fibers and terminals are found in the nucleus accumbens and medial caudate nucleus, the stria terminalis and its bed nucleus, the amygdaloid complex, the cerebral cortex, several brain stem nuclei, and in the substantia gelatinosa of the dorsal horn of the spinal cord and spinal trigeminal nucleus. The substantia gelatinosa immunoreactivity represents the terminals of some of the small-diameter primary afferent neurons (Hökfelt et al., 1976). Neuronal perikarya containing SOM immunoreactivity have been identified in the neocortex, the dentate gyrus, the cortical amygdaloid nucleus, the bed nucleus of the stria terminalis and zona incerta (Hökfelt et al., 1978a, b). The connectivity of these perikarya remains largely unknown.

Centrally acting neuropeptides

Whereas the peptides discussed in the preceding paragraphs were originally characterized as neuroendocrine hormones, several others (i.e., enkephalin, endorphins, substance P) were originally characterized for other properties. However, virtually all the neuroendocrine hormones have also been localized in areas of the nervous system that play no direct role in neuroendocrine regulation; and some of those originally described in other areas have been localized in neuroendocrine systems. The diversity of sites of synthesis and probable release of neuropeptides is reminiscent of the distribution and variety of endocrine and neuronal cells containing catecholamines and most likely suggests a multifunctional role for each neuropeptide, depending mostly upon the site of release of the neuropeptide and the distribution of putative receptors in that vicinity.

Enkephalins and endorphins

The morphinomimetic peptides, leucine- and methionine-enkephalin (L-ENK and M-ENK, respectively) are pentapeptides originally characterized and synthesized by Hughes et al. (1975). β-Endorphin (β-END) is a 31-amino acid peptide and was characterized for its opioid properties (Bradbury et al., 1976; Guillemin et al., 1976; Li and Chung, 1976). These peptides bear an amino acid sequence homology with a portion of the pituitary peptide, β-lipotropin, beginning at its 61st amino acid residue. Recent data from biosynthetic studies in pituitary cells have shown that β-END, β-lipotropin and ACTH immunoreactivity are simultaneously present in a large molecular weight protein (31K daltons) and suggest a common biosynthetic precursor to the peptides (Mains et al., 1977; Roberts and Herbert, 1977). Further substantiation has come from immunohistochemical studies showing the 3 peptides to be simultaneously present in some cells of the anterior pituitary, most cells of the intermediate lobe of the pituitary and in some cells of the hypothalamic arcuate nucleus and their processes (Watson et al., 1978; see also Bloom, this volume). It must be emphasized, however, that the enkephalins do not seem to be contained within the cells described above, making it unlikely that they are derived from the same 31K dalton precursor. Rather, studies of their distribution suggest that they lead an existence independent of β-END, β-lipotropin and ACTH.

The enkephalins are widely distributed in the CNS. Some biochemical evidence suggests a differential distribution of M-ENK and L-ENK. Thus on a regional basis, the ratio of M-ENK to L-ENK ranged from 10 to 30 in one study (Simantov and Snyder, 1976) and from 3 to 12 in another (Yang et al., 1977). We and others (Elde et al., 1976; Hökfelt et al., 1977a; Simantov et al., 1977; Watson et al., 1977) have used immunohistochemical methods to determine the distribution of the two enkephalins. In some cases, the antisera used had only limited cross-reactivity (less than 1%) to the opposite enkephalin. These antisera were also treated with an excess of the opposite enkephalin in order to block any residual affinity for the opposite enkephalin prior to the immunohistochemical procedure. At the level of analysis attainable with the light micrsocope, dramatic differences in the distribution of the two enkephalins have not been seen in the central nervous system. However, antiserum to M-ENK has been shown to localize a substance in many adrenal medullary gland cells, although antisera to L-ENK demonstrate only a small number of such cells (Schultzberg et al., 1978; see also below).

Nerve fibers and terminals containing enkephalin immunoreactivity form striking networks in several structures of the basal ganglia-extrapyramidal system. The most prominent of these is the dense and expansive meshwork of fibers, terminals and perhaps cells in the globus pallidus. More scattered cells, fibers and terminals in the caudate-putamen and substantia nigra contain enkephalin immunoreactivity; fibers and terminals are seen in patches in nucleus accumbens.

Enkephalin immunoreactivity in cells, fibers and terminals is also prominent in limbic system structures, e.g., in the central nucleus of the amygdala, the lateral septal nucleus and nucleus interstitialis stria terminalis. Uhl et al. (1978) have recently described enkephalinergic projections from the amygdaloid complex via the stria terminalis.

Diencephalic structures containing enkephalin immunoreactivity include fibers and terminals in the thalamic intralaminar nuclei and the hypothalamic median eminence. Fibers, terminals and perikarya containing enkephalin immunoreactivity are found in many hypothalamic nuclei, including the medial preoptic nucleus, the paraventricular nucleus-perifornical area, the ventromedial nucleus and the premammillary nuclei.

In the midbrain and lower brain stem, enkephalin immunoreactive perikarya, fibers and terminals are found in numerous sites, including the midbrain periaqueductal grey, nucleus parabrachialis, the medullary raphe and reticular nuclei, the dorsal cochlear nucleus, nucleus tractus solitarius and the substantia gelatinosa of the caudal spinal trigeminal nucleus and the dorsal horn of the spinal cord.

Enkephalin immunoreactive neuronal perikarya have been described in more than 25 nuclear groups of the CNS in the rat (Hökfelt et al., 1977a). Most of these regions also contain nerve fibers and terminals with enkephalin immunoreactivity, possibly indicating that many of these circuits are local in nature. Certainly in the dorsal horn of the spinal cord the enkephalinergic system must be a local circuit, since neither dorsal rhizotomy nor proximal transection of the spinal cord produces a change in immunoreactive enkephalin content (Hökfelt et al., 1977c).

A striking feature of the distribution of the enkephalins is their proximity to the sites of high concentrations of opiate receptors as described by Pert et al. (1976) and Atweh and Kuhar (1977). This juxtaposition of effector substances and receptors supports the proposed neurotransmitter or neuroregulatory role for the enkephalins. However, it should be noted that not all areas of the CNS containing opiate binding sites have been shown to contain enkephalin immunoreactivity. The hippocampus, for example, contains moderate concentrations of opiate binding activity, but contains low amounts of enkephalin immunoreactivity (Simantov et al., 1977). It is possible, therefore, that other endogenous opioid substances may serve as endogenous ligands for these receptors.

The distribution of β-END immunoreactivity is distinctly different from that of the enkephalins. Bloom et al. (1978; see also this volume) have described β-END immunoreactive perikarya in the region of the hypothalamic arcuate nucleus and rather coarse fibers projecting caudally to innervate certain brain stem nuclei down to nucleus parabrachialis, and rostrally to innervate certain thalamic, hypothalamic and septal nuclei. These neurons and their processes seem to simultaneously contain β-lipotropin and corticotropin (ACTH) immunoreactivity (Watson et al., 1978; see also Watson et al., 1977; Zimmerman et al., 1978). Thus, data strongly suggest that, in the brain, as in the pituitary, the 3 substances arise from a common biosynthetic precursor as previously described (Mains et al., 1977; Roberts and Herbert, 1977).

Substance P (SP)

The undecapeptide SP was characterized for its sialogenic activity and synthesized by Chang et al. (1971). However, it was first encountered in a search for acetylcholine in extracts of brain and intestine by von Euler and Gaddum (1931; see Lembeck, 1978, for a historical review). The distribution of SP immunoreactivity, like that of enkephalins, is extensive. Additionally, the immunohistochemical mapping of SP is more completely characterized than that of enkephalins with the recent studies of Cuello and Kanazawa (1978) and Ljungdahl et al. (1978). Thus, only a brief account of the distribution of SP immunoreactivity is presented here, and the reader is urged to consult the two cited studies for details.

In the telencephalon, SP immunoreactive fibers and terminals are present in the corpus striatum and nucleus accumbens, the septal nuclei, the stria terminalis and its bed nucleus, the amygdaloid complex (especially the medial and central nuclei), and in the olfactory bulb and tubercle. Neuronal perikarya with SP immunoreactivity are also present in most of these areas. Projections of some of these neurons have been investigated (Emson et al., 1978).

In the diencephalon SP immunoreactive fibers and terminals are present in the hypothalamic medial preoptic area, the dorsomedial nucleus, the arcuate-ventromedial nucleus, the anterior hypothalamic nucleus, the entopeduncular nucleus, as well as in the thalamus and habenula. Diencephalic perikarya containing SP immunoreactivity include the hypothalamic dorsomedial nucleus, the ventromedial nucleus, the premammillary nuclei, the lateral preoptic nucleus and the medial habenular nucleus.

In the mesencephalon SP immunoreactive fibers and terminals are present in the interpeduncular nucleus, the substantia nigra and periaqueductal grey matter. Immunoreactive cell bodies are especially prominent in the interpeduncular nucleus and periaqueductal grey matter. More caudally, the nucleus parabrachialis, the medullary raphe nuclei, nucleus tractus solitarius and nucleus commissuralis all contain rather dense networks of SP immunoreactive nerve fibers and terminals. The raphe and commissural nuclei also contain SP perikarya. The former neurons are of further interest since they have been shown to simultaneously contain serotonin (Chan-Palay et al., 1978; Hökfelt et al., 1978c). The SP immunoreactive terminals in the substantia gelatinosa of the caudal spinal trigeminal nucleus and spinal cord will be discussed below with the PNS.

Additional neuropeptides

Preliminary reports describe the distribution of several other neuropeptides in the CNS. Rather conflicting reports describe α-melanocyte stimulating hormone ($ACTH_{1-13}$) as being similar to that of β-END/β-lipotropin/ACTH (Dube et al., 1978), or very widely scattered (Swaab and Fisser, 1977; Oliver and Porter, 1978). A peptide similar to the carboxy-terminal octapeptide of cholecystokinin appears to be prominent in the CNS, especially in cortical neurons (Dockray, 1976; Hökfelt et al., 1978b; Innis et al., 1978; Rehfeld, 1978; Robberecht et al., 1978; Straus and Yalow, 1978). Vasoactive intestinal polypeptide immunoreactivity is also found in cortical areas and the hypothalamus (Fuxe et al., 1977). Fibers and terminals are also found in the intermediate and dorsal horn of the spinal cord. Finally, neurotensin, a tridecapeptide originally isolated from the bovine hypothalamus (Carraway and Leeman, 1975), is found in varous hypothalamic and amygdaloid nuclei and in substantia gelatinosa of the spinal cord and caudal spinal trigeminal nucleus (Uhl et al., 1977).

Studies on the regional distribution of neuropeptides reveal some areas such as the hypothalamus, amygdala and nucleus tractus solitarius that contain immunoreactivity related to several of the neuropeptides. Although these areas are rich in peptidergic components, immunohistochemical analyses indicate substantial differences in nerve terminal morphology and target sites within these areas. For example, Hökfelt et al. (1978b) have shown a variety of immunoreactive nerve terminal configurations in the rat central amygdaloid nucleus after incubation with antiserum against somatostatin, substance P, methionine-enkephalin, angiotensin II and vasoactive intestinal polypeptide. Depending upon the peptide studied, terminals range from being scattered throughout the neuropil to densely packed basket configurations surrounding amygdaloid cell bodies. Furthermore, within the nucleus the density of immunoreactive fibers and terminals ranges from being homogeneously distributed to being found in discrete patches. Thus, in spite of some gross overlap in the distribution of specific peptidergic systems, each appears to be uniquely arranged when viewed in more detail.

Peripheral nervous system

The capability of immunohistochemical identification of neuropeptides has demonstrated that the PNS is extremely complex in terms of peptide-specific circuits. Many neuropeptides that are widely distributed in the CNS are also found in the PNS and in cells of the gastro-entero-pancreatic endocrine system (see Pearse, 1978).

The neurotransmitters utilized by primary afferent neurons have been difficult to establish. With the possible exception of glutamate (Johnson, 1977) it has not been possible to make a strong case for any of the classical neurotransmitters in primary afferent pathways. Using an immunohistochemical approach, we have demonstrated the presence of SP and somatostatin immunoreactivity in separate, but parallel populations of small diameter dorsal root ganglion neurons, in their peripheral processes, and in their central processes and terminals in the substantia gelatinosa of the spinal cord (Hökfelt et al., 1976). Preliminary evidence indicates that other neuropeptides may be contained in further separate primary afferent systems. As previously mentioned, the substantia gelatinosa contains interneurons with enkephalin immunoreactivity and, as well, receives descending projections containing vasopressin, oxytocin and SP immunoreactivity. Thus, a very rich network of various peptidergic fibers converges in the substantia gelatinosa where they may regulate functions of nociception and analgesia (see Hökfelt et al., 1977c).

The myenteric and submucous plexuses of the intestinal wall contain nerve terminals with SP and somatostatin immunoreactivity (Hökfelt et al., 1976) and enkephalin immunoreactivity (Elde et al., 1976). Other investigators have demonstrated that some of these terminals represent intrinsic neuronal circuits, since some ganglion cell bodies contain SP (Pearse and Polak, 1975) and somatostatin immunoreactivity (Costa et al., 1977). In addition, vasoactive intestinal polypeptide (Bryant et al., 1976; Larsson et al., 1976; Hökfelt et al.,

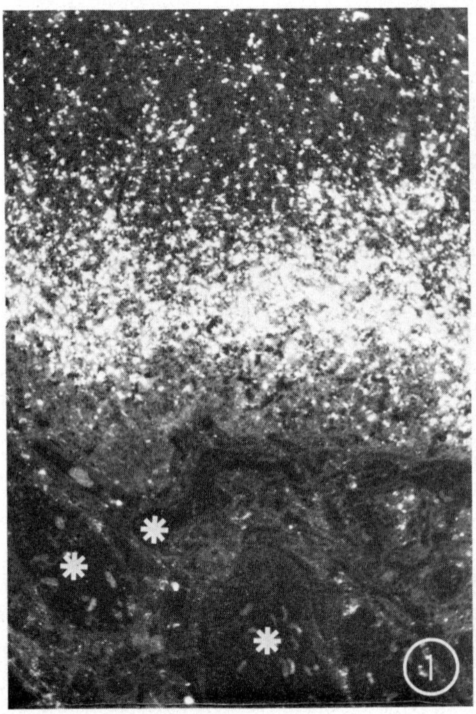

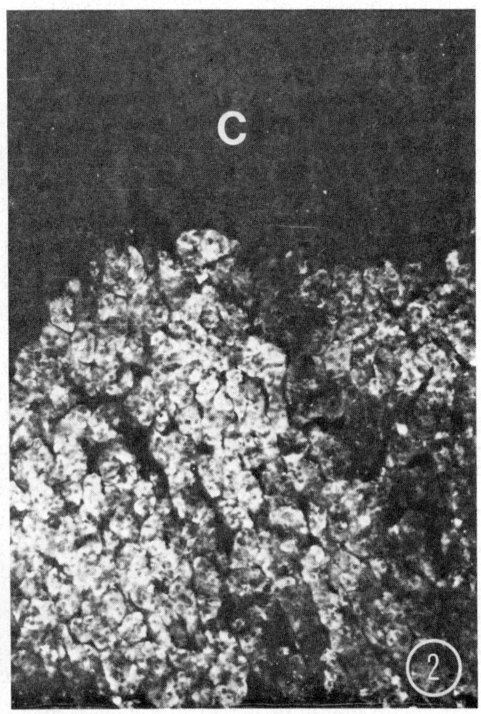

Fig. 1. Immunofluorescence photomicrograph of an ultrathin (100 nm) epoxy section of cat median eminence after inoculation with somatostatin antiserum. This tissue was frozen, dried, fixed by exposure to osmium vapors in vacuo and embedded in Spurr's resin according to Coulter and Terracio (1977), prior to postembedding staining by immunofluorescence. Note the intensely staining zone of somatostatin immunoreactivity in the external layer of the median eminence, near the portal vessels (*). Magnification, × 460.

Fig. 2. Immunofluorescence photomicrograph of a cat adrenal gland after incubation with met-enkephalin antiserum. Note the staining indicating the presence of met-enkephalin immunoreactivity in many medullary cells and the absence of staining in cells of the adrenal cortex (C). Magnification, × 120.

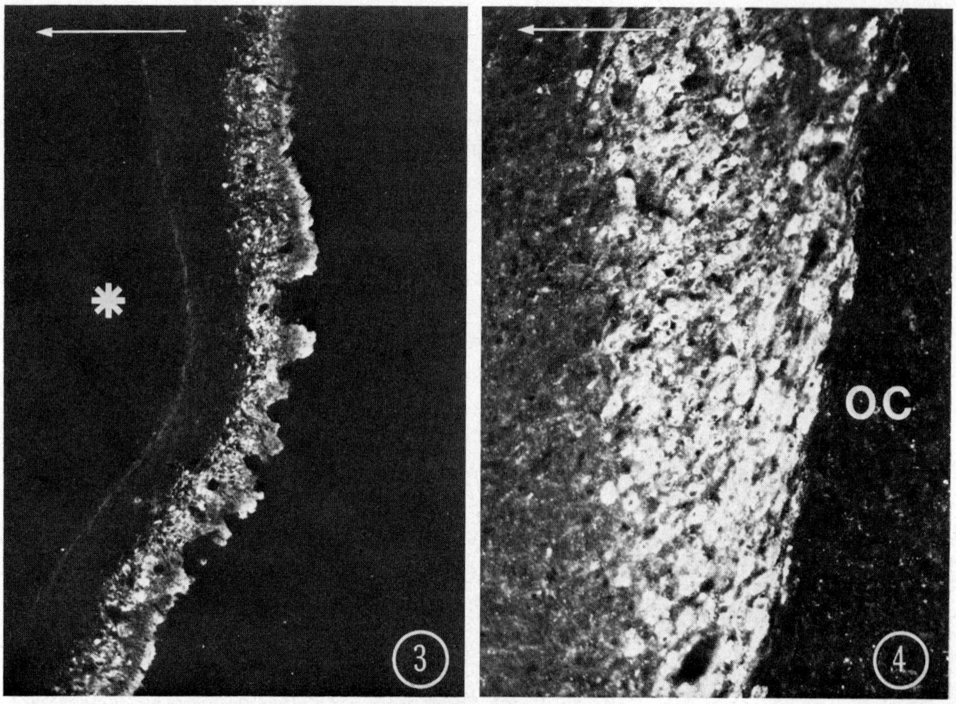

Fig. 3. Immunofluorescence photomicrograph of a portion of the cat median eminence after incubation with met-enkephalin antiserum. Fluorescent dot- and fiber-like staining is apparent especially in the external layer of the median eminence adjacent to the indentations made by portal capillaries. (*) indicates third ventricle; arrow points dorsally. Magnification, × 120.

Fig. 4. Immunofluorescence photomicrograph of the cat supraoptic nucleus after incubation with antiserum to met-enkephalin. Note the concentration of met-enkephalin immunoreactive perikarya in this region of the nucleus and the dot- and fiber-like structures immediately dorsal to the nucleus. OC, optic chiasm; arrow points dorsally. Magnification, × 120.

1978b) and angiotensin II (Hökfelt et al., 1978b) immunoreactivity in cell bodies and terminals are found in these plexuses. Moreover, some sympathetic ganglia (e.g., the inferior mesenteric and superior cervical ganglion) contain adrenergic cell bodies that simultaneously contain somatostatin (Hökfelt et al., 1977b) and enkephalin immunoreactivity (Schultzberg et al., 1979).

Recent studies of the adrenal medulla have revealed that, in addition to the presence of enkephalin immunoreactive terminals, a high proportion of the adrenergic adrenal medullary gland cells in the guinea pig and cat (Fig. 2) contain M-ENK immunoreactivity (Schultzberg et al., 1978). Such cells are not prevalent in the normal rat adrenal medulla, but after interruption of the greater splanchnic nerve, numerous M-ENK immunoreactive adrenergic gland cells are present. The latter findings indicate that the presence of M-ENK immunoreactivity is closely linked to the functional state of the gland cells.

Taken together, the widespread presence of various neuropeptides in the autonomic nervous system suggests a more complex neurotransmitter circuitry than previously appreciated. Furthermore, the neuropeptides, in some cases, seem to simultaneously occur in neurons that utilize classical neurotransmitters. The implications of the latter present new challenges in understanding control mechanisms of neurons containing more than one putative neuroeffector substance.

Phylogenetic and ontogenetic aspects of neuropeptide distribution

The details of the distribution of several neuropeptides in the rat nervous system are now known or are presently under intensive investigation. It is tempting to hypothesize that homologous neural circuits in the brains of other species contain peptides similar to those contained in the rat. While this notion seems to be quite valid, several examples will suggest caution in such hypotheses.

The external layer of the rat median eminence contains virtually no SP immunoreactive terminals (Cuello and Kanazawa, 1978; Hökfelt et al., 1978d). However, it has recently been demonstrated that the external layer of the primate median eminence contains a very high density of SP immunoreactive terminals which suggests that in the primate, SP released at this site may either directly effect the release of pituitary hormones in the manner of a releasing factor, or alternatively, may interact in axo-axonic fashion with median eminence terminals containing true releasing factors (Hökfelt et al., 1978d).

Somewhat similarly, the external layer of the rat median eminence contains only a modest network of enkephalin terminals, while the pituitary stalk and posterior lobe are virtually free of enkephalin immunoreactivity (Hökfelt et al., 1978a). In the cat, on the other hand, an extremely dense pattern of enkephalin immunoreactive fibers is present in the external layer of the median eminence (Fig. 3) and extends into the stalk and posterior pituitary (Micevych and Elde, 1978). Enkephalin immunoreactive perikarya are interspersed among the vasopressin and oxytocin immunoreactive magnocellular perikarya of the supraoptic (Fig. 4) and paraventricular nuclei of the cat.

Finally, De Lanerolle et al. (1979) have recently studied the distribution of enkephalin immunoreactivity in the CNS of the domestic chick using immunohistochemical techniques. Immunoreactive neurons in the chick seem to be, in many cases, projection neurons rather than interneurons, as in the rat. Furthermore, striatal areas in the chick thought to be homologous to the mamallian amygdala, globus pallidus and caudate-putamen are nearly devoid of enkephalin immunoreactive cells, fibers and terminals. Most of the enkephalin immunoreactivity in the chick CNS is found in the diencephalon and lower brain stem. Thus, it is clear that detailed studies of a range of vertebrates are necessary before a hypothetical framework can be constructed to account for the occurrence of neuropeptides in phylogenetically homologous structures.

Little is known concerning the ontogenetic development of peptidergic neurons. Ho et al. (1979) have described the development of somatostatin immunoreactive neurons using immunohistochemical techniques. Somatostatin immunoreactivity was not demonstrable in rat primary afferent neurons until 4 days of postnatal life. The somatostatin neuroendocrine system did not contain detectable quantities of immunoreactivity until the time of partuition. In both cases, it is believed that the neurons have differentiated and sent axonal terminals to their respective targets long before somatostatin immunoreactivity could be demonstrated. This pattern is in striking contrast to monoaminergic neurons, in which the appropriate neurotransmitter in acquired near the "birthdate" of the neuron, before it begins to extend processes to target areas (Olson and Seiger, 1972; Lauder and Bloom, 1974). Thus, the relative role of neuropeptides and monoamines during development may be quite different. It is not known if similar differences persist after development in serving either to maintain synaptic relationships or to regulate neuronal plasticity.

SUMMARY

The distribution of neuropeptides as revealed by immunohistochemical techniques suggests two varieties of neural circuits in which the peptides play a role. The first of these generalized systems is thought to participate in neuroendocrine regulation, since the peptides are found in high concentrations in terminals adjacent to vascular elements that drain either to the anterior pituitary or to systemic circulation. Peptides released from such neurohemal sites may act as hormones upon target cells. Alternatively, they may act via axo-axonic interactions with other peptidergic terminals which liberate "true" hormones.

Neuropeptides are also found in circuits of neurons engaged in interneuronal communication. In the case of the enkephalins, it is especially noteworthy that their distribution in nerve terminals parallels, to a great extent, the distribution of opiate receptors. Thus, it is likely that neuropeptides also play a significant role in interneuronal communication – perhaps as neurotransmitters.

ACKNOWLEDGEMENTS

Work reviewed from the author's laboratory was supported by grants from the Graduate School, University of Minnesota, USPHS DA-02148 and a Scholar in Neuroscience Award to R.E. from the McKnight Foundation. The technical expertise of L. Grouse and T. Mullet and the secretarial assistance of J. L. Mattson are gratefully acknowledged.

REFERENCES

Alpert, L. C., Brawer, J. R., Patel, Y. C. and Reichlin, S. (1976) Somatostatinergic neurons in anterior hypothalamus: immunohistochemical localization. *Endocrinology*, 98: 255–258.

Amoss, M., Burgus, R., Blackwell, R., Vale, W., Fellows, R. and Guillemin, R. (1971) Purification, amino acid composition and N-terminus of the hypothalamic luteinizing hormone releasing factor (LRF) of ovine origin. *Biochem. biophys. Res. Commun.*, 44: 205–210.

Antunes, J. L., Carmel, P. W. and Zimmerman, E. A. (1977) Projections from the paraventricular nucleus to the zona externa of the median eminence of the rhesus monkey: an immunohistochemical study. *Brain Res.*, 137: 1–10.

Arimura, A., Lundquist, G., Rothman, J., Chang, R., Fernandez-Durango, R., Elde, R., Coy, D. H., Meyers, C. and Schally, A. V. (1978) Radioimmunoassay of somatostatin. *Metabolism*, 27 (Suppl. 1): 1139–1144.

Atweh, S. and Kuhar, M. J. (1977) Autoradiographic localization of opiate receptors in rat brain. I. Spinal cord and lower medulla. *Brain Res.*, 124: 53–67.

Barry, J., Dubois, M. P. and Poulain, P. (1973) LRF producing cells of the mammalian hypothalamus. *Z. Zellforsch.*, 146: 351–366.

Bhattacharya, A. N. and Marks, B. H. (1969) Reserpine- and chlorpromazine-induced changes in hypothalamo-hypophyseal-adrenal system in rats in the presence and absence of hypothermia. *J. Pharmacol. exp. Ther.*, 165: 108–116.

Bloom, F., Battenberg, E., Rossier, J., Ling, N. and Guillemin, R. (1978) Neurons containing β-endorphin in rat brain exist separately from those containing enkephalin: immunocytochemical studies. *Proc. nat. Acad. Sci. (Wash.)*, 75: 1591–1595.

Bradbury, A. F., Smyth, D. G. and Snell, C. R. (1976) Lipotropin: precursor to two biologically active peptides. *Biochem. biophys. Res. Commun.*, 69: 950–956.

Brazeau, P., Vale, W., Burgus, R., Ling, N., Butchar, M., Rivier, J. and Guillemin, R. (1973) Hypothalamic polypeptide that inhibits the secretion of immunoreactive pituitary growth hormone. *Science*, 179: 77–79.

Brownstein, M. J. (1977) Biologically active peptides in the mammalian central nervous system. In *Peptides in Neurobiology*, H. Gainer (Ed.), Plenum Press, New York, pp. 145–170.

Brownstein, M. J. (1978) Are "hypothalamic hormones" central neurotransmitters? In *Centrally Acting Peptides*, J. Hughes (Ed.), Macmillan, London, pp. 37–47.

Brownstein, M. J., Palkovits, M., Saavedra, J. M., Bassiri, R. and Utiger, R. D. (1974) Thyrotropin-releasing hormone in specific nuclei of rat brain. *Science*, 185: 267–269.

Brownstein, M. J. Arimura, A., Fernandez-Durango, R., Schally, A. V. and Kizer, J. S. (1977) The effect of hypothalamic deafferentation on somatostatin like activity in the rat brain. *Endocrinology*, 100: 246–253.

Bryant, M. G., Polak, J. M. Modlin, I., Bloom, S. R., Albuquerque, R. H. and Pearse, A. G. E. (1976) Possible dual role for vasoactive intestinal peptide as gastrointestinal hormone and neurotransmitter substance. *Lancet*, 1: 991–993.

Burgus, R., Dunn, T. F., Desiderio, D., Ward, D. N., Vale, W. and Guillemin, R. (1970) Characterization of ovine hypothalamic hypophysiotropic TSH-releasing factor. *Nature (Lond.)* 226: 321–325.

Carraway, R. and Leeman, S. E. (1975) The amino acid sequence of a hypothalamic peptide, neurotensin. *J. biol. Chem.*, 250: 1907–1911.

Chang, M. M., Leeman, S. E. and Niall, H. D. (1971) Amino acid sequence of substance P. *Nature New Biol.*, 232: 86–87.

Chan-Palay, V., Jonsson, G. and Palay, S. L. (1978) Serotonin and substance P coexist in neurons of the rat's central nervous system. *Proc. nat. Acad. Sci. (Wash.)*, 75: 1582–1586.

Choy, V. J. and Watkins, W. B. (1977) Immunohistochemical localization of thyrotropin-releasing factor in the rat median eminence. *Cell Tiss. Res.*, 177: 371–374.

Coons, A. H. (1958) Fluorescent antibody methods. In *General Cytochemical Methods*, J. F. Danielli (Ed.), Academic Press, New York, pp. 399–422.

Costa, M., Patel, Y., Furness, J. B. and Arimura, A. (1977) Evidence that some intrinsic neurons of the intestine contain somatostatin. *Neurosci. Lett.*, 6: 215–222.

Coulter, H. D. and Elde, R. (1979) Neuropeptide immunocytochemistry of frozen-dried nervous tissue. *J. Histochem. Cytochem.*, in press.

Coulter, H. D. and Terracio, L. (1977) Preparation of biological tissues for electron microscopy by freeze-drying. *Anat. Rec.*, 187: 477–494.

Cuello, A. C. and Kanazawa, I. (1978) The distribution of substance P immunoreactive fibers in the rat central nervous system. *J. comp. Neurol.*, 178: 129–156.

Dahlström, A. and Fuxe, K. (1964) Evidence for the existence of monoamine containing neurons in the central nervous system. I. Demonstration of monoamines in the cell bodies of brainstem neurons. *Acta physiol. scand.*, 62 (Suppl. 232): 1–55.

Defendini, R. and Zimmerman, E. A. (1978) The magnocellular neurosecretory system of the mammalian hypothalamus. In *The Hypothalamus*, S. Reichlin, R. J. Baldessarini and J. B. Martin (Eds.), Raven Press, New York, pp. 137–152.

De Lanerolle, N. C., Elde, R. P. and Sparber, S. B. (1979) Distribution of methionine-enkephalin immunoreactivity in the chick brain: an immunohistochemical study. Submitted for publication.

Dockray, G. J. (1976) Immunohistochemical evidence of cholecystokinin-like peptides in brain. *Nature (Lond.)*, 264: 568–570.

Dube, D., Lissitzky, J. C., Leclerc, R. and Pelletier, G. (1978) Localization of α-melanocyte-stimulating hormone in rat brain and pituitary. *Endocrinology*, 102: 1283–1291.

DuVigneaud, V. (1954) Hormones of the posterior pituitary gland: oxytocin and vasopressin. *Harvey Lect.*, Ser. L: 1–26.

Elde, R. and Hökfelt, T. (1978) Distribution of hypothalamic hormones and other peptides in the brain. In *Frontiers in Neuroendocrinology, Vol. 5*, W. F. Ganong and L. Martini (Eds.), Raven Press, New York, pp. 1–33.

Elde, R. P. and Parsons, J. A. (1975) Immunocytochemical localization of somatostatin in cell bodies of the rat hypothalamus. *Amer. J. Anat.*, 144: 541–548.

Elde, R., Hökfelt, T., Johansson, O. and Terenius, L. (1976) Immunohistochemical studies using antibodies to leucine-enkephalin: initial observations on the nervous system of the rat. *Neuroscience* 1: 349–351.

Elde, R. P., Hökfelt, T., Johansson, O., Ljungdahl, Å., Nilsson, G. and Jeffcoate, S. L. (1978) Immunohistochemical localization of peptides in the nervous system. In *Centrally Acting Peptides*, J. Hughes (Ed.), Macmillan, London, pp. 17–35.

Emson, P. C., Jessel, T., Paxinos, G. and Cuello, A. C. (1978) Substance P in the amygdaloid complex, bed nucleus and stria terminalis of the rat brain. *Brain Res.*, 149: 97–105.

Epelbaum, J., Willoughby, J. O., Brazeau, P. and Martin, J. B. (1977) Effects of brain lesions and hypothalamic deafferentation on somatostatin distribution in the rat brain. *Endocrinology*, 101: 1495–1502.

Euler, U. S. von and Gaddum, J. H. (1931) An unidentified depressor substance in certain tissue extracts. *J. Physiol. (Lond.)*, 72: 74–87.

Falck, B., Hillarp, N. A., Thieme, G. and Torp, A. (1962) Fluorescence of catecholamines and related compounds with formaldehyde. *J. Histochem. Cytochem.*, 10: 348–354.

Fuxe, K. (1965) Evidence for the existence of monoamine neurons in the central nervous system. IV. The distribution of monoamine nerve terminals in the central nervous system. *Acta physiol. scand.*, 64 (Suppl. 247): 39–85.

Fuxe, K., Hökfelt, T., Said, S. and Mutt, V. (1977) Evidence for the existence of VIP-containing nerve terminals in the rat brain. *Neurosci. Lett.*, 5: 241–246.

Gainer, H., Sarne, Y. and Brownstein, M. J. (1977) Neurophysin biosynthesis: conversion of a putative precursor during axonal transport. *Science*, 195: 1354–1356.

Guillemin, R. (1978a) Some thoughts on current research with somatostatin. *Metabolism*, 27 (Suppl. 1): 1453–1461.

Guillemin, R. (1978b) Biochemical and physiological correlates of hypothalamic peptides. The new endocrinology of the neuron. In *The Hypothalamus*, S. Reichlin, R. J. Baldessarini and J. B. Martin (Eds.), Raven Press, New York, pp. 155–194.

Guillemin, R., Ling, N. et Burgus, R. (1976) Endorphines, peptides, d'origine hypothalamique et neurohypophysaire à l'activité morphinomimétique. Isolement et structure moléculaire et l'α-endorpine. *C.R. Acad. Sci. (Paris)*, 282: 783–785.

Ho, R., Elde, R. and Sorenson, R. L. (1979) Immunohistochemical and radioimmunoassay studies on the development of somatostatin containing neurons in the rat primary afferent system. Submitted for publication.

Hoffman, G. E., Knigge, K. M., Moynihan-McCourt, J. A., Melnyk, V. and Arimura, A. (1978) Luteinizing hormone-releasing hormone (LH-RH) containing neuronal fields in mouse brain. *Neuroscience*, 3: 219–231.

Hökfelt, T., Efendić, S., Hellerström, C., Johansson, O., Luft, R. and Arimura, A. (1975a) Cellular localization of somatostatin in endocrine-like cells and neurons of the rat with special references to the A_1 cells of the pancreatic islets and to the hypothalamus. *Acta endocr. (Kbh.)*, 200 (Suppl.): 5–41.

Hökfelt, T., Fuxe, K. and Goldstein, M. (1975b) Applications of immunohistochemistry to studies on monoamine cell systems with special references to nervous tissue. *Ann. N.Y. Acad. Sci.*, 254: 407–432.

Hökfelt, T., Fuxe, K., Johansson, O., Jeffcoate, S. and White, N. (1975c) Thyrotropin-releasing hormone (TRH)-containing nerve terminals in certain brain stem nuclei and in the spinal cord. *Neurosci. Lett.*, 1: 133–139.

Hökfelt, T., Fuxe, K., Johansson, O., Jeffcoate, S. L. and White, N. (1975d) Distribution of thyrotropin-releasing hormone (TRH) in the central nervous system as revealed with immunohistochemistry. *Europ. J. Pharmacol.*, 34: 389–392.

Hökfelt, T., Elde, R., Johansson, O., Luft, R., Nilsson, G. and Arimura, A. (1976) Immunohistochemical evidence for separate populations of somatostatin-containing and substance P-containing primary afferent neurons. *Neuroscience*, 1: 131–136.

Hökfelt, T., Elde, R., Johansson, O., Terenius, L. and Stein, L. (1977a) The distribution of enkephalin immunoreactive cell bodies in the rat central nervous system. *Neurosci. Lett.*, 5: 25–31.

Hökfelt, T., Elfvin, L.-G., Elde, R., Schultzberg, M., Goldstein, M. and Luft, R. (1977b) Occurrence of somatostatin-like immunoreactivity in some peripheral sympathetic noradrenergic neurons. *Proc. nat. Acad. Sci. (Wash.)*, 74: 3587–3591.

Hökfelt, T., Ljungdahl, Å., Terenius, L., Elde, R. and Nilsson, G. (1977c) Immunohistochemical analysis of peptide pathways possibly related to pain and analgesia: enkephalin and substance P. *Proc. nat. Acad. Sci. (Wash.)*, 74: 3081–3085.

Hökfelt, T., Elde, R., Fuxe, K., Johansson, O., Ljungdahl, Å., Goldstein, M., Luft, R., Nilsson, G., Said, S., Fraser, H., Jeffcoate, S. L., White, N., Ganten, D. and Rehfeld, J. (1978a) Aminergic and peptidergic pathways in the nervous system with special reference to the hypothalamus. In *The Hypothalamus*, S. Reichlin, R. J. Baldessarini and J. B. Martin (Eds.), Raven Press, New York, pp. 69–135.

Hökfelt, T., Elde, R. P., Johansson, O., Ljungdahl, Å., Schultzberg, M., Fuxe, K., Goldstein, M., Nilsson, G., Pernow, B., Terenius, L., Ganten, D., Jeffcoate, S. L., Rehfeld, J. and Said, S. (1978b) The distribution of peptide containing neurons in the nervous system. In *Psychopharmacology: a Generation of Progress*, M. A. Lipton, A. DiMascio and K. F. Killam (Eds.), Raven Press, New York, pp. 39–66.

Hökfelt, T., Ljungdahl, Å., Steinbusch, H., Verhofstad, A., Nilsson, G., Brodin, E., Pernow, B. and Goldstein, M. (1978c) Immunohistochemical evidence for substance P-like immunoreactivity in some 5-hydroxytryptamine-containing neurons in the rat central nervous system. *Neuroscience,* 3: 517–538.

Hökfelt, T., Pernow, B., Nilsson, G., Welterberg, L., Goldstein, M. and Jeffcoate, S. L. (1978d) Dense plexus of substance P immunoreactive nerve terminals in eminentia medialis of the primate hypothalamus. *Proc. nat. Acad. Sci. (Wash.)*, 75: 1013–1015.

Hughes, J., Smith, F. W., Kosterlitz, H. W., Fothergill, L. H., Morgan, B. A. and Morris, H. R. (1975) Identification of two related pentapeptides from the brain with potent opiate agonist activity. *Nature (Lond.)*, 258: 577–579.

Innis, R. B., Correa, F. M. A. and Snyder, S. H. (1978) Distribution of cholecystokinin octapeptide-like immunoreactivity in the rat brain. *Soc. Neurosci. Abstr.*, 4: 410.

Jackson, I. M. D. and Reichlin, S. (1974) Thyrotropin-releasing hormone (TRH): distribution in hypothalamic and extrahypothalamic brain tissue of mammalian and submammalian chordates. *Endocrinology*, 95: 854–862.

Johnson, J. L. (1977) Glutamic acid as a synaptic transmitter candidate in the dorsal sensory neuron: reconsiderations. *Life Sci.*, 20: 1637–1644.

Krulich, L., Dhariwal, A. P. S. and McCann, S. M. (1968) Stimulatory and inhibitory effects of purified hypothalamic extracts on growth hormone release from rat pituitary in vitro. *Endocrinology,* 83: 783–790.

Larsson, L.-I., Fahrenkrug, J., Schaffalitzky de Muckadell, O., Sundler, F., Hakanson, R. and Rehfeld, J. F. (1976) Localization of vasoactive intestinal polypeptide (VIP) to central and peripheral neurons. *Proc. nat. Acad. Sci. (Wash.)*, 73: 3197–3200.

Lauder, J. M. and Bloom, F. E. (1974) Ontogeny of monoamine neurons in the locus coeruleus, raphe nuclei and substantia nigra of the rat. I. Cell differentiation. *J. comp. Neurol.*, 155: 469–482.

Lembeck, F. (1978) Substance P: a historical account. In *Centrally Acting Peptides,* J. Hughes (Ed.), Macmillan, London, pp. 119–124.

Leonardelli, J., Barry, J. et Dubois, M. P. (1973) Mise en évidence par immunofluorescence d'un constituant immunologiquement apparente au LH-RF dans l'hypothalamus et l'éminence médiane chez les mammifères. *C.R. Acad. Sci. (Paris)*, 276: 2043–2046.

Li, C. H. and Chung, D. (1976) Isolation and structure of an untriakontapeptide with opiate activity from camel pituitary glands. *Proc. natl. Acad. Sci. (Wash.)*, 73: 1145–1148.

Ljungdahl, Å., Hökfelt, T. and Nilsson, G. (1978) Distribution of substance P-like immunoreactivity in the central nervous system of the rat. I. Cell bodies and nerve terminals. *Neuroscience,* 3: 861–943.

Mains, R. E., Eipper, B. A. and Ling, N. (1977) Common precursor to corticotropins and endorphins. *Proc. nat. Acad. Sci. (Wash.)*, 74: 3014–3018.

Micevych, P. and Elde, R. (1978) Comparative immunohistochemistry of met-enkephalin, vasopressin and oxytocin in the median eminence and hypothalamus of the cat. *Soc. Neurosci. Abstr.*, 4: 411.

Nair, R. M. G., Barrett, J. F., Bowers, C. Y. and Schally, A. V. (1970) Structure of porcine thyrotropin releasing hormone. *Biochemistry,* 9: 1103–1106.

Nakane, P. K. (1971) Application of peroxidase-labelled antibodies to the intracellular localization of hormones. In *Karolinska Symposia on Research Methods in Reproductive Endocrinology. Vol. 3. In Vitro Methods in Reproductive Cell Biology,* A. Dickfalusy (Ed.), Forum, Copenhagen, pp. 190–204.

Oliver, C. and Porter, J. C. (1978) Distribution and characterization of melanocyte-stimulating hormone in the rat brain. *Endocrinology,* 102: 697–705.

Oliver, C., Eskay, R. L., Ben-Jonathan, N. and Porter, J. C. (1974) Distribution and concentration of TRH in the rat brain. *Endocrinology,* 96: 540–546.

Olson, L. and Seiger, A. (1972) Early prenatal ontogeny of central monoamine neurons in the rat: fluorescence histochemical observations. *Z. Anat. Entwickl.-Gesch.*, 137: 301–316.

Otsuka, M. and Takahashi, T. (1977) Putative peptide neurotransmitters. *Ann. Rev. Pharmacol. Toxicol.*, 17: 425–439.

Pearse, A. G. E. (1978) Diffuse neuroendocrine system: peptides common to brain and intestine and their relationship to the APUD concept. In *Centrally Acting Peptides,* J. Hughes (Ed.), Macmillan, London, pp. 49–57.

Pearse, A. G. E. and Polak, J. (1975) Immunocytochemical localization of substance P in mammalian intestine. *Histochemistry,* 41: 373–375.

Pease, D. C. (1962) Buffered formaldehyde as a killing agent and primary fixative for electron microscopy. *Anat. Rec.,* 142: 342.

Pert, C. B., Kuhar, M. J. and Snyder, S. H. (1976) Opiate receptor: autoradiographic localization in rat brain. *Proc. nat. Acad. Sci. (Wash.),* 73: 3729–3733.

Rehfeld, J. F. (1978) Immunochemical studies on cholecystokinin. II. Distribution and molecular heterogeneity in the central nervous system and small intestine of man and hog. *J. biol. Chem.,* 253: 4022–4030.

Robberecht, P., Deschodt-Lanckman, M. and Vanderhaeghen, J. J. (1978) Demonstration of biological activity of brain gastrin-like peptidic material in the human: its relationship with the COOH-terminal octapeptide of cholecystokinin. *Proc. nat. Acad. Sci. (Wash.),* 75: 524–528.

Roberts, J. L. and Herbert, E. (1977) Characterization of a common precursor to corticotropin and β-lipotropin: identification of β-lipotropin peptides and their arrangement relative to corticotropin in the precursor synthesized in a cell-free system. *Proc. nat. Acad. Sci. (Wash.),* 74: 5300–5304.

Sachs, H. and Takabatake, Y. (1964) Evidence for a precursor in vasopressin biosynthesis. *Endocrinology,* 75: 939–948.

Schally, A. V., Arimura, A., Baba, Y., Nair, R. M. G., Matsuo, J., Redding, T. W., Debeljuk, L. and White, W. F. (1971) Isolation and properties of the FSH- and LH-releasing hormone. *Biochem. biophys. Res. Commun.,* 43: 393–399.

Schultzberg, M., Lundberg, J. M., Hökfelt, T., Terenius, L., Brandt, J., Elde, R. P. and Goldstein, M. (1978) Enkephalin-like immunoreactivity in gland cells and nerve terminals of the adrenal medulla. *Neuroscience,* 3: 1169–1186.

Schultzberg, M., Hökfelt, T., Terenius, L., Elfvin, L.-G., Lundberg, J. M., Brandt, J., Elde, R. P. and Goldstein, M. (1979) Enkephalin immunoreactive nerve terminals and cell bodies in sympathetic ganglia of the guinea pig and rat. *Neuroscience,* 4: 249–270.

Seybold, V., Elde, R. and Hökfelt, T. (1978) Effects of reserpine on vasopressin and neurophysins in the external layer of the median eminence in the rat. *Soc. Neurosci. Abstr.,* 4: 355.

Silverman, A. J. and Krey, L. C. (1978) The luteinizing hormone-releasing hormone (LHRH) neuronal networks of the guinea pig. I. Intra- and extrahypothalamic projections. *Brain Res.,* 157: 233–246.

Simantov, R. and Snyder, S. H. (1976) Brain-pituitary opiate mechanisms: pituitary opiate receptor binding, radioimmunoassays for methionine enkephalin and leucine enkephalin, and ^{3}H-enkephalin interactions with the opiate receptor. In *Opiates and Endogenous Opioid Peptides,* H. W. Kosterlitz (Ed.), North-Holland, Amsterdam, pp. 41–48.

Simantov, R., Kuhar, M. M., Uhl, G. and Snyder, S. H. (1977) Opioid peptide enkephalin: immunohistochemical mapping in the rat central nervous system. *Proc. nat. Acad. Sci. (Wash.),* 74: 2167–2171.

Sofroniew, M. V. and Weindl, A. (1978) Extra-hypothalamic neurophysin-containing perikarya, fiber pathways and fiber clusters in the rat brain. *Endocrinology,* 102: 334–337.

Steinbusch, H. W. M., Verhofstad, A. A. J. and Joosten, H. W. J. (1978) Localization of serotonin in the central nervous system by immunocytochemistry: description of a specific and sensitive technique and some applications. *Neuroscience,* 3: 811–819.

Sternberger, L. A. (1974) *Immunocytochemistry.* Prentice-Hall, Englewood Cliffs, N.J.

Sternberger, L. A. and Hoffman, G. E. (1978) Immunocytology of luteinizing hormone-releasing hormone. *Neuroendocrinology,* 25: 111–128.

Stillman, M. A., Recht, L. D., Rosario, S. L., Seif, S. M., Robinson, A. G. and Zimmerman, E. A. (1977) The effects of adrenalectomy and glucocorticoid replacement on vasopressin and vasopressin-neurophysin in the zona externa of the median eminence of the rat. *Endocrinology,* 101: 42–49.

Straus, E. and Yalow, R. S. (1978) Species specificity of cholecystokinin in gut and brain of several mammalian species. *Proc. nat. Acad. Sci. (Wash.),* 75: 486–489.

Swaab, D. F. and Fisser, B. (1977) Immunocytochemical localization of α-melanocyte stimulating hormone (α-MSH)-like compounds in the rat nervous system. *Neurosci. Lett.,* 7: 313–317.

Swanson, L. W. (1977) Immunohistochemical evidence for a neurophysin-containing autonomic pathway arising in the paraventricular nucleus of the hypothalamus. *Brain Res.,* 128: 346–353.

Swanson, L. W. (1978) Extra-hypophysial oxytocin-containing pathways in the brain and spinal cord of the rat and monkey. *Soc. Neurosci. Abstr.*, 4: 415.

Uhl, G. R., Kuhar, M. J. and Snyder, S. H. (1977) Neurotensin: immunohistochemical localization in rat central nervous system. *Proc. nat. Acad. Sci. (Wash.)*, 74: 4059–4063.

Uhl, G. R., Kuhar, M. J. and Snyder, S. H. (1978) Enkephalin-containing pathways: amygdaloid efferents in the stria terminalis. *Brain Res.*, 149: 223–228.

Watson, S. J., Barchas, J. D. and Li, C. H. (1977) β-Lipotropin: localization of cells and axons in rat brain by immunocytochemistry. *Proc. nat. Acad. Sci. (Wash.)*, 74: 5155–5518.

Watson, S. J., Akil, H., Richard, C. W. and Barchas, J. D. (1978) Evidence for two separate opiate peptide neuronal systems. *Nature (Lond.)*, 275: 226–228.

Winokur, A. and Utiger, R. D. (1974) Thyrotropin-releasing hormone: regional distribution in rat brain. *Science*, 185: 265–267.

Yang, A.-Y., Hong, J. S. and Costa, E. (1977) Regional distribution of leu- and met-enkephalin in rat brain. *Neuropharmacology*, 16: 303–307.

Zimmerman, E. A., Liotta, A. and Kreiger, D. T. (1978) β-Lipotropin in brain: localization in hypothalamic neurons by immunoperoxidase technique. *Cell Tiss. Res.*, 186: 393–398.

Fiber Connections of the Basal Ganglia

ANN M. GRAYBIEL and CLIFTON W. RAGSDALE, Jr.

Department of Psychology and Brain Science, Massachusetts Institute of Technology, Cambridge, Mass. 02139 (U.S.A.)

INTRODUCTION

The functions of the basal ganglia are still inferred mainly on the basis of clinical syndromes rather than direct physiological study. These syndromes have established the importance of the basal ganglia in the central control of movement and have long suggested a relation of this group of telencephalic nuclei to the purposive as well as to the more mechanical aspects of motor function. It is not yet clear, however, even nearly three-quarters of a century after S. A. Kinnier Wilson coined the term "extrapyramidal system," how the basal ganglia should be fitted into a general framework of the supraspinal motor mechanism considered as a whole. This is partly due to difficulties in undertaking electrophysiological studies of these large subcortical masses and certainly also to the lack, until very recently, of adequate methods for tracing out the anatomical connections linking the basal ganglia with other parts of the brain. But we have entered a new period of intense effort sparked by advances in neuropharmacology and their clinical applications, and given impetus by the development in neuroanatomy of the axon transport techniques. The object of the present review is to incorporate the results of recent work on the anatomy into a general outline of the fiber connections of the basal ganglia. It will be clear that these new findings do not simply represent added facts but are already forcing significant revisions in the outline itself.

TERMINOLOGY

The term, basal ganglia, is used in different ways not only by clinicians but also by classical anatomists. Anatomists tend to include under the designation most or all of the non-cortical gray matter of the telencephalon: the caudate nucleus, the lentiform nucleus (putamen and globus pallidus), the claustrum, the amygdaloid complex and, variably emphasized as belonging to the group, the telencephalic gray matter ventral to the caudate and lentiform nuclei (the so-called fundus striati in and nearby the basal olfactory structures, substantia innominata and nucleus accumbens septi). Clinicians tend to restrict the term basal ganglia on functional grounds to the two nuclear elements of the corpus striatum, the caudate and lentiform nuclei. Because of the clear linkage of these nuclei to the motor system it seems reasonable to follow here the more restrictive clinical usage which further divides the basal ganglia into the *striatum* (caudate nucleus and putamen) and the *pallidum* (globus pallidus) (see Table I). One proviso is necessary, however, because a number of important findings summarized in 1975 by Heimer and Wilson suggest that the nucleus accumbens-olfactory tubercle region properly comprises an extension of the striatum (as Herrick (1926) had recognized by calling this region the olfacto-striatum) while part of the substantia innominata represents a ventral extension of the pallidum. Heimer and Wilson introduced the terms *ventral striatum* and *ventral pallidum* in reference to these districts and their nomenclature will be adopted here.

TABLE I

TERMINOLOGY USED IN REFERENCE TO THE MAIN ELEMENTS OF THE CORPUS STRIATUM

Corpus Striatum	Striatum	Caudate Nucleus	
		Putamen	Lentiform Nucleus
	Pallidum	Globus Pallidus	

We still need a general designation that would encompass, in the "extended family" of the basal ganglia, the substantia nigra and the subthalamic nucleus. For both of these non-telencephalic cell groups are nodal points in the circuitry of the basal ganglia and are, as much as the striatum and pallidum, associated with diseases of the basal ganglia. It would seem unwise to use Kinnier Wilson's term "extrapyramidal system" for the purpose (at least without some form of general consent) since even though Kinnier Wilson did not define the term too closely, it is generally understood to comprise, if not all the elements of the central motor mechanism aside from the pyramidal tract, at least the cerebellum and its allied nuclei in addition to the basal ganglia. It is ironic that although Kinnier Wilson's concept was based on a clinical distinction between the paralytic (pyramidal or corticospinal) and non-paralytic (extrapyramidal) disorders, anatomical findings suggest that the main subcortical input to the pyramidal system comes from the extrapyramidal system by way of trans-thalamic routes from the corpus striatum and cerebellum themselves (Fig. 1).

THE CORPUS STRIATUM

The corpus striatum apparently lies quite far removed from either the immediate "sensory" or "motor" periphery. Nevertheless, the corpus striatum can itself clearly be divided into an input side, the striatum, and an output side, the pallidum. This summary begins with the main afferent pathways and the principal through-conduction route of the system, the pathway from striatum to pallidum to thalamus. Even at the outset, however, it is important to point out that a prominent set of side loops are associated with this classic mainstream of the corpus striatum and that, as will be discussed further, these side loops are by no means dependent fully on the strio-pallido-thalamic pathway for connections with other parts of the brain.

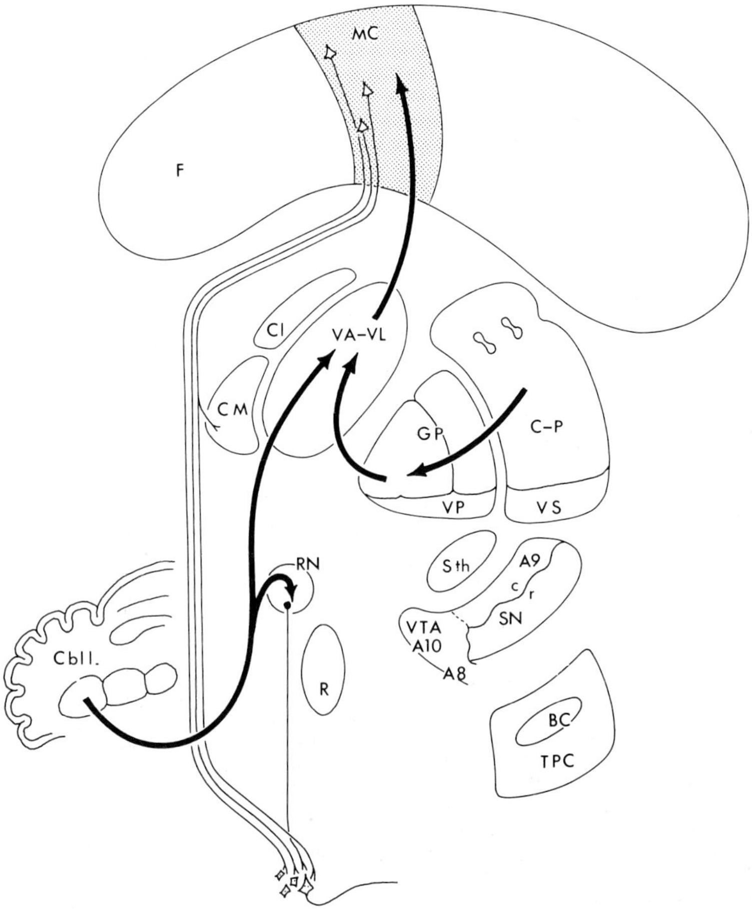

Fig. 1. Schematic diagram illustrating "pyramidal" and "extrapyramidal" motor systems. Cerebral cortex is shown above (F, frontal; MC, motor cortex). Below are the basal ganglia, cerebellum (Cbll.) and their allied nuclei: C-P, caudate-putamen; GP, globus pallidus; VS and VP, ventral striatum and ventral pallidum; Sth, subthalamic nucleus; SN, substantia nigra and related cell groups (r, pars reticulata; c, pars compacta corresponding to dopamine cell group A9; VTA, ventral tegmental area, corresponding to dopamine cell group A10 and partly continuous with dopamine cell group A8). Thalamic correspondents of basal ganglia are VA-VL: nuclei ventralis anterior and ventralis lateralis; and CM: centre médian. In the mesencephalon, red nucleus (RN), dorsal raphe nucleus (R), and the nucleus tegmenti pedunculopontinis (TPC) near the brachium conjunctivum (BC).

The striatum: the caudate nucleus and putamen

The photographs in Fig. 2 were prepared to give some impression of the marked increase in size and change in conformation of the striatum associated with progressive differentiation of the cerebral hemisphere in common laboratory mammals. In small mammals such as rodents (Fig. 2A) the striatum on each side forms a single large mass, the caudoputamen, that is pierced by the dispersed fibers of the internal capsule. In carnivores and primates (Fig. 2B, C) the striatum is relatively speaking much larger and the internal capsule forms a

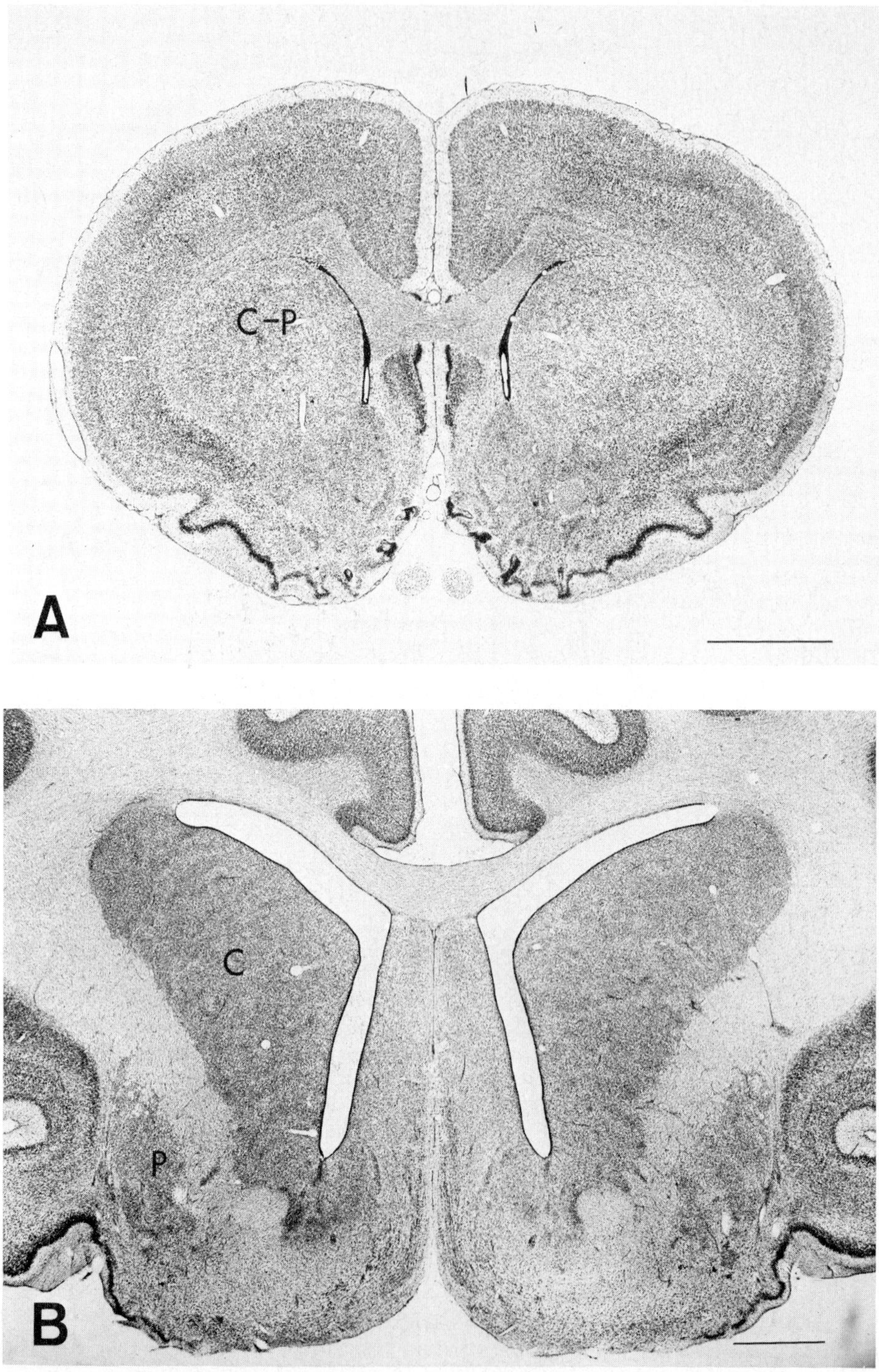

Fig. 2. Photographs illustrating relative differentiation of the striatum in transverse sections from the rat (A), cat (B), and monkey (C). Nissl stain; each bar indicates 2 mm. C-P, caudoputamen; CN, caudate nucleus; P, putamen. In C (an autoradiogram), star at right marks location of patches of labeling resulting from injection of tritiated amino acids into the premotor cortex.

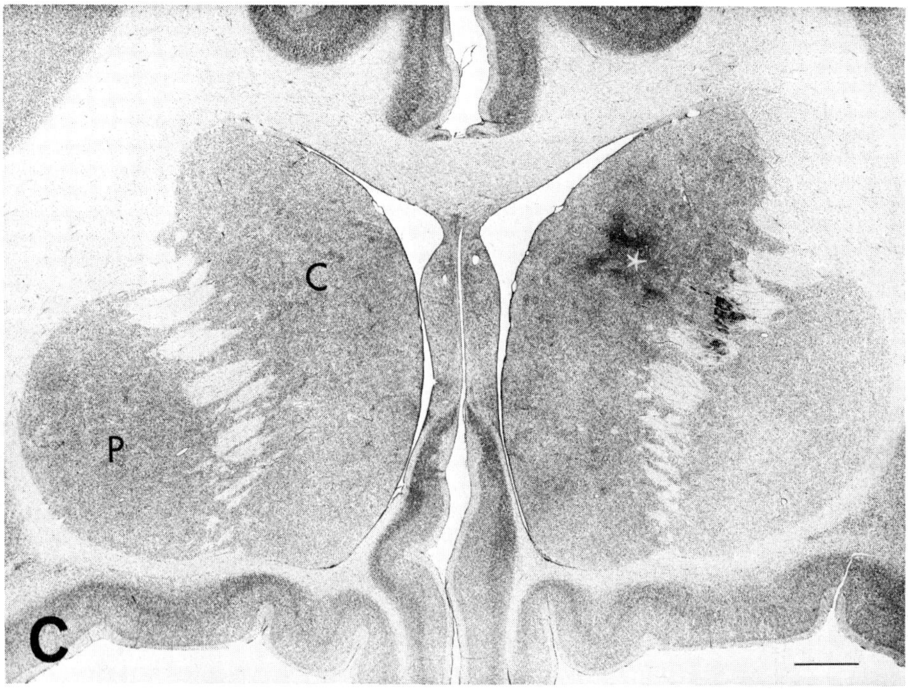

Fig. 2C.

massive fiber plate that almost, but not completely, separates off the caudate nucleus from the putamen. It is the laterally placed putamen that undergoes an apparently disproportionate increase in size in primates in parallel with the progressive development of the lentiform nucleus.

It is not yet known how these different striatal topologies should properly be compared, but this is a matter of some consequence since most neurochemical work and many neuroanatomical studies are performed on the rat, for which the equivalents of caudate nucleus and putamen have not been identified. In fact, the absence of a principled method, anatomical or otherwise, of distinguishing these structures makes it impossible even to establish a sure homology between the "caudate nucleus" of cat and monkey.

Despite these species differences, however, striatal tissue can be defined by at least 3 characteristics that apparently apply equally well to the caudate nucleus, putamen, caudoputamen or, with few qualifications, to the ventral striatum. First, the striatum has a peculiar cellular composition, some 95–98% or more of the neurons being of medium size (12–18 μm in diameter) and, at first glance, of homogeneous distribution; among these are scattered only occasional large or "giant" cells (20–30 μm). Second, the histochemistry of the striatum is unique among regions of the forebrain; this is recognized because of the massive innervation of the dorsal and ventral striatum by dopamine-containing fibers (Dahlström and Fuxe, 1964; Andén et al., 1966; Ungerstedt, 1971) and the extremely high concentration of acetylcholinesterase in these same regions (Koelle, 1954; Jacobowitz and Palkovits, 1974; see Fig. 3). Finally, the striatum can be defined by its fiber connections, for it receives nearly all of the extrinsic afferents of the corpus striatum, but has a limited efferent distribution, projecting only to the pallidum and substantia nigra. As discussed below, this may be a difference between caudate-putamen proper and ventral striatum: unlike the dorsal striatum (caudate-putamen), the ventral striatum apparently has a wide efferent fiber distribution (see below).

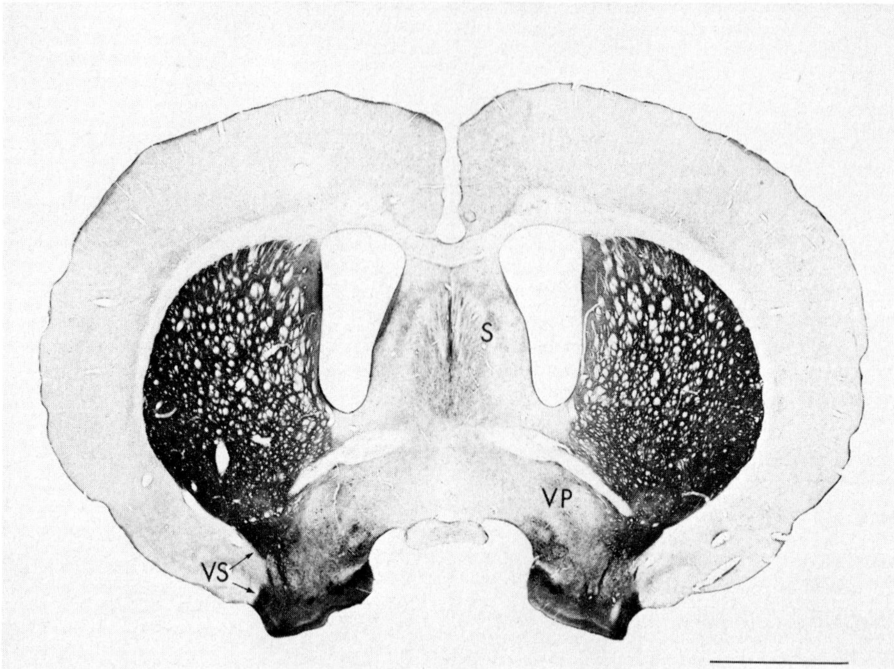

Fig. 3. Photograph of a transverse section from the rat illustrating dense acetylcholinesterase activity in the striatum (caudoputamen, compare with Fig. 2A). Dispersed fibers of internal capsule are not stained. VS, caudal part of ventral striatum; VP, ventral pallidum; S, septum. Geneser-Jensen and Blackstad (1971) reaction. Bar indicates 2 mm.

Afferent connections (Fig. 4)

(a) Cerebral cortex. The largest group of afferents to the striatum comes from the cerebral cortex. Apparently the entire neocortex projects to the caudate nucleus-putamen complex and it is a fundamental recent realization that for the ventral striatum a parallel generalization may hold, namely, that the allocortical formations (hippocampus, piriform cortex) project to the nucleus accumbens-olfactory tubercle region (Heimer and Wilson, 1975).

There is general agreement that the corticostriatal projection must be of cardinal importance in impressing a topography or set of regional subdivisions on the striatum and consequently on the outflow mechanism of the striatum as a whole. The study of this topography has been fraught with difficulties, however, most arising from inadequate techniques but some certainly resulting from the complexities of the sheet-to-solid mapping itself. The extensive work on these fiber projections by the Oxford group using fiber degeneration methods (e.g., Webster, 1961, 1965; Carman et al., 1963, 1965; Cowan and Powell, 1966) was summarized by Kemp and Powell (1970, 1971c). These authors concluded that probably all parts of the caudate nucleus and putamen in the rhesus monkey receive input from more than one cortical area and, conversely, that with only one exception (the second somatic sensory region) all cortical areas project both to the caudate nucleus and to the putamen. Kemp and Powell also confirmed that there is an orderly arrangement of the corticostriatal projection as a whole and that individual cortical inputs must have different weightings because of marked differences in their densities, the projection

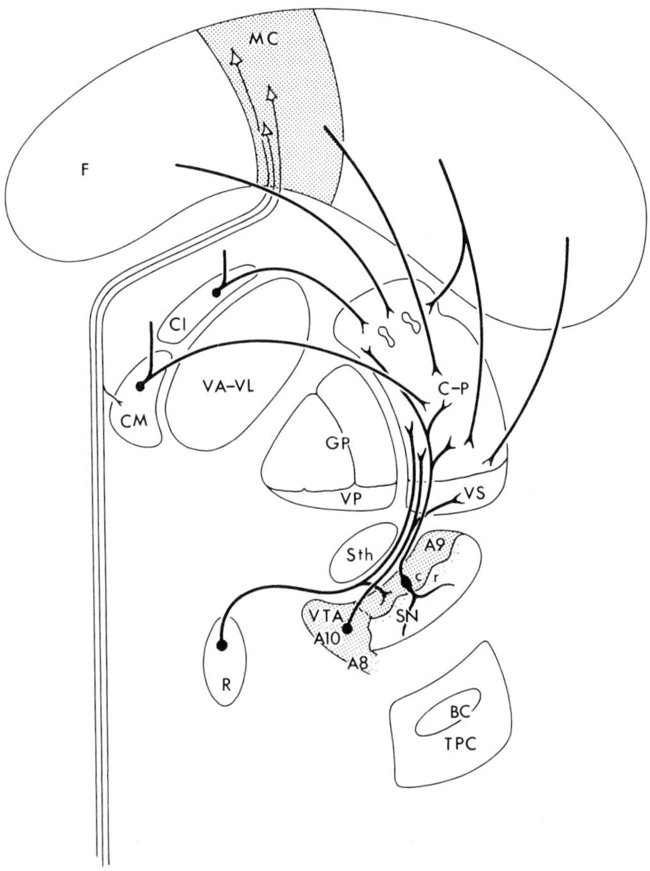

Fig. 4. Schematic diagram illustrating the main afferents of the striatum (abbreviations same as those used in Fig. 1).

from the visual area being notably weak, that from the sensorimotor cortex notably extensive, and that from pericentral cortex bilateral.

It is now clear that the view of corticostriatal organization afforded by fiber degeneration studies will have to be very substantially altered in respect to both the general topography of the projections and their mode of local termination within the striatum. This need for revision was first clearly established as the result of an autoradiographic tracing study by Künzle (1975), who showed that the motor cortex in the rhesus monkey projects almost exclusively to the putamen, rather than in duplicative form to both caudate nucleus and putamen. Künzle further found that the fiber terminations in the putamen were not homogeneously distributed but organized in distinct patches (see Fig. 2C). Künzle concluded, in agreement with certain earlier physiological studies, that despite similarities in their cellular composition, the caudate nucleus and putamen must have a different functional impact on the motor system and identified the putamen as the main striatal staging center for information from the motor cortex. It is noteworthy that Künzle (1977) and others (Jones et al., 1977) have since demonstrated a comparably organized projection to the putamen from the somatic sensory cortex, while Goldman and Nauta (1977) have presented evidence that the monkey's prefrontal cortex projects almost exclusively (and in patches) to the caudate nucleus. This nearly exact complementarity of the striatal affiliations of the prefrontal and sensorimotor cortex raises the question whether a general subdivision of the striatum might obtain, the caudate nucleus being more closely associated with the limbic system, the putamen, with sensorimotor aspects of forebrain effector mechanisms. It need not be concluded on this basis that all cortical areas project exclusively either to the putamen or to the caudate nucleus and in fact recent reports, again in the monkey, suggest that cortical areas in the temporal lobe (Yeterian, 1978) and the premotor cortex (Künzle, 1978) project extensively to both striatal subdivisions.

These new findings suggest a plan of corticostriatal organization dictated by the general functional affiliation of the cortical areas in question rather than simply their physical location. This point of view is strongly supported by Yeterian and Van Hoesen's recent evidence (1978) that cortical areas interconnected by ipsilateral association fibers tend to share common zones of fiber termination within the striatum (Yeterian and Van Hoesen, 1978)*. Work on the logic of these connections has only just begun and of course is limited by our understanding of the cerebral cortex. However differently individual cortical areas may be mapped onto the striatum, all corticostriatal fibers may have a common origin in layer V according to recent retrograde transport studies (Jones et al., 1977; but see also Kitai et al., 1976b). Jones and co-workers concluded that these layer V pyramidal cells do not send axon collaterals elsewhere. This finding argues for a remarkable specificity of the projection and may one day serve as an important clue to its functional nature.

(b) Thalamus. Striatal afferents arising in the thalamus originate mainly from the intralaminar nuclei and are second in density only to the corticostriatal projection. A much less massive fiber projection from the lateral nuclear complex to the caudate and putamen, described in the cat on the basis of degeneration studies (Graybiel, 1973), has been confirmed by autoradiography (Berson and Graybiel, in preparation).

The intralaminar projection (detected by the Vogts, 1941) proved extremely difficult to study by classical anatomical methods, as witnessed by the confusing claims about the boundaries of the nuclei themselves, their afferent connections, the possibility of their projecting to the neocortex, and certainly also their precise relationship to the striatum. Mehler's careful consideration of these problems (1966) resolved a number of the controversies, however, and he, with Powell and Cowan (1956), supported the Vogts' suggestion that the centre médian (the ventrolateral small-celled division of the centre médian-parafascicular complex that is so large in primates) projects densely and selectively to the putamen.

* Topography means place description *(locorum descriptio)*. The term has been used for years in neuroanatomy to indicate an orderliness in the mode of termination of fiber systems whereby the major coordinates of the source region can be correlated with the coordinates of its pattern of fiber termination in a straightforward topological sense (e.g., dorsal A projects to medial B, ventral A projects to lateral B). The usual antonym is "diffuse" meaning A or part of A projects to most or all of B, or vice versa. With the development of electrophysiological methods the description of a projection as "topographic" has come to have, for some workers, the connotation of a much more functionally motivated sort of order: that a functional map (say, retinotopic) is being preserved by the mechanism of an orderly fiber projection from A to B. It certainly is not possible to talk about the corpus striatum in this sense (or for that matter, most of the rest of the brain). Not only do we not know what is being mapped (is there in the striatum a tonotopic map just because the auditory cortex projects there?); we also do not know what the significance is of the afferent and efferent compartmentalization for the process of mapping (see below).

The exclusive termination of this projection within the putamen has been confirmed by Kalil's autoradiographic study in the monkey (1978). It is curious that both the putamen (Künzle, 1975) and the centre médian (Petras, 1969) receive massive inputs from the motor cortex: it is as though the centre médian were part of a transthalamic circuit reiterating the direct motor cortex-to-putamen projection. The centre médian-parafascicular complex fibers terminate in clusters in the striatum both in monkey (Kalil, 1978) and cat (Royce, 1978), as do those from the neocortex. How these two sets of fiber terminations are related is an important question to resolve.

Powell and Cowan (1956, 1967) suggested that the entire intralaminar complex projects to the striatum. They identified (in addition to the centre médian-putamen projection) the parafascicular and central lateral nuclei as projecting to the caudate nucleus, the more rostral parts of the intralaminar complex as projecting to the region of the nucleus accumbens (see also Nauta and Whitlock, 1954). Although the detailed plan of projection of the intralaminar thalamic nuclei still is far from clear, Jones and Leavitt (1974), with the aid of the horseradish peroxidase method, have argued strongly in favor of Murray's (1966) conclusion that the intralaminar projections to the striatum have collateral side-branches innervating the neocortex. Perhaps this fact could be used to work out the topography.

(c) Midbrain. The two remaining afferent systems of the striatum are associated with the biogenic amines serotonin and dopamine. It is important to point out that two terminologies have arisen in association with these aminergic pathways because in fluorescence studies the letter *B* is used for (usually otherwise named) cell groups containing serotonin, the letter *A* for cell groups containing the catecholamines dopamine or norepinephrine (Dahlström and Fuxe, 1964).

A serotonergic pathway to the striatum arises in the midbrain raphe, apparently mainly or even exclusively from the dorsal raphe nucleus (cell group B7 of Dahlström and Fuxe). Recently this pathway has been shown to have an offset terminating in the dopamine-containing pars compacta of the substantia nigra (Bobillier et al., 1976; Azmitia and Segal, 1978; Jacobs et al., 1978). This direct innervation of the pars compacta (and the apparently reciprocal nigro-raphe projection, see below) suggests a complex interplay between the dopamine and serotonin mechanism and should be kept in mind when evaluating supposedly selective effects of neurotoxins on one or the other of these amine systems.

The most intensively investigated afferent system of the striatum is the dopamine-containing nigrostriatal pathway first demonstrated in 1964 in histofluorescence studies carried out by the Swedish school (Dahlström and Fuxe, 1964; Andén et al., 1964, 1965). The original work on this pathway's association with Parkinsonian disorders is rightly celebrated and thoroughly reviewed elsewhere (see Lloyd et al., 1975; Barbeau, 1976).

Soon after the discovery of the dopamine projection, Ungerstedt (1971) showed that it could be divided into two parts: a dopaminergic *nigrostriatal pathway,* originating in the pars compacta proper of the substantia nigra (cell group A9 of Dahlström and Fuxe's nomenclature) and projecting to the caudoputamen; and a dopaminergic *mesolimbic pathway,* originating from cells medial to the pars compacta (in cell group A10, roughly equivalent to the ventral tegmental area of Tsai, 1925). This second part of the ascending dopamine projection was shown to terminate in the nucleus accumbens-olfactory tubercle (that is, the ventral striatum). The "limbic" character of the pathway was deduced both from its origin in the limbic midbrain and also from its innervation of forebrain structures related to the septo-hypothalamic continuum (e.g., septum, amygdala, nucleus of the diagonal band of Broca (Ungerstedt, 1971; for more recent findings see Moore, 1978; Fallon et al., 1978)).

This dual-projection scheme has been influential in generating a large number of behavioral and pharmacological studies, but because the dopamine fibers are resistant to staining by silver impregnation methods (in fact, for a number of years studies by the Nauta technique and its variants did not demonstrate the nigrostriatal pathway at all (see Hedreen and Chalmers, 1972)) it is only recently, since the development of the axon transport methods, that systematic anatomical work could be done (see for example, the paper of Fox and Schmitz (1944), who recognized that the ventral tegmental area projected to the forebrain in a way "similar" to the substantia nigra proper, but had evidence only from retrograde degeneration).

The results of this new work have already yielded 3 major new conclusions:

(1) There exists, in addition to these fiber projections to the striatum, a direct "meso-cortical" dopamine pathway that leads to parts of the frontal, cingulate and entorhinal cortex (Thierry et al., 1973; Fuxe et al., 1974; Hökfelt et al., 1974; Lindvall et al., 1974). The results of horseradish peroxidase experiments suggest that the frontocingulate projection arises in the medial part of the pars compacta (A9) and the adjoining ventral tegmental area (A10) (Beckstead, 1976; see also Divac, 1978). Neurons of this same A10-A9 border zone also provide the dopaminergic innervation of the amygdala (Fallon et al., 1978).

(2) The cells of origin of the ascending dopamine pathways are more widely distributed in the ventral midbrain than previously appreciated. This larger zone includes not only cell groups A9 and A10 (the pars compacta and the ventral tegmental area) but also the third dopamine containing cell group of the midbrain, the A8 cell group of Dahlström and Fuxe. The neurons of A8 lie partly dorsal and partly caudal to the pars compacta, as shown in the maps of Garver and Sladek (1975) in the primate and Dahlström and Fuxe (1964) and Palkovits and Jacobowitz (1974) in the rat; the cell group is, in fact, in partial continuity with both A9 and A10. From the work of Nauta and collaborators in the rat (1978) and Kocsis and Vandermaelan in the cat (1977), it appears that the A8 group (at least as defined by identifying its striatal projection) extends caudally to include the region called the retrorubral nucleus in some cytoarchitectonic studies (see Berman, 1968). Nauta and co-workers (Nauta and Domesick, 1978; Nauta et al., 1978) have introduced the phrase "outlying cell groups of the substantia nigra" to denote the territories whose dopaminergic neurons comprise cell groups A8 and A10 and to emphasize the close ties linking these nuclei to the pars compacta.

(3) The third conclusion of recent anatomical studies on the rat is that the nigrostriatal and mesolimbic dopamine pathways should not be considered fully separate conduction routes because their terminal fields of distribution within the striatum do, after all, overlap to some degree and because they are interlocked. From the work of Nauta et al. (1978) and Fallon and Moore (1978b) in the rat it appears that while A9 distributes its fibers mainly to the caudoputamen, the projections from A10 are not, as originally supposed, limited to the ventral striatum but include also a large part of the medial caudoputamen. Cell group A8 seems to be the partner of A10, judging from the work of Lénárd and Nauta (personal communication), projecting to the ventral striatum and to the lateral part of the caudoputamen. These several findings suggest that there is as precise a topography in the dopamine-containing pathways to the striatum as one would expect to find in non-catecholaminergic pathways and that the 3 dopamine cell groups of origin – A8, A9, A10 – have individually distinct but partly overlapping projections. The matter of overlap, aside from its potential importance to broad formulations of striatal function, recalls the suggestion in a number of reports that there may be, pharmacologically speaking, more than one kind of dopamine fiber terminating in the striatum (Olson et al., 1972) and more than one type of dopamine receptor as well (Tittler et al., 1977; Nagy et al., 1978). It would be of great interest to know whether these two lines of evidence are related.

(d) Sites of termination of afferent fibers within the striatum. Mounting evidence suggests that these diverse afferent fiber systems terminate mainly upon the medium-size neurons of the striatum and specifically on their dendritic spines (Kemp and Powell, 1971b, c; Fox et al., 1971/72a). These are the so-called "spiny neurons" of Fox and colleagues, estimated to comprise from 95% to as much as 98% of all neurons in the caudate nucleus and putamen (see Foix and Nicolesco, 1925; von Namba, 1957; Kemp and Powell, 1971a; Fox et al., 1971/72a). Kemp and Powell (1971e) and Fox and his co-workers (1971/72a) have emphasized (as did Cajal) that the dendritic spines of these neurons form most of the receptive surface of the striatum; the fine afferent fibers terminating on them make en passant, "cross-over" contacts reminiscent of the parallel fiber-to-Purkinje cell model familiar from cerebellar circuitry. Possible exceptions to this characteristic mode of termination on the medium-size neurons have been suggested in the literature: Kemp and Powell (1971b) noted that some cortical afferents terminate on the cell body of the medium-size cells; Tennyson (1975) found that at least some monoamine fibers innervate large striatal neurons; and Fox et al. (1971/72a) noted that some terminals with medium-sized synaptic vesicles (suggested to be dopamine-containing terminals) end on "spidery" (aspiny) neurons. Because the total nigro-striatal path has been estimated to account for only about 10% of the axon terminals in the striatum (Hökfelt and Ungerstedt, 1969) – and because by all estimates there are very few large neurons in the striatum – a sampling problem is clearly to be expected in such studies. It still remains to be resolved whether some fraction of the dopamine or serotonin endings in the striatum can be characterized as non-classical (without synaptic thickenings and other specializations) in the manner demonstrated by Descarries and colleagues for serotonin and norepinephrine terminals in the neocortex (Descarries et al., 1975, 1977). This matter seems important enough to merit painstaking work with serial sections.

On the basis of their physiological studies, Kitai et al. (1976a) have emphasized a remarkable convergence of afferent fibers of different origin on certain medium-size neurons

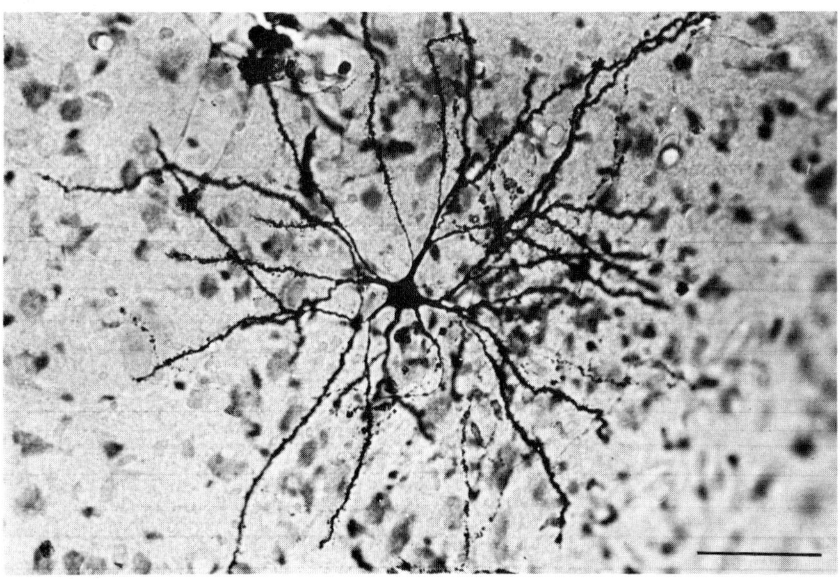

Fig. 5. Photomicrograph illustrating "spiny" neuron from the caudate nucleus of the cat labeled by intracellular injection of HRP. From Kitai et al. (1976a), reproduced with kind permission from the authors. Bar indicates 50 μm.

of the cat's striatum and have further suggested that these afferent fibers are excitatory (but see also Siggins, 1978). Fig. 5 shows a spine-laden medium-size cell stained by the horse-radish peroxidase method following intracellular injection of the marker enzyme during a recording experiment in which Kitai et al. (1976a) identified the neuron as receiving mono-synaptic inputs from the neocortex, intralaminar nuclei and substantia nigra. It is not clear whether the massive convergence suggested by these experiments is the exception or the rule.

Efferent connections

(a) Dorsal striatum (Fig. 6). The impression that the striatum partly has a convergence function is brought to mind not only by the diversity of its afferent connections but also, given this diversity, by the limited scope of its efferent affiliations. Fibers arising in the caudate-putamen complex project, apparently exclusively, to the globus pallidus and to the pars reticulata of the substantia nigra. These striatal efferent fibers are prominent in myelin-stained sections of the primate striatum and since Kinnier Wilson's studies (1914) have been known as "pencil bundles" (probably from the Latin *penecillus,* a small tail or painter's

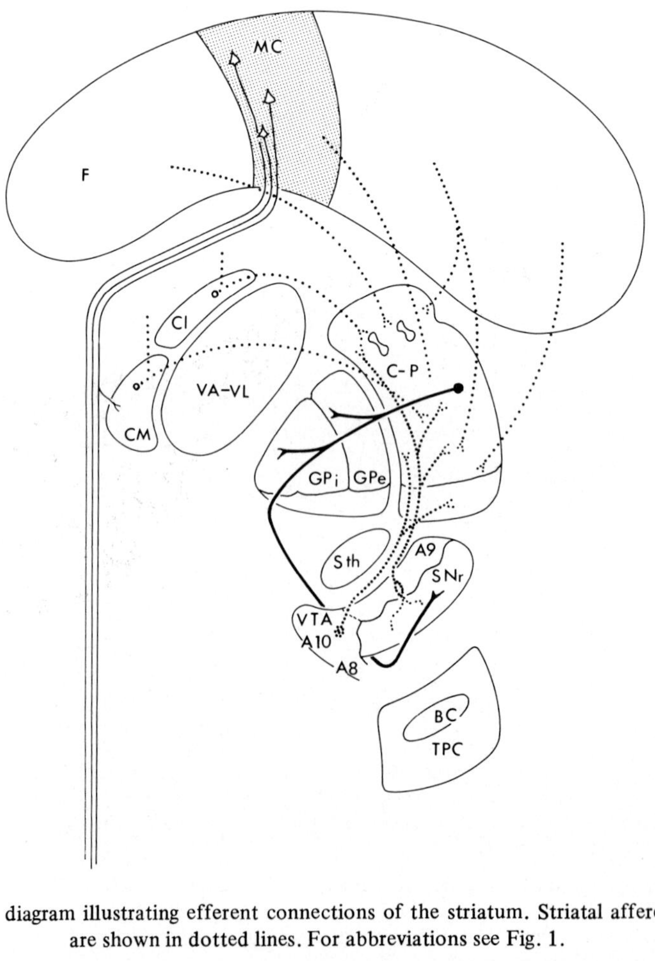

Fig. 6. Schematic diagram illustrating efferent connections of the striatum. Striatal afferents (see Fig. 4) are shown in dotted lines. For abbreviations see Fig. 1.

brush). They converge radially toward the pallidum (in Papez' (1941) often-quoted phrase "like the spokes of a wheel" though of course they do not all lie in a plane); those headed for the substantia nigra can be observed again as the extremely fine myelinated fibers that pierce the cerebral peduncle to form part of the so-called "comb system" (Edinger, 1911) that, in myelin stains in the primate, accounts for the prominent pale streaks in the otherwise darkly stained cerebral peduncle. Electron microscopic study of the terminations of these strionigral fibers indicate that they end on dendrites of pars reticulata neurons (Grofová and Rinvik, 1970; Hattori et al., 1975); there is as yet no convincing evidence for a striatal input to the dopamine-containing pars compacta, even to dopamine-containing dendrites extending into the pars reticulata.

There is fairly good agreement on the basis of fiber degeneration studies that these striatal projections to the pallidum and substantia nigra preserve a general topography and, a point of importance, that both the caudate nucleus and the putamen project to both segments of the pallidum and to the substantia nigra (see Voneida, 1960; Szabo, 1962, 1967, 1970; Cowan and Powell, 1966). Although the subdivision of the pallidum into external and internal segments does not correspond to the striatal subdivision into caudate nucleus and putamen (as one might at first have guessed), Szabo's work in the monkey nevertheless strongly indicates that the projections of these two components of the striatum do not overlap substantially either in the pallidum or in the substantia nigra (Szabo, 1962, 1967, 1970). Not enough work has yet been done by autoradiographic methods in cat or monkey to say more than that in the most general way the triple-projection pattern for caudate and putamen can be confirmed (see Kim et al., 1976). It is not known, for example, whether all parts of the caudate nucleus and putamen project to all 3 striatal targets; the earlier fiber degeneration studies suggested that they may not (see Voneida, 1960).

Yoshida et al. (1974) have suggested that, in the cat, the projections from caudate nucleus to the internal pallidum and substantia nigra are collateral fiber systems, and the careful Golgi observations made by Fox and his colleagues (Fox et al., 1975; Fox and Rafols, 1976) are compatible both with this notion and with the possibility that striatal projections to the two segments of the globus pallidus also are made by collateral branches. Yoshida and his colleagues have concluded on the basis of electrophysiological studies that these projections of the striatum are inhibitory, which fits well with pharmacological evidence that at least the strionigral pathway may use γ-amino butyric acid (GABA) as its neurotransmitter (Kim et al., 1971; Hattori et al., 1973; Fonnum et al., 1974). If this fiber system is a collateral one, this would seem to imply that the striopallidal path uses GABA as well (Obata and Yoshida, 1973).

Until recently most workers accepted the view that the striopallidal and strionigral pathways arose mainly from a restricted subset of neurons in the striatum, the large or "giant" cells (Kemp and Powell, 1971e; Fox et al., 1971/72b). This fitted well with the idea that these large neurons could support heavily collateralized efferent fiber projections to the pallidum and substantia nigra (Fox et al., 1975), and led to the view that most (though not all) of the neurons of medium size represent interneurons with locally ramifying axons. The resulting concept of "information flow" in the striatum ignored many of the complexities of detailed Golgi work on the striatum (see Pasik et al., 1976), stressing instead the rather simple view that the activity of very large numbers of receiving units (the medium-size neurons) could be funneled to a small group of output units (the large neurons) that in turn could control the activity of the globus pallidus and substantia nigra.

There is no doubt now that this view, however attractive for its simplicity, is incorrect. Retrograde cell-labeling experiments with horseradish peroxidase in the rat and cat have

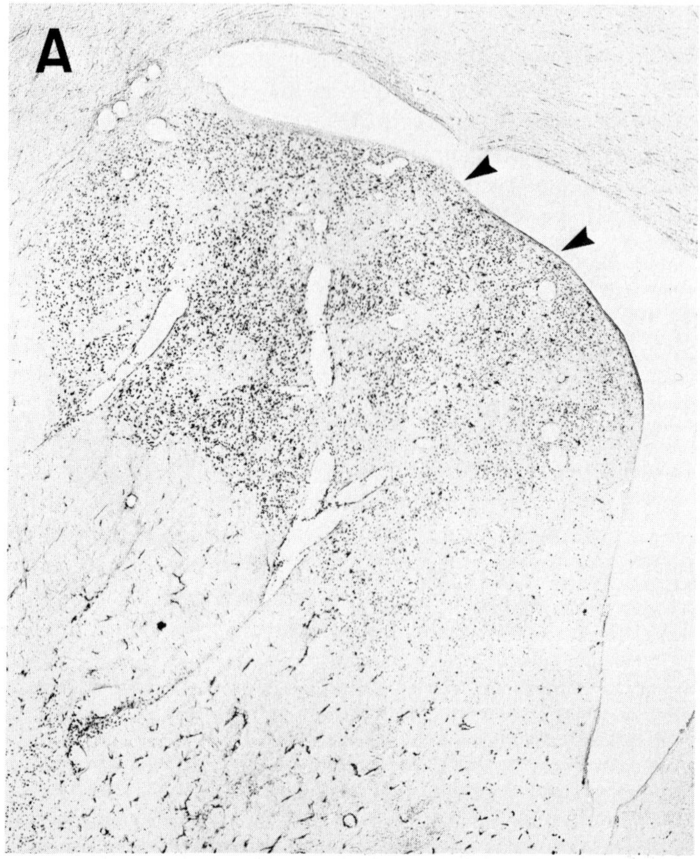

Fig. 7. Matched photographs of adjoining 50 μm thick serial transverse sections through the caudate nucleus of the cat illustrating compartments identified by retrograde transport experiments (A) and enzyme histochemistry (B). A: pattern of retrograde cell labeling that followed injection of horseradish peroxidase into the pallidum; Mesulam's TMB reaction (1978) without counterstain. Note sparsely labeled zones. B: acetylcholinesterase activity (dark) in section stained by Geneser-Jensen and Blackstad's method (1971). Note zones of low enzyme activity (pale) and compare their locations to those of weakly labeled zones in A. Arrows point to two pale zones flanking dark band.

clearly demonstrated that many – if not most – of the medium neurons of the striatum do have long axons that project beyond the confines of the striatum (Grofová, 1975; Bunney and Aghajanian, 1976; Di Figlia et al., 1976; Faull and Mehler, 1976; Bak et al., 1978; Moon Edley et al., 1978; Graybiel et al., 1979). Moreover, these efferent neurons are not uniformly distributed. The experiments of Bunney and Aghajanian (1976) suggest that in the rat a sizable medial part of the caudoputamen does not project to the substantia nigra. In the cat, injections of horseradish peroxidase into the pallidum (or substantia nigra) lead to retrograde labeling of medium-size neurons that are arranged in the striatum so as to form geometrically complex, macroscopically visible fields interrupted by a maze-work of poorly labeled, roughly 0.5 mm wide zones (see Fig. 7). On the basis of these findings it seems clear that the apparent homogeneity of the striatum – at least as compared to the layered and columned neocortex – therefore does not adequately reflect its internal partitioning. Careful observers had in fact previously noticed some provincialization of the cells in the

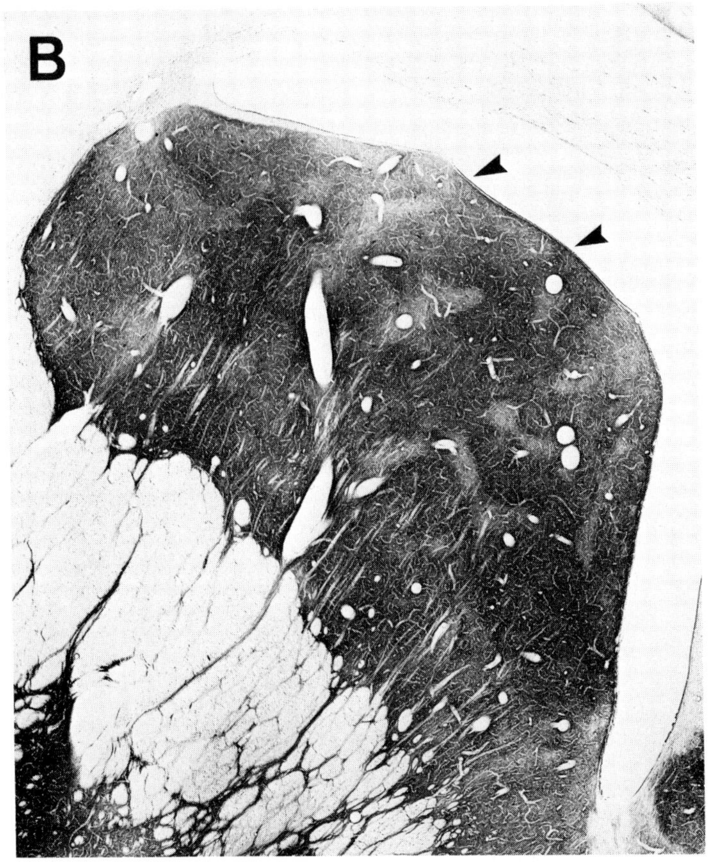

Fig. 7B.

striatum, however, the most prescient, perhaps, being Papez (1929), who said that the cells are organized into "tubular clusters." It is interesting that when this mosaic pattern of retrograde labeling is compared in serial sections to the pattern of acetylcholinesterase staining in the caudate nucleus (Fig. 7B; see below) the zones of slight cell labeling seem to overlap, at least in part, regions of low enzyme activity. The matter of compartmentalization of the striatum is discussed in a separate section. The fact that such compartments in the striatum have only just been identified expresses well how meager current knowledge of the organization of the corpus striatum actually is.

(b) Ventral striatum (Fig. 8). Recent autoradiographic studies of the striatum demonstrate (as Herrick guessed) that the nucleus accumbens does not have the same efferent targets as the caudate-putamen proper but instead, a parallel set of efferent connections (Heimer and Wilson, 1975; Swanson and Cowan, 1975; Conrad and Pfaff, 1976a; Powell and Leman, 1976; Nauta et al., 1978). These include a projection (1) to the ventral extension of the globus pallidus (Heimer and Wilson's "ventral pallidum"), (2) to the A8 and A10 dopamine-containing cell groups of the mesencephalon and, in the rat at least, the adjoining pars compacta of the substantia nigra, and (3) to a surprisingly extensive group of other forebrain

and midbrain components of the limbic system. These findings both extend and significantly modify the "mesolimbic" concept. They suggest a binding together of dorsal and ventral striatum by way of at least one pathway, that from the nucleus accumbens to the substantia nigra's pars compacta and from there to the dorsal striatum (caudate-putamen proper) (Fig. 13). Even more remarkable is the implication that a major input to the pars compacta, and thus to the dopaminergic nigrostriatal system, comes (via the nucleus accumbens) from the limbic system: for, as mentioned above, the nucleus accumbens receives fiber projections from the hippocampus (Fox, 1943; Raisman et al., 1966) and also from the amygdala (De Olmos and Ingram, 1972). Unless the functions of these regions come to be interpreted in a way strikingly different from that now generally accepted, this circuit arrangement must mean that the dopamine mechanism of the substantia nigra's pars compacta, no less than that of cell group A10 (and A8), is driven at least in part by regions of the brain implicated in the general functional realm of mood and affect, in a word, by limbic input*.

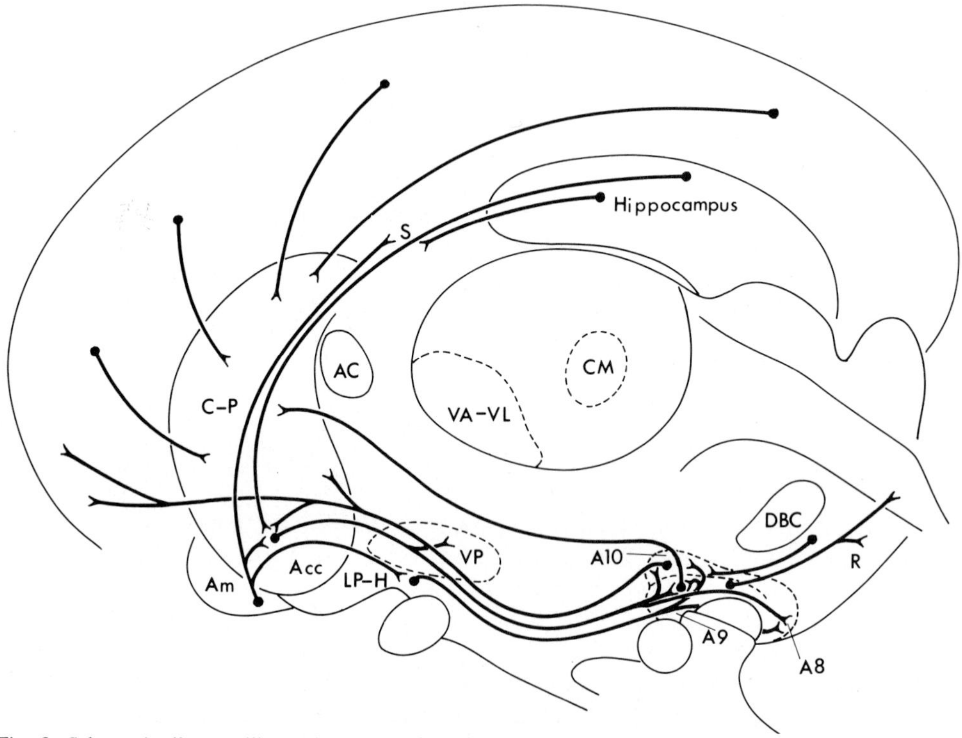

Fig. 8. Schematic diagram illustrating some of the limbic associations of the nucleus accumbens/ventral striatum (Acc) and the dopamine-containing cell groups of the midbrain (A9, A10, A8). Based on drawings by W. J. H. Nauta (see, e.g., Nauta, 1960; Fig. 1-1), with his (Nauta and Domesick, 1978; Nauta et al., 1978) and others' (Heimer and Wilson, 1975; Powell and Lehman, 1975; Swanson and Cowan, 1975; Conrad and Pfaff, 1976a; Fallon and Moore, 1978b) recent findings. S, septum; Acc, nucleus accumbens; Am, amygdaloid complex; LP-H, lateral preoptic-hypothalamic region; VP, ventral pallidum.

---

* Perhaps this should have been expected after Poirier and colleagues found that the pars compacta's efferent fibers travel with the medial forebrain bundle! (Poirier, 1960; Parent and Poirier, 1969).

This conclusion is reinforced by Bunney and Aghajanian's report (1976) that nigral afferents arise in the central nucleus of the amygdaloid complex and also by the finding of Conrad and Pfaff (1976b, c), Swanson (1976) and Nauta and Domesick (1978) that the lateral hypothalamus-preoptic region projects to the pars compacta. Nauta and colleagues (1978) note that the more massive hypothalamic projection to cell group A10 is in part also reflected back to the dorsal striatum by the A10 projection to the medial part of the caudo-putamen (see Fig. 8). It is worth emphasizing a general parallel between these subcortical arrangements and the apparently quite massive input to the inferior parietal lobe from parts of the neocortex implicated in limbic circuitry (Mesulam et al., 1977); it has not escaped the workers in this field that the dividing line between the sensorimotor and affective sides of central nervous processing may in the past have been too boldly drawn.

Compartmentalization

The architecture of the caudate nucleus and putamen is usually described as being homogeneous in comparison to that of the neocortex, and rightly so. While the layers of the cortex are evident at a glance in cell stains, only a hint of cytoarchitectural differentiation is as readily apparent in the striatum and descriptions of marked substructure have invariably resulted from painstaking study (see Papez, 1929; Mensah, 1977). This does not necessarily mean that the striatum lacks subunits comparable to cortical layers; cortical columns are hardly anywhere visible in ordinary Nissl stains (an exception being the barrel fields, Woolsey and Van der Loos, 1970). Even so, it has come as a surprise that according to a variety of recent findings, the caudate nucleus and putamen appear to be composed of subunits that are probably the striatal equivalents of cortical columns or layers. A significant reorientation in thinking about the striatum is likely to result from this new work but in contrast to work on columnar organization, which has preceeded in a quite logical step-by-step fashion since the pioneering observations of Mountcastle (1959) and Hubel and Wiesel (1969), experiments suggesting the existence of comparable subunits in the striatum are diverse, largely independent of one another and so far notably lacking in functional electrophysiology. Some of these findings have already been mentioned above.

(a) Afferents. Autoradiographic evidence (monkey: Künzle, 1975; Goldman and Nauta, 1977; Jones et al., 1977; Yeterian and Van Hoesen, 1978; cat: Ragsdale and Graybiel, in preparation) shows that striatal afferent fibers originating in the cortex terminate in variably shaped "patches" about 0.5–1 mm in diameter. These are visible in cross-sections such as the one illustrated in Fig. 1C. Similar clumping of thalamostriate fibers has been seen as well in the monkey (Kalil, 1978) and cat (Royce, 1978). It is not known whether such afferent fiber clustering also occurs in the rat. At least part of the dopaminergic projection to the striatum apparently also terminates in clusters. This conclusion is based on observations of "islands" of fluorescence, roughly half a millimeter wide, in the caudate nucleus of the fetal human (Nobin and Björklund, 1973), rabbit (Tennyson et al., 1972), and in the neonatal rat (Olson et al., 1972) and on immunohistochemical findings in the rat (Fuxe et al., 1978). Diprenorphine binding studies suggest that opiate receptors also occur in patches in the rat's caudoputamen (Pert et al., 1975). It is not known whether (as seems reasonable) these patches actually mark particular afferent fiber terminations but a relation between opiate receptor marking and dopamine fiber terminations has been claimed (Diamond and Borison, 1978). A more general question still to be answered is whether the clumped patterns of terminal distribution typical of cortical, thalamic and dopaminergic afferents are indicative of a careful segregation of these inputs from one another, or, instead, some form of partial overlap within any given region of the striatum.

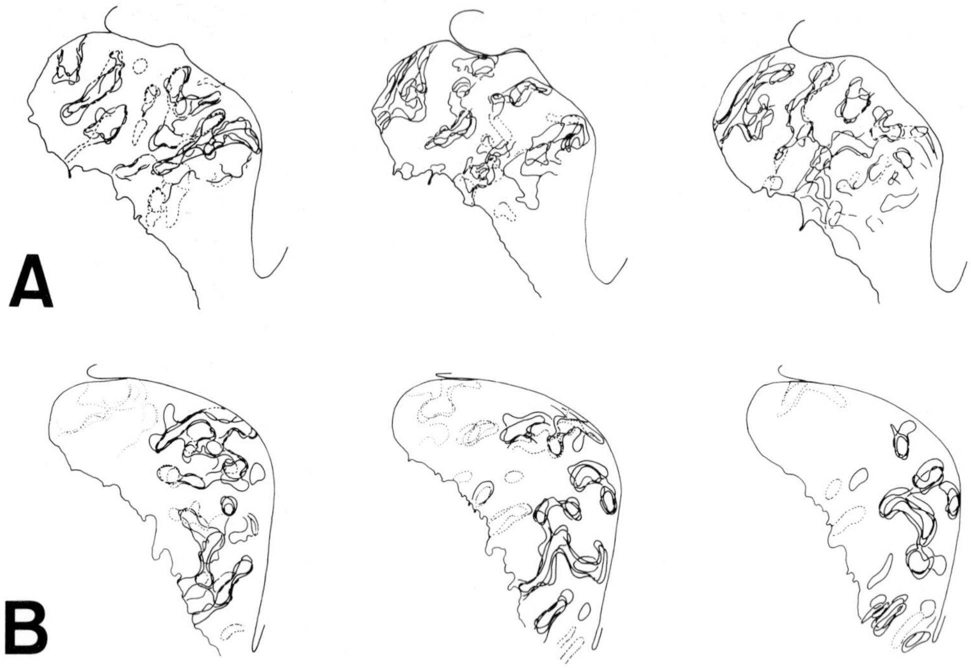

Fig. 9. Illustration of 3-dimensional networks found in caudate nucleus of cat in retrograde labeling experiments (A) and acetylcholinesterase histochemistry (B). A: profiles of weakly labeled zones overlaid (3 serial sections per panel) in register to show continuity from section to section. Sections near that illustrated in Fig. 7A. B: same serial overlay technique has been used to illustrate labyrinths of low cholinesterase activity (Graybiel and Ragsdale, 1978a; Graybiel et al., 1979).

(b) Efferents. Evidence for some form of local subdivision of striatal neurons based on their efferent connections has come from recent retrograde transport experiments in the cat (Moon Edley et al., 1978; Graybiel et al., 1979). As described above, after massive injections of horseradish peroxidase into the pallidum, marked non-uniformities in labeling appear in the caudate nucleus. This finding is illustrated in Fig. 7A, which shows a number of roughly 0.5–0.8 mm wide zones of sparse labeling surrounded by larger regions in which the cell labeling is very dense. When groups of such sections through the caudate nucleus are placed in serial register (Fig. 9) they suggest that the sparsely labeled zones run in continuity from section to section, making tortuous loops and twists over short distances and complicated maze-works over longer distances. Not enough is yet known to say whether this pattern of retrograde labeling indicates a separation of interneurons (in the sparsely labeled gaps) from neurons with extrinsic connections (in the densely labeled fields) or whether, instead, the uneven labeling indicates separate origins of striopallidal and strionigral fibers. There are still technical difficulties in proving the case one way or the other. Even so, this is a crucial point to resolve: for until we understand this organization – and its relation to the afferent clumping just described – it is difficult to imagine how conclusions could be reached about the actual linkages between striatal inputs and outputs.

(c) Acetylcholinesterase histochemistry. A high content of acetylcholinesterase has come to be considered a defining characteristic of the striatum (see Fig. 2). The distribution of this degradative enzyme of the cholinergic mechanism has been carefully mapped in the rat

and has been shown to match remarkably closely the distribution of dopamine histofluorescence in the striatum (Jacobowitz and Palkovits, 1974). The acetylcholinesterase activity, like the dopamine histofluorescence, appears to be quite even in the adult rat's caudoputamen but occurs mainly in patches in the neonatal rat (Butcher and Hodge, 1976). Recently, a detailed analysis of acetylcholinesterase staining in the striatum has been made in cats and primates, and this work suggests a striking difference between these species and the rat (Graybiel and Ragsdale, 1978a, b). In cat, rhesus monkey and human, marked inhomogeneities appear in cholinesterase staining in the adult striatum (particularly in the caudate nucleus) as well as in the striatum of the fetus and newborn (observations in cat and human; Graybiel and Ragsdale, in progress). An example of the adult pattern is shown for the cat in Fig. 7B. In the cross-section illustrated, it is clear that the cholinesterase staining of the caudate nucleus is dense but also that it is interrupted by numerous oblong zones, about 0.5 mm wide, in which the stain is very weak. There is a notable similarity between this discontinuous pattern of cholinesterase labeling and the incomplete pattern of retrograde cell labeling seen after tracer injections into the pallidum (compare Fig. 7A and 7B). Serial section reconstructions (made from overlaid drawings such as those shown in Fig. 9B) indicate that the pale zones seen in single sections, like the sparsely labeled zones in the retrograde labeling experiments (Fig. 9A), actually are parts of complex 3-dimensional arrays. The labyrinths of low enzyme activity are large enough to stretch over at least the several millimeters of striatal tissue so far analyzed in reconstructions of human and cat material. The term, *striosomal organization,* has been introduced in reference to these "striatal bodies," somewhat by analogy to the now familiar "columnar organization" (see Graybiel and Ragsdale, 1978b; Moon Edley et al., 1978).

It is remarkable that, in sharp contrast to this pattern of cholinesterase activity in adult cats and primates, the neonatal pattern in these species (as in the rat, Butcher and Hodge, 1976) is one in which patches of enzyme appear against a pale background of much lower enzyme activity (see below and Fig. 10; also Graybiel and Ragsdale, 1978a). It is not yet known how or for what reason this apparent figure-ground reversal takes place.

(d) Developmental sequence. Very little information is available about the development of the various inhomogeneities just described, but it is clear that quite dramatic changes occur in the striatum early in life: from dopamine patches to a uniform dopamine fluorescence pattern; or again, from acetylcholinesterase patches to a uniform or even reversed pattern in the adult. It is therefore of particular interest that [^{3}H]thymidine pulse-labeling studies of the fetal development of the striatum in the rat (Angevine, 1974) and rhesus monkey (Brand and Rakic, 1978) have recently shown that neurons with similar "birthdays" tend to appear in clusters in the striatum. It will be important to relate this pattern of cellular development to the observations discussed above; it could be that the striosomal organization of the caudate-putamen is crucially dependent on developmental constraints.

The pallidum

The globus pallidus, in contrast to the striatum, is made up almost exclusively of large neurons (Fox et al., 1974). It forms the output side of the corpus striatum and indeed until fairly recently was considered to form the output side of the entire extended circuitry of the basal ganglia. This viewpoint can no longer be accepted as correct because the substantia nigra's pars reticulata is now known to represent another main staging center for outputs from the basal ganglia (see below). The pallidum is nevertheless the logical place to start in considering the efferent side of the basal ganglia first, because it is part of the corpus striatum

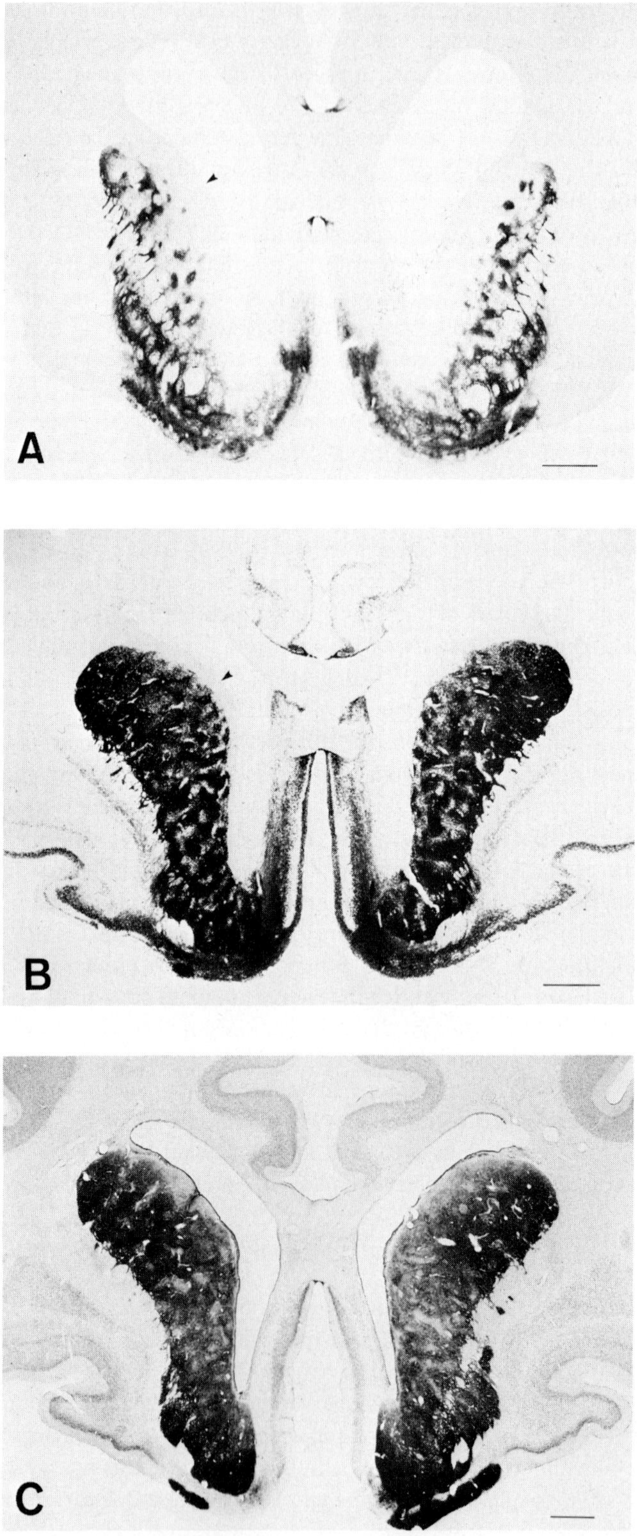

proper and second, because it gives rise to the most massive efferent fiber system of the basal ganglia, the *ansa lenticularis* of von Monakow (1895).

Like the striatum, the pallidum has different conformations in primates and non-primates, but in all species it is divided into two main parts. In primates these are separated by a relatively thin fiber plate (the internal medullary lamina) and are known as the internal and external pallidal segments. In primates and especially in the human the internal pallidum is further divided by an accessory medullary lamina into (apparently unnamed) medial and lateral halves. The two main segments of the globus pallidus are less compact and not so clearly part of a single structure in rodents, carnivores and other non-primates. In these species, the recognized equivalent of the internal pallidal segment is called the entopeduncular nucleus, deriving its name from the fact that its cells are embedded in the cerebral peduncle. The external segment is often simply called the globus pallidus, but this is a confusing nomenclature and should be avoided in favor of the more specific term, external pallidum, so long as the implied homology seems justified. The distinction between the two pallidal segments is important, for even though their afferent connections appear to be similar (and possibly even duplicative), the two segments have different efferent connections.

Afferent connections

The globus pallidus receives massive fiber projections from the caudate nucleus and putamen; these were discussed in a preceding section. The only other clearly identified pallidal afferents arise in the subthalamic nucleus as part of a pallido-subthalamo-pallidal loop (see below). From time to time the suggestion has been made that ascending fibers headed towards the striatum (specifically the dopamine-containing axons) might form synapses en passage while traversing the pallidum, but this has not been convincingly demonstrated. In fiber degeneration studies (Graybiel, 1973; Mehler, in Mehler and Nauta, 1974) a pathway from the region of the mesencephalic tegmentum near the medial geniculate body has been traced as part of a "reverse comb bundle" to the external pallidum (see also Morest, 1964); further, some ascending fibers from the reticular formation of the pons and ponto-medullar border have been followed to the pallidum in autoradiographic experiments (Graybiel, 1977a). The exact origin of these projections is not known and their distributions within the pallidum are too diffuse to be identified with certainty as parts of terminal fields.

Striatal afferents terminate in both pallidal segments but as just discussed it is not clear to what degree the two segments receive different, as opposed to collateral, inputs. These afferent fibers terminate in a highly distinctive fashion, entwining themselves around the long and for the most part smooth dendrites of the large pallidal neurons and encrusting them with a series of boutons en passage. As Fox and Rafols (1976) and Kemp and Powell (1971e) emphasize, this mode of termination conforms to the "longitudinal axodendritic" pattern of Cajal. It seems designed to insure – as is recognized by the familiar model of the cerebellar climbing fiber – a controlling influence by the afferent fibers in question. Heimer

---

◀Fig. 10. Photographs of transverse sections illustrating development of acetylcholinesterase in the striatum of the cat. A: from kitten fetus, taken by laparotomy 15 days before term; B: from kitten 2 days old; C: from 23-day-old kitten. Section in B more darkly stained than those in A and C; all stained by Geneser-Jensen and Blackstad's method (1971), and intensified according to Hardy et al. (1976). In A and B, tip of arrow touches ependyma overlying ganglionic eminence. Bar in each panel indicates 1 mm.

and Wilson (1975) were able to use the distinctive ultrastructural appearance of pallidal synaptic organization in their identification of the ventral pallidum; the synaptic complexes formed there by axons from the ventral striatum are of the same type as those in the pallidum proper.

Efferent connections

(a) External segment (Fig. 11). The external pallidal segment projects massively to the subthalamic nucleus (Vogt and Vogt, 1920; Ranson et al., 1941; Nauta and Mehler, 1966; Carpenter and Strominger, 1967). The fibers forming this connection cut through the cerebral peduncle as part of the comb system and form the middle division of the ansa lenticularis as it was defined by von Monakow (1895); the fiber system is also called the subthalamic fasciculus. According to detailed studies by Carpenter and his colleagues (Carpenter et al., 1976; Kim et al., 1976), this fiber projection is topographic and spares only the medial corner of the subthalamic nucleus. This connection forms part of the pallido-subthalamo-pallidal loop described in a separate section below.

The pallido-subthalamic pathway has been thought by most investigators to be the sole efferent projection of the external segment. The possibility of a pallidonigral connection has been repeatedly mentioned, however, and recently Hattori et al. (1975) have presented light

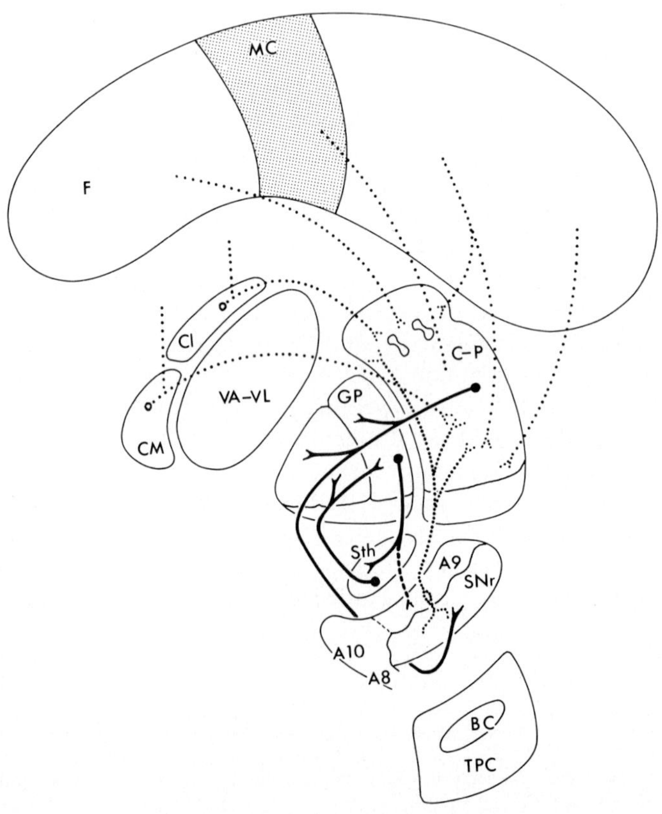

Fig. 11. Schematic drawing illustrating efferent connections of the external pallidal segment. Abbreviations as in Fig. 1.

and electron microscopic autoradiographic evidence suggesting that the external pallidum in the rat projects to dopamine-containing neurons in the substantia nigra's pars compacta. These findings are supported by the observation of labeled neurons in the external pallidum following injections of horseradish peroxidase into the substantia nigra of the cat (Grofová, 1975) and rat (Bunney and Aghajanian, 1976). In the rhesus monkey, Nauta and Mehler (1966) also observed a circumscript distribution field of degenerating fibers within the pars compacta. It should be noted, however, that Faull and Mehler (1976), in their retrograde labeling study in the rat, found labeled neurons in the external pallidum only after (nigral) injections involving the subthalamic nucleus. Moreover, Carpenter's group (Kim et al., 1976), on the basis of autoradiographic findings in the monkey, favors the view that this apparent pallidonigral pathway actually arises in the sublenticular grey matter, a part of the substantia innominata that almost certainly corresponds, at least in part, to the ventral pallidum identified in the rat.

(b) Internal segment (Figs. 12 and 13). All other known pallidal efferents, including the massive pallidothalamic pathway, originate in the internal pallidal segment. These efferent projections are distributed to the thalamus and midbrain, and apparently also to field H of Forel (nucleus campi Foreli) and to the lateral subdivision of the habenula. Certain other efferent connections have been claimed in the literature (see the review by Nauta and Mehler, 1966) but have not been confirmed with axon transport techniques and therefore are not considered here.

The efferent fibers of the internal pallidum form two distinct bundles in the primate that early on were given separate names and that recently have been shown to arise in different parts of the internal segment. One group leaves the pallidum dorsally and medially, makes its way through the internal capsule, and then sweeps over the subthalamic nucleus to join Forel's field H_2; this bundle corresponds to the dorsal division of the ansa as defined by von Monakow (1895) but is now more frequently called the lenticular fasciculus *(fasciculus lenticularis)* after Meynert (1872). The second efferent bundle forms a prominent myelinated tract that runs just alongside the ventral margin of the internal segment and then curves around the medial edge of the internal capsule to enter the subthalamic region. This is von Monakow's ventral division, or the *ansa lenticularis* in Meynert's more restricted use of the term. Oddly enough, these two main efferent bundles join together in field H_2 of Forel and run caudally; most of the fibers then make a remarkable about-face just in front of the red nucleus (in Forel's field H) and head rostrally in field H_1 (the thalamic fasciculus) until they reach the thalamus.

Carpenter's group has presented autoradiographic evidence that the more dorsal lenticular fasciculus arises in the medial part of the internal segment, while the more ventral ansa lenticularis originates in the outer half of the internal segment (Kim et al., 1976). Differential terminations of these two efferent bundles have, with one possible exception (see below), not yet been identified; the fact that a subdivision of the internal segment into medial and lateral halves is so very prominent in the human brain, however, makes the matter of special interest.

(i) Pallidothalamic fibers. By far the most massive efferent connection of the internal segment is its projection to the thalamus. Pallidal fibers terminate (a) in the lateral parts of the VA-VL complex (the nuclei ventralis anterior and lateralis; in the monkey, specifically, VApc, and lateral VLo and VLm) and (b) in the centre médian (CM) (Nauta and Mehler, 1966; Carpenter and Strominger, 1967; Mehler and Nauta, 1974; Kim et al., 1976). The VA-VL connection represents the main link in the path leading from the pallidum toward the motor-premotor cortical field. The CM connection, as discussed below, seems mainly but not

exclusively to comprise part of a loop system leading back to the striatum.

According to the detailed studies of Kim et al. (1976) both of these fiber projections have an orderly place-to-place topography. An interesting suggestion made by these authors on the basis of autoradiographic findings is that the lenticular fasciculus in the monkey carries the majority of pallidal fibers terminating in the subnucleus VLo. A follow-up of this work deserves high priority, for it could mean that there is some form of preferential transthalamic access from the medial part of the internal pallidal segment to the motor cortex receiving VLo inputs. If so, it should be possible by "working backwards" to find out whether the medial part of the internal segment receives, in turn, a unique striatal input (say, from the parts of the putamen that themselves receive cortical afferents from sensorimotor cortex). Aside from this single clue, there is no convincing evidence as to the existence, let alone the identity, of lines of conduction leading from specific parts of the neocortex via the striatum to pallidum and thence to the thalamus.

(ii) Pallidotegmental fibers. In the monkey, fibers from the internal segment terminate in a relatively restricted part of the dorsolateral peribrachial tegmentum named the *nucleus tegmenti pedunculopontis pars compacta* (TPC) in Olszewski and Baxter's (1954) cytoarchitectonic study of the human brain stem. This connection was carefully documented by Nauta and Mehler (1966) in fiber degeneration experiments and has been confirmed in autoradiographic work (Kim et al., 1976). It represents the most caudal fiber projection of the globus pallidus.

It is curious that, in a recent autoradiographic study, Carter and Fibiger (1978) failed to find evidence for such a connection in the rat, and autoradiographic work in progress in the cat (Moon Edley and Graybiel) indicates that the connection may be weak in that species. The apparent variability of this pathway may be indicative of species differences, either in the precise zone of origin of the pathway or in its relative size in different mammals. Rather marked species differences in the degree of cytoarchitectural development of the TPC have also been noted (see Crosby and Woodburne, 1943; Nauta and Mehler, 1966). It is striking that the TPC receives a substantial input from the pars reticulata of the substantia nigra in the cat (Papez, 1941; Graybiel, unpublished autoradiographic findings, see Fig. 17), but, according to an autoradiographic study from Carpenter's group (Carpenter et al., 1976), not in the monkey. This raises the possibility of some form of inverse development of the pallidotegmental and nigrotegmental projections in different mammalian lines.

(iii) Pallido-prerubral fibers. Kinnier Wilson's belief that the red nucleus serves as a direct discharge mechanism for the corpus striatum as well as for the cerebellum has not proven correct. This was shown by the Ransons (1941) and by Nauta and Mehler (1966). However, nearly all recent studies, and several early investigations also (including Kinnier Wilson's, 1914) have demonstrated a quite large accumulation of pallidofugal fibers in the caudal part of the subthalamic region that lies just rostral to the red nucleus and corresponds to the "prerubral field" or nucleus campi Foreli. Just what proportion of these fibers in fact terminate in this region is not easy to judge because it is there that most of the pallidofugal fibers from the internal segment make a U-turn en route to the more rostrally situated VA-VL complex (and CM). Nevertheless, the strength of autoradiographic labeling of the prerubral field after injections of radioactive tracer in the internal pallidum in the cat makes it seem likely that some fibers do terminate in this region (Moon Edley and Graybiel, unpublished observations). This is an important point to settle because the nucleus campi Foreli could be the starting point of pallidal outflow channels still to be identified. To date only one subthalamic efferent system, a projection to the region in and nearby the oculomotor nucleus from the dorsomedial corner of the prerubral field, has been identified (by

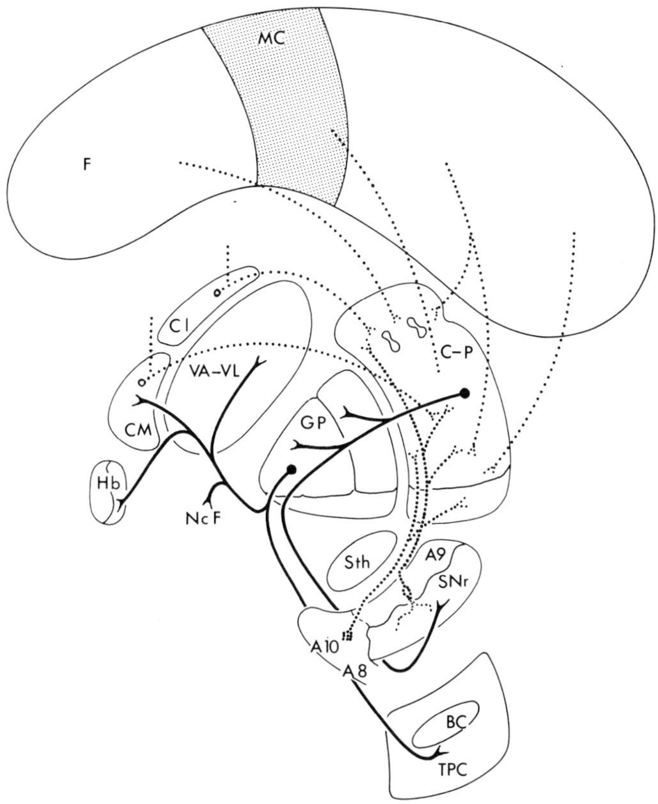

Fig. 12. Schematic drawing illustrating efferent connections of the internal pallidal segment. Abbreviations as in Fig. 1. Hb, habenular complex; NcF, nucleus campi Foreli.

retrograde labeling studies; Graybiel, 1977; Büttner-Ennever and Büttner, 1978). The possibility of synaptic continuity from the pallidum to this apparent source of descending preoculomotor fibers is worth pursuing, as such a path could represent relatively direct access of the pallidum to the oculomotor mechanism and bear some relation to vertical gaze disturbances observed with basal ganglia disease.

(iv) Pallidohabenular fibers. Fibers were traced from the pallidum to the habenular complex in experimental material by Kinnier Wilson (1914), the Ransons (1942), and others and were later described in the extensive monograph written by Nauta and Mehler (1966). However, until the autoradiographic study by Nauta (1974) and other subsequent work (e.g., Filion et al., 1976; Herkenham and Nauta, 1977a), the pathway was always treated with more than the usual suspicion accorded fiber degeneration findings because it seemed to link such disparate structures. The recent autoradiographic and horseradish peroxidase studies strongly support the existence of the pathway nonetheless, although it must be mentioned that Carpenter's group, working in the monkey, favors the alternative view that the connection arises from the sublenticular substantia innominata and displaced neurons of the substantia innominata that invade the internal medullary lamina between the two pallidal segments (Kim et al., 1976). As electrophoretic injections of horseradish peroxidase into the lateral habenula of the rat label large numbers of neurons in the entopeduncular nucleus (Herkenham and Nauta, 1977a), a connection from the presumed

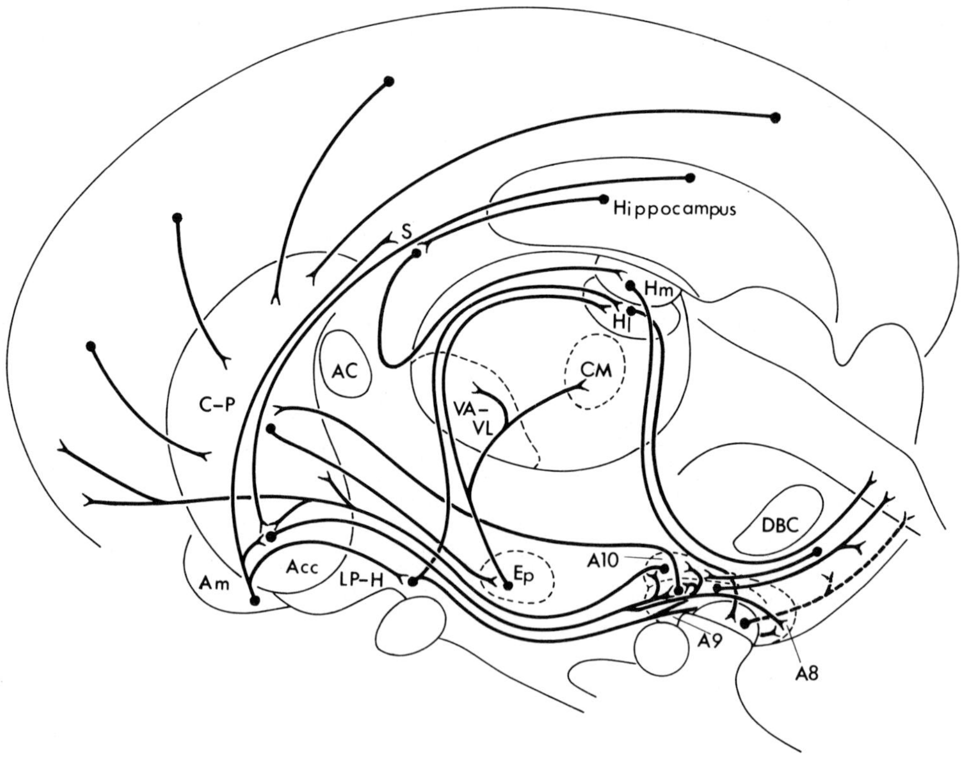

Fig. 13. Links between limbic system and corpus striatum. Some of the connections were illustrated separately in Fig. 8; here, note pallidohabenular connection (Nauta, 1974; Herkenham and Nauta, 1977a) and its transsynaptic extensions into the midbrain. Hm and Hl, medial and lateral subdivisions of habenula; Ep, entopeduncular nucleus.

homologue of the internal pallidum can hardly be denied in rodents. Equally convincing evidence supports the existence in the rat of a major lateral preoptico-hypothalamic projection to the same part of the lateral habenula, so that a direct convergence of pallidal and limbic inputs is strongly indicated. The lateral habenula, in turn, projects to the midbrain raphe, including its serotonin-containing cell groups (Herkenham and Nauta, 1977b). It thus could have a widespread transsynaptic influence not only on limbic structures but also on the substantia nigra, striatum and neocortex as well (see Fig. 13).

(c) Ventral pallidum. The efferent connections of the ventral pallidum are largely unknown. The region has so far been delimited principally by the aid of chartings of its afferents from the ventral striatum such as those originally prepared in the rat by Heimer and Wilson (1975). In the monkey the region can as yet be identified only in a general way as lying in the sublenticular substantia innominata. By inference from fragmentary comments in the literature, it appears that at least some of the efferent connections may parallel those of the dorsal pallidum, as Heimer and Wilson's concept originally suggested. For example, Carpenter and associates (Carpenter et al., 1968; Kim et al., 1976) make special note of the lack of a projection from the external pallidal segment to the medial part of the subthalamic nucleus, while Nauta and Mehler (1966) noted dense fiber degeneration precisely in this

medial part of the subthalamic nucleus after a lesion in the substantia innominata (their case MGB6). Nauta and Mehler's fiber degeneration material, however, like the more recent autoradiographic evidence of Kim et al., indicates that for the most part the sublenticular gray does not contribute to von Monakow's ansa lenticularis (the lenticular fasciculus and ansa lenticularis of Meynert) but rather to pathways more directly related to the hypothalamus.

LOOP SYSTEMS OF THE CORPUS STRIATUM

The neural circuitry of the corpus striatum is characterized by a remarkable set of side paths that appear to represent auxiliaries of the main strio-pallido-thalamic connection. Three such side chains are highly developed in the primate brain: a transthalamic loop leading from striatum to pallidum to centre médian to the striatum (mainly the putamen); a sequence leading from the external pallidum to the subthalamic nucleus and back to the pallidum (both segments); and finally, the strio-nigro-striatal system that engages the midbrain dopamine mechanism. According to findings in the cat (Graybiel, 1977a; Moon Edley and Graybiel, see below) a fourth "loop" involving the nucleus tegmenti pedunculopontis can probably be added to the list.

It is striking that two of the major clinical syndromes of the basal ganglia are associated with pathologies specifically affecting the nodal points in these side-loops: the subthalamic nucleus in hemiballism, and the substantia nigra in Parkinson's disease. Such clinicopathological correlations leave little doubt as to the profound influence of these loops on the functional integrity of the corpus striatum, but at the same time emphasize the paradox of a circuit arrangement in which the loops appear largely as reentrant modulating mechanisms set off from the main stream of strio-pallido-thalamic conduction.

In fact, this paradox is being at least partially resolved by recent work indicating that the nodal points in these circuits – the centre médian, subthalamic nucleus, substantia nigra, and nucleus tegmenti pedunculopontis – are not parts of closed neuronal systems but receive and send information beyond the confines of the loops themselves. Evidence leading to this conclusion, though partly mentioned elsewhere in the text, is brought together here because the recognition of these complications in the extended circuitry of the corpus striatum represents an important recent advance in neuroanatomical study of the basal ganglia.

Substantia nigra

In Nissl stains the substantia nigra can be seen to have two parts: a more dorsal part with closely spaced cell bodies, the *pars compacta,* and a larger ventral part, the *pars reticulata,* in which the neurons are much more widely scattered. Fluorescence studies have clearly demonstrated that most (but not all) dopamine-containing neurons lie in the pars compacta (Dahlström and Fuxe, 1964; Fallon and Moore, 1978b). The neurons of both parts are large and it is surprising, considering the histochemical differences between their neurons, that Golgi studies of the substantia nigra emphasize similarities rather than differences in their cellular composition (Rinvik and Grofová, 1970; Schwyn and Fox, 1974; Juraska et al., 1977). However, Golgi and cytoarchitectonic observations alike point to a predominance of synaptic neuropil in the pars reticulata (Schwyn and Fox, 1974).

The two subdivisions of the substantia nigra lie on opposite sides of a transstriatal circuit, the pars reticulata receiving fiber projections from the caudate-putamen complex, the pars compacta sending dopaminergic fiber projections to the caudate-putamen. This summary statement can be elaborated on the basis of recent work in three important ways.

(1) Intrinsic circuitry

The synaptic interactions that occur within the substantia nigra are likely more complex than the simple subdivision into pars compacta and pars reticulata connotes. The pars reticulata is heavily infiltrated by dendrites of the pars compacta neurons (Cajal, 1911; Rinvik and Grofová, 1970; Schwyn and Fox, 1974; Björklund and Lindvall, 1975; Juraska et al., 1977) and moreover, these dendrites are known both to contain and to release dopamine (Geffen et al., 1976; Korf et al., 1976; Nieoullon et al., 1977; Reubi et al., 1977). If, as some suspect, the released dopamine is capable of influencing pars reticulata neurons or their afferent fibers either by conventional synapses or unconventional "modulation," then the pars compacta could have partial control over one of the main targets of striatal efferents as well as over the striatum. An interesting alternative is that the dopamine release produces some form of self-inhibition (Aghajanian and Bunney, 1973).

(2) Afferent connections

For the first time, fiber projections specifically directed to the pars compacta have been identified, as discussed in some detail above. These include:

(a) afferents from the nucleus accumbens/ventral striatum (Swanson and Cowan, 1975; Conrad and Pfaff, 1976a; Powell and Lehman, 1976; Nauta et al., 1978);

(b) afferents from the central nucleus of the amygdala (Bunney and Aghajanian, 1976; Krettek and Price, 1978);

(c) afferents from the lateral preoptico-hypothalamic region (Conrad and Pfaff, 1976b, c; Swanson, 1976; Nauta and Domesick, 1978);

(d) afferents from the dorsal raphe nucleus (Bobillier et al., 1976; Azmitia and Segal, 1978);

(e) afferents from the region of the nucleus tegmenti pedunculopontinis (Graybiel, 1977a; Moon Edley and Graybiel, in progress; see Fig. 18);

(f) (still a matter of some dispute) afferents issuing from the vicinity of the pallidum (the external pallidal segment according to Grofová, 1975; Hattori et al., 1975; Bunney and Aghajanian, 1976), the sublenticular gray (ventral pallidum?) according to Kim et al. (1976);

(g) afferents from the cerebral cortex (long disputed and finally disclaimed (e.g., Rinvik and Walberg, 1969) but recently reported in an autoradiographic study in the monkey (Künzle, 1978) as arising in areas 6 and 9).

The fact that the first three of these connections arise directly or indirectly from elements of the limbic system has led to the concept of limbic control over the dopaminergic nigro-striatal tract (Figs. 8, 13 and 14). Further limbic system relations of the dopamine mechanism implicate the neighboring cell groups A10 and A8, as reviewed above in the section on striatal afferents.

In sharp contrast to this widespread origin of pars compacta afferents, inputs to the pars reticulata are restricted, only the massive strionigral pathway having been adequately documented. As already discussed, this connection appears to be topographic and may be collateral to the striopallidal connection. The subthalamic nucleus may project to the pars reticulata (see Nauta and Cole, 1974, cf. 1978; Kanazawa et al., 1976) but this is not known for sure; if these were the exclusive (or even main) inputs to the pars reticulata, the parallel between its afferents and those of the pallidum would be exact.

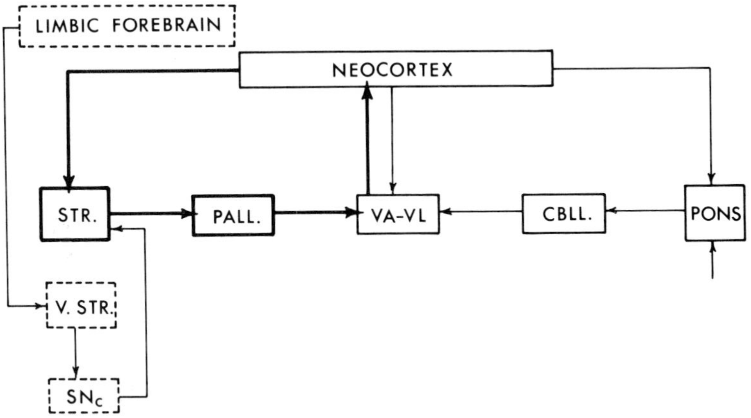

Fig. 14. Highly schematized illustration of some extrapyramidal circuits showing access route from limbic forebrain to the substantia nigra's pars compacta by way of the ventral striatum (V.STR.). Modified from Graybiel, in press.

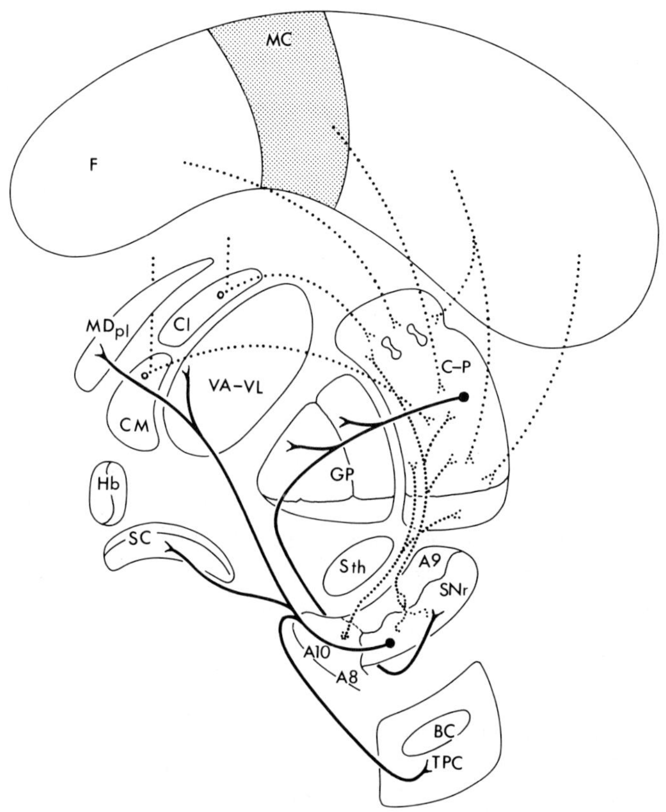

Fig. 15. Schematic diagram illustrating efferent connections of the pars reticulata of the substantia nigra. Abbreviations given in Figs. 1 and 12.

(3) Efferent connections

The efferent connections of the substantia nigra are distributed far more widely than has been previously appreciated. Those from the pars compacta have been reviewed in detail above and will only be briefly mentioned here. The efferent connections of the pars reticulata (like its afferent connections) most closely resemble those of the pallidum. As Fox and his colleagues and others have emphasized, the similarity is not surprising when one considers that the two regions are apparently related embryologically, share the same unusual ultrastructural characteristic of bouton-studded dendritic shafts and are in partial physical continuity (through cell bridges crossing the cerebral peduncle with the comb system and called the fields of Sano (see Schwyn and Fox, 1974)).

(a) Pars compacta (see Figs. 8 and 13)

(i) Nigrostriatal and nigrocortical fibers. These dopamine-containing fibers of the pars compacta lead to certain limbic regions of the neocortex and allocortex as well as to the striatum (see above); they partially overlap and are interlocked with efferent fibers arising in the adjoining dopamine-containing cell groups A10 and A8.

(ii) Nigrotegmental fibers. Beckstead (1977) and Domesick et al. (1976) recently have traced fibers from the pars compacta in a descending direction along two routes. A more lateral, diffuse path sweeps through the lateral tegmentum of the mesencephalon and pons. A more medially disposed group of fibers apparently terminates in quite localized fashion in the dorsal raphe nucleus; this latter connection apparently completes a loop leading from the serotonin-containing dorsal raphe nucleus to the dopamine-containing pars compacta and back again.

(b) Pars reticulata (Fig. 15)

Fibers from the pars reticulata are distributed to the thalamus and midbrain.

(i) Nigrothalamic fibers. The nigrothalamic projection has been studied recently by both anterograde and retrograde transport techniques. Important observations are first, that the connection survives treatment with the dopamine neurotoxin, 6-OHDA, and thus is non-dopaminergic (Hedreen, 1971; Hedreen and Chalmers, 1972). Second, the connection arises from a distinct district of the pars reticulata (Faull and Mehler, 1978). In the rat this is sandwiched between the pars compacta and ventral pars reticulata (Faull and Mehler, 1978); in the monkey (Carpenter et al., 1976) the region apparently forms the rostrolateral part of the pars reticulata. Third, the thalamic zone of distribution of nigral fibers includes the paralamellar part of the mediodorsal nucleus (Carpenter et al., 1976) in addition to the medial part of the VA-VL complex (VM in the rat, Faull and Mehler; VM and medial VA-VL in the cat, Graybiel, unpublished; medial VLm and VAmc in the monkey, Carpenter et al., 1976). The newly described projection to the mediodorsal nucleus implies that the pars reticulata has access to the frontal eye fields (Scollo-Lavizzari and Akert, 1963; Akert, 1964). The restricted projection to the medial part of the VA-VL complex suggests that the nigrothalamic fibers overlap very little, if at all, with pallidothalamic fibers. The thalamocortical projections of this medial sector of the VA-VL complex are not known with certainty in the monkey (presumably they terminate in premotor and/or motor cortex) but an extraordinary recent finding in the rat is that VM projects to nearly the full extent of the neocortex, terminating there in the outer half of layer I (Herkenham, 1976). This observation seems to imply that the caudoputamen (and cerebellum, Faull and Carmen, 1978), while apparently deprived of direct access to the neocortex, can by the intermediary of this thalamic path influence nearly the entire cortical mantle. An equivalent circuit

arrangement has not been demonstrated in the carnivore or primate.

(ii) Nigrotectal fibers. While variously claimed and disclaimed in the early (and even some recent) literature this connection has now been definitively demonstrated in both autoradiographic and horseradish peroxidase experiments. Faull and Mehler (1978) have shown that it arises from the most ventral part of the pars reticulata of the rat; its cells of origin thus overlap very little with the reticulata neurons projecting to the thalamus. Autoradiographic studies have shown that this projection has a remarkable pattern of termination within the intermediate gray layer of the tectum: its terminals are grouped into regularly spaced clusters or "puffs" that appear as more or less discrete patches in cross-section (Fig. 16; Graybiel, 1975; Graybiel and Sciascia, 1975; Jayaraman et al., 1977; Graybiel, 1978) and elongated bands in dorsal view reconstructions (Graybiel, 1978). The finding of these patches could imply some corresponding form of clumping also of the neurons in pars reticulata; so far, however, aside from Golgi observations of a restricted mediolateral spread of nigral dendrites (Rinvik and Grofová, 1970; Schwyn and Fox, 1974; Juraska et al., 1977), the only evidence for compartmentalization of the substantia nigra is at the level of the 3 main dorsal-to-ventral zones identified by Faull and Mehler as projecting to (a) striatum, (b) thalamus, and (c) superior colliculus. Faull and Mehler's findings are comparable, for the substantia nigra, to the original discovery that the two segments of the pallidum have distinct efferent connections.

(iii) Nigrotegmental fibers. Cajal (1911) and many others since (see Rioch, 1929) have described nigrotegmental fibers, which became known by the collective phrase *"courant de la calotte"* and were considered by some to be the main efferent system of the substantia nigra. Only very recently, however, has their existence been established unequivocally. Nigrotegmental fibers arising from the pars compacta apparently comprise a sizable part of this projection system and have been described above but, as Hopkins and Niessen (1976) have emphasized, the pars reticulata contributes fibers to it also. According to Hedreen's experiments in the rat (1971) and more recent autoradiographic evidence in the cat (Graybiel, unpublished observations; see Fig. 17), nigrotegmental fibers from the pars reticulata (like pallidotegmental fibers) terminate in the nucleus tegmenti pedunculopontinis pars compacta (TPC). This pathway was detected by Papez (1941). Amino acid deposits centered in the pars reticulata in the cat also label parts of the dorsolateral central gray substance and nucleus of Darkschewitsch and, variably, the pretectal nucleus of the optic tract (Graybiel, unpublished observations). Two of the nuclei of the accessory optic tract lie pressed against the cerebral peduncle next to the pars reticulata, however, and their involvement (even in quite small injections) could account for some of this labeling (for example, labeling of the nucleus of the optic tract).

The nucleus tegmenti pedunculopontis pars compacta (TPC)

This nucleus is hardly well known. Ever since Nauta and Mehler (1966) identified it as receiving the most caudal projection fibers of the pallidum, however, evidence has been accumulating that the nucleus tegmenti pedunculopontinis is linked by multiple ties to the basal ganglia and, more generally, to the central motor mechanism. The TPC is reported to receive inputs from the substantia nigra's pars reticulata (just reviewed; see Fig. 17), the subthalamic nucleus (Papez, 1941; Nauta and Cole, 1974, 1978) and, in addition, from the motor cortex (Kuypers and Lawrence, 1967) and the red nucleus (Miller and Strominger, 1973).

The efferent connections of the TPC were impossible to work out by the lesion method:

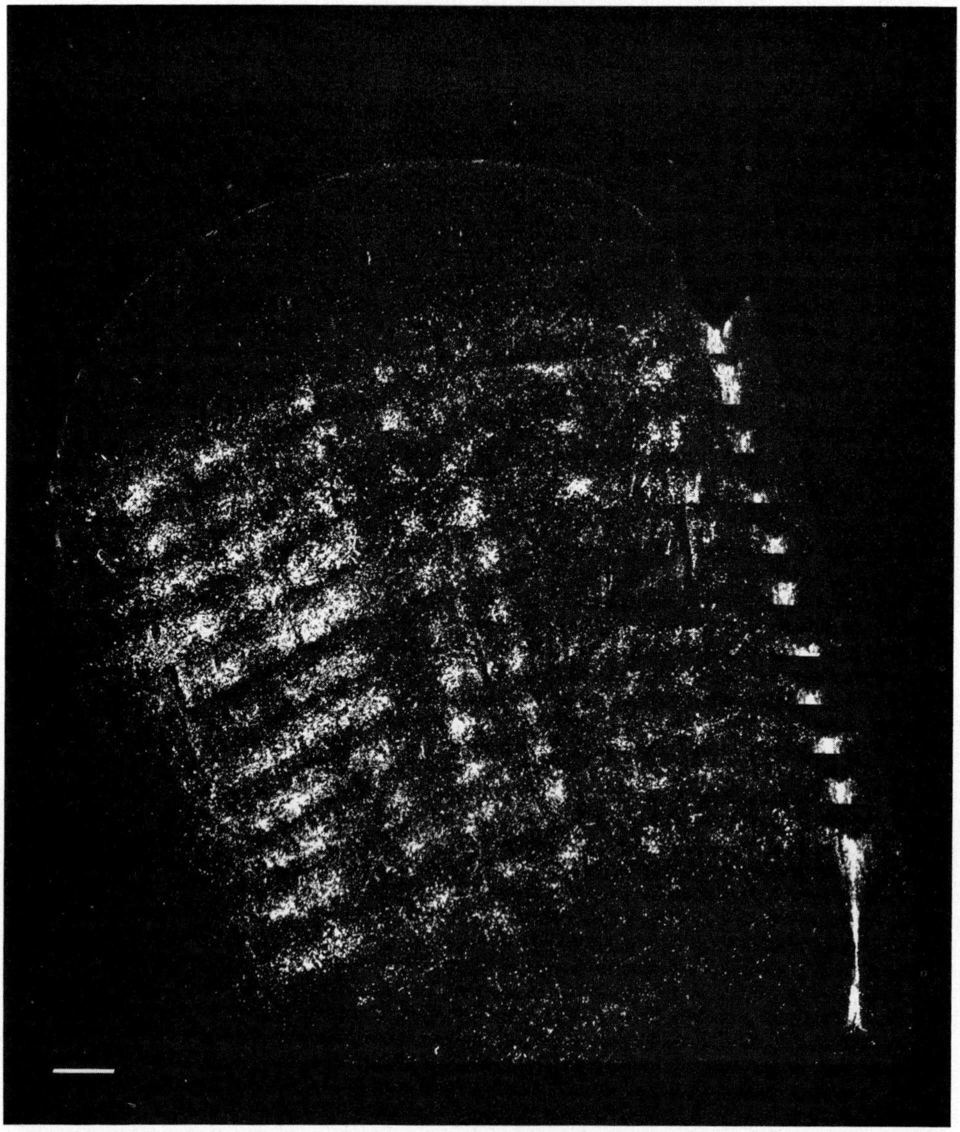

Fig. 16. Photomontage illustrating chain of terminal "puffs" formed by nigrotectal fibers with intermediate gray layer of the superior colliculus in the cat. Photographs of 11 serial sections overlapped in register; medial to the right. From Graybiel, 1978. Bar indicates 0.5 mm.

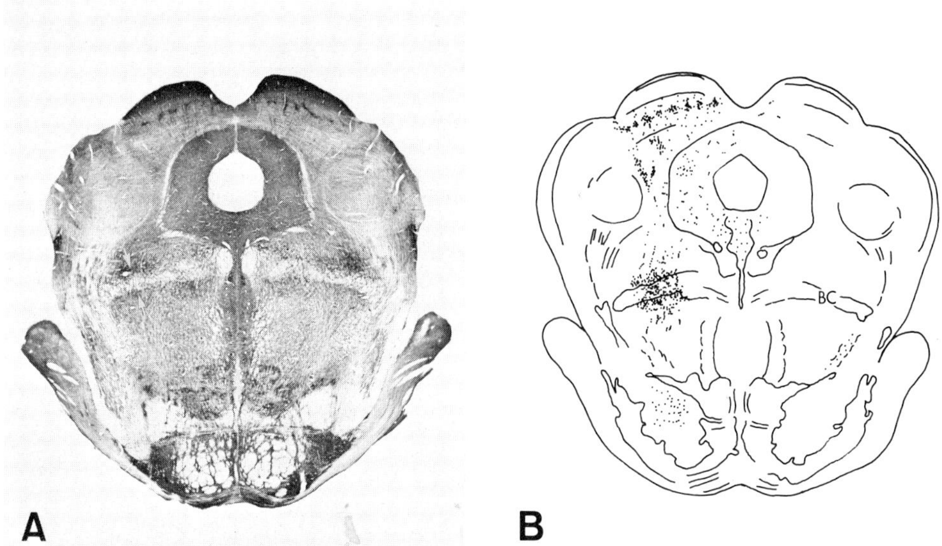

Fig. 17. Photograph of cholinesterase-stained cross-section (A) and charting of autoradiogram (B) at approximately matched transverse levels through the midbrain in the cat. Arrows in A point toward the nucleus tegmenti pedunculopontinis (TPC), which lies in the peribrachial region. B shows labeling of this peribrachial TPC region following an injection of tritiated amino acids into the ipsilateral substantia nigra. Note nigrotectal puffs (and cholinesterase-positive clumps) in intermediate gray layer of superior colliculus.

the nucleus lies embedded in the peribrachial reticular formation of the pontomesencephalic region with its neurons so clustered around the horizontal limb of the brachium conjunctivum that any lesion of TPC would produce massive perforant fiber degeneration. Nevertheless, Mehler was able to deduce that TPC efferents might at least in part be ascending rather than descending (see Mehler and Nauta, 1974). Recent autoradiographic evidence supports this view. Deposits of amino acids into the peribrachial region in the cat (Fig. 18) have been found to produce dense labeling in the pars compacta of the substantia nigra and in the subthalamic nucleus; the largest injections in this region also label the caudal tip of the internal pallidal segment (entopeduncular nucleus) (Graybiel, 1977a; Moon Edley and Graybiel, in progress).

These observations suggest that the nucleus tegmenti pedunculopontinis may represent another member of the family of "loop nuclei" related to the basal ganglia. Whether it in addition has other efferent connections beyond the loops is more difficult to be sure of. For example, because of its position in the pontomesencephalic reticular formation, a natural guess is that the TPC might represent a starting point for descending channels leading from the basal ganglia toward the spinal cord. The nucleus does in fact lie near the so-called "mesencephalic locomotor area" (Grillner and Shik, 1973) and large amino acid injections in this region do label a massive descending path leading into the reticulospinal circuitry of the medulla oblongata (Graybiel, 1977a). Very little such labeling is seen after small injections into the TPC region, however, so that this point is still not settled.

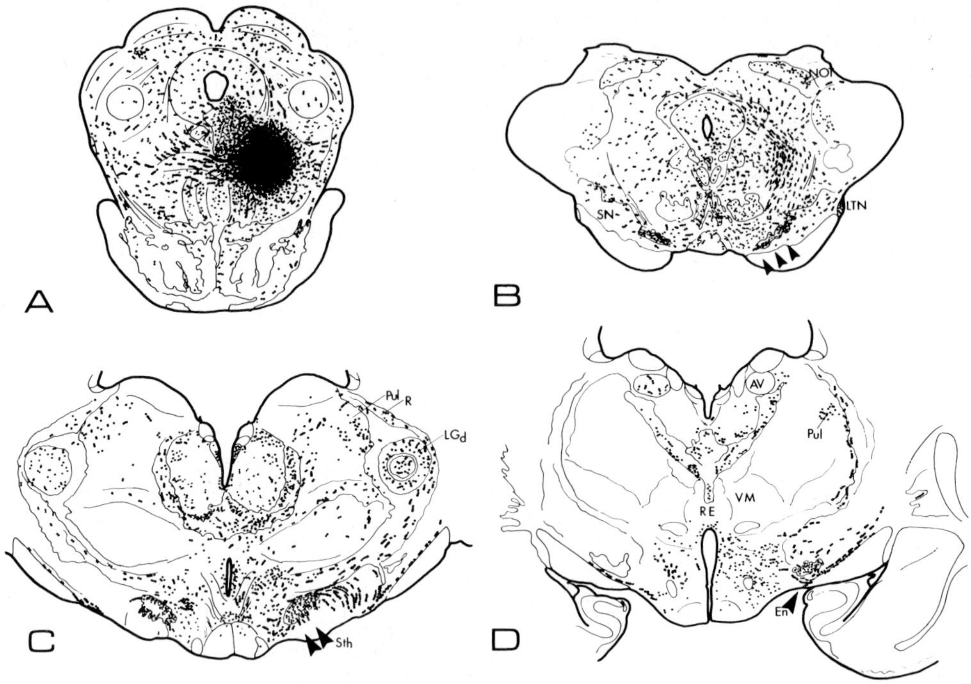

Fig. 18. Chartings of autoradiograms illustrating apparent recurrent pathways traced from peribrachial TPC region (A, injection site black) to more rostral parts of basal ganglia circuitry in the cat: the pars compacta of the substantia nigra (B, 3 arrowheads), the subthalamic nucleus (C, 2 arrowheads), and the caudal tip of the entopeduncular nucleus (D, 1 arrowhead). Modified from Graybiel, 1977a.

The subthalamic nucleus

The subthalamic nucleus is the only part of the subthalamic region with relatively sharply defined cytoarchitectonic borders. It receives apparently all of the massive efferent projection of the external pallidal segment (carried in the subthalamic fasciculus) and is well developed in primates. Its efferent fiber projection to the internal segment of the globus pallidus, coupled with the fact that lesions in the subthalamic nucleus produce the violent dyskinetic "release" syndrome of hemiballism, led some authors to suggest that the subthalamic nucleus functions mainly as an inhibitory intermediate step in the circuit: external pallidum to subthalamic nucleus to internal pallidum (see, e.g., Carpenter and Stromeyer, 1967; Carpenter et al., 1968). The situation is likely more complex. Axon transport evidence (Nauta and Cole, 1978) indicates first that Glees and Wall (1946) were correct in suggesting that the subthalamic nucleus projects to *both* pallidal segments, not to the internal segment only. Furthermore, this projection, in the monkey, is organized into "bands." The subthalamic nucleus also appears to project to the substantia nigra (apparently to the non-dopaminergic neurons) and sparsely (in the monkey) to the TPC (Nauta and Cole, 1978).

The afferent connections of the subthalamic nucleus are also more extensive than the pallidal loop-circuit suggests. Not only does it appear to receive ascending input from the TPC region (Fig. 19) but also, according to the reports by Petras (1969), Künzle (1978) and Hartmann-von Monakow et al. (1978), from the motor cortex. It is interesting that according to the Zurich group (Hartmann-von Monakow et al., 1978; Künzle, 1978) the motor cortex

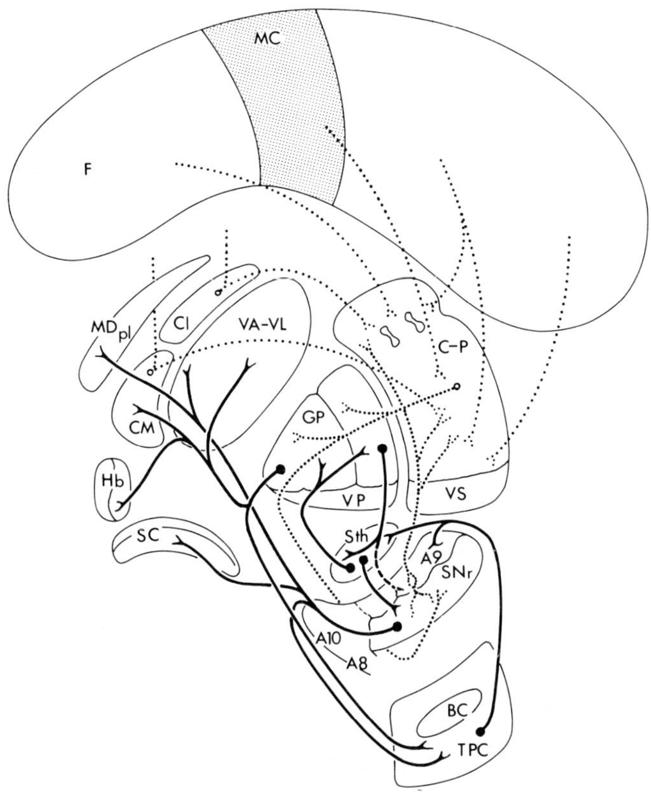

Fig. 19. Schematic diagram putting together some of the pathways illustrated separately in previous figures and emphasizing loop systems of the basal ganglia. Abbreviations given in Figs. 1 and 12.

projects to the lateral part of the subthalamic nucleus while the prefrontal (limbic) cortex projects to the medial part that apparently receives, instead of pallidal input, input from the substantia innominata (Nauta and Mehler, 1966). These findings suggest the possibility that the medial part of the subthalamic nucleus might be the subthalamic equivalent of the ventral pallidum and ventral striatum; it is notable that cytoarchitectural differences between the lateral and medial parts of the nucleus have also been described (see Rafols and Fox, 1976).

The centre médian

Like the other nuclei associated with loop systems of the corpus striatum, this thalamic intralaminar nucleus has connections of two sorts: those that form the loop itself (striatum-pallidum-centre médian-striatum) and those that seem to break the loop on the input or output sides. These connections have been described in preceding sections on the striatum and pallidum and are mentioned briefly here for the sake of clarity.

The only known inputs to centre médian are (1) fibers from the internal pallidal segment, and (2) fibers from the neocortex, principally the motor cortex. The nucleus, despite its quite massive size in primates, is apparently insulated from ascending fiber projections. The known efferent connections of the centre médian are also two in number, namely, its massive projection to the putamen and its apparently much more sparse and diffuse projection to large parts of the neocortex. Retrograde transport and retrograde degeneration experiments alike suggest that the cortical projections are probably collateral offsets of the main centre médian-to-putamen projection (Murray, 1966; Jones and Leavitt, 1974). It is a mystery what the significance may be of the apparently widespread influence of the centre médian on the neocortex. The only other fiber system of the basal ganglia reminiscent of this remarkably broad pallido-thalamo-cortical projection is the path described by Herkenham (1976) from the substantia nigra's pars reticulata to the VM nucleus to layer I of the neocortex in the rat. As the centre médian is poorly developed in the rat (and for that matter, in all non-primates) the nigro-thalamo-cortical pathway conceivably might serve as an alternative to the pallido-thalamo-cortical route involving the centre médian.

CONCLUSIONS

Progress of two types can be identified on the basis of the anatomical studies of the basal ganglia reviewed above: conformations and modifications of earlier findings, and major new conclusions as to the organization of the basal ganglia and their allied nuclei. The importance of the confirmations should not be underestimated. All save a few of the connections of the basal ganglia as traced out by lesion methods were subject to at least some doubt. The use of axon transport methods has greatly reduced this tentativeness, first, with the autoradiographic technique, by removing the fibers-of-passage problem and second, with the retrograde labeling technique, by permitting clear visualization of the cells of origin of many of the pathways. It is only with these techniques that anatomical work on the basal ganglia can proceed with as much solid basis in fact as comparable work on the cerebral cortex. The modifications have in some instances been minor but in others very important: for example, the new findings that the motor cortex projects mainly to the putamen, but prefrontal cortex mainly to the caudate nucleus, indicate that these two subdivisions of the primate striatum may have far more distinctive, if not indeed dissociable, functions than previously realized. Moreover, new work suggests that a large fraction of the neurons in the caudate nucleus and putamen are efferent neurons, not interneurons.

Three major findings can be singled out as representing not simply revisions but conclusions novel enough to reorient some lines of work on the basal ganglia. The first of these is the discovery of a high degree of compartmentalization within the striatum, which at once markedly reduces the contrast between the subcortical and cortical hemisphere and offers the hope that the intrinsic structure of the striatum can be related in a principled way to the logic of its afferent and efferent connections. The second major conclusion is that the nuclei allied to the corpus striatum proper provide not only important points of access into the circuitry of the basal ganglia but also outlets that extend the influence of the basal ganglia well beyond the confines of the traditional outflow channel from corpus striatum to thalamus to motor cortex. The most striking instance is the substantia nigra, now known to be related to widespread parts of the forebrain and midbrain in addition to the striatum. The third (and related) conclusion is that the two great subcortical divisions of the cerebral hemisphere: the corpus striatum and limbic system, are by no means insulated from one another but instead are tied together by pathways that over successive synaptic linkages lose their identities as skeletomotor or limbic. It may well be in part by means of these connections, notably involving the ventral striatum and substantia nigra, that the realm of mood and affect is engrafted onto the exquisitely precise and geometrically ordered sensorimotor topographies of the forebrain.

Insofar as the fundamental challenge of brain science is to relate information about the nervous system to behavior, it is the last named work on the limbic affiliations of the basal ganglia that is likely to yield the greatest gains. In fact, there are already intensive investigations underway, including pharmacological studies, attempting to relate these new findings to the negative signs (akinesias) and "emotionalism" (Kinnier Wilson's term) seen in basal ganglia disorders. In terms of mechanism, it seems probable that study of the compartmented ("striosomal") organization of the striatum, and study of the logic of the loop systems of the basal ganglia, should be pursued further.

But we are far from understanding either the functions of the basal ganglia or the intrinsic logic of their neural circuitry. The finding that the basal ganglia do not stand in relative isolation from other parts of the brain could be said to bring us part way back to Kinnier Wilson's viewpoint, but probably actually not: his idea was that the basal ganglia and cerebellum alike were "extrapyramidal" by virtue of their reliance on brain stem (principally rubrospinal) access, rather than corticospinal access, to the spinal motor apparatus. From recent work it would seem more likely that a parallel between basal ganglia and cerebellum should emphasize that just as the cerebellum is multiply linked to nuclei in the brain stem, so are the basal ganglia multiply linked to nuclei in the forebrain. Perhaps the implied difference (coupled with the many similarities) may be a clue as to why both cerebellum and corpus striatum project so massively into the thalamus-to-motor cortex circuitry. In terms of the circuit arrangements of the basal ganglia, we still lack insight into why all the loops are present or why, in the first place, the entire cortex projects to the striatum (as it does to the cerebellum via the precerebellar nuclei). Such problems as these are clearly not unique to study of the basal ganglia; what is remarkable about recent work on the anatomy is that it has made the basal ganglia accessible, for the first time, to attempts to resolve such fundamental questions about central nervous organization.

ACKNOWLEDGEMENTS

It is a pleasure to thank Mr. H. F. Hall, who is responsible for the photography; Ms. Ree Clark, who typed the manuscript; and the National Science Foundation (BNS75-18758 and BNS78-10549) and the National Institutes of Health (NIH-5-SO7-RR07047-13) which provided financial support for some of the work described. The diagrams are modified from figures prepared for the Society for Neuroscience symposium on the basal ganglia held in 1976 in Toronto (see Graybiel, 1977b).

REFERENCES

Aghajanian, G. K. and Bunney, B. S. (1973) Central dopaminergic neurons: neurophysiological identification and responses to drugs. In *Frontiers in Catecholamine Research,* E. Usdin and S. H. Snyder (Eds.), Pergamon Press, Oxford, pp. 643–648.

Akert, K. (1964) Comparative anatomy of frontal cortex and thalamofrontal connections. In *The Frontal Granular Cortex and Behavior,* J. M. Warren and K. Akert (Eds.), McGraw-Hill, New York, pp. 372–396.

Andén, N.-E., Carlsson, A., Dahlström, A., Fuxe, K., Hillarp, N. A. and Larsson, K. (1964) Demonstration and mapping out of nigro-neostriatal dopamine neurons. *Life Sci.,* 3: 523–530.

Andén, N.-E., Dahlström, A., Fuxe, K. and Larsson, K. (1965) Further evidence for the presence of nigro-neostriatal dopamine neurons in the rat. *Amer. J. Anat.,* 116: 329–333.

Andén, N.-E., Dahlström, A., Fuxe, K., Larsson, K., Olson, L. and Ungerstedt, U. (1966) Ascending monoamine neurons to the telencephalon and diencephalon. *Acta physiol. scand.*, 67: 313–326.

Angevine, Jr., J. B. and McConnell, J. A. (1974) Time of origin of striatal neurons in the mouse: an autoradiographic study. *Anat. Rec.*, 178: 300.

Azmitia, E. C. and Segal, M. (1978) An autoradiographic analysis of the differential ascending projections of the dorsal and median raphe nuclei in the rat. *J. comp. Neurol.*, 179: 641–668.

Bak, I. J., Markham, C. H., Cook, M. L. and Stevens, J. G. (1978) Ultrastructural and immunoperoxidase study of striatonigral neurons by means of retrograde axonal transport of herpes simplex virus. *Brain Res.*, 143: 361–368.

Barbeau, A. (1976) Six years of high-level levodopa therapy in severely akinetic parkinsonian patients. *Arch. Neurol. (Chic.)*, 33: 333–338.

Beckstead, R. M. (1976) Convergent thalamic and mesencephalic projections to the anterior medial cortex in the rat. *J. comp. Neurol.*, 166: 403–416.

Beckstead, R. M. (1977) *Anatomical Observations on the Organization and Interrelationship of the Nigrostriatal, Nigrocortical and Corticostriatal Connections in the Brain of the Rat.* Ph.D. Thesis, Mass. Inst. of Technol., Cambridge, Mass.

Berman, A. L. (1968) *The Brain Stem of the Cat. A Cytoarchitectonic Atlas with Stereotaxic Coordinates.* University of Winconsin Press, Madison, Wisc.

Björklund, A. and Lindvall, O. (1975) Dopamine in dendrites of substantia nigra neurons: suggestions for a role in dendritic terminals. *Brain Res.*, 83: 531–537.

Bobillier, P., Sequin, S., Petitjean, F., Salvert, D., Touret, M. and Jouvet, M. (1976) The raphe nuclei of the cat brain stem: a topographical atlas of their efferent projections as revealed by autoradiography. *Brain Res.*, 113: 449–486.

Brand, S. and Rakic, P. (1978) Time of origin of neurons in primate neostriatum: ^{3}H-thymidine autoradiographic analysis in the rhesus monkey. *Anat. Rec.*, 190: 345–346.

Bunney, B. S. and Aghajanian, G. K. (1976) The precise localization of nigral afferents in the rat as determined by a retrograde tracing technique. *Brain Res.*, 117: 423–436.

Butcher, L. L. and Hodge, G. K. (1976) Postnatal development of acetylcholinesterase in the caudate-putamen and substantia nigra of rats. *Brain Res.*, 106: 223–240.

Büttner-Ennever, J. A. and Büttner, U. (1978) A cell group associated with vertical eye movements in the rostral mesencephalic reticular formation of the monkey. *Brain Res.*, 151: 31–47.

Cajal, S. Ramón y (1911) *Histologie du Système Nerveux de l'Homme et des Vertébrés.* Maloine, Paris.

Carman, J. B., Cowan, W. J. and Powell, T. P. S. (1963) The organization of cortico-striate connections in the rabbit. *Brain*, 86: 525–562.

Carman, J. B., Cowan, W. M., Powell, T. P. S. and Webster, K. E. (1965) A bilateral cortico-striate projection. *J. Neurol. Neurosurg. Psychiat.*, 28: 71–77.

Carpenter, M. B. (1976) Anatomical organization of the corpus striatum and related nuclei. In *The Basal Ganglia*, M. D. Yahr (Ed.), Raven Press, New York, pp. 1–36.

Carpenter, M. B. and Peter, P. (1972) Nigrostriatal and nigrothalamic fibers in the rhesus monkey. *J. comp. Neurol.*, 144: 93–116.

Carpenter, M. B. and Strominger, N. L. (1967) Efferent fibers of the subthalamic nucleus in the monkey. A comparison of the efferent projections of the subthalamic nucleus, substantia nigra and globus pallidus. *Amer. J. Anat.*, 121: 41–72.

Carpenter, M. B., Fraser, R. A. R. and Shriver, J. E. (1968) The organization of pallidosubthalamic fibers in the monkey. *Brain Res.*, 11: 522–559.

Carpenter, M. B., Nakano, K. and Kim, R. (1976) Nigrothalamic projections in the monkey demonstrated by autoradiographic technics. *J. comp. Neurol.*, 165: 401–416.

Carter, D. A. and Fibiger, H. C. (1978) The projections of the entopeduncular nucleus and globus pallidus in the rat as demonstrated by autoradiography and horseradish peroxidase histochemistry. *J. comp. Neurol.*, 177: 113–124.

Chow, K. L. and Pribram, K. H. (1956) Cortical projections of the thalamus ventrolateral nuclear group in monkeys. *J. comp. Neurol.*, 104: 57–75.

Chronister, R. B., Farnell, K. E., Marco, L. A. and White, Z. E. (1976) The rodent neostriatum: a Golgi analysis. *Brain Res.*, 108: 37–46.

Cole, M., Nauta, W. J. H. and Mehler, W. R. (1964) The ascending efferent projections of the substantia nigra. *Trans. Amer. neurol. Ass.*, 89: 74–78.

Conrad, L. C. A. and Pfaff, D. W. (1976a) Autoradiographic tracing of nucleus accumbens efferents in the rat. *Brain Res.*, 113: 589–596.

Conrad, L. C. A. and Pfaff, D. W. (1976b) Efferents from medial basal forebrain and hypothalamus in the rat. I. An autoradiographic study of the medial preoptic area. *J. comp. Neurol.*, 169: 185–220.

Conrad, L. C. A. and Pfaff, D. W. (1976c) Efferents from medial basal forebrain and hypothalamus in the rat. II. An autoradiographic study of the anterior hypothalamus. *J. comp. Neurol.*, 169: 221–262.

Conrad, L. C. A., Leonard, C. M. and Pfaff, D. W. (1974) Connections of the median and dorsal raphe nuclei in the rat: an autoradiographic and degeneration study. *J. comp. Neurol.*, 156: 179–206.

Cowan, W. M. and Powell, T. P. S. (1955) The projections of the midline and intralaminar nuclei of the thalamus of the rabbit. *J. Neurol. Neurosurg. Psychiat.*, 18: 266–279.

Cowan, W. M. and Powell, T. P. S. (1966) Strio-pallidal projections in the monkey. *J. Neurol. Neurosurg. Psychiat.*, 29: 426–439.

Crosby, E. C. and Woodburne, R. T. (1943) The nuclear pattern of non-tectal portions of the midbrain and isthmus in primates. *J. comp. Neurol.*, 78: 441–520.

Dahlström, A. and Fuxe, K. (1964) Evidence for the existence of monoamine-containing neurons in the central nervous system. *Acta physiol. scand.*, 62 (Suppl. 232): 1–55.

De Olmos, J. S. and Ingram, W. R. (1972) The projection field of the stria terminalis in the rat brain. *J. comp. Neurol.*, 146: 303–334.

Descarries, L., Beaudet, A. and Watkins, K. C. (1975) Serotonin nerve terminals in adult rat neocortex. *Brain Res.*, 100: 563–588.

Descarries, L., Watkins, K. C. and Lapierre, Y. (1977) Noradrenergic axon terminals in the cerebral cortex of rat. III. Topometric ultrastructural analysis. *Brain Res.*, 133: 197–222.

Diamond, B. I. and Borison, R. L. (1978) Enkephalins and nigrostriatal function. *Neurology (Minneap.)*, 28: 1085–1088.

Di Figlia, M., Pasik, P. and Pasik, T. (1976) A Golgi study of neuronal types in the neostriatum of monkeys. *Brain Res.*, 114: 245–256.

Divac, I., Björklund, A., Lindvall, O. and Passingham, R. E. (1978) Converging projections from the mediodorsal thalamic nucleus and mesencephalic dopaminergic neurons to the neocortex in three species. *J. comp. Neurol.*, 180: 59–72.

Domesick, V. B., Beckstead, R. M. and Nauta, W. J. H. (1976) Some ascending and descending projections of the substantia nigra and ventral tegmental area in the rat. *Neurosci. Abstr.*, 2: 61.

Edinger, L. (1911) *Vorlesungen über den Bau der nervösen Zentralorgane, Vol. 1.* Vogel, Leipzig (8th ed.).

Fallon, J. H. and Moore, R. Y. (1978a) Catecholamine innervation of the basal forebrain. III. Olfactory bulb, anterior olfactory nuclei, olfactory tubercle and piriform cortex. *J. comp. Neurol.*, 180: 533–544.

Fallon, J. H. and Moore, R. Y. (1978b) Catecholamine innervation of the basal forebrain. IV. Topography of the dopamine projection to the basal forebrain and neostriatum. *J. comp. Neurol.*, 180: 545–580.

Fallon, J. H., Koziell, D. A. and Moore, R. Y. (1978) Catecholamine innervation of the basal forebrain. II. Amygdala, suprarhinal cortex and entorhinal cortex. *J. comp. Neurol.*, 180: 509–532.

Faull, R. L. M. and Carmen, J. B. (1978) The cerebellofugal projections in the brachium conjunctivum of the rat. I. The contralateral ascending pathway. *J. comp. Neurol.*, 178: 495–518.

Faull, R. L. M. and Mehler, W. R. (1976) Studies of the fiber connections of the substantia nigra in the rat using the method of retrograde transport of horseradish peroxidase. *Neurosci. Abstr.*, 2: 62.

Faull, R. L. M. and Mehler, W. R. (1978) The cells of origin of nigrotectal, nigrothalamic and nigrostriatal projections in the rat. *Neuroscience*, 3: 989–1002.

Filion, M., Harnois, C. and Guano, G. (1976) Electrophysiological study of the distribution of axonal branches of individual entopeduncular neurons in the cat. *Neurosci. Abstr.*, 2: 63.

Foix, C. et Nicolesco, J. (1925) *Les Noyaux Gris Centraux et la Région Mésencéphalo-sous-optique.* Masson et Cie, Paris.

Fonnum, F., Grofová, I., Rinvik, E., Storm-Mathisen, J. and Walberg, F. (1974) Origin and distribution of glutamate decarboxylase in substantia nigra of the cat. *Brain Res.*, 71: 77–92.

Fox, C. A. (1943) The stria terminalis, longitudinal association bundle and precommissural fornix in the cat. *J. comp. Neurol.*, 79: 277–295.

Fox, C. A. and Rafols, J. A. (1975) The radial fibers in the globus pallidus. *J. comp. Neurol.*, 159: 177–200.

Fox, C. A. and Rafols, J. A. (1976) The striatal efferents in the globus pallidus and in the substantia nigra. In *The Basal Ganglia*, M. D. Yahr (Ed.), Raven Press, New York, pp. 37–55.

Fox, C. A. and Schmitz, J. T. (1944) The substantia nigra and the entopeduncular nucleus in the cat. *J. comp. Neurol.*, 80: 323–334.

Fox, C. A., Andrade, A., Hillman, D. E. and Schwyn, R. C. (1971/72a) The spiny neurons in the primate striatum: a Golgi and electron microscopic study. *J. Hirnforsch.*, 13: 181–201.

Fox, C. A., Andrade, A. N., Schwyn, R. C. and Rafols, J. A. (1971/72b) The aspiny neurons and the glia in the primate striatum: a Golgi and electron microscopic study. *J. Hirnforsch.*, 13: 341–362.

Fox, C. A., Andrade, A. N., LuQui, I. J. and Rafols, J. (1974) The primate globus pallidus: a Golgi and electron microscope study. *J. Hirnforsch.*, 15: 75–93.

Fox, C. A., Rafols, J. A. and Cowan, W. M. (1975) Computer measurements of axis cylinder diameters of radial fibers and "comb" bundle fibers. *J. comp. Neurol.*, 159: 201–224.

Fuxe, K., Hökfelt, T., Johansson, O., Johnsson, G., Lidbrink, P. and Ljungdahl, Å. (1974) The origin of the dopamine terminals in limbic and frontal cortex. Evidence for meso-cortico dopamine neurons. *Brain Res.*, 82; 349–355.

Fuxe, K., Hökfelt, J., Agnati, L. F., Johannson, O., Goldstein, M., Perez de la Mora, M., Possani, L., Tapia, R., Teran, L. and Palacios, R. (1978) Mapping out central catecholamine neurons: immunohistochemical studies on catecholamine-synthesizing enzymes. In *Psychopharmacology: a Generation of Progress*, M. A. Lipton, A. Di Mascio and K. F. Killam (Eds.), Raven Press, New York, pp. 67–94.

Garver, D. L. and Sladek, Jr., J. R. (1975) Monoamine distribution in primate brain. I. Catecholamine-containing perikarya in the brain stem of *Macaca speciosa*. *J. comp. Neurol.*, 159: 289–304.

Geffen, L. B., Jessell, T. M., Cuello, A. C. and Iversen, L. L. (1976) Release of dopamine from dendrites in rat substantia nigra. *Nature (Lond.)*, 260: 258–260.

Geneser-Jensen, F. A. and Blackstad, J. W. (1971) Distribution of acetyl cholinesterase in the hippocampal region of the guinea pig. I. Entorhinal area, parasubiculum, and presubiculum. *Z. Zellforsch.*, 114: 460–481.

Glees, P. and Wall, P. D. (1946) Fibre connections of the subthalamic region and the centro-median nucleus of the thalamus. *Brain*, 69: 195–208.

Goldman, P. S. and Nauta, W. J. H. (1977) An intricately patterned prefronto-caudate projection in the rhesus monkey. *J. comp. Neurol.*, 171: 369–386.

Graybiel, A. M. (1973) The thalamo-cortical projection of the so-called posterior nuclear group: a study with anterograde degeneration methods in the cat. *Brain Res.*, 49: 229–244.

Graybiel, A. M. (1975a) Anatomical organization of retinotectal afferents in the cat: an autoradiographic study. *Brain Res.*, 96: 1–23.

Graybiel, A. M. (1975b) Wallerian degeneration and anterograde tracer methods. In *The Use of Axonal Transport for Studies of Neuronal Connectivity*, W. M. Cowan and M. Cuénod (Eds.), Elsevier, Amsterdam, pp. 174–216.

Graybiel, A. M. (1977a) Direct and indirect preoculomotor pathways of the brainstem: an autoradiographic study of the pontine reticular formation in the cat. *J. comp. Neurol.*, 175: 37–78.

Graybiel, A. M. (1977b) Basal ganglia in health and disease (A. Barbeau, Chairman). In *Society for Neuroscience, 6th Annual Meeting, Summaries of Symposia (BIS Conference Report No. 45)*. Brain Information Service, Los Angeles, Calif., pp. 41–45.

Graybiel, A. M. (1978) Organization of the nigrotectal connection: an experimental tracer study in the cat. *Brain Res.*, 143: 339–348.

Graybiel, A. M. (1979) Some patterns of connectivity in the central nervous system: a tribute to Rafael Lorente de Nó. In *Integration in the Nervous System*, V. Wilson and H. Asanuma (Eds.), Igaku-Shoin, Tokyo, in press.

Graybiel, A. M. and Ragsdale, Jr., C. W. (1978a) Histochemically distinct compartments in the striatum of human, monkey and cat demonstrated by acetylthiocholinesterase staining. *Proc. nat. Acad. Sci. (Wash.)*, 75: 5723–5726.

Graybiel, A. M. and Ragsdale, Jr., C. W. (1978b) Striosomal organization of the caudate nucleus. I. Acetylcholinesterase histochemistry of the striatum in the cat, rhesus monkey and human being. *Neurosci. Abstr.*, 4: 44.

Graybiel, A. M. and Sciascia, T. R. (1975) Origin and distribution of nigrotectal fibers in the cat. *Neurosci. Abstr.*, 1: 174.

Graybiel, A. M., Ragsdale, Jr., C. W. and Moon Edley, S. (1979) Compartments in the striatum of the cat observed by retrograde cell-labelling. *Exp. Brain Res.*, 34: 189–195.

Grillner, S. and Shik, M. L. (1973) On the descending control of the lumbrosacral spinal cord from the "mesencephalic locomotor region". *Acta physiol. scand.*, 87: 320–333.

Grofová, I. (1975) The identification of striatal and pallidal neurons projecting to substantia nigra. An experimental study by means of retrograde axonal transport of horseradish peroxidase. *Brain Res.*, 91: 286–291.

Grofová, I. and Rinvik, E. (1970) An experimental electron microscopic study on the striatonigral projection in the cat. *Exp. Brain Res.*, 11: 249–262.

Hardy, H., Heimer, L., Switzer, R. and Watkins, D. (1976) Simultaneous demonstration of horseradish peroxidase and acetylcholinesterase. *Neurosci. Lett.*, 3: 1–5.

Hartmann-von Monakow, K., Akert, K. and Künzle, H. (1978) Projections of the precentral motor cortex and other cortical areas of the frontal lobe to the subthalamic nucleus in the monkey. *Exp. Brain Res.*, 33: 395–403.

Hattori, T., McGeer, P. L., Fibiger, H. C. and McGeer, E. G. (1973) On the source of GABA containing terminals in the substantia nigra. Electron microscopic, autoradiographic and biochemical studies. *Brain Res.*, 54: 103–114.

Hattori, T., Fibiger, H. C. and McGeer, P. L. (1975) Demonstration of a pallido-nigral projection innervating dopaminergic neurons. *J. comp. Neurol.*, 162: 487–504.

Hedreen, J. C. (1971) Separate demonstration of dopaminergic and non-dopaminergic projections of substantia nigra in the rat. *Anat. Rec.*, 169: 338.

Hedreen, J. C. and Chalmers, J. P. (1972) Neuronal degeneration in rat brain induced by 6-hydroxydopamine; a histological and biochemical study. *Brain Res.*, 47: 1–36.

Heimer, L. and Wilson, R. D. (1975) The subcortical projections of the allocortex: similarities in the neural associations of the hippocampus, the piriform cortex, and the neocortex. In *Golgi Centennial Symposium*, M. Santini (Ed.), Raven Press, New York, pp. 177–193.

Herkenham, M. (1976) The nigro-thalamic-cortical connection mediated by the nucleus ventralis medialis thalami: evidence for a wide cortical distribution in the rat. *Anat. Rec.*, 184: 426.

Herkenham, M. and Nauta, W. J. H. (1977a) Afferent connections of the habenular nuclei in the rat. A horseradish peroxidase study, with a note on the fiber-of-passage problem. *J. comp. Neurol.*, 173: 123–146.

Herkenham, M. and Nauta, W. J. H. (1977b) Projections of the habenular nuclei in the rat. *Anat. Rec.*, 187: 603.

Herrick, C. J. (1926) *Brains of Rats and Men.* University of Chicago Press, Chicago, Ill.

Hökfelt, T. and Ungerstedt, U. (1969) Electron and fluorescence microscopical studies on the nucleus caudatus putamen of the rat after unilateral lesions of ascending nigro-neostriatal dopamine neurons. *Acta physiol. scand.*, 76: 415–426.

Hökfelt, T., Ljungdahl, Å., Fuxe, K. and Johansson, O. (1974) Dopamine nerve terminals in the rat limbic cortex: aspects of the dopamine hypothesis of schizophrenia. *Science*, 184: 177–179.

Hopkins, D. A. and Niessen, L. W. (1976) Substantia nigra projections to the reticular formation, superior colliculus and central gray in the rat, cat and monkey. *Neurosci. Lett.*, 2: 253–259.

Hubel, D. H. and Wiesel, T. N. (1969) Anatomical demonstration of columns in monkey striate cortex. *Nature (Lond.)*, 221: 747–750.

Jacobowitz, D. M. and Palkovits, M. (1974) Topographic atlas of catecholamine and acetylcholinesterase-containing neurons in the rat brain. I. Forebrain (telencephalon, diencephalon). *J. comp. Neurol.*, 157: 13–28.

Jacobs, B. L., Foote, S. L. and Bloom, F. E. (1978) Differential projections of neurons within the dorsal raphe nucleus of the rat: a horseradish peroxidase (HRP) study. *Brain Res.*, 147: 149–153.

Jayaraman, A., Batton, III, R. R. and Carpenter, M. B. (1977) Nigrotectal projections in the monkey: an autoradiographic study. *Brain Res.*, 135: 147–152.

Jones, E. G. and Leavitt, R. Y. (1974) Retrograde axonal transport and the demonstration of non-specific projections to the cerebral cortex and striatum from the thalamic intralaminar nuclei in the rat, cat and monkey. *J. comp. Neurol.*, 154: 349–378.

Jones, E. G., Coulter, J. D., Burton, H. and Porter, R. (1977) Cells of origin and terminal distribution of corticostriatal fibers arising in the sensory-motor cortex of monkeys. *J. comp. Neurol.*, 173: 53–80.

Juraska, J. M., Wilson, C. J. and Groves, P. M. (1977) The substantia nigra in the rat: a Golgi study. *J. comp. Neurol.*, 172: 585–600.

Kalil, K. (1978) Patch-like termination of thalamic fibers in the putamen of the rhesus monkey: an autoradiographic study. *Brain Res.*, 140: 333–339.

Kanazawa, I., Marshall, G. R. and Kelly, J. S. (1976) Afferents to the rat substantia nigra studied by horseradish peroxidase, with special reference to fibres from the subthalamic nucleus. *Brain Res.*, 115: 485–491.

Kataoka, K., Bak, I. J., Hassler, R., Kim, J. S. and Wagner, A. (1974) L-Glutamate decarboxylase and choline acetyltransferase activity in the substantia nigra and striatum after surgical interruption of strio-nigral fibers of the baboon. *Exp. Brain Res.*, 19: 217–227.

Kemp, J. M. (1970) The termination of striopallidal and strionigral fibers. *Brain Res.*, 17: 125–128.

Kemp, J. M. and Powell, T. P. S. (1970) The cortico-striate projection in the monkey. *Brain,* 93: 525–546.

Kemp, J. M. and Powell, T. P. S. (1971a) The structure of the caudate nucleus of the cat: light and electron microscopy. *Phil. Trans. B,* 262: 383–401.

Kemp, J. M. and Powell, T. P. S. (1971b) The synaptic orgnization of the caudate nucleus. *Phil. Trans. B,* 262: 403–412.

Kemp, J. M. and Powell, T. P. S. (1971c) The site of termination of afferent fibers in the caudate nucleus. *Phil. Trans. B,* 262: 413–427.

Kemp, J. M. and Powell, T. P. S. (1971d) The termination of fibres from the cerebral cortex and thalamus upon the dendritic spines in the caudate nucleus: a study with the Golgi method. *Phil. Trans. B,* 262: 429–439.

Kemp, J. M. and Powell, T. P. S. (1971e) The connexions of the striatum and globus pallidus: synthesis and speculation. *Phil. Trans. B,* 262: 441–457.

Kim, J. S., Bak, I. J., Hassler, R. and Okada, Y. (1971) Role of γ-aminobutyric acid (GABA) in the extrapyramidal motor system. 2. Some evidence for the existence of a type of GABA-rich strio-nigral neurons. *Exp. Brain Res.,* 14: 95–104.

Kim, R., Nakano, K., Jayaraman, A. and Carpenter, M. B. (1976) Projections of the globus pallidus and adjacent structures: an autoradiographic study in the monkey. *J. comp. Neurol.,* 169: 263–290.

Kitai, S. T., Kocsis, J. D., Preston, R. J. and Sugimori, M. (1976a) Monosynaptic inputs to caudate neurons identified by intracellular injection of horseradish peroxidase. *Brain Res.,* 109: 601–606.

Kitai, S. T., Kocsis, J. D. and Wood, J. (1976b) Origin and characteristics of the cortico-caudate afferents: an anatomical and electrophysiological study. *Brain Res.,* 118: 137–141.

Kitai, S. T., Sugimori, M. and Kocsis, J. D. (1976c) Excitatory nature of dopamine in the nigro-caudate pathway. *Exp. Brain Res.,* 24: 351–363.

Kocsis, J. D. and Vandermaelan, C. P. (1977) The caudate projection of the retrorubral nucleus and its relationship to the substantia nigra. *Anat. Rec.,* 187: 628–629.

Kocsis, J. D., Sugimori, M. and Kitai, S. T. (1977) Convergence of excitatory synaptic inputs to caudate spiny neurons. *Brain Res.,* 124: 403–413.

Koelle, G. B. (1954) The histochemical localization of cholinesterase in the central nervous system of the rat. *J. comp. Neurol.,* 100: 211–236.

Korf, J., Zieleman, M. and Westerink, B. H. C. (1976) Dopamine release in substantia nigra? *Nature (Lond.),* 260: 257–258.

Krettek, J. E. and Price, J. L. (1978) Amygdaloid projections to subcortical structures within the basal forebrain and brainstem in the rat and cat. *J. comp. Neurol.,* 178: 225–254.

Kristensson, K. and Olsson, Y. (1971) Retrograde axonal transport of protein. *Brain Res.,* 29: 363–365.

Künzle, H. (1975) Bilateral projections from precentral motor cortex to the putamen and other parts of the basal ganglia. *Brain Res.,* 88: 195–210.

Künzle, H. (1977) Projections from the primary somatosensory cortex to basal ganglia and thalamus in the monkey. *Exp. Brain Res.,* 30: 481–492.

Künzle, H. (1978) An autoradiographic analysis of the efferent connections from premotor and adjacent prefrontal regions (areas 6 and 9) in *Macaca fascicularis. Brain Behav. Evol.,* 15: 185–234.

Künzle, H. and Akert, K. (1977) Efferent connections of cortical area 8 (frontal eye field) in *Macaca fascicularis.* A reinvestigation using the autoradiographic method. *J. comp. neurol.,* 173: 147–164.

Kuo, J.-S. and Carpenter, M. B. (1973) Organization of pallidothalamic projections in the rhesus monkey. *J. comp. Neurol.,* 151: 201–236.

Kuypers, H. G. J. M. and Lawrence, D. G. (1967) Cortical projections to the red nucleus and the brain stem in the rhesus monkey. *Brain Res.,* 4: 151–188.

LaVail, J. H. and LaVail, M. M. (1972) Retrograde axonal transport in the central nervous system. *Science,* 176: 1416–1417.

Lindvall, O., Björklund, A., Moore, R. Y. and Stenevi, U. (1974) Mesencephalic dopamine neurons projecting to neocortex. *Brain Res.,* 81: 325–331.

Lloyd, K. G., Davidson, L. and Hornykiewicz, O. (1975) The neurochemistry of Parkinson's disease: effect of L-dopa therapy. *J. Pharmacol. exp. Ther.,* 195: 453–464.

Mehler, W. R. (1966) Further notes on the center median nucleus of Luys. In *The Thalamus,* D. P. Purpura and M. D. Yahr (Eds.), Columbia University Press, New York, pp. 109–128.

Mehler, W. R. and Nauta, W. J. H. (1974) Connections of the basal ganglia and of the cerebellum. *Confin. neurol. (Basel),* 36: 205–222.

Mensah, P. L. (1977) The internal organization of the mouse caudate nucleus: evidence for cell clustering and regional variation. *Brain Res.,* 137: 53–66.

Mesulam, M.-M. (1978) Tetramethyl benzidine for horseradish peroxidase neurohistochemistry: a non-carcinogenic blue reaction-product with superior sensitivity for visualizing neural afferents and efferents. *J. Histochem. Cytochem.*, 26: 106–117.

Mesulam, M.-M., Van Hoesen, G. W., Pandya, D. N. and Geschwind, N. (1977) Limbic and sensory connections of the inferior parietal lobule (area PG) in the rhesus monkey: a study with a new method for horseradish peroxidase histochemistry. *Brain Res.*, 136: 393–414.

Meynert, Th. (1872) Vom Gehirne der Säugethiere. In *Handbuch der Lehre von den Geweben,* S. Stricker (Ed.), Engelmann, Leipzig.

Miller, R. A. and Strominger, N. L. (1973) Efferent connections of the red nucleus in the brainstem and spinal cord of the rhesus monkey. *J. comp. Neurol.*, 152: 327–346.

Monakow, C. von (1895) Experimentelle und pathologische-anatomische Untersuchungen über die Haubenregion, den Sehhügel und die Regio subthalamica, nebst Beiträgen zur Kenntnis früherworbener Gross- und Kleinhirndefekte. *Arch. Psychiat. Nervenkr.*, 27: 1–128.

Moon Edley, S., Graybiel, A. M. and Ragsdale, Jr., C. W. (1978) Striosomal organization of the caudate nucleus. II. Evidence that neurons in the striatum are grouped in highly branched mosaics. *Neurosci. Abstr.*, 4: 47.

Moore, R. Y. (1978) The catecholamine innervation of the basal forebrain. I. The septal area. *J. comp. Neurol.*, 177: 665–684.

Morest, D. K. (1964) The lateral tegmental system of the midbrain and the medial geniculate body: study with Golgi and Nauta methods in cat. *J. Anat. (Lond.)*, 99: 611–634.

Mountcastle, V. B. (1957) Modality and topographic properties of single neurons of cat's somatic sensory cortex. *J. Neurophysiol.*, 20: 408–434.

Murray, M. (1966) Degeneration of some intralaminar thalamic nuclei after cortical removals in the cat. *J. comp. Neurol.*, 127: 344–368.

Nagy, J. I., Lee, T., Seeman, P. and Fibiger, H. C. (1978) Direct evidence for presynaptic and postsynaptic dopamine receptors in brain. *Nature (Lond.)*, 274: 278–281.

Namba, M. von (1957) Cytoarchitektonische Untersuchungen am Striatum. *J. Hirnforsch.*, 13: 181–201.

Nauta, H. J. W. (1974) Evidence of a pallidohabenular pathway in the cat. *J. comp. Neurol.*, 156: 19–28.

Nauta, H. J. W. and Cole, M. (1974) Efferent projections of the subthalamic nucleus. *Trans Amer. neurol. Ass.*, 99: 170–173.

Nauta, H. J. W. and Cole, M. (1978) Efferent projections of the subthalamic nucleus: an autoradiographic study in the monkey and cat. *J. comp. Neurol.*, 180: 1–16.

Nauta, W. J. H. (1960) Some neural pathways related to the limbic system. In *Electrical Studies on the Unanesthetized Brain,* E. R. Ramey and D. S. O'Doherty (Eds.), Hoeber (Harper), New York, pp. 1–16.

Nauta, W. J. H. and Domesick, V. B. (1978) Crossroads of limbic and striatal circuitry: hypothalamo-nigral connections. In *Limbic Mechanisms,* K. E. 'Livingston and O. Hornykiewicz (Eds.), Plenum Press, London, pp. 75–93.

Naura, W. J. H. and Mehler, W. R. (1966) Projections of the lentiform nucleus in the monkey. *Brain Res.*, 1: 3–42.

Nauta, W. J. H. and Whitlock, D. G. (1954) An anatomical analysis of the non-specific thalamic projection system. In *Brain Mechanisms and Consciousness,* J. F. Delafresnaye (Ed.), Thomas, Springfield, Ill., pp. 81–116.

Nauta, W. J. H., Smith, G. P., Faull, R. L. M. and Domesick, V. B. (1978) Efferent connections and nigral afferents of the nucleus accumbens septi in the rat. *Neuroscience,* 3: 385–401.

Nieoullon, A., Cheramy, A. and Glowinski, J. (1977) Release of dopamine in vivo from cat substantia nigra. *Nature (Lond.)*, 266: 375–377.

Nobin, A. and Björklund, A. (1973) Topography of the monoamine neuron systems in the human brain as revealed in fetuses. *Acta physiol. scand.*, 88 (Suppl. 388): 1–40.

Obata, K. and Yoshida, M. (1973) Caudate-evoked inhibition and actions of GABA and other substances on cat pallidal neurons. *Brain Res.*, 64: 455–459.

Olson, L., Seiger, Å and Fuxe, K. (1972) Heterogeneity of striatal and limbic dopamine innervation: highly fluorescent islands in developing and adult rats. *Brain Res.*, 44: 283–288.

Olszewski, J. and Baxter, D. (1954) *Cytoarchitecture of the Human Brain Stem.* Lippincott, Philadelphia, Pa.

Palkovits, M. and Jacobowitz, D. M. (1974) Topographic atlas of catecholamine and acetylcholinesterase-containing neurons in the rat brain. II. Hindbrain (mesencephalon, rhombencephalon). *J. comp. Neurol.*, 157: 29–42.

Papez, J. W. (1929) *Comparative Neurology*. Thomas Y. Crowell, New York.

Papez, J. W. (1941) A summary of fiber connections of the basal ganglia with each other and with other portions of the brain. In *The Diseases of the Basal Ganglia,* T. J. Putnam, A. M. Frantz and S. W. Ranson (Eds.), Williams and Wilkins, Baltimore, Md., pp. 21–68.

Parent, A. and Poirier, L. J. (1969) The medial forebrain bundle (MFB) and ascending monoaminergic pathways in the cat. *Canad. J. Physiol. Pharmacol.,* 47: 781–785.

Pasik, P., Pasik, T. and DiFiglia, M. (1976) Quantitative aspects of neuronal organization in the neostriatum of the Macaque monkey. In *The Basal Ganglia,* M. D. Yahr (Ed.), Raven Press, New York, pp. 57–90.

Pert, C. B., Kuhar, M. J. and Snyder, S. H. (1976) Opiate receptor: autoradiographic localization in rat brain. *Proc. nat. Acad. Sci. (Wash.),* 73: 3729–3733.

Petras, J. M. (1969) Some efferent connections of the motor and somatosensory cortex of simian primates and felid, canid and procyonid carnivores. *Ann. N.Y. Acad. Sci.,* 167: 469–505.

Poirier, L. J. (1960) Experimental and histological study of midbrain dyskinesia. *J. Neurophysiol.,* 23: 534–551.

Powell, E. W. and Leman, R. B. (1976) Connections of the nucleus accumbens. *Brain Res.,* 105: 389–403.

Powell, T. P. S. and Cowan, W. M. (1956) A study of thalamo-striate relations in the monkey. *Brain,* 79: 364–390.

Powell, T. P. S. and Cowan, W. M. (1967) The interpretation of the degenerative changes in the intralaminar nuclei of the thalamus. *J. Neurol. Neurosurg. Psychiat.,* 30: 140–153.

Rafols, J. A. and Fox, C. A. (1971/72) Further observations on the spiny neurons and synaptic endings in the striatum of the monkey *(Saimiri sciureus). J. Hirnforsch.,* 13: 299–308.

Rafols, J. A. and Fox, C. A. (1976) The neurons in the primate subthalamic nucleus: a Golgi and electron microscope study. *J. comp. Neurol.,* 168: 75–112.

Raisman, G., Cowan, W. M. and Powell, T. P. S. (1966) An experimental analysis of the efferent projection of the hippocampus. *Brain,* 89: 83–108.

Ranson, S. W. and Ranson, Jr., S. W. (1942) Efferent fibers of the corpus striatum. In *The Diseases of the Basal Ganglia,* T. J. Putnam, A. M. Frantz and S. W. Ranson (Eds.), Williams and Wilkins, Baltimore, Md., pp. 69–76.

Ranson, S. W., Ranson, Jr., S. W. and Ranson, M. (1941) Fiber connections of the corpus striatum as seen in Marchi preparations. *Arch. Neurol. Psychiat. (Chic.),* 46: 230–249.

Reubi, J.-C., Iversen, L. L. and Jessell, T. M. (1977) Dopamine selectively increases ^{3}H-GABA release from slices of rat substantia nigra in vivo. *Nature (Lond.),* 268: 652–654.

Rinvik, E. (1975) Demonstration of nigrothalamic connections in the cat by retrograde transport of horseradish peroxidase. *Brain Res.,* 90: 313–318.

Rinvik, E. and Grofová, I. (1970) Observations on the fine structure of the substantia nigra in the cat. *Exp. Brain Res.,* 11: 229–248.

Rinvik, E. and Walberg, F. (1969) Is there a cortico-nigral tract? A comment based on experimental electron microscopic observations in the cat. *Brain Res.,* 14: 742–744.

Rinvik, E., Grofová, I. and Ottersen, O. P. (1976) Demonstration of nigrotectal and nigroreticular projections in the cat by axonal transport of proteins. *Brain Res.,* 112: 388–394.

Rioch, D. M. (1929) Studies on the diencephalon of carnivora. Part II. Certain nuclear configurations and fiber connections of the subthalamus and midbrain of the dog and cat. *J. comp. Neurol.,* 49: 121–153.

Royce, G. J. (1978) Autoradiographic evidence for a discontinuous projection to the caudate nucleus from the centromedian nucleus in the cat. *Brain Res.,* 146: 145–150.

Schwyn, R. C. and Fox, C. A. (1974) The primate substantia nigra: a Golgi and electron microscopic study. *J. Hirnforsch.,* 15: 95–126.

Scollo-Lavizzari, G. and Akert, K. (1963) Cortical area 8 and its thalamic projection in *Macaca mulatta. J. comp. Neurol.,* 121: 259–269.

Siggins, G. R. (1978) Electrophysiological role of dopamine in striatum: excitatory or inhibitory? In *Psychopharmacology: a Generation of Progress,* M. A. Lipton, A. DiMascio and K. F. Killam (Eds.), Raven Press, New York, pp. 143–158.

Swanson, L. W. (1976) An autoradiographic study of the efferent connections of the preoptic region in the rat. *J. comp. Neurol.,* 167: 227–256.

Swanson, L. W. and Cowan, W. M. (1975) A note on the connections and development of the nucleus accumbens. *Brain Res.,* 92: 324–330.

Szabo, J. (1962) Topical distribution of the striatal efferents in the monkey. *Exp. Neurol.,* 5: 21–36.

Szabo, J. (1967) The efferent projections of the putamen in the monkey. *Exp. Neurol.,* 19: 463–476.

Szabo, J. (1970) Projections from the body of the caudate nucleus in the rhesus monkey. *Exp. Neurol.,* 27: 1–15.

Tennyson, V. M. (1975) Fluorescence and electron microscope studies of the caudate nucleus following chronic isolation. In *Local Circuit Neurons, Report of NRP Work Session, June 7–9, 1973,* P. Rakic (Ed.), *Neurosci. Res. Progr. Bull.,* 13: 381–385.

Tennyson, V. M., Barrett, R. E., Cohen, G., Côté, L., Heikkila, R. and Mytilineou, C. (1972) The developing neostriatum of the rabbit: correlation of fluorescence histochemistry, electron microscopy, endogenous dopamine levels, and [^{3}H]dopamine uptake. *Brain Res.,* 46: 251–285.

Tennyson, V. M., Heikkila, R., Mytilineou, C., Côté, L. and Cohen, G. (1974) 5-Hydroxydopamine "tagged" neuronal boutons in rabbit neostriatum: interrelationship between vesicles and axonal membrane. *Brain Res.,* 82: 341–348.

Thierry, A. M., Blanc, G., Sobel, A., Stinus, L. and Glowinski, J. (1973) Dopaminergic terminals in the rat cortex. *Science,* 182: 499–501.

Tittler, M., Weinreich, P. and Seeman, P. (1977) New detection of brain dopamine receptors with [^{3}H]dihydroergocryptine. *Proc. nat. Acad. Sci. (Wash.),* 74: 3750–3753.

Troiano, R. and Siegal, A. (1978) Efferent connections of the basal forebrain in the cat: the nucleus accumbens. *Exp. Neurol.,* 61: 185–197.

Tsai, C. (1925) The optic tracts and centers of the opossum, *Didelphys virginiana. J. comp. Neurol.,* 39: 173–216.

Ungerstedt, U. (1971) Stereotaxic mapping of the monoamine pathways in the rat brain. *Acta physiol. scand.,* 197 (Suppl. 367): 1–48.

Vogt, C. und Vogt, O. (1920) Zur Lehre der Erkrankungen des striären Systems. *J. Psychol. Neurol. (Lpz.),* 25: 627–846.

Vogt, C. und Vogt, O. (1941) Thalamusstudien I–III. I. Zur Einführung. II. Homogenität und Grenzgestaltung der Grisea des Thalamus. III. Das Griseum centrale (centrum medianum Luys). *J. Psychol. Neurol. (Lpz.),* 50: 31–154.

Voneida, T. J. (1960) An experimental study of the course and destination of fibers arising in the head of the caudate nucleus in the cat and monkey. *J. comp. Neurol.,* 115: 75–87.

Webster, K. E. (1961) Cortico-striate interrelations in the albino rat. *J. Anat. (Lond.),* 95: 532–545.

Webster, K. E. (1965) The cortico-striatal projection in the cat. *J. Anat. (Lond.),* 99: 329–337.

Wilson, S. A. K. (1912) Progressive lenticular degeneration: a familial nervous disease associated with cirrhosis of the liver. *Brain,* 34: 295–509.

Wilson, S. A. K. (1914) An experimental research into the anatomy and physiology of the corpus striatum. *Brain,* 36: 427–492.

Woolsey, T. A. and Van der Loos, H. (1970) The structural organization of layer IV in the somatosensory region (SI) of mouse cerebral cortex. *Brain Res.,* 17; 205–242.

Yeterian, E. H. (1978) Widespread cortico-striate projections from the temporal lobe in the rhesus monkey. *Anat. Rec.,* 190: 589.

Yeterian, E. H. and Van Hoesen, G. W. (1978) Cortico-striate projections in the rhesus monkey: the organization of certain cortico-caudate connections. *Brain Res.,* 139: 43–63.

Yoshida, M., Rabin, A. and Anderson, M. (1974) Monosynaptic inhibition of pallidal neurons by axon collaterals of caudato-nigral fibers. *Exp. Brain Res.,* 15: 333–347.

Biochemical Interactions in the Basal Ganglia

P. L. McGEER, E. G. McGEER and T. HATTORI

Kinsmen Laboratory of Neurological Research, Department of Psychiatry, University of British Columbia, Vancouver, B.C. V6T 1W5 (Canada)

INTRODUCTION

So far, 8 distinct biochemical neuronal types have been identified in the extrapyramidal system. They are dopamine, noradrenaline, serotonin, GABA, acetylcholine, glutamate, substance P and enkephalin containing neurons. They all serve major systems within the basal ganglia. However, they do not account for all of the neuronal pathways described in the previous chapter by Graybiel. Major neurotransmitters remain to be identified.

It is convenient to think of the pathways serving the basal ganglia as composed of input, processing and output pathways. Most of those which have been biochemically identified are illustrated in Fig. 1, along with some of their suggested interconnections.

The massive projection from the neocortex to the neostriatum is at least partly a glutamate pathway. Three known pathways form the input from the midbrain to the neostriatum. The major one is the well known nigrostriatal dopaminergic tract. The second is the serotonergic tract which comes mainly from the dorsal raphe. A third, minor input, is noradrenergic from the locus coeruleus and possibly other noradrenergic cell groups. A second, chemically unidentified, nigrostriatal tract has been suggested from physiological and axonal transport data. The transmitter for the final major input, which comes from the thalamus, is unknown but is presumed on physiological grounds to be excitatory.

Within the neostriatum, more than half of the neurons are interneurons. Many are cholinergic and some are GABAnergic. Other interneuronal types may exist as well. Some, for example, may contain angiotensin II.

The principal output pathways from the neostriatum are to the globus pallidus and to the substantia nigra. The only type so far known to extend from the neostriatum to the globus pallidus is enkephalin, although some evidence supports a descending GABA pathway. At least two neuronal types serve the striatonigral pathway. From the more rostral aspects of the neostriatum, substance P cells descend. From the more caudal aspects, GABA neurons descend. The transmitter for one of the globus pallidus output pathways from the external globus pallidus to the subthalamic nucleus is thought to be GABA but it is not known what completes the circuit back to the internal globus pallidus (entopeduncular nucleus). The transmitter for the major output from the internal globus pallidus to the thalamus is unknown. There are other pathways to the lateral habenula (which appears to be a GABA pathway) and to the pedunculopontine nucleus.

Output pathways from the pars reticulata of the substantia nigra go to the thalamus and the superior colliculi and probably consist, at least in part, of GABAnergic fibers.

The interconnections which have been suggested are the following (Fig. 1): ascending nigrostriatal dopaminergic neurons with cholinergic interneurons of the neostriatum; descending GABA neurons with dopaminergic neurons in the substantia nigra; and cortico-striatal glutamate neurons with a variety of neostriatal neuronal types including acetylcholine, GABA, substance P and enkephalin neurons.

The interactions of these neurons may extend beyond the classical concept of axodendritic movement of transmitters. There is evidence that dopamine is synthesized, stored and released from nigral dopaminergic dendrites to act on receptors on GABAnergic nerve endings. There is also evidence that acetylcholine is synthesized and stored in cholinergic neostriatal dendrites and is released to act at nicotinic sites on dopaminergic nerve endings. It is hypothesized, therefore, that reverse, or dendroaxonic, neurotransmission takes place in the extrapyramidal system in addition to the regular axodendritic transmission.

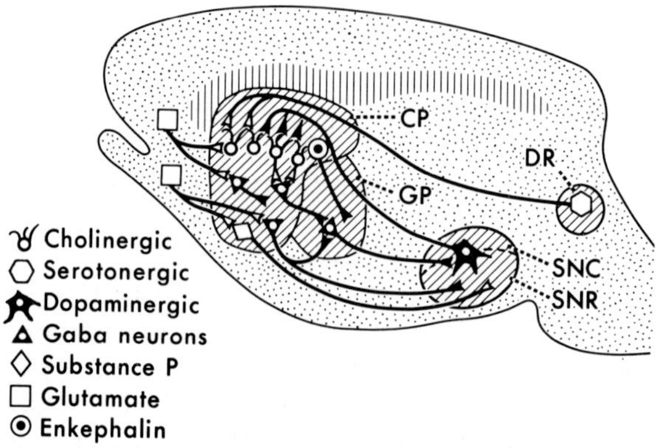

Fig. 1. Diagram indicating the transmitter attributed to many of the pathways of the extrapyramidal system. There is evidence for serotonergic innervation of the substantia nigra and a GABA nigrotectal tract which are not shown. CP = caudate-putamen; DR = dorsal raphe; GP = globus pallidus; SNC = zona compacta of the substantia nigra; SNR = zona reticulata of the substantia nigra.

(A) DETAILED DESCRIPTION OF BIOCHEMICAL PATHWAYS OF THE BASAL GANGLIA

(1) The nigrostriatal dopaminergic tract

This system is now one of the most widely studied pathways in the brain. The A9 cell group, which gives rise to it, is located in the zona compacta of the substantia nigra. The pathway was first described by Dahlström and Fuxe (1964) using the histofluorescent method for catecholamines developed by Falck and Torp (1961). The pathway has since been studied by using the glyoxalic acid method for catecholamines (Lindvall and Björklund, 1974); immunohistochemistry for tyrosine hydroxylase (TH) (Pickel et al., 1976); degeneration following lesions (Moore et al., 1971) and 6-OHDA administration (Maler et al., 1973); and anterograde axoplasmic flow with protein (Fibiger et al., 1972) and catecholamines (E. G. McGeer et al., 1975). The dendrites of the dopaminergic cells extend for a considerable distance into the zona reticulata of the substantia nigra (Björklund and Lindvall, 1975). By electron microscopy the cell bodies are seen to have a very prominent

Golgi apparatus and a nucleus with a smooth envelope. The axons are lightly myelinated and proceed rostrally in a prominent bundle that traverses the lateral hypothalamus just dorsolateral to the medial forebrain bundle. The dopaminergic nerve endings, verified by axoplasmic flow, contain mildly pleomorphic vesicles and make asymmetrical contact with dendritic spines of neostriatal neurons (Fig. 2A) (E.G. McGeer et al., 1975).

(2) The dorsal raphe-striatal pathway

The cells of origin of this pathway are primarily from the B9 cell group in the dorsal raphe described by Dahlström and Fuxe (1964). Some may also come from the B7 and B8 cell groups (Fuxe and Johnsson, 1974). The axons move rostrally in the medial forebrain bundle. Serotonergic innervation of the substantia nigra is also indicated by physiological and chemical evidence, and it has been suggested that this pathway branches to serve the substantia nigra.

Very little is known about the fine morphology of serotonin terminals. The best information about their detailed morphological nature comes from degeneration following specific serotonin toxins such as *p*-chloramphetamine and uptake studies of [^{3}H]serotonin in various brain areas. An electron micrograph of the type of nerve ending of the neostriatum labeled after the administration of [^{3}H]serotonin intraventricularly in rats is shown in Fig. 2B (Hattori et al., 1976a).

(3) The corticostriatal glutamate pathway

Neither histochemical nor immunohistochemical methods exist for identifying glutamate pathways in brain. Nor is there a really satisfying specific physiological antagonist. Consequently, glutamate remains a putative rather than a proven transmitter. Nevertheless, glutamate itself, when applied iontophoretically, acts like an ionotropic excitatory transmitter substance. An ionotropic transmitter acts by opening ionic gates, thus increasing the conductance of the postsynaptic membranes. (For a description of ionotropic and metabotropic transmitters, see P. L. McGeer et al., 1978.) Moreover, a high affinity uptake system, characteristic of neurotransmitter substances, exists for glutamate.

Lesioning of certain pathways in brain will cause a decrease in this high affinity glutamate uptake in the terminal fields. Among the most prominent of these pathways is the corticostriatal pathway. P. L. McGeer et al. (1977b) and Divac et al. (1977) have both lesioned this pathway and have found a drop of 40–50% in high affinity glutamate uptake in the synaptosomal fraction of the ipsilateral striatum. Since aspartate and glutamate seem to have identical high affinity uptake systems, this method is not capable of distinguishing between these two putative neurotransmitters. However, there is an approximately 6:1 ratio of glutamate over aspartate in the neostriatum, which strongly suggests the pathway is glutamatergic. Furthermore, lesioning of the corticostriatal pathway will produce a drop in glutamate levels in the striatum but not in other amino acids including aspartate (Kim et al., 1977).

Fig. 2C shows rat neostriatal terminals labeled by axoplasmic transport following the administration of [^{3}H]proline to the neocortex. Such terminals, which make asymmetric contacts and contain common round vesicles typical of excitatory synapses, are found to make preferential contacts with degenerating terminals following kainic acid administration (E.G. McGeer et al., 1979). Since degeneration following kainic acid administration relies upon glutamate receptors, this is a further indication that this type of nerve ending is a glutamate nerve ending.

(4) The noradrenergic input to the neostriatum

A minor noradrenergic input extends from the locus coeruleus, and possibly other noradrenergic cell groups, to the neostriatum (Lindvall and Björklund, 1978). Noradrenaline is present in only low concentration in the caudate-putamen but has a considerably higher concentration in the nucleus accumbens.

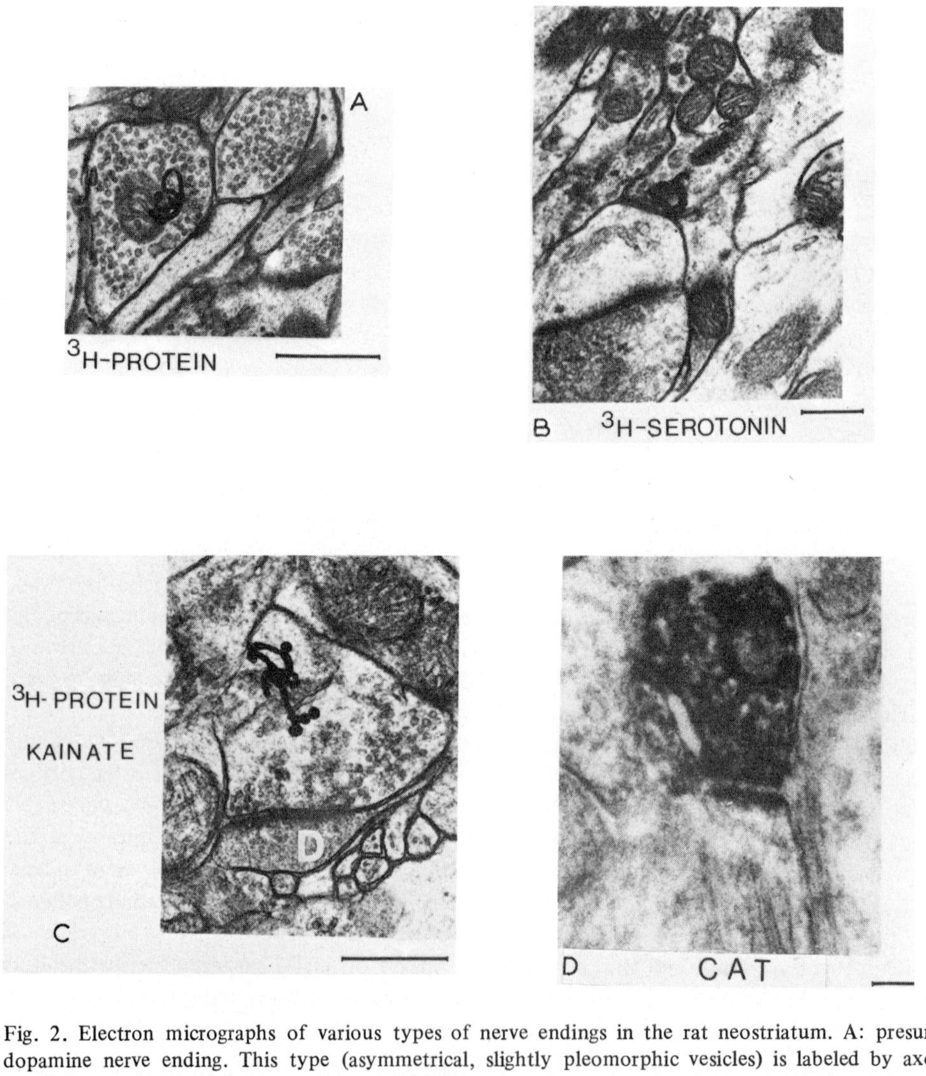

Fig. 2. Electron micrographs of various types of nerve endings in the rat neostriatum. A: presumed dopamine nerve ending. This type (asymmetrical, slightly pleomorphic vesicles) is labeled by axonal transport of [^{3}H]protein (shown) or noradrenaline from the substantia nigra or by degeneration with 6-OHDA. B: presumed serotonin nerve ending, synapses of this type (symmetrical, relatively few, highly pleomorphic vesicles of varying sizes) are preferentially labeled by intraventricularly injected [^{3}H]serotonin and degenerated by the action of *p*-chloramphetamine. C: presumed glutamate nerve ending labeled by [^{3}H]protein transported from the frontal cortex. This type (asymmetrical, closely packed, common round vesicles) is very similar to the type (D) which has been identified as cholinergic since it stains for choline acetyltransferase (CAT).

(5) Neostriatal cholinergic interneurons

Lesioning of all the known afferents to the neostriatum fails to bring about any major reduction in acetylcholine, choline acetyltransferase (CAT) or acetylcholinesterase (AChE) indicating that these inputs are not mainly responsible for the cholinergic activity of the neostriatum. Furthermore, lesioning the known efferents to the globus pallidus and substantia nigra also fails to bring about a reduction in cholinergic levels in either the neostriatum or target areas (P. L. McGeer et al., 1971). Immunohistochemistry for CAT indicates a large population of medium sized neurons staining for this synthetic enzyme. The probability that these are interneurons is consistent with the staining seen for CAT by electron microscopy where asymmetric nerve endings with common round vesicles are observed (Hattori et al., 1976b) (Fig. 2D).

(6) GABA interneurons

Evidence for GABA interneurons rests to date on the finding that lesioning of all of the known afferents and efferents of the neostriatum fails to bring about a reduction in glutamic acid decarboxylase (GAD), the synthetic enzyme for GABA. The reasoning is similar to that for cholinergic interneurons (McGeer and McGeer, 1975).

(7) Angiotensin-containing interneurons

Intrastriatal injections of kainic acid cause a marked loss of angiotensin converting enzyme (ACE) in the neostriatum of rats (Singh and McGeer, 1978) similar to the losses reported in Huntington's disease (Arregui et al., 1977). This enzyme converts angiotensin I to angiotensin II which has been proposed as a neurotransmitter. The losses in the neostriatum in Huntington's disease and the kainic acid "model" are consistent with, but not conclusive of, a neuronal localization. Since hemitransections and lesions of the thalamus and cortex do not affect ACE activity in the neostriatum (E. G. McGeer, unpublished observations), some ACE-containing neurons might be interneurons.

(8) Descending GABA pathways from the neostriatum and globus pallidus

The globus pallidus and substantia nigra contain the highest levels of GABA and GAD in brain (Fahn and Côté, 1968; Chalmers et al., 1970). Hemitransections between the globus pallidus and substantia nigra cause sharp drops in GAD in the substantia nigra (Kim, 1971; E.G. McGeer et al., 1973; Fonnum et al., 1974; Mroz et al., 1977; Jessell et al., 1978). Large lesions of the caudate-putamen will also cause a decrease in nigral GAD (Kim et al., 1971; Fonnum et al., 1974, 1978b). This suggests that descending GABA pathways extend from the globus pallidus and the caudal neostriatum to the substantia nigra. Elegant immunohistochemical staining for GAD has established the presence of many GAD nerve endings in the substantia nigra (Ribak et al., 1977a). Fonnum et al. (1978a) have also lesioned the globus pallidus in cats and found drops in GAD in the subthalamic nucleus. This indicates that the pallidosubthalamic tract is GABAnergic.

Kim et al. (1971) have suggested that the descending GABA pathway from the striatum to the nigra sends axonal branches into the pallidum. P. L. McGeer et al. (1974a) and Fonnum et al. (1978b) found that hemitransections between the neostriatum and globus pallidus led to drops in GAD in the globus pallidus. This suggests a descending GABA pathway extending from the neostriatum to the pallidus but further work is required to establish this pathway and its relationship to other descending striatal GABA pathways.

(9) The striatonigral substance P pathway

Following lesions to the striatonigral tract, sharp drops in substance P levels are found in the substantia nigra (Kanazawa et al., 1977b; Mroz et al., 1977). The substance P cell bodies are evidently located in the most rostral parts of the neostriatum because there is no difference in the degree of deficit of substance P in the substantia nigra as hemitransections are made more caudally in the neostriatum. Such is not the case for GAD levels, where the more caudal the hemitransection, the greater the drop in nigral GAD.

Further evidence of a descending substance P striatonigral tract comes from decreased nigral levels of substance P in Huntington's chorea, where neostriatal but not nigral cells are damaged (Kanazawa et al., 1977a). Similar losses of nigral substance P are found after injections of kainic acid in the caudate, particularly the anterior portion (Hong et al., 1977c). Cell bodies containing substance P have also been noted in the globus pallidus (Cuello and Kanazawa, 1978) and there appears to be a separate pallidonigral substance P containing pathway (Jessell et al., 1978).

(10) The neostriato-pallidal enkephalin tract

By far the highest levels of met-enkephalin in rat brain are found in the caudate nucleus and globus pallidus (10 and 76 ng/mg protein, respectively) (Hong et al., 1977b). The globus pallidus, for example, contains more than 10 times the concentration of met-enkephalin of the hypothalamus and 100 times that of the cerebellum. At least 5 groups have utilized immunohistochemistry for visualization of enkephalins at the cellular level (Elde et al., 1976; Bloom et al., 1977; Sar et al., 1977; Simantov et al., 1977; Watson et al., 1977). Most of the immunohistochemical staining in the globus pallidus appears to be in nerve endings from cell bodies located in the caudate-putamen (Watson et al., 1977). This is consistent with the finding of decreased enkephalin levels in the globus pallidus following caudate lesions (Hong et al., 1977a). Considering the much higher levels of enkephalin which exist in the basal ganglia as compared with other areas of brain, it might be anticipated that drugs which interact with the opiate receptor would have extremely prominent effects on motor performance. It remains a puzzle that this does not appear to be the case.

(11) The entopeduncular habenula tract

A significant pathway appears to extend from the entopeduncular nucleus (internal globus pallidus in primates) to the lateral habenula (Nauta, 1974). Lesion studies would suggest this is a GABA pathway (P. L. McGeer et al., 1977a; Nagy et al., 1978).

(12) The nigro-tectal GABA tract

Lesions of the pars reticulata cause a 40% drop in GAD in the ipsilateral superior colliculus with no change in CAT, or in the uptake of glycine or aspartate (Vincent et al., 1978). Furthermore, injections of [^{3}H]leucine into the nigra lead to rather specific labeling in the tectum of nerve endings identical in morphology to the Purkinje cell terminals in the deep cerebellar nuclei labeled by radioactive GABA transport (P. L. McGeer et al., 1975).

(B) BIOCHEMICAL INTERCONNECTIONS IN THE EXTRAPYRAMIDAL SYSTEM

One of the most significant interrelationships in the extrapyramidal system from a physiological point of view is the one between dopaminergic and cholinergic neurons.

Drugs which affect these neurons produce opposite reactions. Thus, dopaminergic and muscarinic agonists have contrasting effects, as do dopaminergic and muscarinic antagonists (P. L. McGeer et al., 1961). Dopaminergic agonists bring about an increase in striatal acetylcholine levels, while dopaminergic antagonists produce a reduction (P. L. McGeer et al., 1974b; Sethy and Van Woert, 1974). Thus, anatomical connections of the type shown in Fig. 3 had long been suspected. The technique for establishing the connection between these two neuronal systems was through the combined use of 6-hydroxydopamine (6-OHDA) administered intrathecally to cause degeneration of dopaminergic nerve endings and immunohistochemical staining to localize cholinergic neuronal processes.

Fig. 3 illustrates the interconnection. It shows degenerating dopaminergic nerve endings making contact with dendrites and dendritic spines of CAT containing cells in the neostriatum.

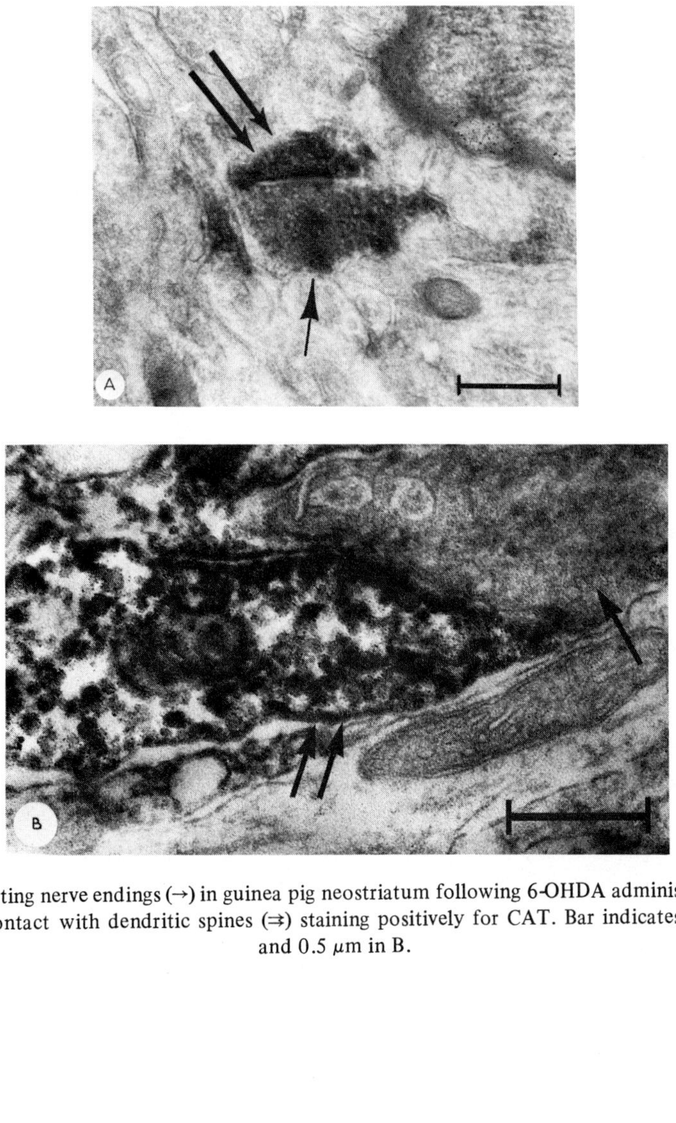

Fig. 3. Degenerating nerve endings (→) in guinea pig neostriatum following 6-OHDA administration making asymmetrical contact with dendritic spines (⇉) staining positively for CAT. Bar indicates 0.25 μm in A and 0.5 μm in B.

These electron micrographs provide positive proof of the direct relationship of dopaminergic and cholinergic structures in the basal ganglia (Hattori et al., 1976b). The implications of the dense dendritic staining for neurotransmitter synthetic enzymes will be discussed in a later section.

A similar direct connection has been demonstrated between descending GABA pathways from the pallidum, and to a lesser extent from the neostriatum, with dopaminergic dendrites in the substantia nigra. In these experiments, the cell bodies were made to degenerate by the same technique of intrathecal administration of 6-OHDA. Nerve endings of descending pathways to the nigra were identified by anterograde axoplasmic flow either of protein following the injection of [^{3}H]leucine into the neostriatum or pallidum (Hattori et al., 1975) or of [^{3}H]GABA injected into the pallidum (P. L. McGeer et al., 1974a). In the case of protein transport, the ratio of grains making contact with degenerating, as opposed to normal, dendrites in the substantia nigra was much higher following pallidal than caudate-putamen injections. Thus, pallidal afferents are much more likely to make contact with dopaminergic dendrites than are neostriatal afferents. This relationship is shown in Fig. 4 where a labeled protein molecule transported from the pallidum is shown in a nerve ending on a dopaminergic dendrite degenerating after 6-OHDA treatment.

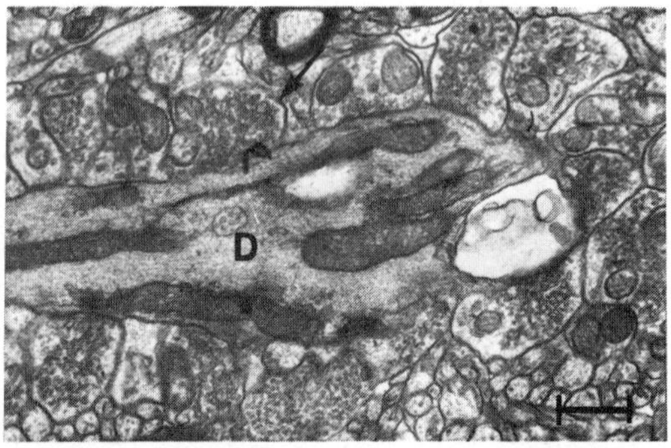

Fig. 4. Labeled bouton (→) synapsing with degenerating dendrite (D) in the substantia nigra following intrathecal 6-OHDA administration and injection of [^{3}H]leucine into the globus pallidus. Bar = 0.5 μm.

There are presumed glutamate interconnections with striatal acetylcholine, GABA, substance P and enkephalin neurons. Kainic acid is one of a series of glutamate analogs that has powerful excitatory actions on central neurons. When kainic acid is injected locally into various areas of brain, acute necrotizing lesions, involving initially dendritic structures, can be observed within 1–3 hr of administration. Olney (1978) has proposed the term "excitotoxin" to describe the action of kainic acid and has offered as an hypothesis of its neuronal toxicity the concept that persistent depolarization due to overexcitation of glutamate receptors is responsible for neuronal death. A problem with this simple excitotoxic hypothesis is the fact that an intact glutamate pathway seems to be required for kainic acid to exert its maximum neurotoxic effect. Striatal injections of kainic acid will cause degeneration of all neuronal elements in the striatum (while sparing nerve endings and axons of passage). However, it has been found that when the corticostriatal pathway, which is apparently a glutamate pathway, is sectioned, the neurotoxicity of kainic acid is reduced by about two orders of magnitude (Biziere and Coyle, 1978; E.G. McGeer et al., 1978). As a result of these experiments, modified hypotheses have been put forward as to the mechanism of kainic acid neurotoxicity. One possibility is that kainic acid excites extrajunctional glutamate receptors and the synergistic effects of excitatory glutamate input lead to persistent depolarization and death of postsynaptic cells (McGeer and McGeer, 1979).

If kainic acid is injected into the striatum in animals with an intact corticostriatal tract, there is a severe loss of GABA, acetylcholine, substance P and enkephalin containing neurons. These losses duplicate the biochemical findings found in the inherited neurological disease, Huntington's chorea (Coyle et al., 1978). In both kainic acid injected animals and Huntington's disease, the myelinated axons of the internal capsule and the nigrostriatal dopaminergic system are relatively preserved. GABA levels, GAD and substance P are all decreased in the substantia nigra, indicative of the loss of descending pathways. The apparent requirement of glutamate input for the neurotoxicity of kainic acid to be exerted therefore suggests the possibility that glutamate nerve endings may contact all of the neuronal types so far identified in the striatum.

(C) EVIDENCE FOR DENDRO-AXONIC TRANSMISSION IN THE EXTRAPYRAMIDAL SYSTEM

One of the most firmly held tenets in all of neuroscience is that neuronal action is unidirectional. Within the neuron, electrical impulses travel from dendrites to somata to axons. Across the synapse, neurotransmitters are chemical transducers carrying the message from axonal tips to dendrites or soma to influence postsynaptic electrical activity. The possibility that there could be reverse neurotransmission, with molecules being released from dendrites to affect axonal endings has not so far been seriously considered. Histochemical or immunohistochemical methods for most of the neurotransmitters described in this chapter have demonstrated that the neurotransmitters and their synthetic enzymes are concentrated in dendrites as well as axonal tips. For example, histofluorescent localization of serotonin and the catecholamines show them to occur in dendrites extending a considerable distance from the neuronal perikarya (Dahlström and Fuxe, 1964; Björklund and Lindvall, 1975). Similarly, immunohistochemical localizations for the synthetic enzymes TH (Pickel et al., 1975, 1976), dopa decarboxylase (Goldstein et al., 1972), tryptophan hydroxylase (Pickel et al., 1976), and CAT (Hattori et al., 1976b) show that these enzymes all exist in dendrites. The same holds true for GAD under special circumstances where axonal transport has been inhibited (Ribak et al., 1977b).

If the presence of these neurotransmitters in dendrites is for the purpose of reverse neurotransmission, then it should be possible to demonstrate a storage apparatus for the synthesized neurotransmitters, their release upon stimulation, the presence of receptors for them on axonal endings, and evidence of physiological action at the presynaptic site.

The nigrostriatal dopaminergic system can be used as a model to test this hypothesis. Information is available regarding interconnections of this system and methods exist for damaging these interconnections selectively. The concentration of receptor sites can be measured under various circumstances, thus yielding information regarding the pre- and postsynaptic localization.

(1) Interaction between dopaminergic dendrites and GABA nerve endings

As already described, the dendrites of dopaminergic cells of the substantia nigra prominently contain dopamine (Björklund and Lindvall, 1975) and TH (Pickel et al., 1976).

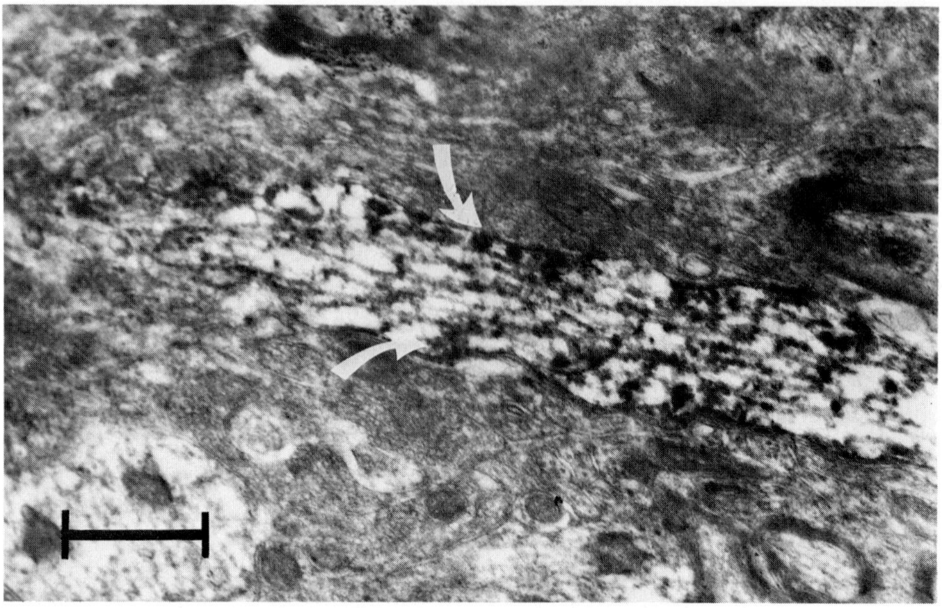

Fig. 5. Cross-section of rat substantia nigra dendrite stained heavily (1/20 dilution of serum) for tyrosine hydroxylase. Note association of stain with microtubules and postsynaptic surface (arrows). Bar = 0.5 μm.

More precise details of this localization are shown in the electron micrographs of Figs. 5 and 6.

Fig. 5 is an electron micrograph prepared using the immunohistochemical technique for TH (Pickel et al., 1976). Microtubules stained for TH can be seen in such pictures and these microtubules are sometimes observed to approach or to contact the surface of the dendrite at the point of a postsynaptic thickening.

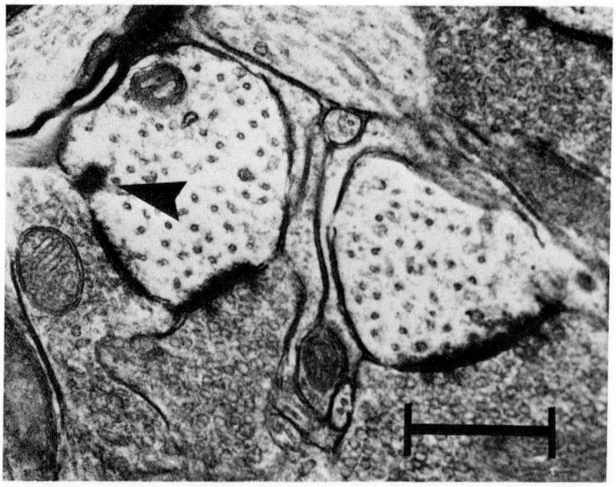

Fig. 6. Cross-section of rat substantia nigra dendrite showing large dense-core vesicle (arrow) apparently attached to postsynaptic surface following administration of 5-OHDA. Bar = 0.5 μm.

Fig. 6 shows the storage apparatus for dopamine in dendrites. 5-Hydroxydopamine (5-OHDA) is an agent which has been used successfully to identify binding sites of catecholamines (Tranzer and Thoenen, 1967). Following the intraventricular administration of this material, the smooth endoplasmic reticulum, as well as large vesicles, can be seen to contain electron-dense material. Thus, in dopaminergic dendrites of the substantia nigra, the synthetic apparatus seems to be primarily associated with microtubules and the storage apparatus with smooth endoplasmic reticulum. Both organelles approach or make contact with the dendritic or supposedly postsynaptic surface. What evidence exists for the release of the dendritic dopamine?

It has previously been reported that electrical stimulation of the medial forebrain bundle region in vivo leads to antidromic invasion of nigral cell bodies and the appearance of dopamine and its metabolites in the extracellular nigral fluid (Korf et al., 1976; Nieoullon et al., 1977). Stimulation of substantia nigra slices in vitro by a high potassium concentration also causes the appearance of dopamine and its metabolites in extracellular fluid. This evoked release is dependent on calcium and inhibited by magnesium, just as is the exocytotic release of vesicle-bound transmitter from presynaptic nerve endings (Geffen et al., 1976). Furthermore, dopamine is recaptured by dendrites through an active uptake process (Sotelo, 1971; Geffen et al., 1976) such as occurs in dopaminergic nerve endings. Thus, dopamine appears to be released upon stimulation and recaptured by dendrites in fashions comparable to those in nerve endings.

Does the released dopamine act on presynaptic receptor sites? In order to test this possibility, we measured the specific binding of the dopaminergic receptor binding agent [^{3}H]spiroperidol in the substantia nigra under two conditions. The first was following destruction of GABA and other afferent nerve endings from the striatum through the use of kainic acid. The second was following destruction of dopaminergic dendrites through the use of 6-OHDA. Differing amounts and combinations of the toxic agents were used so that dose-response relationships could be obtained.

The results are shown in Fig. 7. As the figure shows, there was a drop in spiroperidol binding following kainic acid administration in which the afferent input was decreased, but

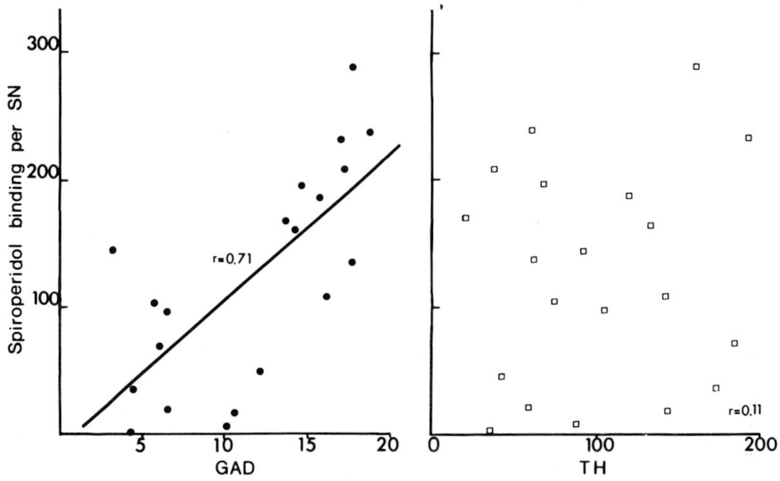

Fig. 7. Saturable [^{3}H]spiroperidol binding (counts/min/SN) in substantia nigra plotted against the average GAD and TH activities in the corresponding striata (2–3 SN combined for each point).

not following 6-OHDA where the dopaminergic dendrites were destroyed. TH and GAD measurements in the striatum were used as indices of the integrity of the dopaminergic and descending systems and the experiments do not demonstrate whether the binding is only to GABA neurons, to substance P neurons or to both.

It has been previously reported that dopamine sensitive adenylate cyclase activity in the substantia nigra disappears when brain lesions are performed which eliminate descending afferents from the neostriatum (Gale et al., 1977; Spano et al., 1977). Adenylate cyclase is believed to be the second messenger for dopamine. Thus, not only dopamine binding sites but the second messenger receptor system exists on striatal afferents to the substantia nigra. Dopamine added to nigral slices will promote the release of bound [^{3}H]GABA suggesting this may be the action of dendritically released dopamine (Reubi et al., 1977).

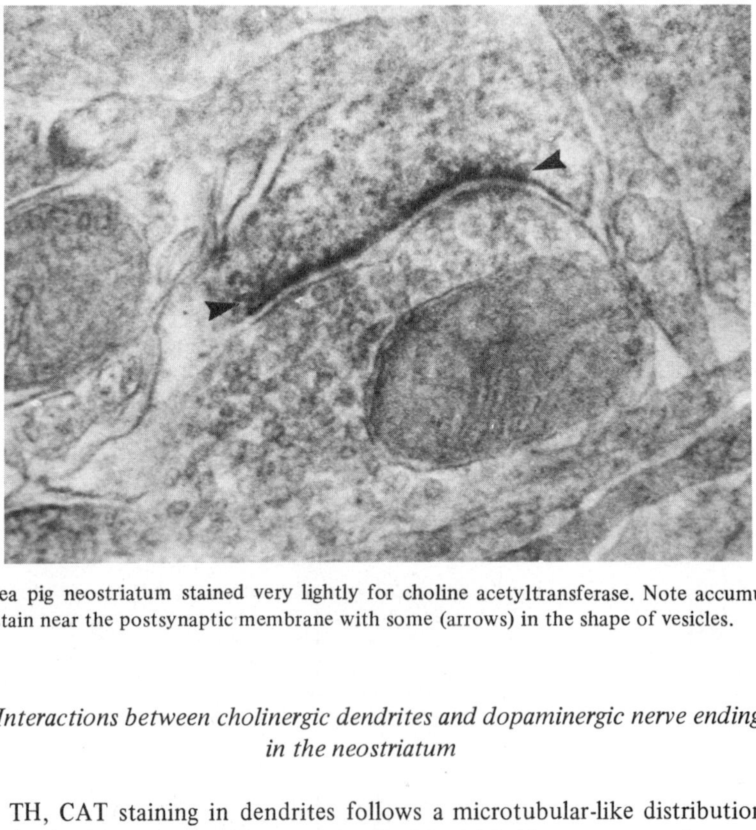

Fig. 8. Guinea pig neostriatum stained very lightly for choline acetyltransferase. Note accumulation of stain near the postsynaptic membrane with some (arrows) in the shape of vesicles.

(2) Interactions between cholinergic dendrites and dopaminergic nerve endings in the neostriatum

As with TH, CAT staining in dendrites follows a microtubular-like distribution but, in addition, at the dendritic spine level it is associated with vesicle-like structures of approximately the same size as presynaptic vesicles (Fig. 8). These positively stained vesicular structures are situated underneath the postsynaptic membrane of asymmetrical type synapses similar to the type shown in Fig. 3. The morphological basis thus exists for synthesizing acetylcholine in the dendritic spines which make contact with dopaminergic nerve endings.

We explored the possible location of acetylcholine receptor sites in the striatum by measuring the specific receptor binding of the muscarinic agent [^{3}H]QNB and of the nicotinic agent [^{125}I]α-bungarotoxin (α-BTX) under conditions which would selectively destroy pre- or postsynaptic sites. The presynaptic dopaminergic nerve endings were selectively destroyed by intrathecal administration of 6-OHDA. The postsynaptic sites were destroyed through

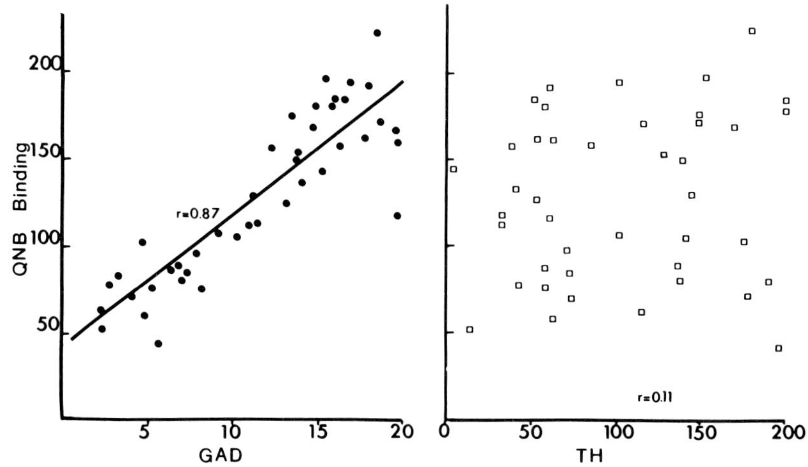

Fig. 9. [^{3}H]QNB binding (counts/min/20 μg protein) in rat neostriatum as a function of GAD (in μm/hr/100 mg protein) and TH (in nm/hr/100 mg protein) activities.

the use of intrastriatal kainic acid. TH was used as a measure of the integrity of dopaminergic nerve endings, and GAD and CAT were used as indices of the extent of kainic acid-induced neurotoxicity. Again, varying amounts and combinations of 6-OHDA and kainic acid were used so that dose-response relationships could be assessed.

The results are shown in Figs. 9 and 10. Fig. 9 shows the QNB binding versus residual GAD and TH activities in the neostriatum of rats. The figure demonstrates that there is no correlation between QNB binding and TH levels indicating that an appreciable population of muscarinic receptor sites probably does not exist on dopaminergic afferents to this structure. The figure indicates, however, a strong correlation between QNB binding and GAD levels, suggesting that most of the muscarinic binding sites are on neurons destroyed by the kainic acid injections.

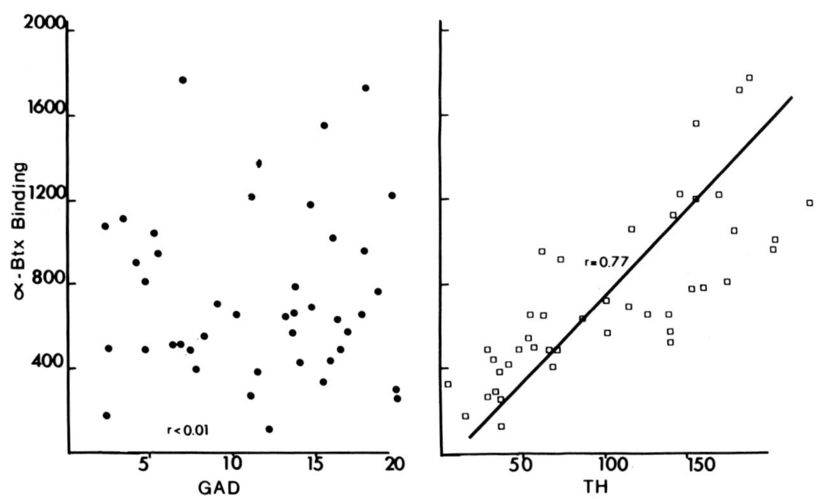

Fig. 10. Saturable [^{125}I]α-BTX binding (counts/min/2 mg protein) in rat neostriatum as a function of GAD and TH activities.

CAT levels dropped in parallel with GAD levels in these animals (correlation coefficient (r) 0.88). Thus, it is not possible to distinguish which neuronal population contains the muscarinic receptors.

The results with α-BTX on individual striata were quite different. Fig. 10 shows that there was a strong correlation between residual TH activity and binding whether or not the rats received kainic acid; there was no significant correlation with residual GAD (or CAT) activities.

There was no significant loss in α-BTX binding in the striatum after thalamic lesions but there seemed to be about a 15% loss after cortical lesions. Scatchard plots suggest that the reduction in α-BTX binding following 6-OHDA injections (or cortical lesions) was not due to a reduction in affinity but in the numbers of receptors. Thus, it would appear as if nicotinic cholinergic receptors exist on dopaminergic afferents to the striatum but not on postsynaptic neurons destroyed by kainic acid.

Is there any evidence suggesting a direct influence of acetylcholine on dopaminergic nerve endings in the striatum? In isolated striatal slices, it has been shown that acetylcholine increases the release of [^{3}H]dopamine previously synthesized from [^{3}H]tyrosine (Giorguieff et al., 1976, 1977) and that this is a nicotinic effect (De Belleroche and Bradford, 1978). Since the dopaminergic nerve endings are cut from their cell bodies in such slices, the data cannot be explained on the basis of interneuronal loops acting back on the substantia nigra. Nor can the data be explained on the basis of axo-axonic synapses since these have never been observed in the striatum. But they can be explained on the basis of dendritically released acetylcholine acting directly on dopaminergic nerve endings. The apparent association of α-BTX binding sites in the striatum with dopaminergic nerve endings is consistent with this explanation.

The quantities of α-BTX and spiroperidol that are bound in the striatum and substantia nigra respectively would suggest that far fewer receptor sites exist on nerve endings for dendritically released transmitters than on dendrites for axonally released transmitters. For example, the maximal amount of α-BTX bound in the striatum, presumably to presynaptic binding sites, was 16–24 fmoles/mg of protein. This may be compared to 600 fmoles/mg protein for QNB binding which is presumably to postsynaptic sites. Similarly, the maximal spiroperidol binding in the substantia nigra was approximately 20 fmoles/mg of protein while in the striatum it was roughly 400 fmoles. The 20–30-fold difference implies a bias in the direction of transmitter movement. Such a bias might account for the paucity of storage vesicles seen in dendrites as opposed to nerve endings. The numbers of molecules that would need to be released from the dendritic side in order to saturate the available receptors on axonal tips would be far fewer in number than those required to be released from nerve endings to saturate dendritic receptors.

ACKNOWLEDGMENT

This work was supported by grants from the Medical Research Council of Canada. We thank Dr. Menek Goldstein of New York University Medical Center for giving us the tyrosine hydroxylase antiserum.

REFERENCES

Arregui, A., Bennett, J. P. and Bird, E. D. (1977) Huntington's chorea: selective depletion of activity of angiotension converting enzyme in the corpus striatum. *Ann. Neurol.,* 2: 294–298.

Biziere, K. and Coyle, J. T. (1978) Influence of cortico-striatal afferents on striatal kainic acid neurotoxicity. *Neurosci. Lett.,* 8: 303–310.

Björklund, A. and Lindvall, O. (1975) Dopamine in dendrites of substantia nigra neurons: suggestions for a role in dendritic terminals. *Brain Res.,* 83: 531–537.

Bloom, F., Rossier, J., Battenberg, E., Vargo, T., Minik, S., Ling, N. and Guillemin, R. (1977) Regional distribution of β-endorphin and enkephalin in rat brain. *Neurosci. Abstr.,* 7: 907.

Chalmers, A., McGeer, E. G., Wickson, V. and McGeer, P. L. (1970) Distribution of glutamic acid decarboxylase in the brains of various mammalian species. *Comp. Gen. Pharmacol.,* 1: 385–390.

Coyle, J. T., McGeer, E. G., McGeer, P. L. and Schwarcz, R. (1978) Neostriatal injections: a model for Huntington's chorea. In *Kainic Acid as a Tool in Neurobiology,* E. G. McGeer, J. W. Olney and P. L. McGeer (Eds.), Raven Press, New York, pp. 139–160.

Cuello, A. C. and Kanazawa, I. (1978) The distribution of substance P immunoreactive fibers in the rat central nervous system. *J. comp. Neurol.,* 178: 129–156.

Dahlström, A. and Fuxe, K. (1964) Evidence for the existence of monoamine-containing neurons in the central nervous system. *Acta physiol. scand.,* 62 (Suppl. 232): 1–55.

De Belleroche, J. and Bradford, H. F. (1978) Biochemical evidence for the presence of presynaptic receptors on dopaminergic nerve terminals. *Brain Res.,* 142: 53–68.

Divac, I., Fonnum, F. and Storm-Mathisen, J. (1977) High affinity uptake of glutamate in terminals of cortico-striatal axons. *Nature (Lond.),* 266: 377–378.

Elde, R., Hökfelt, T., Johansson, O. and Terenius, L. (1976) Immunohistochemical studies using antibodies to leucine-enkephalin: initial observations on the nervous system of the rat. *Neuroscience,* 1: 349–355.

Fahn, S. and Côté, L. (1968) Regional distribution of γ-aminobutyric acid (GABA) in brain of rhesus monkey. *J. Neurochem.,* 15: 209–213.

Falck, B. and Torp, A. (1961) A fluorescence method for histochemical demonstration of noradrenaline in the adrenal medulla. *Med. Exp.,* 5: 428–432.

Fibiger, H. C., Pudritz, R. E., McGeer, P. L. and McGeer, E. G. (1972) Axonal transport in nigrostriatal and nigro-thalamic neurons: effects of medial forebrain bundle lesions and 6-hydroxydopamine. *J. Neurochem.,* 19: 1697–1708.

Fonnum, F., Grofová, I., Rinvik, E. and Storm-Mathisen, J. (1974) Origin and distribution of glutamate decarboxylase in the substantia nigra of the cat. *Brain Res.,* 71: 77–92.

Fonnum, F., Grofová, I. and Rinvik, E. (1978a) Origin and distribution of glutamic acid decarboxylase in the nucleus subthalamus of the cat. *Brain Res.,* 153: 370–375.

Fonnum, F., Gottesfeld, Z. and Grofová, I. (1978b) Distribution of glutamate decarboxylase, choline acetyltransferase and aromatic amino acid decarboxylase in the basal ganglia of normal and operated rats. Evidence for striatopallidal, striatoentopeduncular and striatonigral GABAergic fibers. *Brain Res.,* 143: 125–128.

Fuxe, K. and Johnsson, G. (1974) Further mapping of central 5-hydroxytryptamine neurons: studies with the neurotoxic dihydroxytryptamines. In *Advances in Biochemical Pharmacology, Vol. 10,* E. Costa, G. L. Gessa and M. Sandler (Eds.), Raven Press, New York, pp. 1–12.

Gale, K., Guidotti, A. and Costa, E. (1977) Dopamine sensitive adenylate cyclase location in substantia nigra. *Science,* 195: 503–505.

Geffen, L. B., Jessell, T. M., Cuello, A. C. and Iversen, L. L. (1976) Release of dopamine from dendrites in rat substantia nigra. *Nature (Lond.),* 260: 258–260.

Giorguieff, M. F., Le Floc'h, M. L., Westfall, T. C., Glowinski, J. and Besson, M. J. (1976) Nicotinic effect of acetylcholine on the release of newly synthesized [^{3}H]dopamine in rat striatal slices and cat caudate nucleus. *Brain Res.,* 106: 117–131.

Giorguieff, M. F., Le Floc'h, M. L., Glowinski, J. and Besson, M. J. (1977) Involvement of cholinergic presynaptic receptors of nicotinic and muscarinic types in the control of the spontaneous release of dopamine from striatal dopaminergic terminals in the rat. *J. Pharmacol. exp. Ther.,* 200: 535–544.

Goldstein, M., Fuxe, K. and Hökfelt, T. (1972) Characterization and tissue localization of catecholamine synthesizing enzymes. *Pharmacol. Rev.,* 24: 293–309.

Hattori, T., Fibiger, H. C. and McGeer, P. L. (1975) Demonstration of a pallidonigral projection innervating dopaminergic neurons. *J. comp. Neurol.*, 162: 487–504.

Hattori, T., McGeer, P. L. and McGeer, E. G. (1976a) Synaptic morphology in the neostriatum of the rat: possible serotonergic synapse. *Neurochem. Res.*, 1: 451–467.

Hattori, T., Singh, V. K., McGeer, E. G. and McGeer, P. L. (1976b) Immunohistochemical localization of choline acetyltransferase containing neostriatal neurons and their relationship with dopaminergic synapses. *Brain Res.*, 102: 164–173.

Hong, J. S., Yang, H.-Y. and Costa, E. (1977a) On the location of methionine enkephalin neurons in rat striatum. *Neuropharmacology*, 16: 451–453.

Hong, J. S., Yang, H.-Y., Fratta, W. and Costa, E. (1977b) Determination of methionine enkephalin in discrete regions of rat brain. *Brain Res.*, 134: 383–386.

Hong, J. S., Yang, H.-Y., Racagni, G. and Costa, E. (1977c) Projections of substance P containing neurons from neostriatum to substantia nigra. *Brain Res.*, 122: 541–544.

Jessell, T. M., Emson, P. C., Paxinos, G. and Cuello, A. C. (1978) Topographic projections of substance P and GABA pathways in the striato- and pallidonigral system. *Brain Res.*, 152: 487–498.

Kanazawa, I., Bird, E., O'Connell, R. and Powell, D. (1977a) Evidence for a decrease in substance P content of substantia nigra in Huntington's chorea. *Brain Res.*, 120: 387–392.

Kanazawa, I., Emson, P. C. and Cuello, A. C. (1977b) Evidence for the existence of substance P-containing fibers in striato-nigral and pallido-nigral pathways in rat brain. *Brain Res.*, 119: 447–453.

Kim, J. S., Bak, I. J., Hassler, R. and Okada, Y. (1971) Role of γ-aminobutyric acid (GABA) in the extrapyramidal motor system. *Exp. Brain Res.*, 14: 95–104.

Kim, J. S., Hassler, R., Haug, P. and Paik, K. S. (1977) Effect of frontal cortex ablation on striatal glutamic acid level in rat. *Brain Res.*, 132: 370–374.

Korf, J., Zieleman, M. and Westerink, B. H. C. (1976) Dopamine release in substantia nigra? *Nature (Lond.)*, 260: 257–258.

Lindvall, O. and Björklund, A. (1974) The organization of the ascending catecholamine neuron system in the rat brain. *Acta physiol. scand.*, 412 (Suppl.): 1–48.

Lindvall, O. and Björklund, A. (1978) Organization of catecholamine neurons in the rat CNS. In *Chemical Pathways in the Brain*, L. L. Iversen, S. D. Iversen and S. H. Snyder (Eds.), Plenum Press, New York, pp. 139–231.

Maler, L., Fibiger, H. C. and McGeer, P. L. (1973) Demonstration of the nigrostriatal projection by silver staining after nigral injections of 6-hydroxydopamine. *Exp. Neurol.*, 40: 505–515.

McGeer, E. G., Fibiger, H. C., McGeer, P. L. and Brooke, S. (1973) Temporal changes in amine synthesizing enzymes of rat extrapyramidal structures after hemitransections or 6-hydroxydopamine administration. *Brain Res.*, 52: 284–300.

McGeer, E. G., Hattori, T. and McGeer, P. L. (1975) Electron microscopic localization of labeled norepinephrine transported in nigro-striatal neurons. *Brain Res.*, 86: 478–482.

McGeer, E. G., McGeer, P. L. and Singh, K. (1978) Kainic acid-induced degeneration of neostriatal neurons: dependency upon cortico-striatal tract. *Brain Res.*, 139: 381–383.

McGeer, E. G., McGeer, P. L. and Hattori, T. (1979) Glutamate in the striatum. In *Biochemistry and Physiology of Glutamic Acid*, S. Garattini (Ed.), Raven Press, New York, pp. 187–201.

McGeer, P. L. and McGeer, E. G. (1975) Evidence for glutamic acid decarboxylase containing interneurons in the neostriatum. *Brain Res.*, 91: 331–335.

McGeer, P. L. and McGeer, E. G. (1979) Use of the neurotoxic agents kainic acid and tetanus toxin in the extrapyramidal system. In *Neurotoxins: Tools in Neurobiology*, B. Ceccarelli and F. Clementi (Eds.), Raven Press, New York, pp. 437–446.

McGeer, P. L., Boulding, J. C., Gibson, W. C. and Foulkes, R. G. (1961) Drug-induced extrapyramidal reactions. *J. Amer. med. Ass.*, 177: 665–670.

McGeer, P. L., McGeer, E. G., Fibiger, H. C. and Wickson, V. (1971) Neostriatal choline acetylase and acetylcholinesterase following selective brain lesions. *Brain Res.*, 35: 308–314.

McGeer, P. L., Fibiger, H. C., Maler, L., Hattori, T. and McGeer, E. G. (1974a) Evidence for descending pallido-nigral GABA-containing neurons. In *Advances in Neurology, Vol. 5*, F. H. McDowell and A. Barbeau (Eds.), Raven Press, New York, pp. 153–160.

McGeer, P. L., Grewaal, D. S. and McGeer, E. G. (1974b) Influence of noncholinergic drugs on rat striatal acetylcholine levels. *Brain Res.*, 80: 211–217.

McGeer, P. L., Hattori, T. and McGeer, E. G. (1975) Chemical and autoradiographic analysis of γ-aminobutyric acid transport in Purkinje cells of the cerebellum. *Exp. Neurol.*, 47: 26–41.

McGeer, P. L. McGeer, E. G. and Hattori, T. (1977a) Transmitters in the basal ganglia. In *Amino Acids as Chemical Transmitters*, F. Fonnum (Ed.), Raven Press, New York, pp. 123–142.

McGeer, P. L., McGeer, E. G., Scherer, U. and Singh, K. (1977b) A glutamatergic corticostriatal path? *Brain Res.*, 128: 369–373.

McGeer, P. L., Eccles, J. C. and McGeer, E. G. (1978) *Neurobiology of the Mammalian Brain.* Plenum Press, New York.

Moore, R. Y., Bhatnagar, R. K. and Heller, A. (1971) Anatomical and chemical studies of a nigro-neostriatal projection in the cat. *Brain Res.*, 30: 119–135.

Mroz, E., Brownstein, M. J. and Leeman, S. E. (1977) Evidence for substance P in the striato-nigral tract. *Brain Res.*, 125: 305–311.

Nagy, J. I., Carter, D. A., Lehmann, J. and Fibiger, H. C. (1978) Evidence for a GABA-containing projection from the entopeduncular nucleus to the lateral habenula in the rat. *Brain Res.*, 145: 360–364.

Nauta, W. J. H. (1974) Evidence of a pallidohabenula pathway in the cat. *J. comp. Neurol.*, 156: 19–28.

Nieoullon, A., Chéramy, A. and Glowinski, J. (1977) Release of dopamine in vivo from cat substantia nigra. *Nature (Lond.)*, 266: 375–377.

Olney, J. W. (1978) Neurotoxicity of excitatory amino acids. In *Kainic Acid as a Tool in Neurobiology*, E. G. McGeer, J. W. Olney and P. L. McGeer (Eds.), Raven Press, New York, pp. 95–122.

Pickel, V. M., Tong, H. J., Field, P. M., Becker, C. G. and Reis, D. J. (1975) Cellular localization of tyrosine hydroxylase by immunohistochemistry. *J. Histochem. Cytochem.*, 23: 1–12.

Pickel, V. M., Tong, H. J. and Reis, D. J. (1976) Monoamine synthesizing enzymes in central dopaminergic, noradrenergic and serotonergic neurons. *J. Histochem. Cytochem.*, 24: 792–806.

Reubi, J. C., Iversen, L. L. and Jessel, T. M. (1977) Dopamine selectively increases ^{3}H-GABA release from slices of rat substantia nigra in vitro. *Nature (Lond.)*, 268: 652–654.

Ribak, C. E., Vaughn, J. E., Saito, K., Barber, R. and Roberts, E. (1977a) Immunocytochemical localization of glutamate decarboxylase in rat substantia nigra. *Brain Res.*, 116: 287–298.

Ribak, C. E., Vaughn, J. E., Saito, K., Barber, R. and Roberts, E. (1977b) Glutamate decarboxylase localization in neurons of the olfactory bulb. *Brain Res.*, 126: 1–18.

Sar, M., Stumpf, W. B., Miller, R. J., Chang, K. J. and Cuatrecasas, P. (1977) Immunohistochemical localization of enkephalins in rat brain. *Neurosci. Abstr.*, 7: 966.

Sethy, V. H. and Van Woert, M. H. (1974) Modification of striatal acetylcholine concentration by dopamine receptor agonists and antagonists. *Res. Commun. Chem. Pathol. Pharmacol.*, 8: 13–28.

Simantov, R., Kuhar, M. J., Uhl, G. R. and Synder, S. H. (1977) Opioid peptide enkephalin: immunohistochemical mapping in rat central nervous system. *Proc. nat. Acad. Sci. (Wash.)*, 74: 2167–2171.

Singh, E. A. and McGeer, E. G. (1978) Angiotensin converting enzyme in kainic acid injected striata. *Ann. Neurol.*, 4: 85–95.

Sotelo, C. (1971) The fine structural localization of norepinephrine-^{3}H in the substantia nigra and area prostrema of the rat. An autoradiographic study. *J. ultrastruct. Res.*, 36: 824–841.

Spano, P. F., Trabucchi, M. and Di Chiara, G. (1977) Localization of nigral dopamine-sensitive adenylate cyclase on neurons originating from the corpus striatum. *Science*, 196: 1343–1345.

Tranzer, J. P. and Thoenen, H. (1967) Electron microscopic localization of 5-hydroxydopamine (3,4,5-trihydroxyphenylethylamine), a new false sympathetic transmitter. *Experientia (Basel)*, 23: 743–745.

Vincent, S. R., Hattori, T. and McGeer, E. G. (1978) The nigrotectal projection: a biochemical and ultrastructural characterization. *Brain Res.*, 151: 159–164.

Watson, S. J., Akil, H., Sullivan, S. and Barchas, J. D. (1977) Immunocytochemical localization of methionine enkephalin. *Life Sci.*, 21: 733–738.

Recent Advances in the Morphological Localization of γ-Aminobutyric Acid Receptors in the Cerebellum by Means of [^{3}H]Muscimol

VICTORIA CHAN-PALAY

Department of Neurobiology, Harvard Medical School, Boston, Mass. 02115 (U.S.A.)

INTRODUCTION

γ-Aminobutyric acid (GABA) is a major inhibitory neurotransmitter in the mammalian central nervous system, and deficits of GABA have been implicated in certain neurological and psychiatric disorders, such as Huntington's chorea, Parkinson's disease and schizophrenia. Considerable interest attaches to the identification of GABA-containing neurons and receptor sites for GABA. Although cells and processes with GABA-synthesizing enzymes and with GABA uptake systems have been identified morphologically (Hökfelt and Ljungdahl, 1970; McLaughlin et al., 1974; Barber and Saito, 1976; Ribak et al., 1976; Chan-Palay, 1977), the receptor binding sites for GABA have been visualized only recently, in various parts of the central nervous system at the light and electron microscope level and also in cultures of the mammalian spinal cord (Chan-Palay, 1978a, b; Chan-Palay and Palay, 1978; Chan-Palay et al., 1978).

In the mammalian cerebellum, the cortical neurons that have been demonstrated to have immunoreactivity for antibody against glutamic acid decarboxylase (GAD), the GABA-synthesizing enzyme, are stellate cells, basket cells, Golgi cells, and Purkinje cells and their various dendritic and axonal processes. These neurons and some small neurons in the deep cerebellar nuclei have also been demonstrated to have uptake capacity for [^{3}H]GABA by autoradiography (reviewed in Chan-Palay, 1977). Fig. 1a indicates schematically the GABA-containing neurons (stipple) of the cerebellum. Granule cells, Lugaro cells, the large cerebellar nuclear neurons and other small nuclear neurons have not been demonstrated to be GABA-containing. GABA receptor sites have been localized by only one method so far. This approach is to manipulate the GABA system pharmacologically by using molecules structurally related to it that can specifically simulate the action of the transmitter. Muscimol (3-hydroxy-5-aminomethylisoxazole) is one of a group of compounds that have been reported to be GABA receptor agonists in the central nervous system (Krogsgaard-Larsen et al., 1975; Johnston et al., 1976; Enna et al., 1977; Krogsgaard-Larsen, 1978). It is a psychotomimetic compound isolated from the mushroom *Amanita muscaria* (Eugster, 1969) and is structurally analogous to GABA according to X-ray crystallography (Brehm et al., 1972); it appears to be a powerful GABA agonist at bicuculline-sensitive postsynaptic receptors (Curtis et al., 1971), weakly inhibits high-affinity uptake of GABA in brain slices, is not a substrate for GABA:2-oxoglutarate aminotransferase (Beart and Johnston, 1973), and has a dissociation constant of approximately 2 nM.

Studies comparing the binding of [^{3}H]muscimol ([^{3}H]M) with that of [^{3}H]GABA in rat brain homogenates indicate that the high-affinity binding characteristics of both substances are similar, although not identical. The regional distributions of [^{3}H]M receptor binding and [^{3}H]GABA uptake are comparable: cerebellum > cerebral cortex > hippocampus > corpus striatum > midbrain and hypothalamus > medulla and spinal cord (Enna et al., 1978). Furthermore, it has been indicated (Beaumont et al., 1978) that [^{3}H]M is displaced stereospecifically only by drugs or related amino acids known to interact with the synaptic GABA receptor and is unaffected by other agents that activate or inhibit other neurotransmitter receptors.

In the present situation, muscimol was used in its tritiated form as a histochemical marker for GABA receptor sites. Tritiated muscimol ([^{3}H]M) has a free amino group that enables the substance, when it is bound to receptor sites in tissue constituents, to be covalently linked by aldehyde fixation. Subsequent manipulations are then possible for autoradiographic visualization of the bound [^{3}H]M. At the light microscope level the quantitative analysis of resulting autoradiograms provides data on the distribution of [^{3}H]M binding sites in the cerebellum both in a laminar display across the layers of the cerebellar cortex and nuclei, and in a cellular manner. It is also imperative to know the subcellular locations of these [^{3}H]M binding sites and this ultrastructural definition can be provided by electron microscopic autoradiography.

The major questions to be addressed include whether or not GABA receptors are associated with (i) membranes of neuronal or neuroglial elements, (ii) synaptic sites, (iii) specific cellular types, or (iv) unusual non-synaptic relationships.

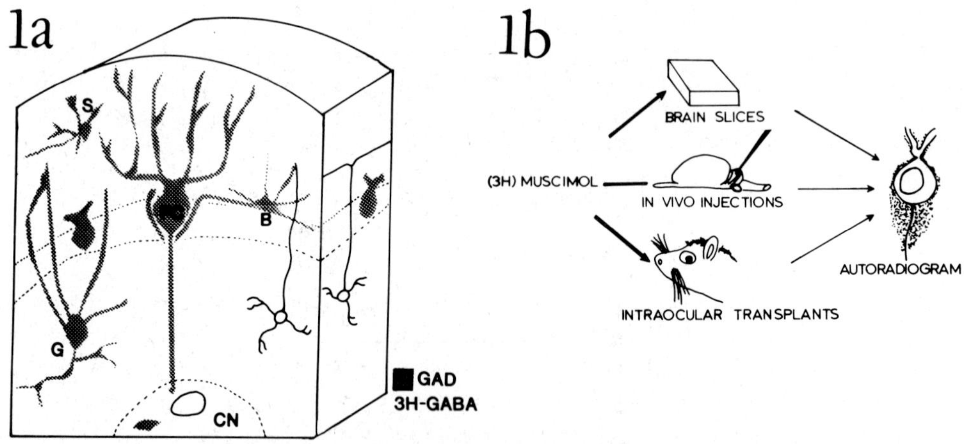

Fig. 1. a: the cerebellar cortical and nuclear neurons with GAD immunoreactivity and uptake capacities for [^{3}H]GABA are indicated by stippling. These are the stellate (S), basket (B), Purkinje cells (PC), Golgi cells (G) of the cortex and some small neurons in the deep cerebellar nuclei (CN). b: 3 experimental modes utilized for studies with [^{3}H]M autoradiography: brain slices, in vivo intracortical injections and intraocular transplants.

MATERIALS AND METHODS

All experiments were performed on tissues from adult 200 g rats (Sprague-Dawley, Charles River Laboratories). Three experimental procedures were used: brain slices, intracortical injections and intraocular transplants (see Fig. 1b).

Brain slices

Thin (0.5 mm) slices of freshly dissected cerebellar cortex and nuclei were individually incubated for 60 min in artificial cerebrospinal fluid (pH 7.3 at 20°C), maintained with 95% O_2/5% CO_2. The medium contained [^{3}H]M (New England Nuclear, Boston; custom synthesis, purity >98% by chromatography, specific activity 10.3 Ci/mmol) at a concentration of 2 nM. [^{3}H]M was checked for purity by silica gel thin-layer co-chromatography with unlabeled purified muscimol in butanol/glacial acetic acid/water (4:1:1) and detected with 5% (w/v) ferric chloride. The muscimol was labeled in the ring as indicated in the formula

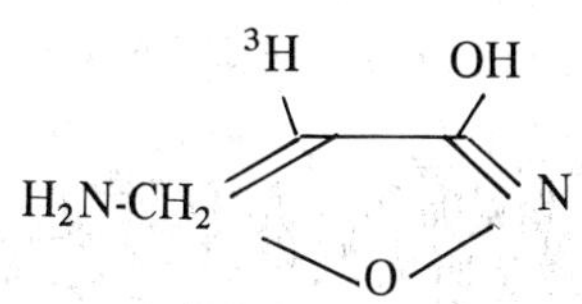

After incubation, the slices were fixed by immersion in aldehyde mixtures.

Intracerebellar injections

[^{3}H]M (at 2 nM) was injected, via glass capillary micropipettes with a tip diameter of 4 μm, into the cerebellum. Each injection was carefully placed to include the deep cerebellar nuclei and numerous cortical folia. After each penetration, a total of 1 μl was injected during the withdrawal of the micropipette. Five separate penetrations were made into each cerebellum. The stereotaxic locations of these tracks were recorded. Sixty minutes after the last injection, the animals were fixed by vascular perfusion through the heart with aldehyde mixtures, and the tissues were dissected carefully into sagittal slabs including the entire trajectories of the injections and processed for embedding in epoxy resin.

Intraocular transplants

Cerebellar *Anlagen* from 13 mm embryos were transplanted into the anterior chamber of the eyes of adult female rats and allowed to grow for 4 weeks prior to experimentation. Ten μl of [^{3}H]M (2 nM) were injected into the anterior chamber. One hour after the injection the animals were fixed by perfusion with aldehyde mixtures and the tissue was processed for embedding in epoxy resin.

Controls

(1) Nipecotic acid and guvacine as uptake inhibitors prior to administration of [^{3}H]M. (–)Nipecotic acid hydrate (Krogsgaard-Larsen and Johnston, 1975) or guvacine hydrobromide (Johnston et al., 1975), dissolved in artificial cerebrospinal fluid to a concentration of 10 μM, was used for a brief incubation (10 min) of slices of cerebellar cortex and cerebellar nuclei. After this, the tissues were incubated in [^{3}H]M for 60 min, as described above.

(2) Intravenous injections of unlabeled muscimol followed by incubation of brain slices in [^{3}H]M. Adult female 200 g rats were anesthetized by intraperitoneal injections of 35% chloral hydrate (0.1 ml/100 g of body weight) and given unlabeled muscimol by injection into the femoral vein (1 mg/100 g body weight in sterile saline). One hour later, thin slices of cerebellar cortex and nuclei were removed, incubated in [^{3}H]M for 60 min, and then fixed.

(3) Incubation of slices in unlabeled muscimol (10^{-5} M) for 15 min, followed by incubation in [^{3}H]M for 1 hr prior to fixation.

(4) Incubation of slices in GABA (10^{-5} M) for 15 min with or without aminooxyacetic acid (AOAA) followed by incubation in [^{3}H]M for 1 hr prior to fixation.

(5) Incubation of slices in THIP (isoxazole 16) or in isoguvacine, two GABA agonists (10^{-5} M), for 15 min followed by incubation in [^{3}H]M for 1 hr prior to fixation.

(6) Bicuculline (10^{-5} M) and picrotoxin (10^{-5} M) as GABA antagonists used in pretreatment of tissue slices prior to incubation with [^{3}H]M and then fixation.

Tissue preparation for high-resolution autoradiography

All tissues were fixed with 1% glutaraldehyde and 1% formaldehyde in phosphate buffer, pH 7.3. Tissue slices after incubation in [^{3}H]M were fixed by immersion for 1–18 hr. These tissues and those obtained by perfusion were postfixed in 2% osmium tetroxide in phosphate buffer, dehydrated, stained en bloc with uranyl acetate, and embedded in epoxy resin (Palay and Chan-Palay, 1974). Epoxy embedding was selected because of the better tissue preservation and the possibility of using this material for both light and electron microscope autoradiography. Autoradiograms for light microscopy were prepared from 1 to 2 μm thick sections of each tissue slice by using Kodak NTB-2 emulsion, exposure durations of 8–21 days, and development in D-19 (Chan-Palay, 1977). These sections were counterstained lightly with toluidine blue and observed with dark-field and bright-field optics.

Quantitation of silver grains in autoradiograms

Five separate regions taken from two specimen blocks from two animals were used for grain counts. Areas of the vermal cerebellar cortex containing all 3 cortical laminae, dentate nucleus and white matter, were selected, photographed and enlarged 2240-fold. A grid of 1 cm squares was laid over each field and every silver grain within every grid square was counted manually and recorded. Each square represented 20 μm^2 of cerebellum, and grains over a total of 2×10^7 μm^2 of tissue were counted. In all, the samples were selected to include: large and small cerebellar dentate nucleus neurons, neuroglial cells, and the neuropil; granular layer with numerous glomerular islets, granule cells, several Golgi cells and neuroglial cells; 14 Purkinje cells and several Golgi epithelial (neuroglial) cells; molecular layer containing the dendritic expansions of at least 3 Purkinje cells, 15 basket and stellate neurons and 10 neuroglial cells. From these data the cumulative grain count over horizontal strips of the cerebellar cortex and nuclei provided a quantification of the laminar distribution of silver grains. Separate counts of grains over individual neurons and neuroglial cells and over the basket around the initial segment of the Purkinje cell were also obtained in order to quantify binding of [^{3}H]M on specific cell types.

Quantitative electron microscope autoradiography

The animals were perfused with 1% (v/v) glutaraldehyde and 1% (w/v) formaldehyde in 0.12 M phosphate buffer, pH 7.4. The tissue slices containing the injected sites were postfixed in osmium tetroxide, stained en bloc, and embedded in epoxy resin (Palay and Chan-Palay, 1974). Autoradiograms at the light microscopic level provided the means to study large areas of entire folia of cerebellar cortex and nuclei (Chan-Palay, 1978a). For ultrastructural study, we selected certain areas that were well oriented in the sagittal plane and contained several Purkinje cell somata and dendritic fields, molecular layer, granular layer and regions of the dentate nucleus. Electron microscopic autoradiograms were prepared from 150 serial thin sections by using the parlodion-coated slide/film-stripping technique (Chan-Palay, 1975, 1977). The slides were coated with Ilford L4 emulsion (1:4) and exposures of up to 5 weeks were used. Phenidone was selected as the best developer (Lettré and Paweletz, 1966) after comparative trials with Microdol-X and physical developers (Chan-Palay, 1977). The phenidone grains were small, round, and well suited to the precise localization of [^{3}H]M radiation sources. The other major technical concern was to keep the background to a minimum by careful selection of exposure and development times in these procedures. All sections were examined in a Philips EM-300. Approximately 350 electron micrographs containing silver grains were obtained. The position of every grain in every micrograph was quantitatively analyzed with respect to its relationship to the nearest adjacent membrane. Because of the harsh procedures used in the preparation of these autoradiograms, it was difficult to study the cytoplasmic morphology of axons. The identification of other cellular elements was made on the basis of their location and structure and the known connections of the various cell types. The selectivity of the method and the paucity of silver grains developed (in order to reduce background) made it impossible to estimate the true density of GABA receptor sites by means of the number of silver grains. The ratio of grains to receptor site density is not 1:1; nevertheless, the presence of a silver grain indicates the presence of labeled receptors.

RESULTS

A differential distribution of [^{3}H]M binding was displayed in the cerebellar cortex and nuclei (Figs. 2 and 4); a laminar distribution with the highest density of autoradiographic signal around, but not including, the Purkinje cell somata and in basket and stellate neurons of the molecular layer. There was binding of [^{3}H]M throughout the cerebellar neuropil, highest in the molecular layer and in the granular layer, low in the cerebellar nuclei and insignificant over the white matter.

Examination of the autoradiograms in stained sections readily revealed the identity of the various structures labeled (Fig. 3). Counts of the silver grains over selected fields that sample the molecular, Purkinje cell and granular layers of the cortex, dentate nucleus and

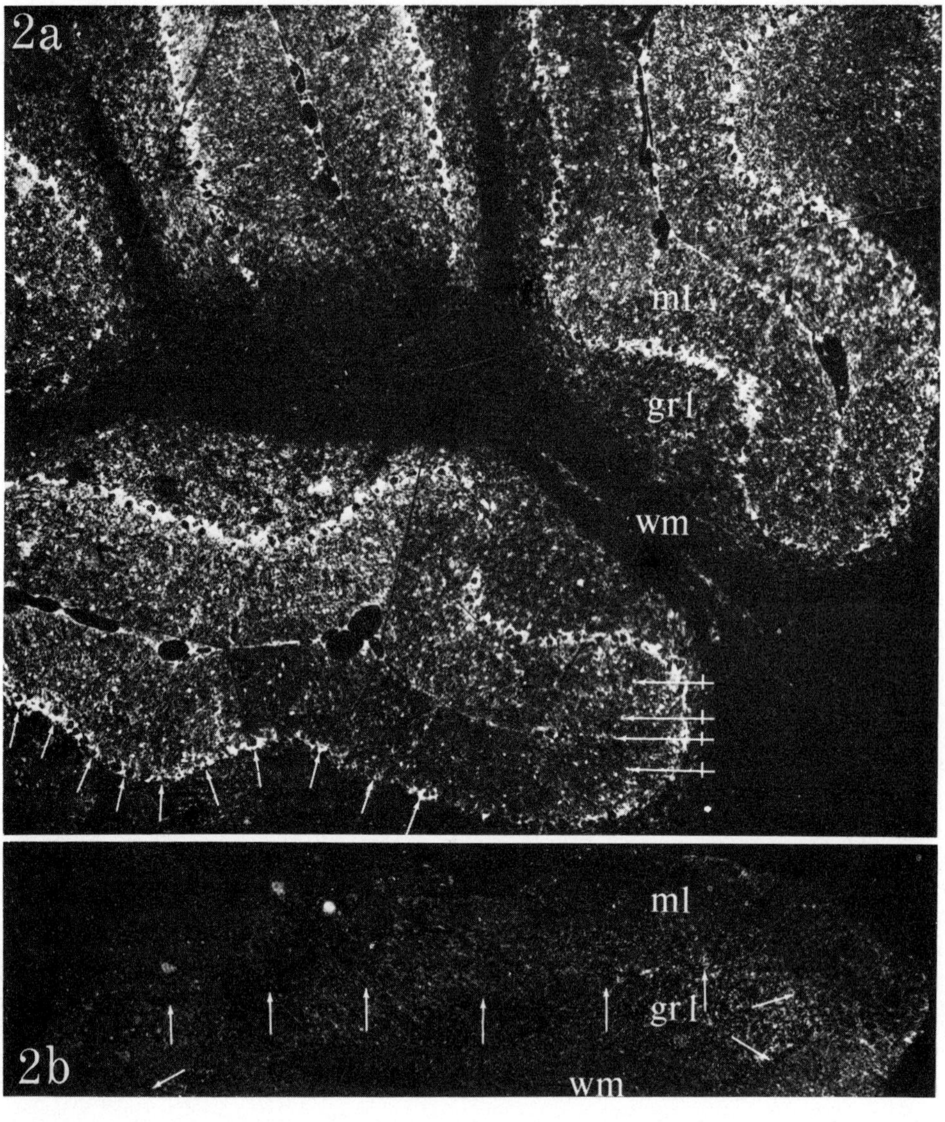

Fig. 2. Sites of GABA receptors in the cerebellar cortex demonstrated by [^{3}H]M autoradiography. Upper: after exposure to [^{3}H]M. Low-magnification (× 100) dark-field microscopy of several cortical folia in the sagittal plane of the cerebellum (1 μm epoxy section). Silver grains are generally distributed over the neuropil of the molecular layer (ml), over the granular layer (grl) and the white matter (wm) is virtually label-free. Intracortical neurons of the molecular layer are heavily labeled (horizontal arrows). The highest amount of silver grain deposition is over the basket axon formation around the Purkinje cell body and the axonal initial segment (vertical arrows). Lower: systemic injection of unlabeled muscimol 1 hr prior to administration of [^{3}H]M causes a significant loss of [^{3}H]M binding and autoradiographic label throughout the cerebellar cortical layers, particularly over intracortical neurons and the basket axon formations over Purkinje cell somata and axonal initial segments (arrows). Sagittal plane of rat cerebellum, 1 μm epoxy section, × 100.

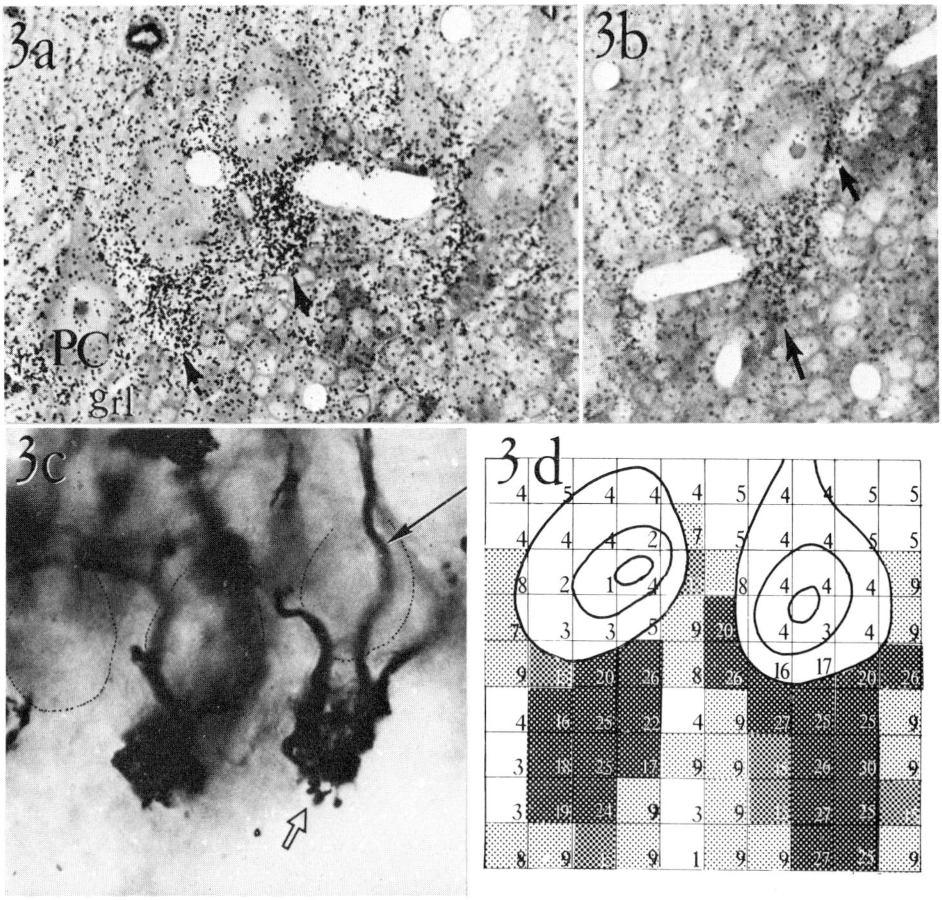

Fig. 3. a, b: Purkinje cell layer and basket axonal formations around the cells' somata heavily labeled (triangles) after [^{3}H]M binding. 1 μm epoxy section, × 600. c: basket axons around the Purkinje cell somata (dotted lines) descend as thick fibers (solid arrow) and form a basket of axonal branches (open arrow) around the initial segment of the Purkinje cells. Rapid Golgi preparation, adult rat; 90 μm sagittal section, × 600. d: diagram of distribution of GABA receptors, indicated in absolute numbers of autoradiographic silver grains after [^{3}H]M binding within 20 μm^2 squares of a grid placed over the basket formation of two Purkinje cell somata. The Purkinje cell somata have minimal grains per unit area (0–5), the region surrounding the basket formation has 5–10, and within the basket itself the grain counts rise considerably from 10 to 35.

white matter provided a quantitative display of the laminar distribution of the autoradiographic signal generated by [^{3}H]M binding. The highest binding of [^{3}H]M occurred on the Purkinje cell somatic surface, in the basket axon formation surrounding the Purkinje cell body and its axon initial segment. Neuroglial cells of the cortex have no [^{3}H]M binding capacity; some glial cells in the cerebellar nuclei do. The role of these glial cells in GABA receptor-mediated mechanisms remains to be clarified. The data are summarized in Fig. 4 where, together, the graph and the cellular diagrams show that the distribution of GABA receptors indicated by [^{3}H]M binding differs from the cellular distribution of reported

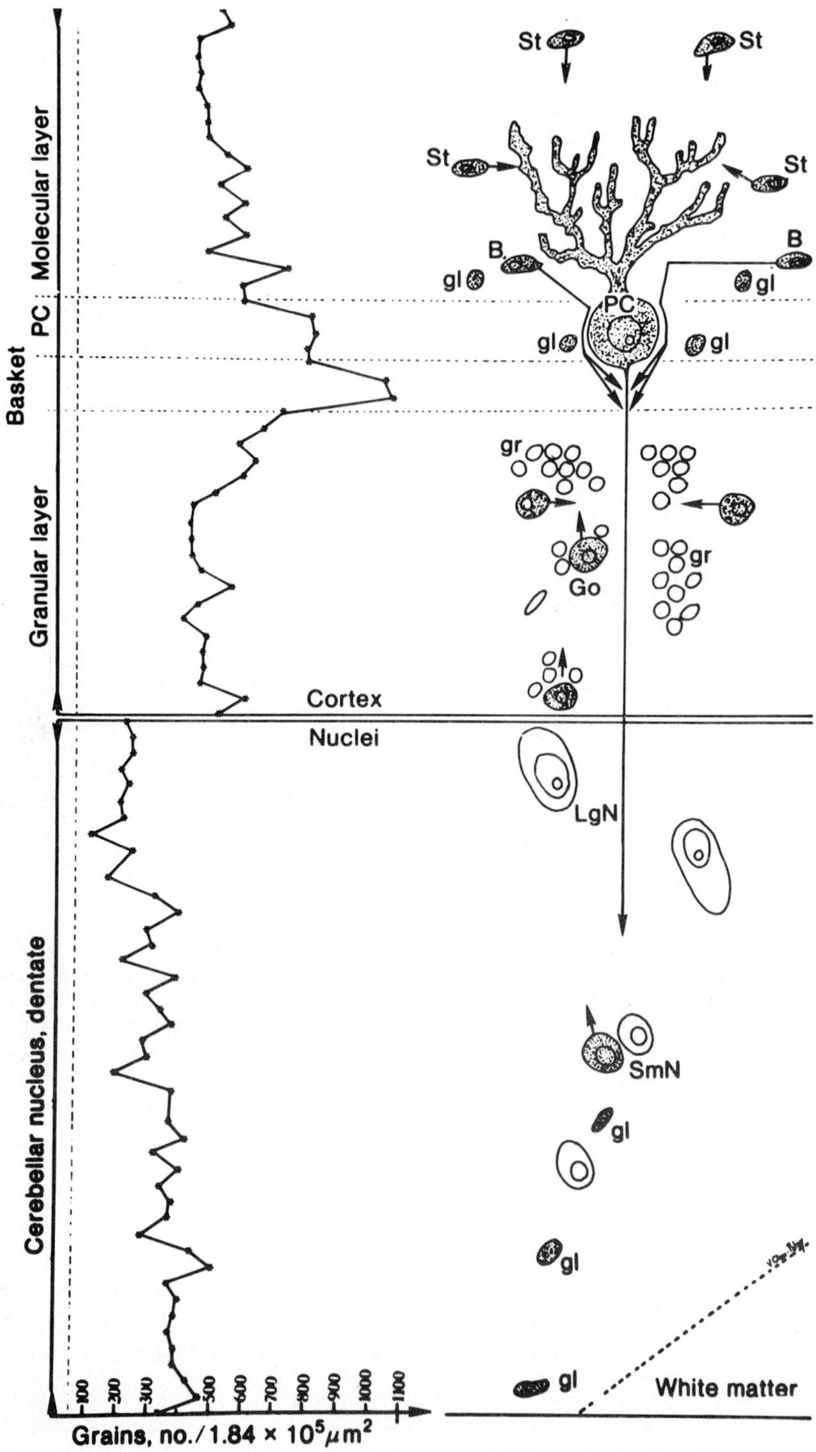
Molecular layer
PC
Basket
Granular layer
Cerebellar nucleus, dentate
Cortex
Nuclei
St
B
gl
PC
gr
Go
LgN
SmN
White matter
100
200
300
500
600
700
800
900
1000
1100
Grains, no./1.84 × 10^5 μm^2

4

Cell type	Grains per unit area
Cortex	
Basket/stellate cells	25
Purkinje cell	
Primary and secondary dendrites	12
Somata	5
Initial segment/basket	35
Neuroglial cells	0–3
Granule cells	5
Golgi cells	5–10
Neuropil of molecular and granular layers	5
Nuclei	
Large neurons	3
Small neurons	3
Neuroglial cells	15
Neuropil	5
White matter	0–3

Fig. 5. Relative distributions of autoradiographic grains over the cells and neuropil of the cerebellar cortex and nuclei.

[^{3}H]GABA and GABA synthesizing and degradative enzyme sites. Fig. 5 compares the relative distribution of autoradiographic grains over identified cells within the cerebellar cortex and nuclei. In the cortex, almost all basket and stellate cells were heavily labeled; Purkinje cell dendritic surfaces and the somatic surface surrounded by basket axons were well labeled but the cell body itself was not. The highest density of label was found in the region of the Purkinje cell initial axonal segment.

Specificity of [^{3}H]M binding was indicated by control experiments summarized in Fig. 6. In order to examine whether [^{3}H]M binding could be attributable in part to the GABA uptake and transport system, it was necessary to pretreat brain slices with inhibitors of GABA uptake before incubation with [^{3}H]M. (–)Nipecotic acid, and guvacine, a psychoactive agent found in betel nuts, are potent inhibitors of GABA uptake and combine with the carrier. When cerebellar slices were incubated with either of these substances for 10 min prior to incubation with [^{3}H]M, there was no detectable change in the pattern of distribution or quantity of silver grains in the autoradiograms. These results indicate that the [^{3}H]M binding to GABA receptors is not interfered with by GABA transport- or uptake-inhibitors and thus that the binding of [^{3}H]M is selective for receptors.

◀ Fig. 4. Schema showing the quantitative distribution (left side) of silver grains in autoradiograms after [^{3}H]M binding in laminae of the cerebellar cortex, in the dentate nucleus and in white matter. The estimated background level is indicated by the vertical dotted line. Each point on the chart was obtained by counting the grains overlying 1.84×10^5 μm^2 of tissue. The cerebellar neurons and neuroglial cells present in each layer are indicated on the right. Cells with previously reported [^{3}H]GABA uptake or containing GABA-synthesizing or degradative enzymes are indicated by stippling. Abbreviations: B, basket cell; gl, neuroglial cell; Go, Golgi cell; gr, granule cell; LgN, large neuron in dentate nucleus; PC, Purkinje cell; SmN, small neuron in dentate nucleus; St, stellate cell.

Substance	*Action*	*Negative [³H]M binding*	*Positive [³H]M binding*
(–)Nipecotic acid	Uptake Inhibitors		+
Guvacine			+
Bicuculline	Antagonists	+	
Picrotoxin		+	
Cold muscimol (systemic)	GABA Agonists	+	
Cold muscimol		(±)	
THIP (isoxazole 16)		+	
Isoguvacine		+	
Cold GABA		+	
Cold GABA/AOAA		+	

Fig. 6. Summary of control experiments on brain slices with pretreatment using GABA uptake inhibitors, agonists or antagonists prior to incubation in [^{3}H]M followed by preparation of autoradiograms.

The GABA receptor antagonists bicuculline and picrotoxin were equally effective in preventing subsequent binding with [^{3}H]M and no autoradiographic label occurred. Pretreatment with non-radioactive GABA also effectively prevents further binding with [^{3}H]M and no label occurs in the autoradiograms.

Systemic administration of muscimol can cause a number of behavioral changes including lethargy and hallucinations, an observation that suggests that the substance penetrates the blood/brain barrier. However, the possibility exists that the effects elicited may be the result of the action of metabolites of muscimol. In the present study, unlabeled muscimol administered intravenously 1 hr prior to exposure of cerebellar slices to [^{3}H]M produced a significant decrease in autoradiographic silver grains. In the cerebellum, the sites most severely affected were the basket and stellate cells of the molecular layer and the basket axon formation around Purkinje cells, which are the sites with the highest binding of [^{3}H]M (Fig. 2). These results show that muscimol administered parenterally can enter the brain and bind to available receptor sites, blocking most of these sites from subsequently binding to [^{3}H]M. Thus, unlabeled muscimol or its metabolites are effective competitors in vivo for receptors of [^{3}H]M subsequently introduced in vivo or in vitro into brain tissue. On the other hand, pretreatment in vitro with non-radioactive muscimol directly upon brain slice prior to incubation with [^{3}H]M can partially inhibit binding with the radioactive [^{3}H]M, presumably because some exchange between bound and unbound M and [^{3}H]M occurs. Pretreatment of cerebellar slices with cold GABA in the presence or absence of AOAA inhibits binding with [^{3}H]M and no labeling occurs in autoradiograms. The same result occurs with pretreatment with two GABA agonists THIP (isoxazole 16) and isoguvacine. These pharmacological/morphological tests for specificity of binding suggest that [^{3}H]M binding indicates binding at GABA receptor sites.

Several interesting observations deserve comment at this point. (1) The failure to obtain significant autoradiographic labeling in the brain after systemic intravenous injections of [^{3}H]M suggests that the majority of the injected material may be metabolized in blood plasma with only minute quantities possibly binding in the brain sites examined. (2) [^{3}H]M binding on certain neuroglial cells in the deep cerebellar nuclei needs to be further examined for possible GABA receptor-mediated mechanisms. (3) The discrepancy in the relative distribution between the M binding GABA receptor sites and the distribution of GAD and [^{3}H]GABA uptake sites needs further examination. For instance, although the terminals of Purkinje cells have considerable GAD content and capacity to take up [^{3}H]GABA, the amount of [^{3}H]M binding in the deep cerebellar nuclei is low. Several possible explanations can be entertained, first that these regions were less accessible to autoradiographic labeling because of their distance from the injection sites. Repeated injections into the cerebellar nuclei have not changed this result, suggesting that the technical approach is an unlikely explanation. Secondly, it can be proposed that there may be more than one class of GABA receptors, one that can be demonstrated by muscimol, and others that cannot under the present experimental conditions. Thirdly, that the conditions for the visualization procedures used here may have favored the demonstration of only a portion of the GABA receptor binding sites; perhaps others are masked by the presence of endogenous GABA; or can only be demonstrated by the use of [^{3}H]M in concentrations other than the 2 nM range.

Thus it appears reasonable at this time to conclude that [^{3}H]M autoradiography is useful for the morphological demonstration of GABA receptors. Nevertheless, a possibility remains that the receptors detected by M may be only one of a set of different GABA receptors. The characteristics and locations of others may be discovered by the application of similar procedures with different GABA mimetics. The fundamental aim of all these studies is to define and visualize the sites at which GABA acts in order to discover safe pharmacological tools for the treatment of those nervous and mental disorders in which GABA may be deficient.

ULTRASTRUCTURAL LOCALIZATION OF γ-AMINOBUTYRIC ACID RECEPTORS

Cellular localization

The deposition of phenidone-developed silver grains was selectively localized to the plasma membranes of several neuronal types and their processes. Background label was low. Serial section autoradiograms exposed for 3 weeks exhibited half the number of silver grains encountered in those exposed for 5 weeks; however, the grains were on comparable structures in adjacent serial sections exposed for the two durations. Silver grains in the cerebellar cortex were associated with plasma membranes of the following structures: (i) somata and primary dendrites of basket and stellate cells in the molecular layers; (ii) somata and primary and secondary dendritic shafts of Purkinje cells; (iii) axons and axon terminals of basket cells in the pinceau region; (iv) initial axonal segments and myelinated axons of Purkinje cells; (v) the dendrites of granule cells and Golgi cells in the granular layer; (vi) somata and dendritic shafts of large and small neurons in the cerebellar nuclei.

These data correspond well to the distribution and density of GABA receptors on cells in the cerebellar cortex and nuclei in light microscopic autoradiograms (Chan-Palay, 1978a). In almost all cases the label was associated with neuronal plasma membranes and not with the neuroglial investment. However, one example was found of label on the membranes of opposing axon and neuroglial cell in the dentate nucleus. Furthermore, the label occurred in relation to the cellular surface membranes and not to internal cytoplasmic membranes.

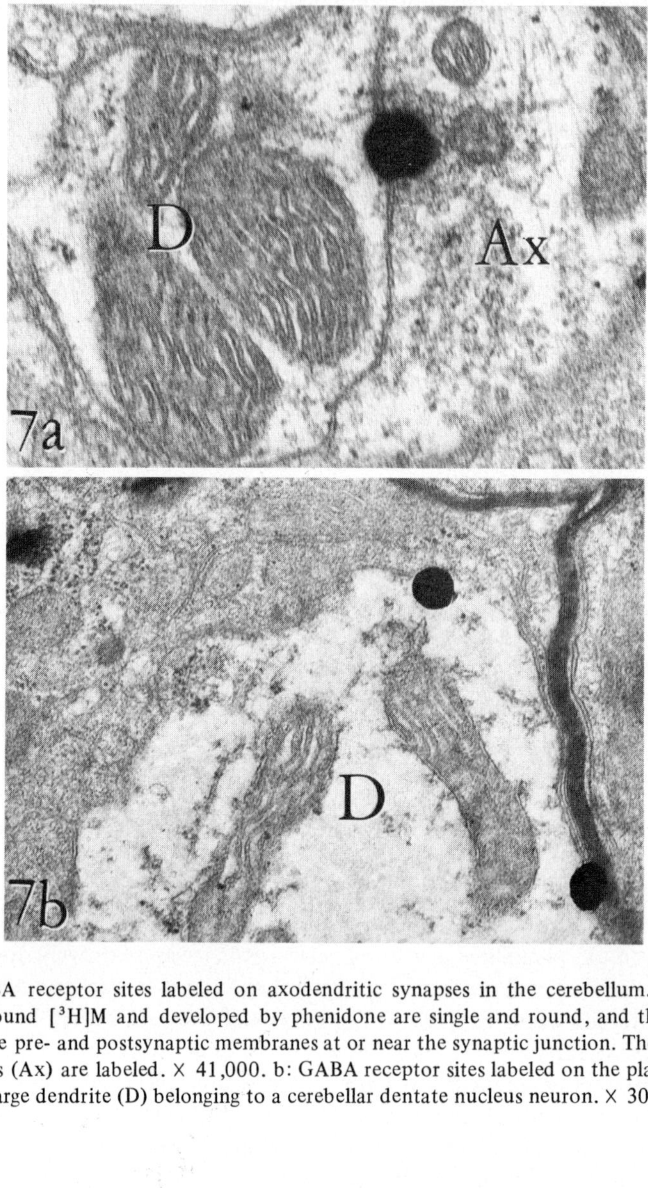

Fig. 7. a: GABA receptor sites labeled on axodendritic synapses in the cerebellum. The silver grains produced by bound [^{3}H]M and developed by phenidone are single and round, and they are selectively deposited on the pre- and postsynaptic membranes at or near the synaptic junction. The dendrite (D) and axonal terminals (Ax) are labeled. × 41,000. b: GABA receptor sites labeled on the plasma membrane of a large dendrite (D) belonging to a cerebellar dentate nucleus neuron. × 30,000.

Synaptic terminal localization

One hundred and thirty-five electron microscopic autoradiograms were obtained in which silver grains were deposited on membranes belonging to axonal varicosities and to postsynaptic elements bearing visible synaptic junctions (Fig. 7a). In 88.9% of these examples, the label was associated with axodendritic synapses on Purkinje cells and in 11.1% the label was associated with axosomatic synapses on Purkinje, stellate and basket cells.

Of the 135 examples of labeled synaptic terminals, 24% had the silver grain directly upon the opposing pre- or postsynaptic membrane at or near the synaptic junction. The remaining examples had silver grains scattered on either the pre- or postsynaptic side, close to the

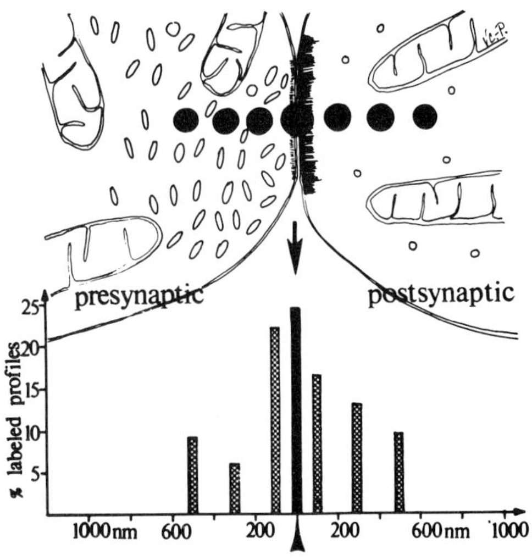

Fig. 8. Diagram summarizing the distribution of phenidone-developed autoradiographic silver grains produced by bound [^{3}H]M on the membranes of profiles bearing synaptic junctions. The sample includes 135 profiles, 24% of which have grains on the synaptic interfaces; the remaining 37.5% and 38.5% were disposed on pre- and postsynaptic sides, respectively, within 500 nm of the synaptic interfaces. This scatter of grains is within the limits of resolution of the autoradiographic method for a tritium source and the Ilford L4 emulsion.

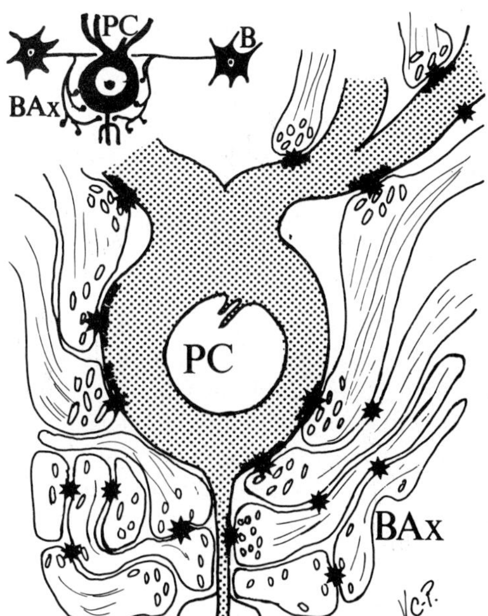

Fig. 9. Summary of the location and relative density of GABA receptor sites detected on surfaces of the Purkinje cell soma, dendrites and initial axonal segment by [^{3}H]M autoradiography. The basket cell (B) – Purkinje cell (PC) relationships are diagrammed in the Inset. GABA receptor sites (*) are found on the membranes of the Purkinje cell as well as on the membranes between basket axons (BAx). The diagram aims to show only the relative density of receptors, not the absolute number.

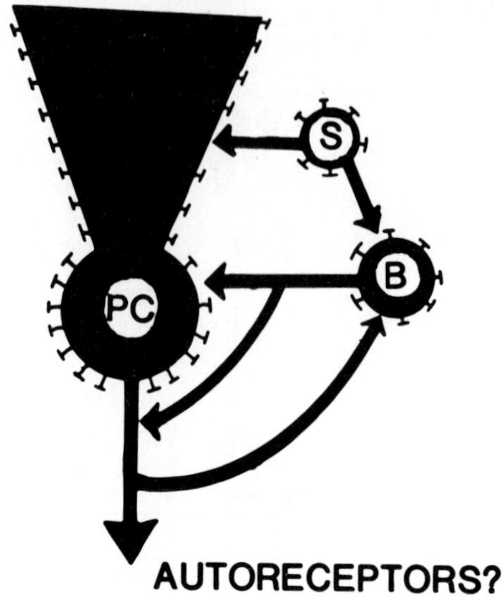

Fig. 10. Schema illustrating the concept of GABA autoreceptors on Purkinje cells, basket and stellate cells of the cerebellar cortex.

synaptic membranes. Of the original population, 37.5% had label on the presynaptic side, 22.2% of which contained silver grains within the first 100 nm of the synaptic junction; the remaining 15.3% had silver grains within 450 nm of the synaptic function. Of the original population, 38.5% had silver grains on the postsynaptic side, all of which lay within the first 500 nm of the synaptic membranes. These results are summarized diagrammatically in Fig. 8. The data show that the silver grains were clearly localized upon and near synaptic junctions. The spread of grains reported here reflects the scatter of β particles from the bound [^{3}H]M. The 500 nm maximal spread is well within the limits of resolution of this technique utilizing tritium and Ilford L4 emulsion (Fertuck and Salpeter, 1976).

The diameters of silver grains ranged from 110 to 150 nm. The neuronal plasma membrane was approximately 8 nm wide and the extracellular space between neuronal appositions was 20–25 nm wide. At symmetric synapses the synaptic cleft was 20–25 nm wide, whereas at asymmetric synapses the cleft was usually widened to 30 nm (Peters et al., 1976). Therefore, the diameter of one silver grain is 3–4 times the combined widths of pre- and postsynaptic membranes and the synaptic cleft. *Thus, although the electron microscope autoradiographic technique indicates that labeling occurs directly in conjunction with membranes at or near synapses, it is not possible to decide whether or not the source for the label, i.e., [^{3}H]M bound to GABA receptors, is associated with either the pre- or postsynaptic membrane.*

Non-synaptic locations

Sixty-four examples of neuronal profiles were obtained with silver grains located on plasma membranes of structures without visible synaptic contacts. Of these, 66% were on plasma membranes between axons and 34% were on dendrites (Fig. 7b).

The basket region around the Purkinje cell body and initial axon segment presented the most examples of silver grains over axonal plasma membranes. Here, the axons belonging to the GABA-containing basket cells of the molecular layer are complexly intertwined with one another, with some neuroglial processes between them (Palay and Chan-Palay, 1974). Few, if any, true axo-axonal synapses exist, although specialized, septate-like junctions have been described (Gobel, 1971; Mugnaini, 1972; Sotelo and Llinás, 1972; Palay and Chan-Palay, 1974). The label over the pinceau was found on the membranes between apposed basket axons that were bare of neuroglia and not at any specialized junction, as summarized in Fig. 9. These observations confirm the earlier report from light microscopic autoradiograms that the basket region around Purkinje cells was most densely labeled with [^{3}H]M binding GABA receptor sites (Chan-Palay, 1978a).

The absence of GABA receptors on the membranes of GABA-containing axons raises the obvious question of their function. Do the basket axon terminals within this region release GABA at non-synaptic locations? If so, does binding of GABA to the receptors in the basket produce self-inhibition of the basket and consequently a self-regulated inhibition of discharges from the Purkinje cell axon that it surrounds or does it produce a presynaptic facilitation? Because the basket formation around each Purkinje cell consists of axon collaterals from a number of different basket cells (Eccles et al., 1967; Palay and Chan-Palay, 1974), the effect of activation of any one basket cell axon is difficult to predict. It could result in inhibition of the other members of the basket and thus a reduction of the effect. Alternatively, is is conceivable that the membrane events in the terminals could lead to synchronized activation of the whole formation and to reinforcement of the effect of exciting a single basket cell. Moreover, is it possible that presynaptic suppression of inhibitory action of basket cell on the Purkinje cell could result? The inhibitory effect of basket cell activation on Purkinje cell discharges builds up and decays relatively slowly (Eccles et al., 1966, 1967). Some aspects of these electrical properties may be explainable by the general distribution of GABA receptors throughout the axons of the basket formation. The present findings suggest that re-examination of the physiology of the complicated synapse between basket and Purkinje cells would be useful.

Several issues will be brought up at this point for discussion. The present studies demonstrate that [^{3}H]M or a labeled metabolite can be utilized to demonstrate the location and distribution of a GABA receptor which will be termed the muscimol receptor of GABA. This receptor appears to be most heavily distributed over the molecular layer interneurons, basket and stellate cells and especially over the basket cell axon membrane relations with the Purkinje cell. Although the muscimol GABA receptor can also be found in the granular layer neuropil within and around glomeruli and in the cerebellar nuclear neuropil, it is not the predominant receptor visualization.

GABA autoreceptors

Although GABA-synthesizing enzymes and [^{3}H]GABA uptake have been consistently demonstrated in basket and stellate cells, the demonstration of these mechanisms in the Purkinje cell body has been less consistent. For example, [^{3}H]GABA uptake has been shown only in immature Purkinje cells in culture (Sotelo et al., 1972), in intraocular transplants (Ljungdahl et al., 1973), and inconsistently in the mature cerebellar cortex in vivo (Chan-Palay, 1977); GAD immunoreactivity is more readily demonstrable after the application of colchicine (Ribak et al., 1976). In the light of the muscimol GABA receptor distribution demonstrated here, it appears that many GABA-containing cerebellar neurons, in particular the basket, stellate, and Purkinje cells, have receptors for the same transmitter on their various membrane surfaces. These may be regarded as examples of identified GABA autoreceptors (Fig. 10).

Superfusion of cerebellar cortex with [^{3}H]muscimol

Data have been obtained from preliminary experiments with superfusion of [^{3}H]M over the vermal cerebellar cortical surface (unpublished experiments in collaboration with Dr. R. Llinás). The experiments were performed on adult Sprague-Dawley rats anesthetized with 40% urethane, with tracheal cannulation, curarization and artificial respiration. The cerebellar cortex in the vermis was exposed and an antidromic stimulating electrode (As) for activation of Purkinje cells was placed in the white matter at a depth of 3–4 mm. A concentric stimulating electrode (LOC) was placed on the surface of the cerebellar folium that was found by a wandering surface electrode to give a large response to antidromic stimulation. A recording glass microelectrode (RE) with a resistance of about 1.5 MΩ was inserted into the middle of the cerebellar folium approximately 1 mm lateral to the surface stimulating electrode so as to be in the beam of excited parallel fibers. The cerebellar surface was then flooded with sterile saline and with push-pull cannulae in place, the cortex was covered with 2% agar. Control physiological records were obtained from the cortex with saline, then the saline was removed and the cortex was superfused by a solution containing 2 nM [^{3}H]M for further recording. Evoked potentials were recorded at approximately 400 μm from the

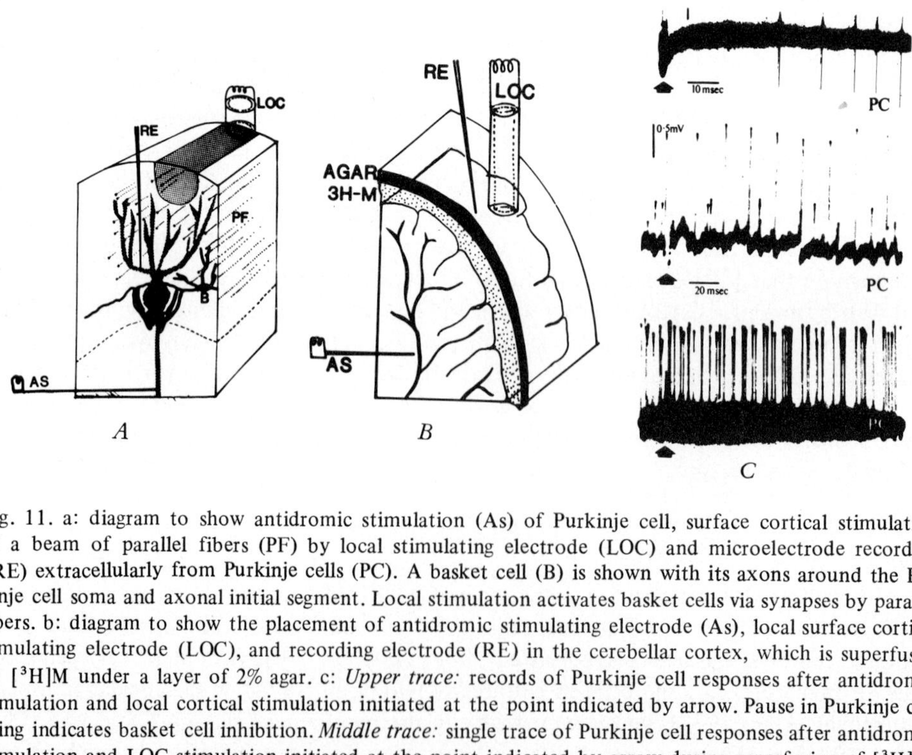

Fig. 11. a: diagram to show antidromic stimulation (As) of Purkinje cell, surface cortical stimulation of a beam of parallel fibers (PF) by local stimulating electrode (LOC) and microelectrode recording (RE) extracellularly from Purkinje cells (PC). A basket cell (B) is shown with its axons around the Purkinje cell soma and axonal initial segment. Local stimulation activates basket cells via synapses by parallel fibers. b: diagram to show the placement of antidromic stimulating electrode (As), local surface cortical stimulating electrode (LOC), and recording electrode (RE) in the cerebellar cortex, which is superfused by [^{3}H]M under a layer of 2% agar. c: *Upper trace:* records of Purkinje cell responses after antidromic stimulation and local cortical stimulation initiated at the point indicated by arrow. Pause in Purkinje cell firing indicates basket cell inhibition. *Middle trace:* single trace of Purkinje cell responses after antidromic stimulation and LOC stimulation initiated at the point indicated by arrow during superfusion of [^{3}H]M. No effective basket cell inhibition is present. *Lower trace:* superimposed traces of Purkinje cell responses after antidromic stimulation and LOC stimulation initiated at the point indicated by arrow during superfusion of [^{3}H]M. No effective basket cell inhibition is present.

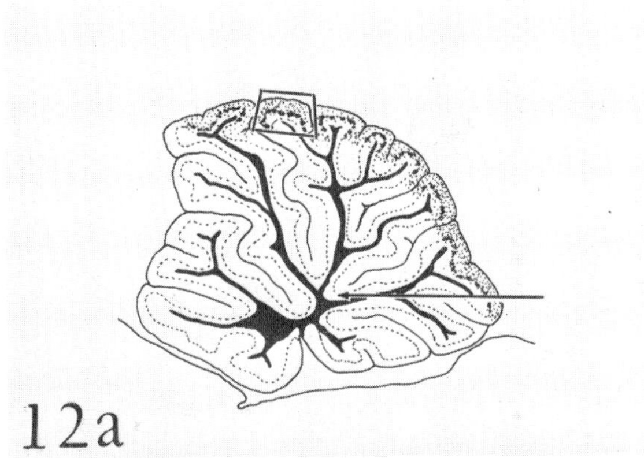

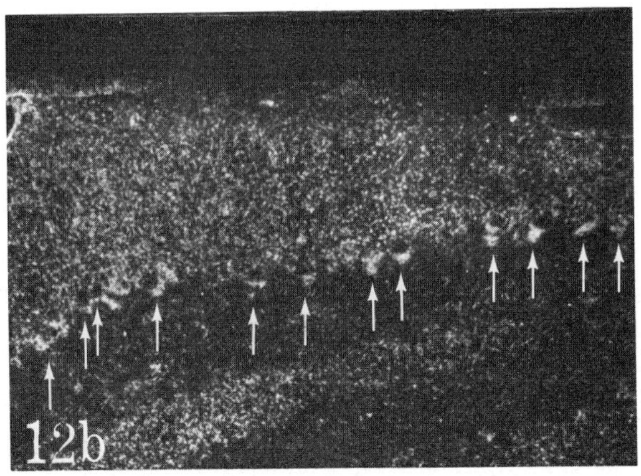

Fig. 12. a: diagram showing the distribution of autoradiographic label in the [^{3}H]M superfused cerebellar cortex and the AS electrode track (arrow). Box area is enlarged in figure. b: Dark-field micrograph of an autoradiogram of [^{3}H]M binding in cerebellar cortical surface after superfusion with [^{3}H]M. Intense labeling occurs in the basket axon area around Purkinje cells (arrows) and lighter significant label occurs in the molecular layer. × 50.

surface and with stimulus duration of 200 μsec. At the end of the physiological experiments, the animals were perfused with mixtures of aldehydes (see Materials and Methods) and sagittal serial sections of the cerebella were prepared for autoradiography in the usual manner (see Fig. 11a–c).

Preliminary results indicate that in the control experiments with physiological saline superfused over the cortex, Purkinje cell responses after antidromic stimulation could be inhibited by local stimulation of parallel fibers and activation of basket cell inhibition as previously described (Eccles et al., 1966, 1967). However, in the records obtained from cortex superfused with [^{3}H]M, the Purkinje cell responses from antidromic stimulation were not affected by local stimulation of parallel fibers and basket cells (see traces in Fig. 11c). These results suggest that basket cell stimulation by the local stimulating electrode may not be effective in inhibition of Purkinje cell responses because the muscimol GABA receptor sites are already occupied by [^{3}H]M available from the superfusate. Correlating data to support this interpretation were obtained when the cerebella were prepared for autoradiography after the recording experiments. [^{3}H]M binding was detectable over all cortical surfaces exposed to the superfusate and intense labeling was found over the basket axon-Purkinje cell axon initial segment area and less intensely over the molecular layer (Fig. 12a, b). Further studies are needed to clarify the details of the functional interaction of muscimol on cerebellar neurons.

SUMMARY

Muscimol, a structural analogue and potent agonist of γ-aminobutyric acid (GABA), was used in its tritiated form for the autoradiographic localization of GABA receptors in the rat cerebellum. [^{3}H]Muscimol ([^{3}H]M) was incubated with brain slices or was injected intracortically or into intraocular brain transplants. As indicated by [^{3}H]M binding and autoradiographic silver grains, GABA receptors display a laminar distribution over the cerebellar cortex. Specificity was indicated in control experiments by inhibition of binding by [^{3}H]muscimol after pretreatment with GABA, GABA and aminooxyacetic acid or the GABA analogues, THIP (isoxazole 16) and isoguvacine, or with receptor antagonist bicuculline and picrotoxin. Pretreatment with the GABA uptake and transport inhibitors (−)nipecotic acid and guvacine did not affect binding with [^{3}H]M. Systemic administration of unlabeled muscimol interfered with binding of [^{3}H]M subsequently administered in vitro, indicating that muscimol or a metabolite of it traverses the blood/brain barrier and binds to receptor sites, possibly in a manner competitive with [^{3}H]M. [^{3}H]M binding was greatest in the cerebellum. Systemic administration of [^{3}H]M does not produce binding in the cerebellum in sufficient quantity to produce effective autoradiograms. Quantitative analyses of the distribution of autoradiographic silver grains in the cerebellar cortex and dentate nucleus showed a general distribution of GABA receptors in the neuropil: molecular layer $>$ granular layer $>$ cerebellar nuclei $>$ white matter. The highest binding of [^{3}H]M occurred on the Purkinje cell somatic surface, in the basket axon formation surrounding the cell body and its axon initial segment, and somewhat less on basket and stellate cell somata. Neuroglial cells of the cortex have no [^{3}H]M binding capacity; some glial cells in the cerebellar nuclei do bind [^{3}H]M. The role of glial cells in GABA uptake, metabolism, and GABA receptor-mediated mechanisms remains to be clarified. The distribution of GABA receptors as indicated by [^{3}H]M binding differs from the distribution of [^{3}H]GABA uptake and GABA-synthesizing and degradative sites.

Tritiated muscimol binding and electron microscope autoradiography (Ilford L4 emulsion and phenidone development) localized GABA receptor sites in the cerebellum of the rat. In the cerebellar cortex, silver grains were associated with somata and dendrites of basket and stellate cells in the molecular layer; with somata and primary and secondary dendritic shafts of Purkinje cells; with axons and terminals of basket cells in the pinceau or basket, initial axonal segments and myelinated axons of Purkinje cells; with dendrites of granule and Golgi cells in the granular layer, and with somata and dendritic shafts of large and small cells in the cerebellar nuclei. Label over GABA receptor sites can be localized to the plasma membranes between pre- and postsynaptic elements at synaptic junctions, of which 88.9% of the samples are axodendritic and the remaining 11.1% are axosomatic. GABA receptor sites are also found along axonal membranes of the GABA-containing basket cell, within the basket surrounding Purkinje cells, where true axo-axonal synapses are rare. It is speculated that GABA receptors in the basket may be related to synchronization of basket cells, either self-inhibition or facilitation within the basket formation, or presynaptic suppression of the inhibitory action of basket cell on Purkinje cell. The presence of GABA autoreceptors in the cerebellum is proposed on the basis of the findings presented here. It is also suggested that GABA receptors other than the muscimol type demonstrated here may exist and may be localized by means of other GABA agonists.

ACKNOWLEDGMENTS

This work was supported in part by Research Grant NS03659 from the U.S. Public Health Service, the Parkinson's Disease project at the Massachusetts General Hospital, and an Alfred P. Sloan Fellowship in Neuroscience.

REFERENCES

Barber, R. and Saito, K. (1976) Light microscopic visualization of GAD and GABA-T in immunocytochemical preparations of rodent CNS. In *GABA in Nervous System Function,* E. Roberts, T. N. Chase and D. B. Tower (Eds.), Raven Press, New York, pp. 113–131.

Beart, P. M. and Johnston, G. A. R. (1973) GABA uptake in rat brain slices: inhibition by GABA analogues and by various drugs. *J. Neurochem.,* 20: 319–324.

Beaumont, K., Chilton, W., Yamamura, H. I. and Enna, S. J. (1978) Muscimol binding in rat brain: association with synaptic GABA receptors. *Brain Res.,* 148: 153–162.

Brehm, L., Hjeds, H. and Krogsgaard-Larsen, P. (1972) The structure of muscimol, a GABA analogue of restricted conformation. *Acta chem. scand.,* 26: 1298–1299.

Chan-Palay, V. (1975) Fine structure of labeled axons in the cerebellar cortex and nuclei of rodents and primates after intraventricular infusions with tritiated serotonin. *Anat. Embryol.,* 148: 235–265.

Chan-Palay, V. (1977) *Cerebellar Dentate Nucleus, Organization, Cytology, and Transmitters.* Springer, Berlin, 548 pp.

Chan-Palay, V. (1978a) Autoradiographic localization of γ-aminobutyric acid receptors in the rat central nervous system using ^{3}H-muscimol. *Proc. nat. Acad. Sci. (Wash.),* 75: 1024–1028.

Chan-Palay, V. (1978b) Quantitative visualization of γ-aminobutyric acid receptors in the hippocampus and area dentata demonstrated by ^{3}H-muscimol autoradiography. *Proc. nat. Acad. Sci. (Wash.),* 75: 6281–6284.

Chan-Palay, V. and Palay, S. L. (1978) Ultrastructural localization of γ-aminobutyric acid receptors in the mammalian central nervous system by means of ^{3}H-muscimol binding. *Proc. nat. Acad. Sci. (Wash.),* 75: 2977–2980.

Chan-Palay, V., Yonezawa, T., Yoshida, S. and Palay, S. L. (1978) Gamma-aminobutyric acid receptors visualized in spinal cord cultures by [^{3}H]muscimol autoradiography. *Proc. nat. Acad. Sci. (Wash.),* 75:6281–6284.

Curtis, D. R., Duggan, A. W., Felix, D. and Johnston, G. A. R. (1971) Bicuculline, an antagonist of GABA and synaptic inhibition in the spinal cord of cat. *Brain Res.,* 32: 69–96.

Eccles, J. C., Llinás, R. and Sasaki, K. (1966) The inhibitory interneurons within the cerebellar cortex. *Exp. Brain Res.,* 1: 1–16.

Eccles, J. C., Ito, M. and Szentágothai, J. (1967) *The Cerebellum as a Neuronal Machine.* Springer, Berlin.

Enna, S. J., Collins, J. F. and Snyder, S. H. (1977) Stereospecificity and structure-activity requirements of GABA receptor binding in rat brain. *Brain Res.,* 124: 185–190.

Enna, S. J., Beaumont, K. and Yamamura, H. I. (1978) Comparison of ^{3}H-muscimol and ^{3}H-GABA receptor binding in rat brain. In *Amino Acids as Chemical Transmitters, NATO Advanced Study Inst. Symp.,* F. Fonnum (Ed.), Plenum Press, New York, pp. 487–492.

Eugster, C. H. (1969) Chemie der Wirkstoffe aus dem Fliegenpilz *(Amanita muscaria). Fortschr. Chem. Org. Naturstud.,* 27: 261–321.

Fertuck, H. C. and Salpeter, M. M. (1976) Quantitation of junctional and extrajunctional acetylcholine receptors by electron microscope autoradiography after ^{125}I-α-bungarotoxin binding at mouse neuromuscular junctions. *J. Cell Biol.*, 69: 144-158.

Gobel, S. (1971) Axo-axonic septate junctions in the basket formations of the cat cerebellar cortex. *J. Cell Biol.*, 51: 328–333.

Hökfelt, T. and Ljungdahl, Å. (1970) Cellular localization of labeled gamma-aminobutyric acid ([^{3}H]-GABA) in rat cerebellar cortex: an autoradiographic study. *Brain Res.*, 22: 391–396.

Johnston, G. A. R., Krogsgaard-Larsen, P. and Stephanson, A. (1975) Betel nut constituents as inhibitors of γ-aminobutyric acid uptake. *Nature (Lond.)*, 258: 627–628.

Johnston, G. A. R., Krogsgaard-Larsen, P., Stephanson, A. L. and Twitchin, B. (1976) Inhibition of the uptake of GABA and related amino acids in rat brain slices by the optical isomers of nipecotic acid. *J. Neurochem.*, 26: 1029–1032.

Krogsgaard-Larsen, P. (1978) GABA agonists and uptake inhibitors of restricted conformations: structure activity relations. In *Amino Acids as Chemical Transmitters, NATO Advanced Study Inst. Symp.*, F. Fonnum (Ed.), Plenum Press, New York, pp. 305–322.

Krogsgaard-Larsen, P. and Johnston, G. A. R. (1975) Inhibition of GABA uptake in rat brain slices by nipecotic acid, various isoxazoles, and related compounds. *J. Neurochem.*, 25: 797–802.

Krogsgaard-Larsen, P., Johnston, G. A. R., Curtis, D. R., Game, C. J. A. and McCulloch, R. M. (1975) Structure and biological activity of a series of conformationally restricted analogues of GABA. *J. Neurochem.*, 25: 803–809.

Lettré, H. and Paweletz, N. (1966) Problem der elektronenmikroskopischen Autoradiographie. *Naturwissenschaften*, 53: 268–271.

Ljungdahl, Å., Seiger, Å., Hökfelt, T. and Olson, L. (1973) [^{3}H]GABA uptake in growing cerebellar tissue: autoradiography of intraocular transplants. *Brain Res.*, 61: 379–384.

McLaughlin, B., Wood, J. G., Saito, K., Barber, R., Vaughn, J. E., Roberts, E. and Wu, J.-Y. (1974) The fine structural localization of glutamate decarboxylase in synaptic terminals of rodent cerebellum. *Brain Res.*, 76: 377–391.

Mugnaini, E. (1972) The history and cytology of the cerebellar cortex. In *The Comparative Anatomy and Histology of the Cerebellum: the Human Cerebellum, Cerebellar Connections and Cerebellar Cortex*, O. Larsell and J. Jansen (Eds.), Univ. of Minnesota Press, Minneapolis, Minn., pp. 201–265.

Palay, S. L. and Chan-Palay, V. (1974) *Cerebellar Cortex, Cytology and Organization.* Springer, Berlin.

Peters, A., Palay, S. L. and Webster, H. de F. (1976) The fine structure of the nervous system. In *The Cells and their Processes*, 2nd edition, Saunders, Philadelphia, Pa.

Ribak, C. E., Vaughn, J. E. and Saito, K. (1978) Immunocytochemical localization of glutamic acid decarboxylase in neuronal somata following colchicine inhibition of axonal transport. *Brain Res.*, 140: 315–332.

Sotelo, C. and Llinás, R. (1972) Specialized membrane junctions between neurons in the vertebrate cerebellar cortex. *J. Cell Biol.*, 53: 271–289.

Sotelo, C., Privat, A. and Drian, M. J. (1972) Localization of [^{3}H]GABA in tissue culture of rat cerebellum using electron microscopy radioautography. *Brain Res.*, 45: 302–308.

Calcium Conductances in Purkinje Cell Dendrites: their Role in Development and Integration

R. LLINÁS and M. SUGIMORI

Department of Physiology and Biophysics, New York University Medical Center, New York, N.Y. 10016 (U.S.A.)

INTRODUCTION

It has become evident in recent years that the presence of voltage- and ion-dependent membrane conductance changes is a crucial parameter in determining the integrative properties of central neurons. In addition, the issue of neuronal integration has in itself been modified by the quantitative characterization of the cable properties of their dendritic and axonic processes (cf., Jack et al., 1975) and by the discovery that the former cellular processes respond, electrically, in a non-linear manner (cf., Llinás, 1975). With improved techniques for in vitro study of mammalian CNS, long-term intracellular recordings can now be obtained. Studies are presently determining the nature of these membrane conductances and the ionic species involved. In the present paper we will attempt a short review of the role of calcium in both the integrative properties of neurons and in their role as modulators of other cell biological parameters.

Voltage-dependent calcium conductance changes large enough to be self-regenerative have been observed in a multitude of neuronal elements, most of the work having been obtained in invertebrate neurons (Geduldig and Junge, 1968; Geduldig and Gruener, 1970; Wald, 1972; Kostyuk et al., 1974a, b; Kleinhaus and Prichard, 1975; Standen, 1975a, b; Eckert and Lux, 1976; Horn, 1977; Kostyuk and Krishtal, 1977). In vertebrates, action potentials have been demonstrated in several types of central and peripheral neurons (Koketsu and Nishi, 1969; Hirst and Spence, 1973; Dichter and Fischbach, 1977; Moolenaar and Spector, 1977). In most cases the inward calcium current has occurred at the somatic level while the axon is for the most part devoid of such conductance.

DENDRITIC ELECTRORESPONSIVENESS; CALCIUM SPIKES

Present evidence is clearly supportive of the fact that dendrites are capable of electroresponsive behavior. While such properties had already been envisioned from the early paper of Lorente de Nó and Condouris (1959) (cf., Purpura, 1967; Llinás, 1975), it is only in the last decade that direct intradendritic recordings have been obtained from vertebrate neurons. An example of the differences between intradendritic and intrasomatic recordings from a Purkinje cell may be seen in Fig. 1. At the somatic level the action potentials evoked either anti- or orthodromically have the typical shape first observed in motoneurons (cf., Eccles, 1957). The duration is approximately 1 msec and the rising phase consists of two parts: the so-called IS or initial segment and the SD or somadendritic component. These two main components of the somatic spike may be separated by either repetitive stimulation or by hyperpolarization, demonstrating that the SD component is generated near or at the site of penetration. Somatic action potentials, in addition, often show after-potentials which may

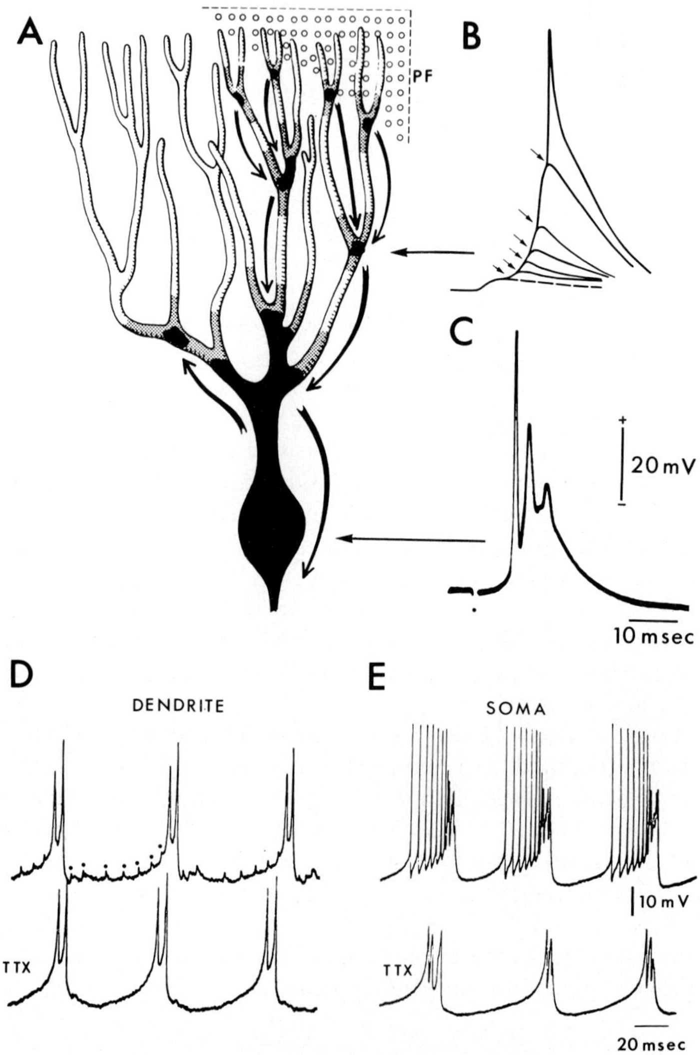

Fig. 1. Dendritic and somatic action potentials from Purkinje cells. A: diagram of dendritic spike generation. Each all-or-none dendritic spike component (B, arrow) is generated by a different hot spot, probably at or near dendritic bifurcations (dark areas in A). Somatic spikes (C) are activated by electrotonically conducted dendritic spikes and synaptic potentials. Dendritic spikes are largely calcium-dependent. Intradendritic spikes from in vitro mammalian Purkinje cells (D) are not blocked by tetrodotoxin (lower record), while fast somatic spikes (E) are abolished (lower record). (Somatic spikes are passively conducted into dendrites (dots in D) and are blocked by tetrodotoxin.) Similar results are found after removing sodium from the bathing solution.

be depolarizing and follow directly the falling phase of the action potential, as in Fig. 1C. These after-depolarizations are themselves followed by after-hyperpolarizations which generally last for tens or hundreds of milliseconds.

Intradendritic recordings, on the other hand, are characterized by their comparatively long duration (generally 10 msec or longer) (cf., Llinás and Nicholson, 1971). In the case illustrated in Fig. 1B, the spike may decompose into several components (arrows) if the dendrite impaled is hyperpolarized by current through the recording microelectrode. This hyperpolarizing current produces a blockage of the action potentials such that the largest is the first to disappear (i.e. closest to the site of impalement). With increasing hyperpolarizations the action potentials which follow in height are successively deleted (i.e. they are generated at increasing distances from the recording site), leaving finally a small potential which cannot be shifted by further current injection.

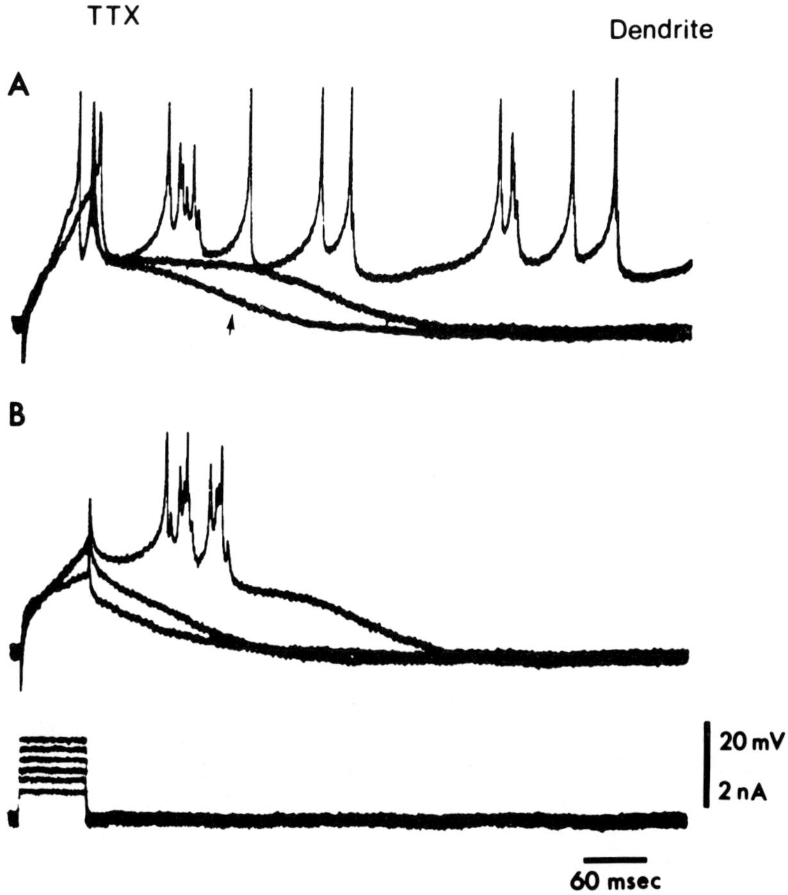

Fig. 2. Intradendritic recording from adult guinea pig cerebellum in vitro. A and B show responses to direct stimulation with current pulses of increasing amplitude (last trace). In A the 3 largest pulses evoked prolonged depolarizations (arrow) which outlasted the duration of the stimulus. In the highest trace this prolonged depolarization generated calcium spikes which lasted for a period of over 700 msec. The lower two records show depolarizations of decreasing duration but similar height. In B further decrease of the current injection shows the all-or-none character of this calcium-dependent local response which, in the uppermost trace in B, generated a set of calcium-dependent dendritic spikes of varying heights (Llinás and Sugimori, unpublished observations).

More relevant to the present discussion is the fact that dendritic spikes are predominantly generated by calcium currents. In fact, dendritic calcium-dependent spikes have recently been demonstrated by direct somatic and dendritic recording from Purkinje cells (Llinás and Hess, 1976; Llinás et al., 1977) and confirmed in hippocampus pyramidal cells (Schwartzkroin and Slawsky, 1977; Wong and Prince, 1977; Wong et al., 1979). Calcium-dependent dendritic spikes in Purkinje cells have also been demonstrated in rat and guinea pig in vitro cerebellar slices (Llinás and Sugimori, 1978, and unpublished observations). These spikes (Fig. 1D) are not blocked by tetrodotoxin or by the total removal of extracellular sodium. They are blocked, however, by cadmium chloride 1 mM, or by removal of extracellular calcium. As indicated in Fig. 1A, somatic spikes do not invade antidromically the dendritic tree. Thus, as initially proposed from current density analysis (Llinás and Nicholson, 1969), *somatic spikes are passively conducted towards the dendrites.* This is shown in D where the large intradendritic calcium spikes are recorded together with the small somatic spikes (dots). It is also clear from D and E that the Purkinje cell "bursting" often found in the in vitro preparation is not modified by addition of tetrodotoxin to the medium, indicating that this voltage-dependent bursting (blocked by hyperpolarization) is calcium-dependent. The hyperpolarization which follows each spike is most probably due to the calcium-dependent potassium conductance change (Krnjević and Lisiewicz, 1972; Meech, 1972, 1974; Jansen and Nicholls, 1973; Nishi and North, 1973; Clusin et al., 1975; Lux and Schubert, 1975; Meech and Standen, 1975; Barrett and Barrett, 1976; Heyer and Lux, 1976) since both the calcium spiking and the after-depolarization are blocked by cadmium chloride or by removal of extracellular calcium.

In addition to the all-or-none calcium spikes shown in dendrites, another form of prolonged conductance change has also been observed. This long-lasting all-or-none depolarization (Fig. 2, arrow) is blocked by cadmium chloride and by low extracellular calcium but is tetrodotoxin-insensitive and may be seen both at the dendrite and at the soma level. Such electroresponsiveness is also produced by a calcium conductance change which in this case is probably not predominate in dendrites but also present in the soma. This conductance has a low enough channel density per unit area as to produce only prolonged local responses. The rather low level of this all-or-none depolarization (10–20 mV) indicates, in addition, that it must be accompanied by a sizeable and simultaneous outward potassium current.

ELECTROPHYSIOLOGY OF PURKINJE CELLS DURING DEVELOPMENT

A further in vitro study of cerebellar cortex at different stages of postnatal embryogenesis has yielded some relevant results (Llinás and Sugimori, 1978). In contrast to the view that calcium precedes sodium conductances in immature cells, our results suggest that at 1 day after birth, when Purkinje cells are characterized by filopodia and axons but no dendrites (Fig. 3), their electroresponsive properties are basically dominated by sodium currents. In the days that follow, the Purkinje cells continue to behave similarly until the third or fourth day, at which time *some* Purkinje cells demonstrate clear calcium responses, as shown in Fig. 4C and D. Using horseradish peroxidase as a marker (Llinás and Sugimori, 1978), it was found that the particular cells demonstrating calcium conductances had, invariably, the beginnings of the main dendrite and a prominent dendritic growth cone (Fig. 4). This finding strongly suggests a relationship between the calcium current and the generation of the dendritic tree. Often such cells demonstrate climbing fiber synaptic potentials (Fig. 4A) but, due to our inability to activate the climbing fiber afferent for many of these cells

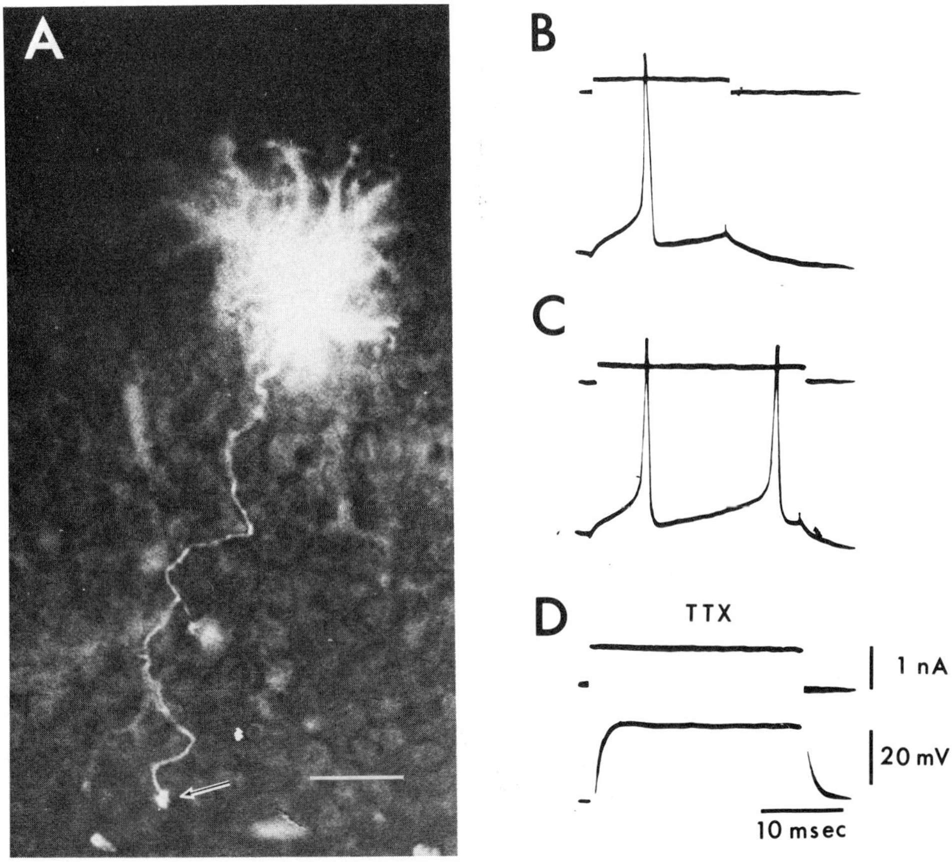

Fig. 3. Recording from a Purkinje cell in a cerebellar slice of a 1-day-old rat, in vitro. A: horseradish peroxidase injection of a Purkinje cell showing filopodia, axon and growth cone (arrow). Calibration 10 μm. B and C: typical simple spikes evoked by direct, stimulation through the recording electrode. D: the addition of tetrodotoxin to the bath completely blocks *all* electroresponsive properties in this cell (Llinás and Sugimori, unpublished observations).

(probably due to the orientation of the cerebellar slice), we cannot determine unequivocally whether the generation of the dendrite and its calcium conductance go pari passu with the presence of the climbing fiber synapse. This is nevertheless a very attractive possibility which would suggest that the climbing fiber may be responsible for the triggering of calcium conductance change in the plasma membrane. As described below, we seriously believe that this calcium conductance property of growing dendrites is probably general to all systems demonstrating growth cones.

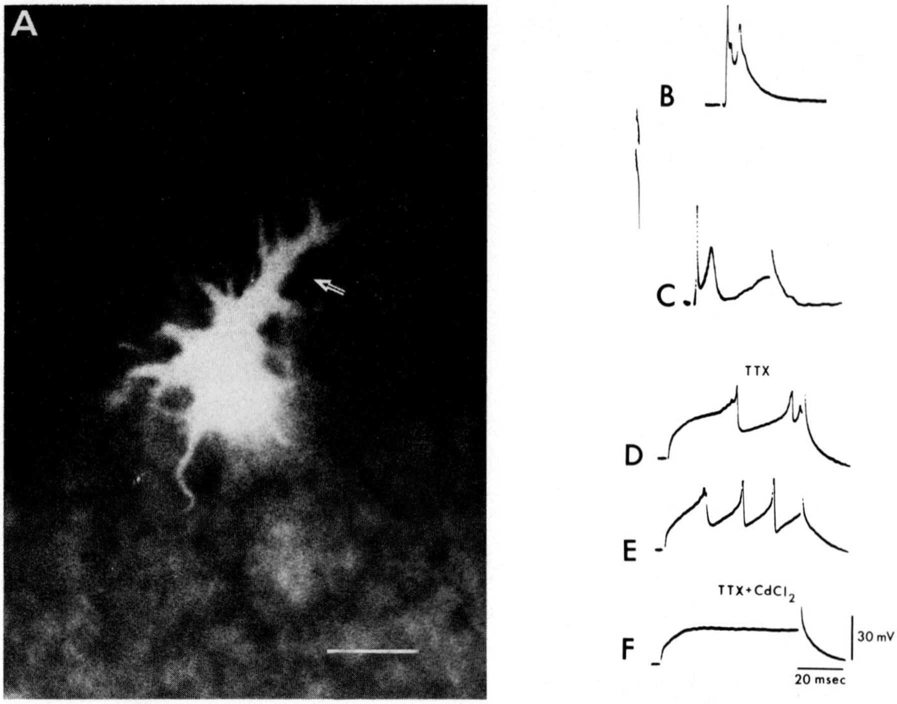

Fig. 4. Intracellular recording from Purkinje cell in a cerebellar slice of a 5-day-old rat, in vitro. A: horseradish peroxidase injection showing the beginning of an apical dendrite (arrow). Calibration 10 μm. B: white matter stimulation demonstrates antidromic as well as climbing fiber activation. C: direct stimulation produced an initial fast sodium-dependent action potential followed by a slower calcium-dependent spike and a distinct after-hyperpolarization. D and E: following the addition of tetrodotoxin to the bath, the early response in C disappears but the slow-rising action potentials remain. F: addition of cadmium chloride and tetrodotoxin to the bath produces a complete blockage of the slow calcium-dependent spike (Llinás and Sugimori, unpublished observations).

POSSIBLE ROLES OF DENDRITIC CALCIUM SPIKES

The entry of calcium into dendrites can serve many biological functions (see Fig. 5): first and most obviously, as shown in Figs. 1 and 3, a charge carrier system. In fact, Traub and Llinás (1977, 1979) have demonstrated that the magnitude and precise distribution of calcium conductances is a significant variable in the integrative properties of nerve cells. In addition to the actual movement of calcium itself, this current can, as stated above, activate calcium-dependent potassium conductance changes which will produce very significant changes in the electrophysiological properties of neurons.

Beyond its charge carrier function, calcium may be regarded as triggering the release of intracellular substances from dendrites, thus becoming a central issue in the problem of local circuit function. That calcium does trigger transmitter release from dendrites is clear from the work on, for instance, the olfactory bulb (Getchell and Shepherd, 1975). In addition, it is possible that such calcium may play a role in the release of substances other than transmitter from dendrites; e.g. peptides and neurohormones (cf., Barker and Smith, 1977). The

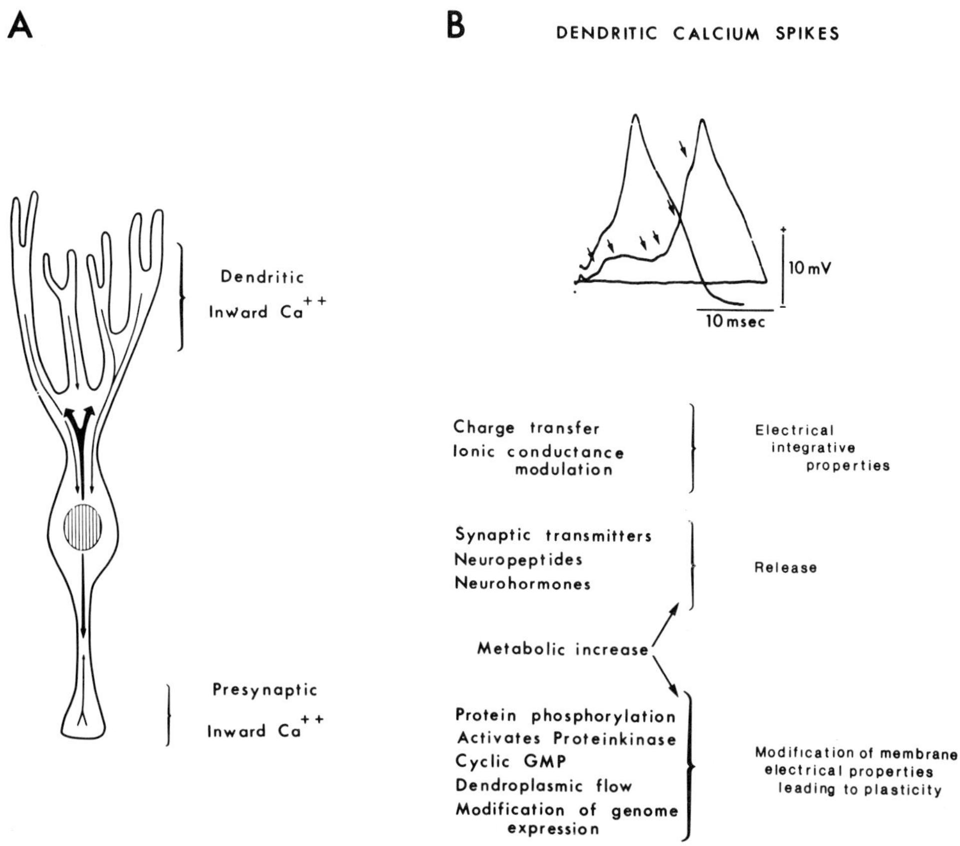

Fig. 5. Dendritic calcium spikes. A: dendritic and presynaptic calcium currents are assumed to activate a set of events leading to a modification of genome expression (centripetal arrows). The product of nuclear transcription is envisaged as distributed centrifugally via axoplasmic and dendroplasmic flow back to the somatic, dendritic, axonic and presynaptic plasmalemmal membrane (thick arrows). B: Purkinje cell dendritic calcium spikes following blockage of sodium currents with tetrodotoxin. Note the presence of multiple sites for spike origin (arrows). The table suggests different actions of calcium spikes in cell function. (From Llinás, 1979.)

functional advantage of this particular scheme is that such release would be actively regulated by the functional state of the dendrites themselves and would not necessarily depend on somatic or axonic firing. Furthermore, it is quite possible that calcium also regulates the metabolic level of the cell (Landowne and Ritchie, 1971; Kretsinger, 1976) which would be of importance in maintaining dendritic release and in the possible plastic effects subserved by electrical activity.

Beyond this, calcium probably plays a similar role in dendrites as it does in peripheral nerve as far as axoplasmic flow is concerned. It is now apparent from various studies (Ochs, 1972; Edström, 1974; Dravid and Hammerschlag, 1975; Hammerschlag et al., 1975, 1976, 1977; Dravid, 1977; Ochs et al., 1977) that calcium regulates axoplasmic flow. It seems reasonable, therefore, that dendroplasmic flow (Kreutzberg et al., 1973) may also be regulated, to a certain extent, by such a mechanism, i.e., the speed with which substances would flow along the intradendritic compartment may be modulated as in axons (Badr and

McLean, 1975) by the membrane's electric field via the voltage-dependent inward calcium current. Also, inasmuch as calcium is now being considered as a trigger for cyclic nucleotide synthesis (in particular, cyclic GMP) (Rasmussen, 1970; Schultz et al., 1973; Bloom, 1975; Guidotti et al., 1975; Ferendelli et al., 1976; Rasmussen and Goodman, 1977; Greengard, 1978), the possibility becomes very attractive that synaptic input, through either direct or voltage-dependent calcium inflow, may be part of the second messenger system as indicated by Schulman and Greengard (1978) who have shown that this ion can produce phosphorylation directly and activate protein kinases independently from its action on cyclic GMP.

The most far reaching possibility, of course, is that calcium, by acting as a second messenger and in conjunction with the other properties mentioned above, may modify transcription by altering genome expression, as recently shown for cartilage (Rodan et al., 1978), and thus serve as a feedback system regulating the nuclear production of membrane proteins. In this sense then, the system would work as envisaged by Palade (1975) for the generation of gamma-globulin or, in more direct relation to the present problem, as envisaged by Fambrough and Devroetes (1978) who have shown that ACh receptors are found at the perinuclear Golgi apparatus before being inserted in the membrane.

Beyond the examples of dendritic calcium spiking, it is possible to imagine a more basic theme underlying these phenomena.

SYNAPTIC TRANSMISSION AND PLASTICITY AS DIFFERENT ASPECTS OF "ISOMETRIC CALCIUM-DEPENDENT GROWTH"

The present hypothesis was first presented at the Neuroscience Research Program's 1977 meeting in Boulder and was written for *The Neurosciences: Fourth Study Program* to be published in 1979. As stated in that paper (Llinás, 1979), calcium has a long evolutionary history as a cell regulator and thus the functional themes in which calcium may be involved are probably diverse and may involve many levels of organization. Our own bias is that calcium, which regulates cell motility (Porter, 1976), could through this action regulate growth. The actual mechanism would be one where calcium controls the rate of addition of new membrane at growth cones, probably by promoting fusion between intracellular vesicles or subcisternal systems and the plasma membrane, in a manner similar to that hypothesized for chemical synaptic transmission. Support for this view is provided by our own study on Purkinje cell ontogeny outlined above (Llinás and Sugimori, 1978). Through this membrane addition, then, newly minted proteins would be inserted into the plasmalemma membrane and intracellular substances released.

The teleology behind this view, given that growth cones may have a significant voltage-dependent calcium conductance, is that calcium would, in addition to promoting membrane fusion, (a) reduce intracellular viscosity by regulating the fluidity of the axoplasm (Hodgkin and Katz, 1949) or dendroplasm, and (b) activate axo- or dendroplasmic flow, probably by acting on the endoskeletal filamentous structures (Droz et al., 1975; Smith et al., 1975; Mannherz and Goody, 1976) or on the submembranous cisternae (Wood et al., 1974; Wood and McLaughlin, 1976). This would allow the high mobility which a growth cone is known to possess.

Following from the above, synaptic terminals may be regarded as a modified growth cone where growth is largely subdued and actually becomes *isometric,* i.e., membranes are introduced into the plasmalemma by synaptic vesicles, only to be taken up again by a recycling mechanism such as postulated by Heuser and Reese (1973). That an actual increase in the surface area in synaptic terminals occurs with synaptic release has been shown by Frontali et al. (1976) in the neuromuscular junction and by Schaeffer and Raviola (1975) and Ripps et al. (1977) in the retina.

Furthermore, dendrites may have such properties as well. One may assume that the growth cone that generates the dendrite is vestigially represented by a membrane turnover for the release of intracellular substances and, in addition, as a mechanism to introduce new proteins into surface membrane. In this respect, presynaptic terminals and dendritic arborizations (especially the remote dendrites) may be modified growth cones and plasticity nothing other than a modification of the general growth theme.

SUMMARY

The presence of calcium-dependent electroresponsive properties of dendrites in mammalian Purkinje cells in in vitro cerebellar slices is reviewed. It is shown that these spikes are preferentially recorded at dendritic level and play an important role in neuronal integration. Besides the all-or-none calcium dendritic action potentials, prolonged calcium-dependent local responses may also be seen in somas and dendrites. The ontogeny of this voltage-dependent membrane conductance indicates that the calcium component appears with the development of the dendritic trees. A general hypothesis is proposed for the role of calcium currents in neuronal function.

ACKNOWLEDGMENT

Research was supported by United States Public Health Service Grant NS-13742 from NINCDS.

REFERENCES

Badr, G. G. and McLean, W. G. (1975) The effect of electrical stimulation on the distribution of labelled proteins in isolated segments of rabbit vagus nerve. *J. Neurochem.*, 25: 921–923.

Barker, J. L. and Smith, Jr., T. G. (1977) Peptides as neurohormones. In *Society for Neuroscience Symposia, Vol. 2,* W. M. Cowan and J. A. Ferrendelli (Eds.), Soc. for Neuroscience, Bethesda, Md., pp. 340–373.

Barrett, E. F. and Barrett, J. N. (1976) Separation of two voltage-sensitive potassium currents, and demonstration of a tetrodotoxin-resistant calcium current in frog motoneurones. *J. Physiol. (Lond.)*, 255: 737–774.

Bloom, F. E. (1975) The role of cyclic nucleotides in central synaptic function. *Rev. Physiol. Biochem. Pharmacol.*, 74: 1–103.

Clusin, W., Spray, D. C. and Bennett, M. V. L. (1975) Activation of a voltage-insensitive conductance by inward calcium current. *Nature (Lond.)*, 256: 425–427.

Dichter, M. A. and Fischbach, G. D. (1977) The action potential of chick dorsal root ganglion neurones maintained in cell culture. *J. Physiol. (Lond.)*, 267: 281–298.

Dravid, A. R. (1977) Role of calcium in the initiation of fast axonal transport of protein: effects of divalent cations. *J. Neurobiol.*, 8: 439–451.

Dravid, A R. and Hammerschlag, R. (1975) Axoplasmic transport of proteins in vitro in primary afferent neurons of frog spinal cord: effect of Ca^{2+}-free incubation conditions. *J. Neurochem.*, 24: 711–718.

Droz, B., Rambourg, A. and Koenig, H. L. (1975) The smooth endoplasmic reticulum: structure and role in the renewal of axonal membrane and synaptic vesicles by fast axonal transport. *Brain Res.*, 93: 1–13.

Eccles, J. C. (1957) *The Physiology of Nerve Cells.* John Hopkins Press, Baltimore, Md.

Eckert, R. and Lux, H. D. (1976) A voltage-sensitive persistant calcium conductance in neuronal somata of *Helix. J. Physiol. (Lond.),* 254: 129–151.

Edström, A. (1974) Effects of Ca^{2+} and Mg^{2+} on rapid axonal transport of proteins in vitro in frog sciatic nerves. *J. Cell Biol.,* 61: 812–818.

Fambrough, D. M. and Devroetes, P. N. (1978) Newly synthesized acetylcholine receptors are located in the Golgi apparatus. *J. Cell Biol.,* 76: 237–244.

Ferendelli, J. A., Rubin, E. H. and Kinscherf, D. A. (1976) Influence of divalent cations on regulation of cyclic GMP and cyclic AMP levels in brain tissue. *J. Neurochem.,* 26: 741–748.

Frontali, N., Ceccarelli, B., Gorio, A., Mauro, A., Siekevitz, P., Tzeng, M.-C. and Hurlbut, W. P. (1976) Purification from black widow spider venom of a protein factor causing the depletion of synaptic vesicles at neuromuscular junctions. *J. Cell Biol.,* 68: 462–479.

Geduldig, D. and Gruener, R. (1970) Voltage clamp of the *Aplysia* giant neurone early sodium and calcium currents. *J. Physiol. (Lond.),* 211: 217–244.

Geduldig, D. and Junge, D. (1968) Sodium and calcium components of action potentials in the *Aplysia* giant neurone. *J. Physiol. (Lond.),* 199: 347–365.

Getchell, T. V. and Shepherd, G. M. (1975) Short-axon cells in the olfactory bulb: dendrodendritic synaptic interactions. *J. Physiol. (Lond.),* 251: 523–548.

Greengard, P. (1978) Phosphorylated proteins as physiological effectors. *Science,* 199: 146–152.

Guidotti, A., Biggio, G. and Costa, E. (1975) 3-Acetylpyridine: tool to inhibit tremor and increase of cGMP content in cerebellar cortex elicited by harmaline. *Brain Res.,* 96: 201–205.

Hammerschlag, R., Dravid, A. R. and Chiu, A. Y. (1975) Mechanism of axonal transport: proposed role for calcium ions. *Science,* 188: 273–275.

Hammerschlag, R., Chiu, A. Y. and Dravid, A. R. (1976) Inhibition of fast axonal transport of [^{3}H]-protein by cobalt ions. *Brain Res.,* 114: 353–358.

Hammerschlag, R., Bakhit, C., Chiu, A. Y. and Dravid, A. R. (1977) Role of calcium in the initiation of fast axonal transport of protein: effects of divalent cations. *J. Neurobiol.,* 8: 439–451.

Heuser, J. E. and Reese, T. S. (1973) Evidence for recycling of synaptic vesicle membrane during transmitter release at the frog neuromuscular junction. *J. Cell. Biol.,* 57: 315–344.

Heyer, C. B. and Lux, H. D. (1976) Properties of a facilitating calcium current in bursting pacemaker neurons of the snail, *Helix pomatia. J. Physiol. (Lond.),* 262: 319–348.

Hirst, G. D. S. and Spence, I. (1973) Calcium action potentials in mammalian peripheral neurones. *Nature New Biol.,* 243: 54–56.

Hodgkin, A. L. and Katz, B. (1949) The effect of calcium on the axoplasm of giant nerve fibres. *J. exp. Biol.,* 26: 292–294.

Horn, R. (1977) Tetrodotoxin-resistant divalent action potentials in an axon of *Aplysia. Brain Res.,* 133: 177–182.

Jack, J. J. B., Noble, D. and Tsien, R. W. (1975) *Electric Current Flow in Excitable Cells.* Oxford Univ. Press, London.

Jansen, J. K. S. and Nicholls, J. G. (1973) Conductance changes, an electrogenic pump and the hyperpolarization of leech neurones following impulses. *J. Physiol. (Lond.),* 229: 635–655.

Kleinhaus, A. L. and Prichard, J. W. (1975) Calcium-dependent action potentials produced in leech Retzius cells by tetraethylammonium chloride. *J. Physiol. (Lond.),* 246: 351–361.

Koketsu, K. and Nishi, S. (1969) Calcium and action potentials of bullfrog sympathetic ganglion cells. *J. gen. Physiol.,* 53: 608–623.

Kostyuk, P. G. and Krishtal, O. A. (1977) Separation of sodium and calcium currents in the somatic membrane of mollusc neurones. *J. Physiol. (Lond.),* 270: 545–568.

Kostyuk, P. G., Krishtal, O. A. and Doroshenko, P. A. (1974a) Calcium currents in snail neurones. I. Identification of calcium current. *Pfluegers Arch. ges. Physiol.,* 348: 83–93.

Kostyuk, P. G., Krishtal, O. A. and Doroshenko, P. A. (1974b) Calcium currents in snail neurones. II. The effect of external calcium concentration on the calcium inward current. *Pfluegers Arch. ges. Physiol.,* 348: 95–104.

Kretsinger, R. H. (1976) Calcium-binding proteins. *Ann. Rev. Biochem.,* 45: 239–266.

Kreutzberg, G. W., Schubert, P., Tóth, L. and Rieske, E. (1973) Intradendritic transport to postsynaptic sites. *Brain Res.,* 62: 399–405.

Krnjević, K. and Lisiewicz, A. (1972) Injections of calcium ions into spinal motoneurones. *J. Physiol. (Lond.),* 225: 363–390.

Landowne, D. and Ritchie, J. M. (1971) On the control of glycogenolysis in mammalian nervous tissue by calcium. *J. Physiol. (Lond.)*, 212: 503–517.

Llinás, R. (1975) Electroresponsive properties of dendrites in central neurons. In *Physiology and Pathology of Dendrites (Advances in Neurology, Vol. 12)*, G. W. Kreutzberg (Ed.), Raven Press, New York, pp. 1–13.

Llinás, R. (1979) The role of calcium in neuronal function. In *The Neurosciences: Fourth Study Program*, F. O. Schmitt and F. G. Worden, M.I.T. Press, Cambridge, Mass., pp. 555–571.

Llinás, R. and Hess, R. (1976) Tetrodotoxin-resistant dendritic spikes in avian Purkinje cells. *Proc. nat. Acad. Sci. (Wash.)*, 73: 2520–2523.

Llinás, R. and Nicholson, C. (1969) Electrophysiological analysis of alligator cerebellum: a study on dendritic spikes. In *Neurobiology of Cerebellar Evolution and Development*, R. Llinás (Ed.), American Medical Ass., Chicago, Ill., pp. 431–465.

Llinás, R. and Nicholson, C. (1971) Electrophysiological properties of dendrites and somata in alligator Purkinje cells. *J. Neurophysiol.*, 34: 534–551.

Llinás, R. and Sugimori, M. (1978) Dendritic calcium spiking in mammalian Purkinje cells: in vitro study of its function and development. *Soc. Neurosci. Abstr.*, 4: 66.

Llinás, R., Sugimori, M. and Walton, K. (1977) Calcium dendritic spikes in the mammalian Purkinje cells. *Soc. Neurosci. Abstr.*, 3: 58.

Lorente de Nó, R. and Condouris, G. A. (1959) Decremental conduction in peripheral nerve. Integration of stimuli in the neuron. *Proc. nat. Acad. Sci. (Wash.)*, 45: 592–617.

Lux, H. D. and Schubert, P. (1975) Some aspects of the electroanatomy of dendrites. In *Physiology and Pathology of Dendrites (Advances in Neurology, Vol. 12)*, G. W. Kreutzberg (Ed.), Raven Press, New York, pp. 29–44.

Mannherz, H. G. and Goody, R. S. (1976) Proteins in contractile systems. *Ann. Rev. Biochem.*, 45: 428–465.

Meech, R. W. (1972) Intracellular calcium injection causes increased potassium conductance in *Aplysia* nerve cells. *Comp. Biochem. Physiol.*, 42A: 493–499.

Meech, R. W. (1974) Sensitivity of *Helix aspersa* neurons to injected calcium ions. *J. Physiol. (Lond.)*, 237: 259–277.

Meech, R. W. and Standen, N. B. (1975) Potassium activation in *Helix aspersa* neurones under voltage clamp: a component mediated by calcium influx. *J. Physiol. (Lond.)*, 249: 211–239.

Moolenaar, W. H. and Spector, I. (1977) Membrane currents examined under voltage clamp in cultured neuroblastoma cells. *Science*, 196: 331–336.

Nishi, S. and North, R. A. (1973) Intracellular recording from the myenteric plexus of the guinea-pig ileum. *J. Physiol. (Lond.)*, 231: 471–491.

Ochs, S. (1972) Fast transport of material in mammalian nerve fibers. *Science*, 176: 252–260.

Ochs, S., Worth, R. M. and Chan, S.-Y. (1977) Calcium requirement for axoplasmic transport in mammalian nerve. *Nature (Lond.)*, 270: 748–750.

Palade, G. (1975) Intracellular aspects of the process of protein synthesis. *Science*, 189: 347–358.

Porter, K. R. (1976) Motility in cells. In *Cell Motility, Cold Spring Harbor Conf. on Cell Proliferation, Vol. 3*, R. Goldman, T. Pollard and J. Rosenbaum (Eds.), Long Island Biol. Ass., Long Island, N.Y., pp. 1–28.

Purpura, D. P. (1967) Comparative physiology of dendrites. In *The Neurosciences: a Study Program*, G. C. Quarton, T. Melnechuk and F. O. Schmitt (Eds.), Rockefeller Univ. Press, New York, pp. 372–393.

Rasmussen, H. (1970) Cell communication, calcium ion and cyclic adenosine monophosphate. *Science*, 170: 404–412.

Rasmussen, H. and Goodman, D. B. P. (1977) Relationships between calcium and cyclic nucleotides in cell activation. *Physiol. Rev.*, 57: 421–509.

Ripps, H., Shakib, M. and MacDonald, E. D. (1977) On the fate of synaptic vesicle membrane in photoreceptor terminals of the skate retina. *Biol. Bull.*, 153: 443–444.

Rodan, G. A., Bourret, L. A. and Norton, L. A. (1978) DNA synthesis in cartilage cells is stimulated by oscillating electric fields. *Science*, 199: 690–692.

Schaeffer, S. F. and Raviola, E. (1975) Ultrastructural analysis of functional changes in the synaptic endings of turtle cone cells. *Cold Spr. Harb. Symp. quant. Biol.*, 40: 521–528.

Schulman, H. and Greengard, P. (1978) Stimulation of brain membrane protein phosphorylation by calcium and an endogenous heat-stable protein. *Nature (Lond.)*, 271: 478–479.

Schultz, G., Hardman, J. G., Schultz, K., Baird, C. E. and Sutherland, E. W. (1973) The importance of calcium ions for the regulation of guanosine 3',5'-cyclic monophosphate levels. *Proc. nat. Acad. Sci. (Wash.)*, 70: 3889–3893.

Schwartzkroin, P. A. and Slawsky, M. (1977) Probable calcium spikes in hippocampal neurons. *Brain Res.*, 135: 157–161.

Smith, D. S., Järlfors, U. and Cameron, B. F. (1975) Morphological evidence for the participation of microtubules in axonal transport. *Ann. N.Y. Acad. Sci.*, 253: 472–506.

Standen, N. B. (1975a) Calcium and sodium ions as charge carriers in the action potential of an identified snail neurone. *J. Physiol. (Lond.)*, 249: 241–252.

Standen, N. B. (1975b) Voltage-clamp studies of the calcium inward current in an identified snail neurone: comparison with the sodium inward current. *J. Physiol. (Lond.)*, 249: 253–268.

Traub, R. D. and Llinás, R. (1977) Spatial distribution of ionic conductances in normal and axotomized motoneurons. *Neuroscience*, 2: 829–849.

Traub, R. D. and Llinás, R. (1979) Hippocampal pyramidal cells: significance of dendritic ionic conductances for neuronal function and epileptogenesis. *J. Neurophysiol.*, 42: 476–496.

Wald, F. (1972) Ionic differences between somatic and axonal action potentials in snail gaint neurones. *J. Physiol. (Lond.)*, 220: 267–281.

Wong, R. K. S. and Prince, D. A. (1977) Burst generation and calcium mediated spikes in hippocampus neurons. *Soc. Neurosci. Abstr.*, 3: 148.

Wong, R. K. S., Prince, D. A. and Basbaum, A. I. (1979) Intradendritic recordings from hippocampal neurons. *Proc. nat. Acad. Sci. (Wash.)*, 76: 986–990.

Wood, J. G. and McLaughlin, B. J. (1976) Cytochemical studies of lectin binding sites in smooth membrane cisternae of rat brain. *Brain Res.*, 118: 15–26.

Wood, J. G., McLaughlin, B. J. and Barber, R. P. (1974) Visualization of concanavalin A binding sites in Purkinje cell somata and dendrites of rat cerebellum. *J. Cell Biol.*, 63: 541–549.

In Vitro Models of Neural Growth and Differentiation

A. PRIVAT*, A. M. MARSON and M. J. DRIAN

Laboratoire de Culture de Tissu Nerveux, INSERM U-106, 42, rue Desbassyns de Richemont, 92150 Suresnes (France)

INTRODUCTION

Tissue culture, whatever the technique used, is a time consuming and expensive process, which should be undertaken only in the cases in which "in situ" experiments are not fully adequate. The study in isolation of a given region of the nervous system can indeed provide information that could hardly be obtained by any other technique; however, the decision for a given technique of culture – organotypic, dissociated, permanent line – should be carefully taken in connection with the question raised.

Some of the basic problems of neural differentiation may be – and have been – fruitfully addressed by tissue culture techniques. One just needs to list the unchallenged possibilities of in vitro systems, and present them with the problem to which they apply:

- Isolation of minute regions and possibility of further recombination.
- Continuous observation under light microscope, and easy access to microsurgery and microphysiology.
- Use of a controlled environment (medium, temperature, etc. . .).
- Factors governing neural connectivity, intrinsic program and cellular interactions.
- Time dimension and precise chronology in developmental events.
- Close anatomo-physiological correlation.
- Biochemical and biophysical parameters of development.

This short list does not pretend to be exhaustive, but simply gives a broad outline of the fields in which tissue culture techniques may be a necessary tool. In the 4-step scheme provided by Vrensen (1978) for the visual system, tissue culture techniques apply best to the analysis of the initial steps of growth and recognition (macrostructural and partly microstructural), and not at all to the last steps of organization influenced by the function.

In the present paper, we shall review data gathered in this field in our laboratory and in collaboration with others, and open some perspectives with ongoing projects.

---

* Reprints request: A. Privat, address as above.

CEREBELLUM

(1) Organotypic cultures

Organotypic cultures of nervous tissue in the Maximov assembly have been extensively worked out during the last 30 years (Murray, 1965) and they represent a satisfactory compromise between the complex interactions prevailing "in situ", and the extreme status of isolation represented by dissociated cells grown in monolayers. Of the several regions of the CNS grown in organotypic cultures, cerebellum offers the unique example of a highly geometric neuronal array, whose constituents and interactions have been extensively worked out "in situ" (reviewed in Palay and Chan-Palay, 1974). However, our goal was not to reproduce "in vitro" the "in situ" condition, which would have been a waste of time and money, but to examine the behavior of easily recognizable neurons in a modified environment. Indeed, in addition to the non-specific alteration involved in any tissue culture system, a slice of cerebellum from a newborn rat undergoes deprivation from the extraneous afferents, the climbing and mossy fibers. Our attention was focused at first on synaptogenesis, as we estimated that it was the most specific evidence of differentiation. And, as we knew that synapses were already present at the time of explantation in our cerebellar slices (Del Cerro and Snider, 1972), we looked for "de novo" synaptogenesis in the outgrowth zone readily constituted after explantation by the migration of external granule cells and the elongation

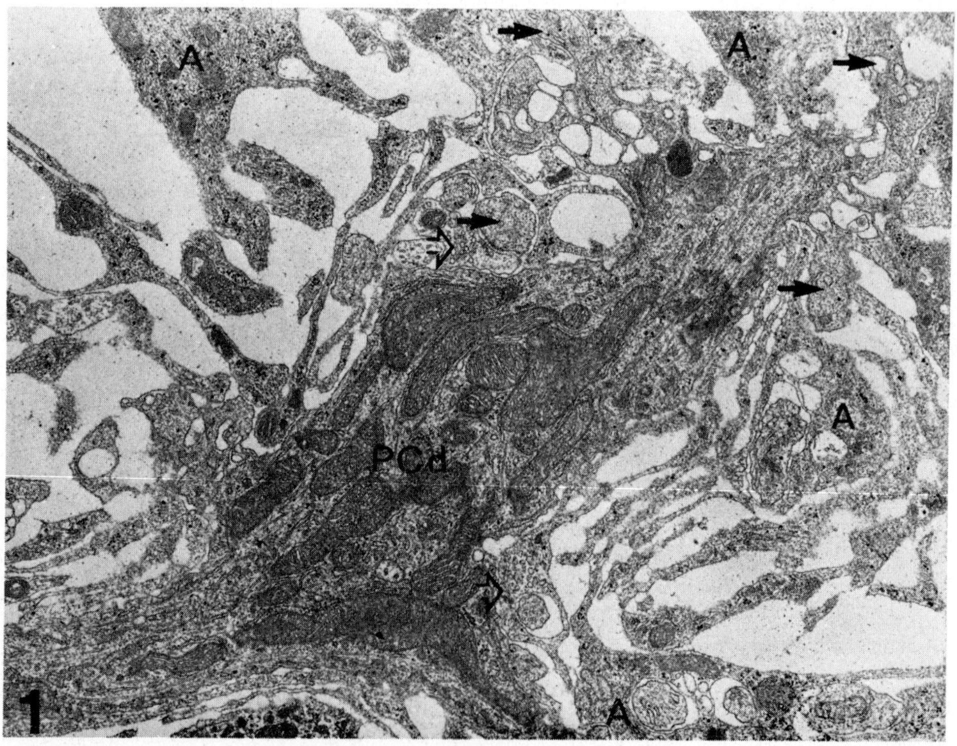

Fig. 1. Newborn rat cerebellum 10 days in vitro (DIV). In the outgrowth, a Purkinje cell dendrite (PCd) is surrounded by astrocyte processes filled with gliofilaments and glycogen (A). The dendritic growth cone, filled with mitochondria, is studded with spine-like appendages (arrows), some of which are contacted by axonal boutons (large arrows). × 21, 000.

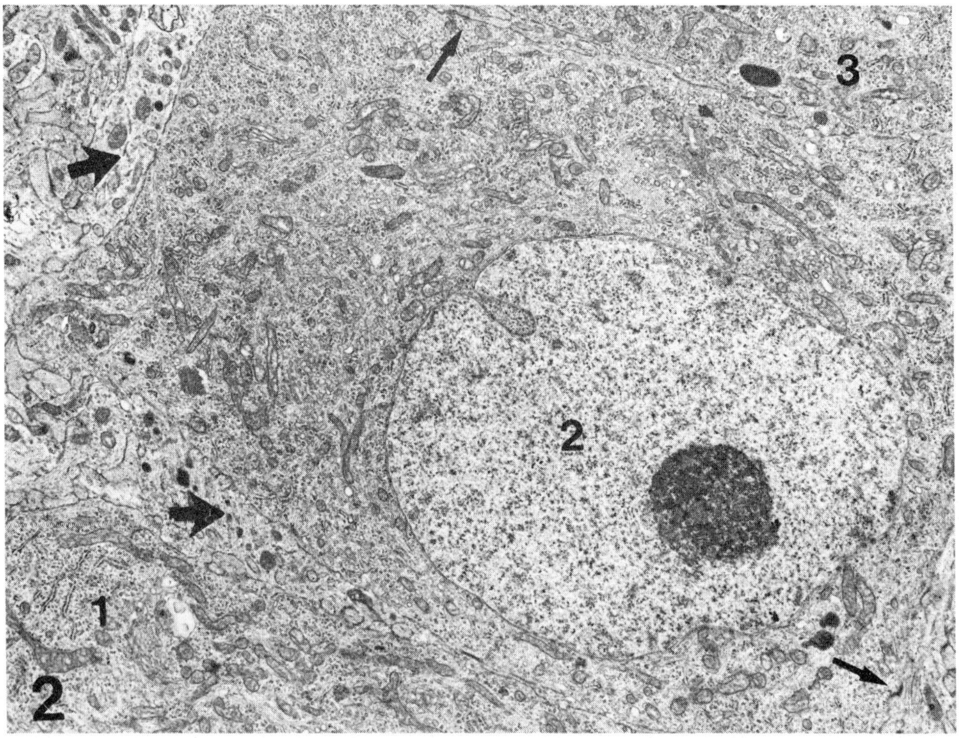

Fig. 2. Newborn rat cerebellum, 20 DIV. In the explant, 3 Purkinje cells (1, 2, 3) display the typical appearance of these cells in vitro, with somatic synapses of the "en passant" type (arrows) and abundance of somatic spines embedded in astrocyte cytoplasm (large arrows). × 8000.

of neurites whose parent cells remained in the explant (Privat et al., 1973). We found, as early as 48 hr after the explantation, membrane specializations suggestive of early synaptic interactions appearing, usually as postsynaptic membrane thickenings, with a densification of the extracellular space, and discrete (if any) presynaptic dense projections in the supposedly axonal neurite. Synaptic vesicles appeared slightly later, first sparsely, then in increasing number as the paramembranous densities acquired a mature appearance (Figs. 4 and 5). Axodendritic as well as axosomatic synapses were readily found, though the former appeared far more numerous. Worth noting was the fact that these early synapses were always found (Privat et al., 1974) on, or in the close vicinity of, growth cones, both on dendrites and axons (Fig. 1). This prompted us to a closer analysis of growth cone motility and behavior, which can best be analyzed in dissociated cultures, and will be dealt with in the corresponding paragraph.

Another issue arising from the study of this outgrowth was the migrating ability of the external granule cells, whose sliding along astrocyte fibers was analyzed in vivo by Rakic (1971). We found, in our in vitro conditions, that granule cells were also able to slide on bundles of neurites, which led us to the hypothesis that the apposition in-between migrating neuroblasts and radial glial fibers is merely a casual one, providing a low resistance pathway across a field of orthogonally directed fibers; moreover, freeze-fracture study of the migrating granule cell "in situ" has not disclosed any membrane specialization suggestive of active

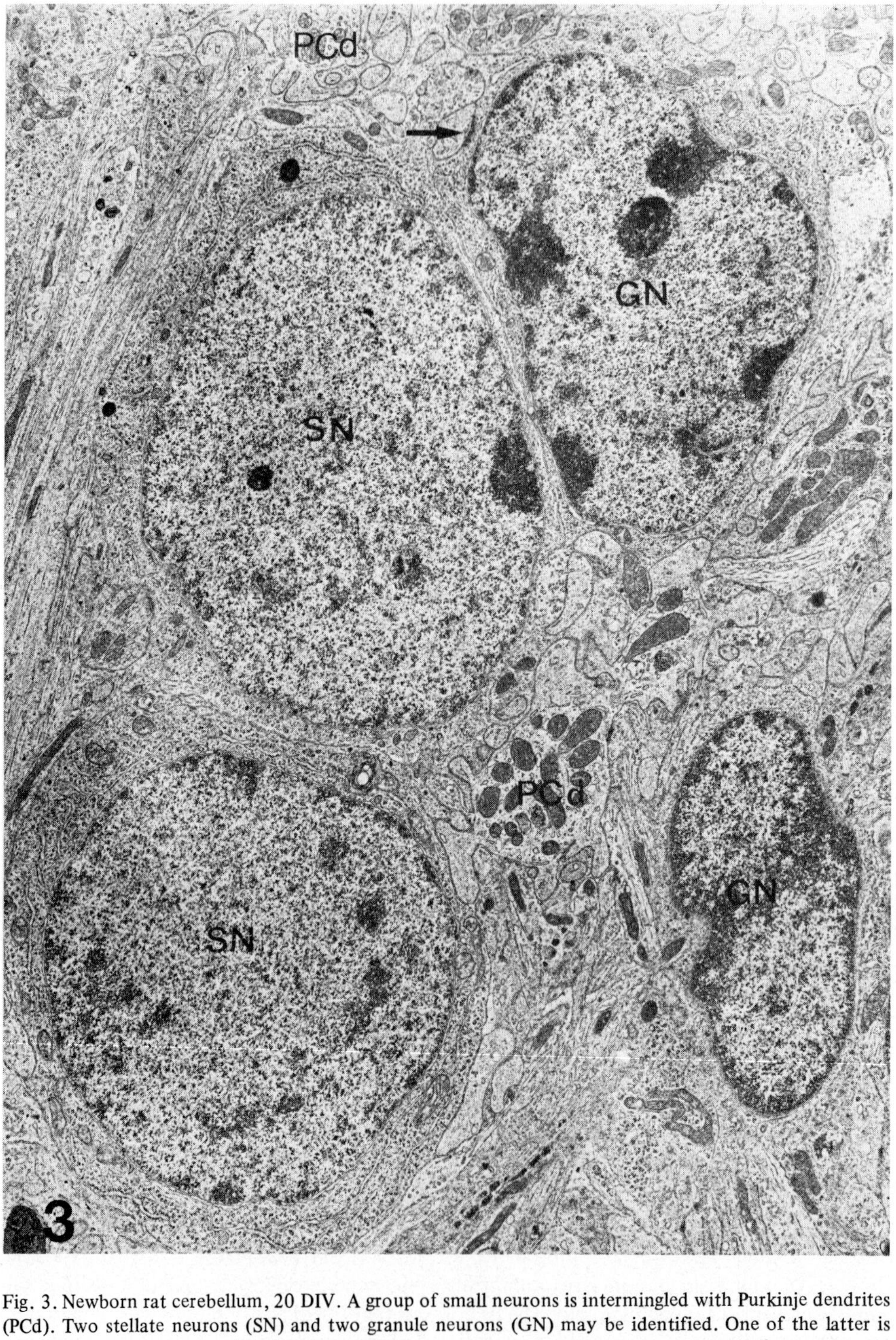

Fig. 3. Newborn rat cerebellum, 20 DIV. A group of small neurons is intermingled with Purkinje dendrites (PCd). Two stellate neurons (SN) and two granule neurons (GN) may be identified. One of the latter is presynaptic to a presumptive Purkinje spine (arrow). Many of these spines are devoid of synapses, and some bear isolated postsynaptic densities: notice the absence of glomeruli. × 10,500.

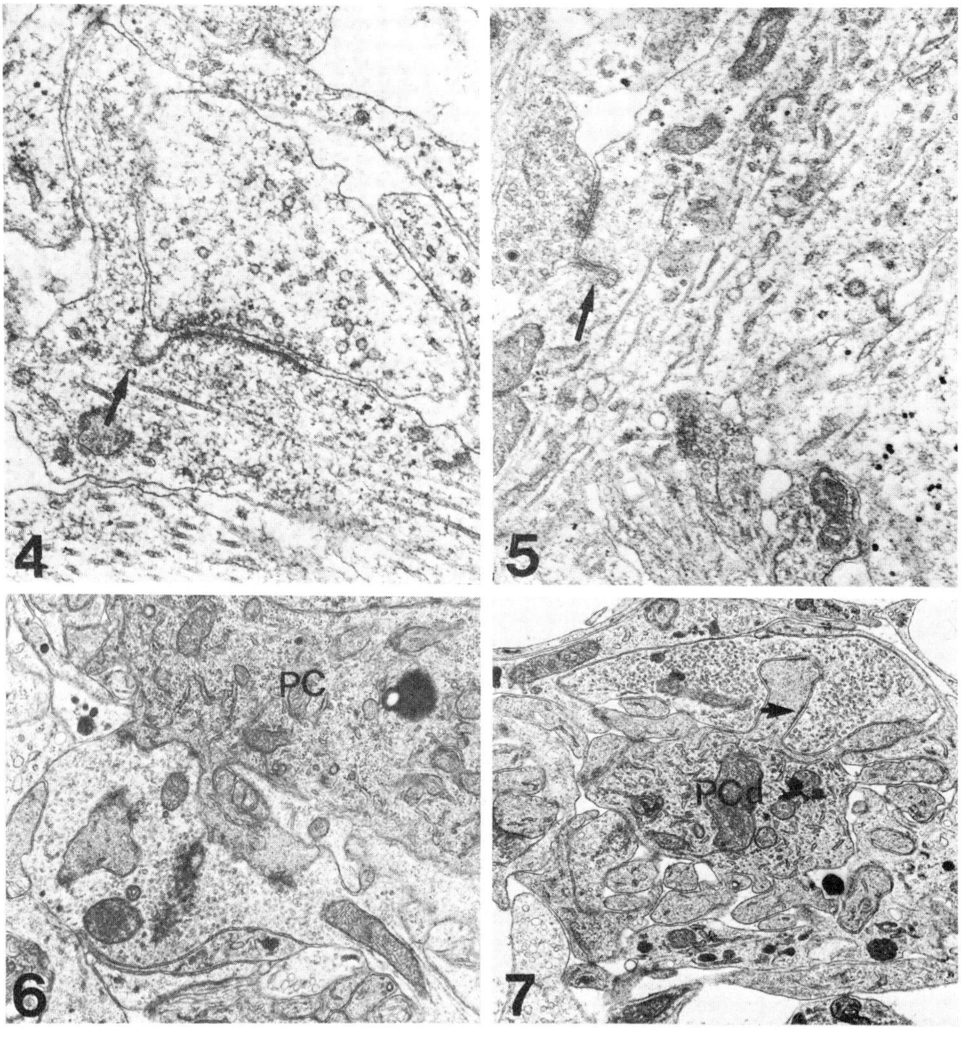

Fig. 4. Newborn rat cerebellum, 4 DIV. An immature synapse upon a small Purkinje dendrite is located close to a filopodium; an omega-shaped coated vesicle is in continuity with the postsynaptic thickening (arrow), a common feature of immature synapses. (From Privat and Drian, 1976.) × 40,000.

Fig. 5. Newborn rat cerebellum, 4 DIV. Synapse "en passant" on a large Purkinje dendrite, with an omega-shaped coated vesicle, similar to that of Fig. 4; this latter image is suggestive of membrane sequestration rather than membrane addition. (From Privat and Drian, 1976.) × 32,000.

Fig. 6. Newborn rat cerebellum, treated with MAM, 19 DIV. The somatic spines of a Purkinje cell (PC) are capped by a large bouton containing pleomorphic vesicles, tentatively identified as a Purkinje axon collateral. Such collaterals can arise from the same Purkinje cell (autapse) or from neighboring cells. × 18,000.

Fig. 7. Newborn rat cerebellum, treated with MAM, 20 DIV. A Purkinje cell dendrite (PCD) has several of its spines capped by a large bouton, similar with that of Fig. 6. Notice that one of the postsynaptic densities (arrow) is not facing an active zone of the bouton, suggesting a late occupation of previously formed postsynaptic sites. × 20,000.

interaction with neighboring cells and processes (Privat, in preparation). In addition, it has been shown in another system, the transmedial migration of oculomotor neuroblasts (Puelles and Privat, 1977), that astrocyte processes were absent along migrating neuroblasts.

We then focused our attention on the maturation of the Purkinje cells in various conditions of culture, in order to discriminate between the intrinsic program of the cell and the influence of the tissue milieu. In the "standard" cerebellar slice, as stated above, the cerebellum is deprived of its two extracerebellar afferents, the climbing and mossy fibers. It had been reported (Kornguth and Scott, 1972; Hamori, 1973) that climbing fibers were responsible for the elongation of the Purkinje dendrite. Our finding was that the elongation of the Purkinje cell dendrite occurred in our cultures, in the absence of climbing fibers, but the geometrical extension of spiny branchlets was missing (Privat, 1975) and the large dendritic trunks were studded with spines. Since the multiplication, survival and migration of granule cells are reduced in our conditions of culture, we estimated that parallel fibers could indeed be responsible for the geometrical growth of the Purkinje cell dendrite. Many synapses were found on the soma and dendrites of Purkinje cells (Fig. 2) and they generally mimicked their "in situ" counterpart: parallel fibers synapsed on spines, whereas stellate cells' axon boutons occupied preferentially the shafts, and basket axons the soma, together with a few recurrent collaterals of Purkinje axons. However, some spines remained unoccupied, due to the limited survival of granule cells in vitro, and a few of them nevertheless exhibited postsynaptic densities (Fig. 3). In order to test the point of postsynaptic differentiation in the absence of specific afferents, we devised a culture system devoid of granule cells, by the application of the drug MAM (methyl-azoxy-methanol), known to interfere with granule cell multiplication (Shimada and Langman, 1970). As a result, the outgrowth of the Purkinje cell dendritic tree was not inhibited, but it appeared more random than in the preceding condition, with many primary trunks stemming from the perikaryon. An unexpected finding was the presence, on the soma as well as on the dendrites, of many large axonal boutons tentatively identified as recurrent collaterals of the Purkinje axon (Figs. 6 and 7). The identity of these axons was later confirmed by Calvet et al. (1976) on the same material, with the use of intracellularly injected Procion yellow dye which showed a profusion of recurrent branches to the Purkinje cell and its neighbors. Thus, Purkinje cells behaved as if their vacant postsynaptic sites exerted an attraction upon the only axons present in the system and promoted the establishment of synapses. That these synapses were functional was shown by Calvet et al. (1974) who found a high order of electrical connectivity and inhibition between neighboring Purkinje cells in these cultures.

In order to test the specificity of the climbing fiber-Purkinje cell synapses, we devised another culture system, where the cerebellar plate and attached half pons and medulla were explanted altogether from 16–17-day embryos. We found that climbing fibers were growing in the cerebellum, and that they synapsed on the soma of Purkinje cells after 10 days in vitro, i.e., with the same timing as in situ. However, the somatic synapses were still present after 24 days in vitro, an observation at variance with the in situ condition. Some climbing boutons were, nevertheless, found on dendritic shafts, whose growth and architecture were not different from those found in the standard culture (Fig. 10).

From this series of experiments, we can propose that Purkinje cells have the intrinsic program for the growth of their dendrites and axons. In the absence of the oriented field of parallel fibers, dendritic growth is random, and proceeds by several primary trunks. It is likely that the initial dendritic outgrowth also occurs at random "in situ" (stage of "Capuchon" of Cajal), and that a resorption of spine-like appendages, precursors of dendrites, occurs everywhere but at the apex of the cell, where parallel fibers are present. Climbing

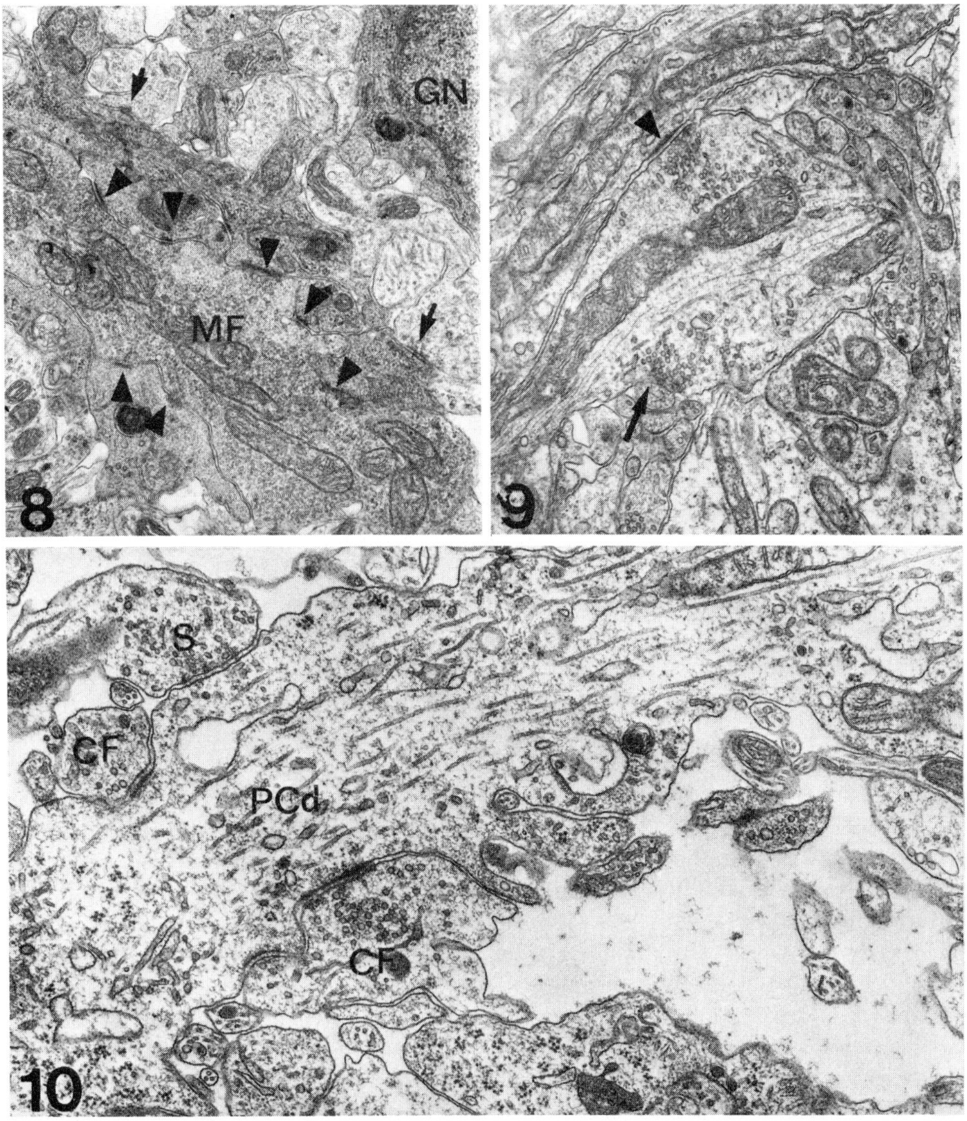

Figs. 8–10. Fetal rat cerebellum, with attached pons and medulla.

Fig. 8. 18 DIV. A mossy fiber is surrounded by granule cell dendritic claws, making a typical glomerulus. The arrowheads point to synaptic active zones; at the periphery of the glomerulus, Golgi II axons synapse upon granule cell dendrites (arrows). × 18,000.

Fig. 9. 15 DIV, treated with MAM. A mossy fiber (MF) synapse with a presumptive Purkinje cell spine (arrow), and with an unidentified dendrite; such heterologous synapses are found in agranular cerebella in vivo. × 21,000.

Fig. 10. 28 DIV. A Purkinje dendrite is contacted by a climbing fiber varicosity (CF) which makes a type I synapse. Close to it, a type II synapse is contributed by a stellate or recurrent basket bouton (S). × 24,000.

fibers synapsing upon the somatic spines are withdrawn from those spines which are spontaneously abortive, and follow in their course the apical ones which extend over the molecular layer, among parallel fibers. It may be speculated that the outgrowth of spiny branchlets is triggered and directed by the field of parallel fibers, which are prevented synapsing upon the main dendritic trunks by the presence of climbing fibers. Indeed, when the latter are absent few if any spiny branchlets are found and the parallel fibers synapse upon the profuse spines of the main trunk. This profusion of spines on the large trunks seems to be directly dependent upon the absence of climbing fibers, as, in an experimental system, Sotelo et al. (1975) have triggered the outgrowth of the supernumerary spines by removal of climbing fibers. Postsynaptic differentiations were found to arise in the absence of presynaptic axons, as already reported in agranular cerebella (Hirano and Dembitzer, 1973; Llinás et al., 1973), thus suggesting that the Purkinje cell is programmed for the production of synaptic receptors, in the absence of afferents. Here again, the number of sites and their geometry must be modulated by the afferent system.

For the Purkinje cell axon, it appears that the intense sprouting and profuse innervation found after treatment with MAM are concomitant with the presence of unoccupied synaptic sites on Purkinje cell dendrites. More than 50 years ago, Cajal pointed to the existence of numerous Purkinje cell axon collaterals at early stages of cerebellum morphogenesis, which later disappeared. It is likely that, together with a true sprouting, the absence of specific afferents on Purkinje cells have favored a survival of these supernumerary axons.

As to the biochemical aspect of Purkinje cell maturation, we have evidenced with high resolution radioautography the specific uptake of labeled GABA by Purkinje cells after 7 days in vitro (Sotelo et al., 1972; Privat, 1976). This ability to take up the putative neurotransmitter seems to be independent of the presence of the specific target, as it occurred even when cerebellar nuclei were absent from the explant.

Our next step in the study of cerebellar morphogenesis was to examine the formation of the cerebellar glomerulus "in vitro". In standard cultures, devoid of extracerebellar afferents, we have not seen any evidence of glomerular formation. However, several reports (Kim, 1971; Hendelman et al., 1977) questioned this issue. As a possible species difference was involved (mouse vs. rat), we cultivated some mouse cerebellum in the same conditions as our rat explants, and indeed we did find a few glomerular-like formations in some of the explants. This discrepancy with our results obtained with rat material may be explained by a somewhat different location of vestibular and other brain stem nuclei, which could be incorporated in mouse cerebellar explants.

In explants incorporating the cerebellar plate and the attached pons and medulla, obtained from 17-day rat fetuses, many glomeruli were formed around ingrowing mossy fibers (Fig. 8). The sequence was similar to that reported by Larramendi (1969) in situ, with the only difference being that, even after 1 month in vitro, their architecture remained relatively simple, without the complex intertwining described by Palay and Chan-Palay (1974).

When the cerebellar plate was separated from the pons-medulla by a scalpel cut at the time of explantation, and the two tissue blocks left to reaggregate at random, typical glomeruli were again found in all the cultures, suggesting that there exists a specificity in the mossy fiber-granule cell synapse. A similar phenomenon was found "in situ" by Chan-Palay (1972) for arrested granule cells in the molecular layer. However, when the drug MAM was incorporated into the medium of these complex cultures with the resulting absence of granule cells, some mossy fibers were seen synapsing directly upon Purkinje dendrites, as reported in agranular cerebella "in vivo" (Fig. 9).

(2) Dissociated cell cultures

In order to appreciate other parameters of growth and differentiation, we prepared cell suspensions by mechanical dissociation of 17th day cerebellar plates. These were plated onto collagen coated coverslips in the Maximov assembly.

As early as 24 hr after plating, cells were found to reaggregate into small clumps of spherical cells, devoid of processes. Rapidly thereafter, neurites grew out of these clumps, and after 4 days (Fig. 11) numerous bundles of neurites extended between the small

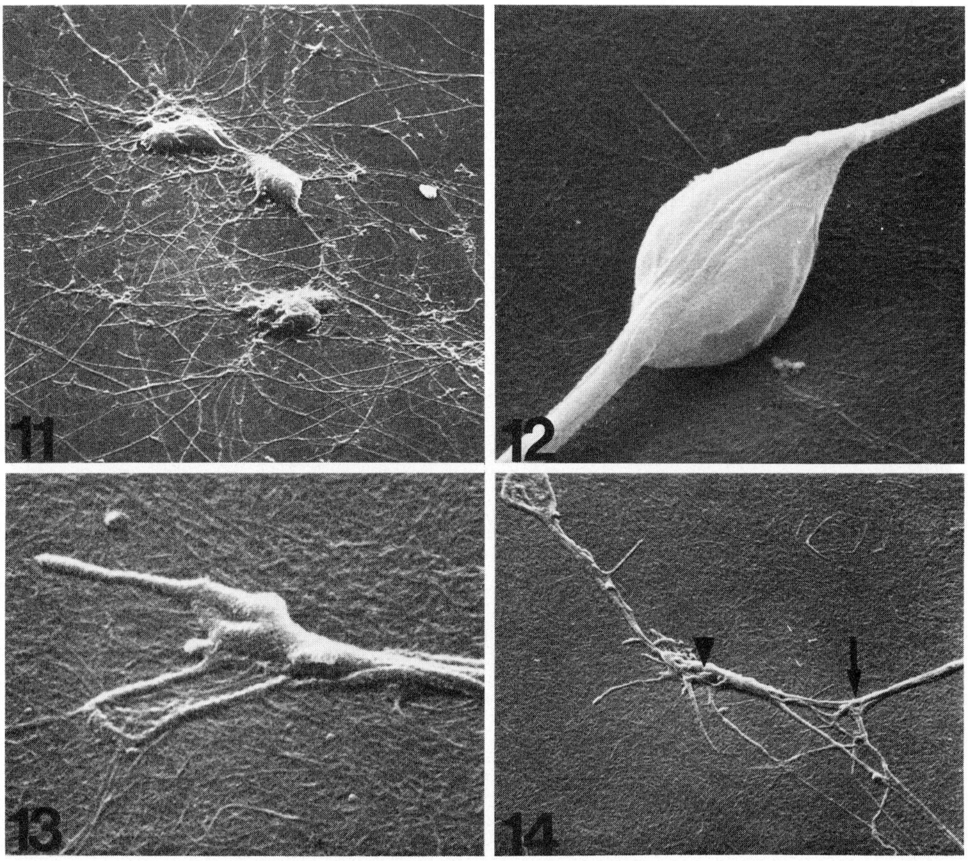

Figs. 11–14. Dissociated fetal cerebellum.

Fig. 11. 4 DIV. On this scanning electron micrograph, small clumps of cells are linked by a dense network of neurites. × 3200.

Fig. 12. 4 DIV. This migrating bipolar neuroblast, presumably a granule neuroblast, is sliding on a bundle of thin neurites. × 6500.

Fig. 13. 4 DIV. The tip of a bundle of neurites shows the varicosity of the growth cone (arrow), and attached filopodia. See for comparison the transmission EM picture of Fig. 15. × 25,000.

Fig. 14. 4 DIV. A bundle of neurites, at the right of the picture, bifurcates upon crossing another bundle (arrow). At the arrowhead is a growth cone whose filopodia extend on the crossed neurites. × 8000.

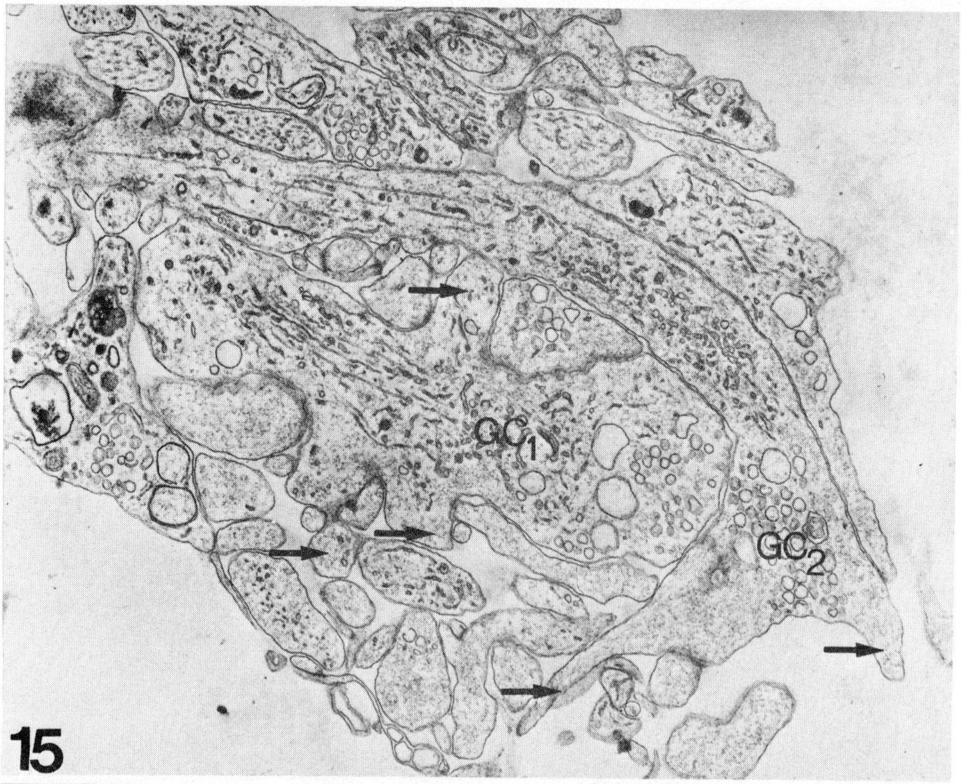

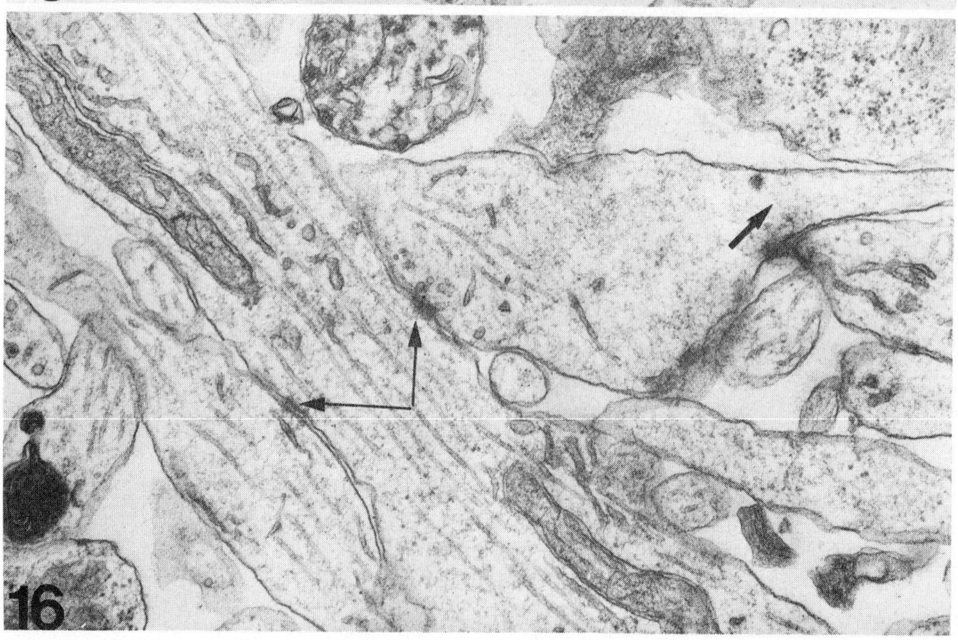

Figs. 15–16. Fetal dissociated cerebellum.

Fig. 15. 4 DIV. The tip of a bundle of neurites shows the typical appearance of two growth cones (GC1, GC2) with their large varicosity filled of vesicular and tubular membranes, their filopodia containing a filamentous matrix (arrows). × 20,000.

Fig. 16. 4 DIV. An incipient synapse is found in a small aggregate, the presynaptic neurite being endowed with a filopodium, as seen on growth cones. × 30,000.

aggregates. Then, bipolar cells migrated upon these bundles (Fig. 12) and progressively established a compact network of cells and processes over the whole coverslip.

Ultrastructural examination of aggregates and bundles of processes revealed a striking similarity with the outgrowth zones of organotypic cultures (Fig. 15). Synapses were found after 4 days of culture (Fig. 16), and granule as well as stellate/basket neurons were readily identified. However, despite careful examination, we were unable to identify safely a Purkinje cell. Some large, multipolar neurons were tentatively recognized as deep nuclear neurons, but none exhibited the typical perikaryon and dendrite of a Purkinje cell.

Time-lapse study of growth cone behavior of the profuse neurites (Figs. 13 and 14) revealed that filopodia are not only acting in promoting the elongation of neurites, but also in surface recognition. Two different behaviors were apparent upon inter-neuritic or neurite-soma encounter: following an initial, very short contact of one filopodium, there

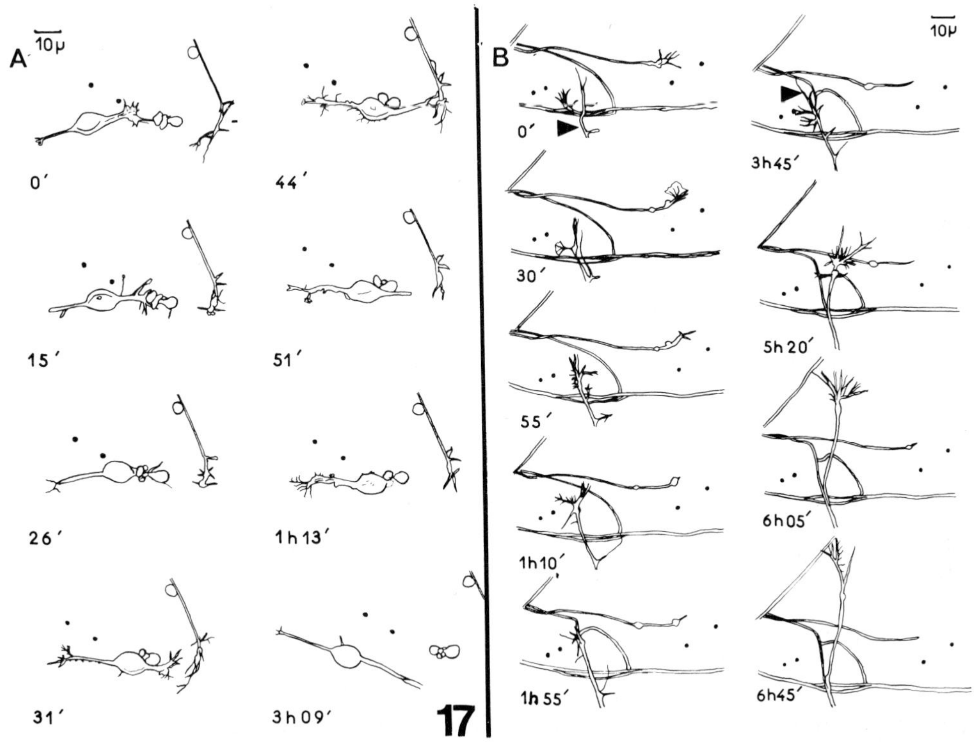

Fig. 17. Fetal dissociated cerebellum. These drawings are made from time lapse pictures illustrating the early interactions occurring between migrating cells and bundles of neurites 4 days after plating. Two examples have been selected which are supposed to be positive and negative recognition phenomena. A: this sequence shows an example of negative recognition. The bipolar cell at the left of the field emits a large process towards a bundle of neurites provided with a growth cone. The whole cell moves towards the right, and its growth cone contacts the bundle of neurites. Following intense palpation with filopodia, the growth cone is retracted, the cell moves back, and the tip of the bundle of neurites takes another direction. The duration of the whole process is 3 hr. B: this sequence shows an example of positive recognition. A bundle of neurites growing from the bottom of the field (arrowhead) crosses a field of horizontally directed neurites. After a protracted period of palpation with filopodia, it gives off a branch towards the left (3 hr 45 min), then the main bundle moves upwards and crosses another bundle of neurites (6 hr 45 min). When similar regions are then examined with electron microscopy, they very often show immature synapses such as those of Fig. 16.

follows either an extensive palpation by several filopodia and a spreading over the target (Fig. 17B), or a retraction of the whole neurite or bundle of neurites, and a further extension with marked angulation (Fig. 17A); following positive recognition by one neurite, several growth cones are often seen to proceed along the same pathway, and to spread over the presumptive target.

In summary, then, such cultures revealed the same order of events as seen in the outgrowth (Privat et al., 1974) (Figs. 4 and 5) and studied in greater detail by Rees et al. (1976). Work is now in progress to positively identify the cells and processes involved in these recognition phenomena and to correlate them with biochemical events.

(3) Prospective

Our studies of cerebellar morphogenesis "in vitro" have recently expanded into 3 directions:

In the first one, we tried to interfere specifically, by immunological techniques, with the maturation and synaptogenesis of Purkinje cells. Antibodies were raised by J. Mallet against Purkinje cells, and their specificity was tested by immunochemical and immunocytochemical techniques (Mallet et al., 1976). Purified immunoglobulins (IgG) were incorporated in the culture nutrient from the time of explantation onwards. Preliminary results seem to indicate that Purkinje cells react in two different ways: some of them undergo a progressive necrosis, starting from the Golgi apparatus and endoplasmic reticulum, whereas other remain apparently alive, however with stunted dendritic spines, and rarefaction of synapses. However, granule cells were also severely affected in most cases, and we were unable to decide if it was a direct toxic effect or an indirect one "en cascade" (Sotelo, 1975). We are now reproducing these experiments with antibodies previously reacted out on liver and forebrain membranes.

The second direction (explored in collaboration with B. Pessac), is the obtention of permanent cell lines, realized by transformation by SV40 viruses of cultivated dissociated cerebellar neurons. Previous attempts to obtain cloned nerve cells were performed irrespective of the nature of the original cell. We estimated that it was of paramount importance to have on hand cell lines which could be traced to the parent cell, as we can identify it in primary cultures. Several clones have been obtained, and they are presently characterized by morphological, biochemical and enzymological techniques. Clones of putative granule cells have been obtained from transformation of cultivated 11-day cerebellum and clones of larger cells, which may be either deep nuclei neurons or Purkinje cells, have been isolated from transformed 15-day fetal cerebellum.

In the third direction (in collaboration with I. Victorov), we have raised organotypic cultures from 3–4-day weaver mice cerebellum.

Previous work with dissociated cultures of weaver cerebellum yielded conflicting results, as Messer and Smith (1977) claimed a normal survival of granule cells in *Wv/Wv*, whereas Trenkner (cited in Wolf, 1977) evidenced a degeneration of granule cells in small aggregates, except when the serum was delipidated. Both works pointed to the absence of fiber bundles between cell clumps, and Wolf (1977) assumed that a deficiency of astrocytes was responsible for this absence of fibers.

In our work the whole litter, including at least 8 pups obtained from J. L. Guenet, Pasteur Institute, was used, half of each cerebellum being prepared for light and electron microscopy, respectively, in order to identify "a posteriori" the pups as *+/+*, *W/+* or *W/W*. Preliminary results indicate a poor survival of granule cells and a high incidence of myelinated perikarya of interneurons in *W/W*. Astrocytes were present and appeared similar with those of control cultures.

Our interpretation is that the *Wv*/mutation is directed to the granule cell rather than to the Bergmann astrocyte (Sotelo and Changeux, 1974). The absence of fiber bundles in dissociated cultures reported by Trenkner (cited in Wolf, 1977), could as well be secondary to the defect of elongation of granule cell neurites, which in the outgrowth zone of our explant cultures constitute the bulk of fiber bundles (Privat et al., 1973). Work is now in progress to analyze more specifically in co-cultures the ability of *WW* granule neurons to survive and migrate on a carpet of control astrocytes/fibroblasts.

(4) Conclusion

The cerebellum, then, appears a good choice for the "in vitro" study of the basic mechanisms of cell growth and connectivity. The main advantage of this structure is that all the cells and their connections have been extensively worked out "in vivo" (Palay and Chan-Palay, 1974), providing a solid morphological background which is a prerequisite for any culture study. The stereotyped, repetitive structure is another advantage, together with the well identified input and output of this "en dérivation" structure.

We can therefore "dissect" the intricate events of cerebellar morphogenesis by the use of simplified systems, where the influence of isolated parameters can best be studied. Thus, we could observe that each cell type is provided with an intrinsic program which, if it is not modulated by that of neighboring cells, would result in a structure very different from the "in vivo" condition; migration of granule cells, growth of the Purkinje dendrite, extension of mossy fibers are modulated by their tissue environment, and mutual affinity leading to synapse formation is one of these modulating elements.

These results are, up to now, essentially descriptive. Our hope is, through the new approaches listed above (prospective), to enter into the intimate mechanisms of these interactions.

RETINA

Dissociated cell cultures of chick neuroretina provide another interesting model for the study of neuronal differentiation and of synapse formation "in vitro". Chick neuroretina has already been extensively used for the analysis of cell aggregation mechanisms, and the maturation and differentiation of cell aggregates is well documented (Stefanelli et al., 1967; Sheffield and Moscona, 1970). Our own purpose was to describe the behavior of immature neuroretina cells plated as a monolayer.

Though remote from the brain, neuroretina is part of the central nervous system and, as with the cerebellum, its repetitive structure is fairly well understood (Dowling and Boycott, 1965). Moreover, chick embryo neuroretina can easily be dissected from other structures and, being avascular, is free of mesenchymal cells; at variance with the cerebellum the retina receives little, if any, afferent innervation, so that one can imagine that its initial organization and differentiation is more largely governed by an intrinsic program.

After gentle dissociation with trypsin, cells suspended in PBS appear as single cells or tiny clumps. They rapidly settle on the bottom of the petri dish, and after 2 days processes begin to grow and to connect small groups of cells.

After 4 days two types of cells are evident: large cells flattened upon the substrate show, under the electron microscope, bundles of filaments and tubules, and are linked by attachment plates; smaller, spherical cells, emit long and rectilinear processes, containing microtubules.

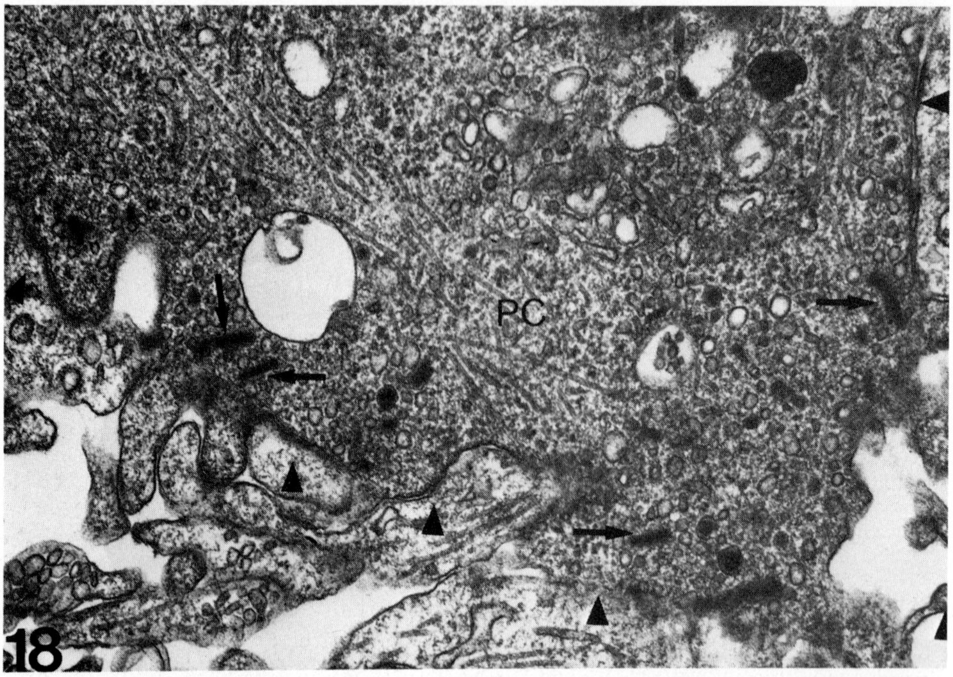

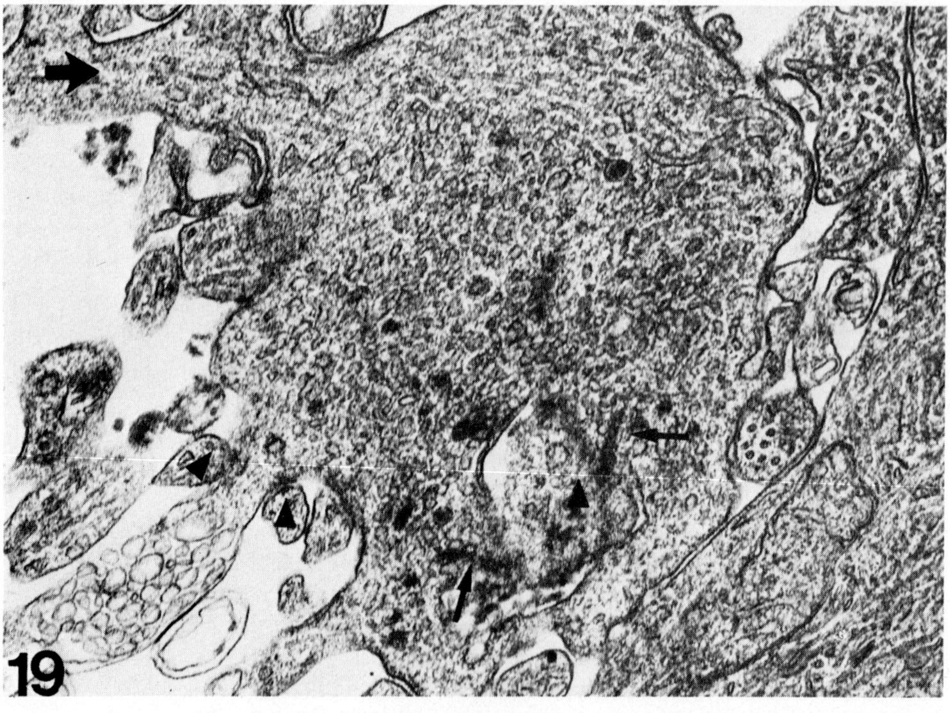

Figs. 18–19. Seven days dissociated chick embryo neuroretina.

Fig. 18. 8 DIV. Portion of a photoreceptor (PC) shows several synaptic ribbons (arrows), surrounded by vesicles, and facing light profiles of presumptive bipolar and horizontal cells. At the arrowheads are the active zones of the synapses. × 36,000.

Fig. 19. 21 DIV. In a region of neuropile reminiscent of the inner plexiform layer, a thin process (large arrow) ends up as a varicosity containing a few ribbons (small arrows), and numerous vesicles facing light profiles (arrowheads); this varicosity may correspond to a bipolar cell ending. × 60,000.

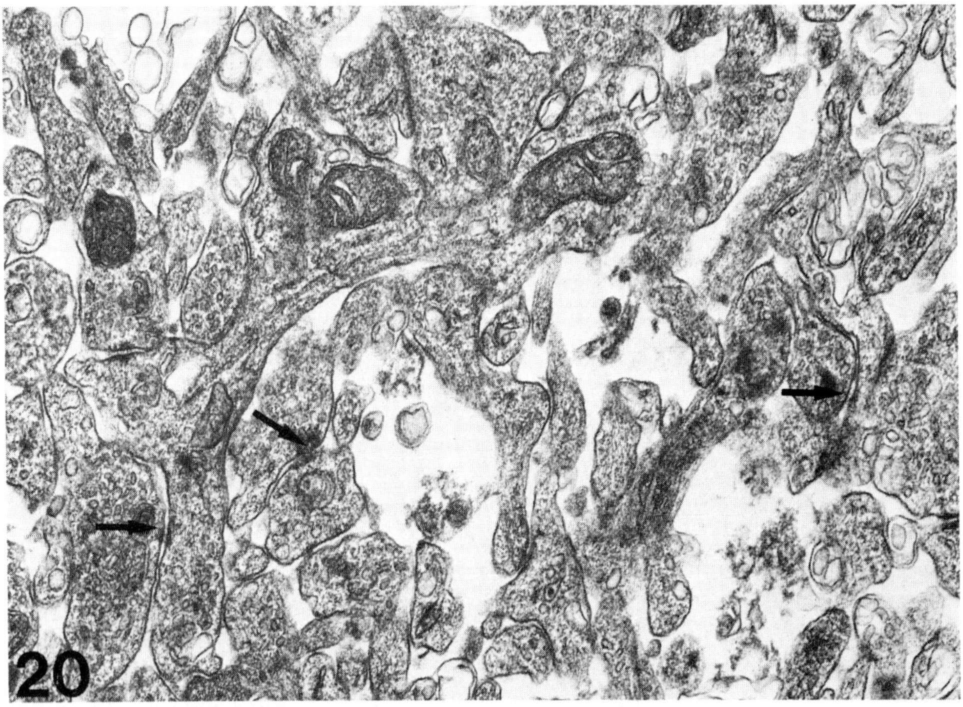

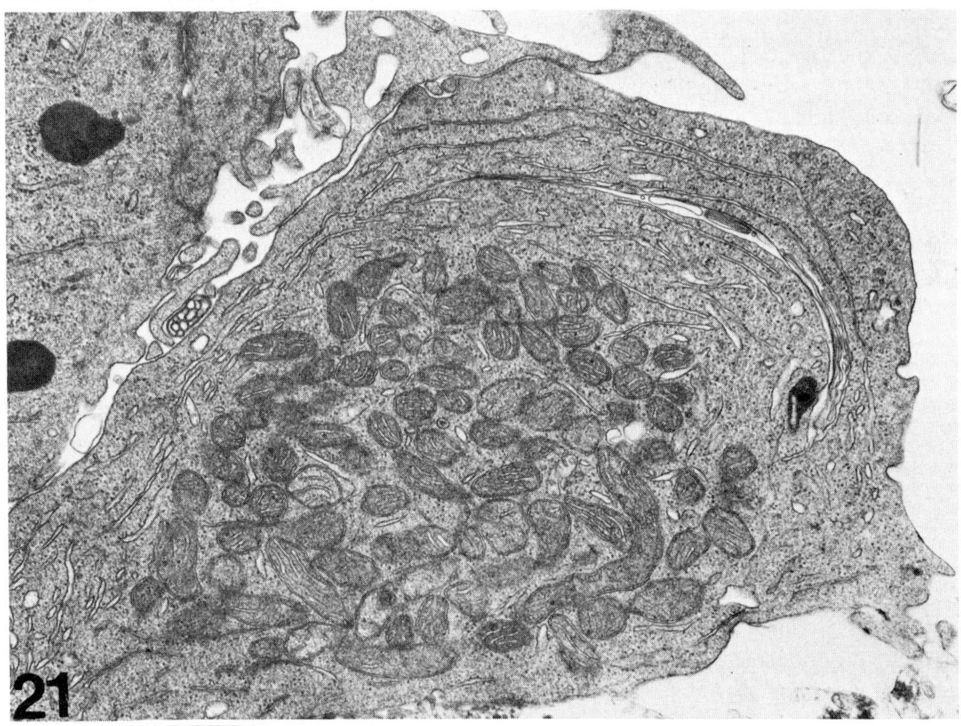

Figs. 20–21. Chick neuroretina.

Fig. 20. Cell culture, 21 DIV. Regions of neuropile enclosed in small cell clumps are reminiscent of plexiform layers, with a complex meshwork of processes and synapses (arrows). × 48,000.

Fig. 21. Organ culture, 18 DIV. A rudimentary outer segment of photoreceptor is seen budding from the external limiting membrane. × 20,000.

After 8 days, photoreceptors may be identified on the presence of synaptic ribbons. However, triads are rare, the postsynaptic elements appearing as small profiles clumped in the vicinity of the ribbon (Fig. 18).

Areas of neuropile are frequently enclosed within a group of cells. There may be found all kinds of synapses normally present in the inner plexiform layer (Figs. 19 and 20). The bottom of the dish is now covered with a continuous layer of flattened cells, which we tentatively identify as Müller cells. After a longer time "in vitro" (15, 20 days), the number of synapses increases, and most of the cells now have a mature appearance. However, their identification is more difficult than those of the cerebellum, and we only tentatively identified a few ganglion cells.

A parallel biochemical study (Crisanti Combes et al., 1978) has shown by the measurement of choline acetyltransferase activity, a simultaneous maturation of the cholinergic system.

Moreover, it was found that the timing of both morphological and biochemical landmarks of maturation were similar "in vitro" to those found "in situ" (Crisanti Combes et al., 1977, 1978). However, besides quantitative data which cannot be easily appreciated "in vitro", some qualitative differences were evident: the outer segments of photoreceptors did not differentiate in our cultures, and various attempts to obtain this maturation in other culture systems were largely unsuccessful. Only in organ cultures of retina that were maintained in agitation in Erlenmeyer flasks could we find rudimentary outer segments consisting of a bulbous expansion containing crowded mitochondria and stacked membrane (Fig. 21). Similarly, the survival and differentiation of ganglion cells appeared rather limited in our cultures.

Nevertheless, it appears that, despite the disruption of all pre-existing anatomical relationships, neurons of the retina are able to differentiate both morphologically and biochemically, and to establish synapses qualitatively similar to those prevailing "in situ". Moreover, the timing of this differentiation is strictly scheduled, as testified to by the day of appearance of synaptic complexes on the one hand, and the enzymatic machinery of cholinergic transmission on the other. Experiments are in progress with co-cultures of mouse retina and lateral geniculate body to study the specificity of the retinogeniculate projections "in vitro" and to evaluate an eventual feedback effect on retinal differentiation of this projection.

In addition, the finding that retinal cells showed a large degree of intrinsic program for their differentiation prompted us (in collaboration with B. Pessac) to try to obtain permanent cell lines by viral transformation. Preliminary attempts (Pessac et al., in preparation) allowed the obtention of several permanent cell lines, some of which showed high activities of choline acetyltransferase and of glutamic acid decarboxylase coincident with some morphological evidence of neuronal differentiation.

In conclusion, then, cultures of neuroretina appear to be a powerful tool for the study of cell differentiation and connectivity, besides the basic problems of cell adhesion, for which they have been a choice material for many years. They are complementary to cerebellar cultures, as the main problem here is the organization of the efferents, whereas that of the cerebellum is the integration of afferents.

HYPOTHALAMUS

The third and last model we would like to discuss in this review is the organotypic culture of hypothalamus. It is our opinion that this can provide the best tool for the study of the differentiation of the secretory function of the neuron. Magnocellular neurosecretory neurons of the hypothalamus differ from other neurons by the exacerbation of synthesis and release mechanisms, and the relative simplification of other characteristics, such as the multiplicity of afferents and efferents. Moreover, the relative ease of assay of synthetized and released neurophysins, oxytocin and vasopressin "in vitro" may help in the analysis of the response of various receptors to various stimuli.

The first question we addressed this system to was the ability of neurosecretory neurons to differentiate in the absence of a specific target or feedback stimulus. Therefore, pieces of hypothalamus including either the supraoptic or the paraventricular nucleus were explanted from 40-day guinea-pig embryos, where it has been demonstrated (Pearson et al., 1975; Silverman, 1975) that synthesis of neurophysins and peptides is not detectable. At this stage, in the anlage of neurosecretory nuclei, the neurons appear poorly differentiated, with a restricted Golgi zone, no neurosecretory granule and no axosomatic afferent synapse. After 10 days in vitro afferent synapses are found, and after 15 days neurosecretory granules are

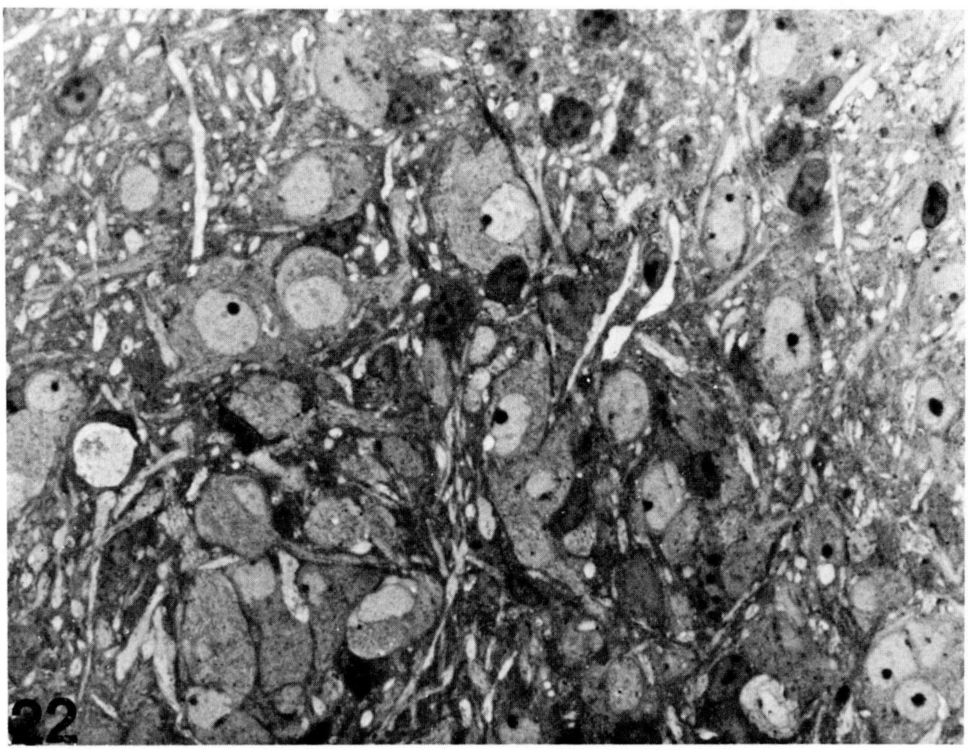

Figs. 22–23. Fetal guinea-pig hypothalamus.

Fig. 22. 40 DIV. In this I section, a group of magnocellular neurons is easily identified upon the size of the cells, the large light nucleus often eccentrically located, the prominent nucleolus, the frequence of astrocyte satellites. × 1000.

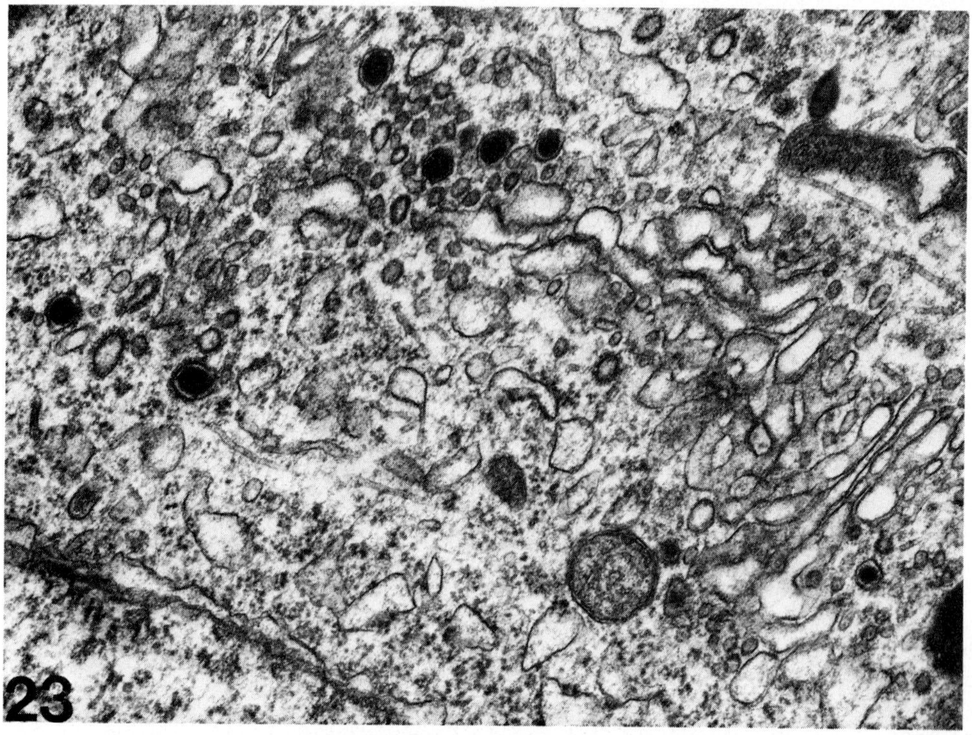

Fig. 23. 40 DIV. Detail of a magnocellular neuron showing the well developed Golgi zone, with several dense-core granules, 100–170 nm in diameter. × 50,000.

present in the Golgi region. After 40 days in vitro (Fig. 22) the neurons have a mature appearance, with a large perikaryon, a spherical nucleus with a prominent nucleolus, abundance of organelles and a variable amount of neurosecretory granules (Fig. 23). They bear numerous afferent synapses, and the neuropile contains, besides conventional synapses, axo-axonic ones where the postsynaptic element is a neurosecretory axon containing typical granules. Many profiles in the neuropile contain neurosecretory granules, but these profiles have not been found to occupy a preferential location in the explant. This preliminary work thus indicates, on morphological grounds, that, as well as being "classical" neurons, neurosecretory cells have in the intrinsic program for differentiation of their main function, neurosecretion, and that it can be maintained for long periods "in vitro". Work is now in progress to evaluate with radioimmunoassays the quantitative aspects of synthesis and release, and their variation under the influence of various stimuli. In addition, the existence in this culture system of cholinergic and GABAergic afferents to magnocellular neurons is being investigated by specific uptake of labeled transmitters.

Finally, there exists more and more evidence that hypothalamic peptides could act as classical neurotransmitters in several brain regions (Buijs, 1978). Co-cultures of hypothalamus with various systems could provide some insight into these hypothetical functions.

GENERAL CONCLUSIONS

The purpose of this review was to attempt to delineate, through several culture systems used in our laboratory, the possibilities and the limitations of our approach towards the understanding of the principles of neuronal organization.

Starting with an essentially morphological approach, we have been able to show that there exists a high degree of specificity in the establishment of neural connections, but that this specificity is not an absolute one, and we proposed that there might be a gradient of affinity between different pre- and postsynaptic elements (Privat and Drian, 1976).

Moreover, the precise geometry of the cells and their processes depends upon the orderly interaction of the different elements, each of them being a depository of a rudimentary program (maximal extent of growth, and perhaps maximal number of receptor or effector sites) which is modulated by those of the afferents and efferents. These interactions may be positive as well as negative; one can imagine that a contact and a positive recognition (Fig. 17) may trigger further growth and further contacts, whereas the absence of recognition may trigger a retraction, and eventually, after several negative experiments, the degeneration of a supernumerary process. The poor survival of ganglion cells in neuroretina cultures might be the expression of such an absence of recognition (McLoon and Hughes, 1978), whereas the apparent sprouting of Purkinje cell axon collaterals in MAM-treated cerebellum would result from an absence of repression by climbing and parallel fibers.

Regarding the chemical specificity of cell differentiation, i.e., essentially the neurotransmitter synthesis and release, all the indirect evidence we have obtained by uptake experiments and measurements of enzyme activities points to the feeling that the synthesis of neurotransmitter is part of the intrinsic program of the central neuron, which would then differ from those of the PNS (see Patterson, this volume). An alternative explanation, however, could be that our conditions of culture do not realize a state of isolation which allows the cells to express other potentialities. More work is certainly needed to obtain clear evidence on this point, but here we are limited by the poor differentiation and survival of isolated CNS neurons. The use of permanent cell lines (Pessac et al., 1978) will certainly allow further progress in this direction. Similarly, permanent cell lines could provide further insight into the intimate mechanisms of cell recognition, for which we have obtained only descriptive data. If we know that growth cones are actively involved in this process (Pfenninger and Rees, 1975; Bunge et al., 1977) and that actual contact is needed (Fig. 17), the absence of specific intramembranous structures, as seen on freeze-fractures (Pfenninger and Bunge, 1974), suggests the involvement of cell coat components in cell recognition (Pfenninger and Maylié-Pfenninger, this volume). Cell recognition and synaptogenesis appear closely related, chronologically and spatially, as synapses are first seen in the close vicinity of growth cones (Privat et al., 1974; Vaughn and Grieshaber, 1974). Whether or not the neurotransmitters are involved in this process is still an enigma, though static ultrastructural data would suggest a relatively late involvement, at least for their vesicular component. The use of antibodies directed specifically against synaptic sites will possibly resolve some of these points (Mallet et al., in preparation).

As for the functional aspect of neuronal activity, as can be explored by electrophysiological techniques, it also appears specific for a given cell type (Calvet, 1976; Gähwiler and Dreifuss, this volume), the "in situ" recorded activity being really the result of the modulation by various afferents of the basic intrinsic activity of the cell which can be recorded "in vitro", as well as the geometric growth of the Purkinje dendrite being the result of the influence of parallel and climbing fibers on the intrinsic program for the growth of the dendrite.

Finally, in the great debate about nature and nurture in CNS organization, it is worth noting that all our studies apply to only one level of organization, that of the initial wiring of brain circuitry, upon which may be superimposed "in vivo" the subtle imprinting of the environment. At this basic level of initial wiring, the genetic program seems to prevail, through the complex and orderly interaction of the cells and their processes, each of which is coded for a limited program. However, even at this level, tissue culture techniques cannot answer all of the questions, and the results obtained by these techniques must be compared with those using other approaches, "in situ" (Privat, 1978; Sotelo and Privat, 1978) or "in vitro" (Llinás and Sugimori, this symposium).

ACKNOWLEDGMENTS

The authors acknowledge the help and advice of Drs. J. E. Gruner, B. Pessac, J. Mallet and M. C. Calvet.

This work was supported by INSERM Grant No. 29-76-61 and D.G.R.S.T.

REFERENCES

Buijs, R. M. (1978) Intra- and extrahypothalamic vasopressin and oxytocin pathways in the rat. *Cell Tiss. Res.*, 192: 423–435.

Bunge, R., Johnson, M. and Ross, C. D. (1978) Nature and nurture in development of the autonomic neuron. *Science*, 199: 1409–1416.

Calvet, M. C., Drian, M. J. and Privat, A. (1974) Spontaneous electrical patterns in cultured Purkinje cells grown with an antimitotic agent. *Brain Res.*, 79: 285–290.

Calvet, M. C., Lepault, A. M. and Calvet, J. (1976) A Procion yellow study of cultured Purkinje cells. *Brain Res.*, 111: 399–406.

Chan-Palay, V. (1972) Arrested granule cells and their synapses with mossy fibers in the molecular layer of the cerebellar cortex. *Z. Anat. Entwickl.-Gesch.*, 139: 11–20.

Crisanti Combes, P., Privat, A., Pessac, B. and Calothy, G. (1977) Differentiation of chick embryo neuroretina cells in monolayer cultures. An ultrastructural study. *Cell Tiss. Res.*, 185: 159–173.

Crisanti Combes, P., Pessac, B. and Calothy, G. (1978) Choline acetyltransferase in chick embryo neuroretinas during development "in ovo" and in monolayer culture. *Develop. Biol.*, 65: 228–232.

Del Cerro, M. P. and Snider, R. S. (1972) Axo-somatic and axo-dendritic synapses in the cerebellum of the newborn rat. *Brain Res.*, 54: 581–586.

Dowling, J. and Boycott, B. (1965) Neural connections of the retina: fine structure of the inner plexiform layer. *Cold Spr. Harb. Symp. quant. Biol.*, 30: 393–402.

Hamori, J. (1973) Developmental morphology of dendritic postsynaptic specializations. In *Recent Developments of Neurobiology in Hungary*, Akademiai Kiado, Budapest, pp. 9–32.

Hendelman, W. J., Marshall, K. C., Aggerwal, A. S. and Wojtowicz, J. M. (1977) Organization of pathways in cultures of mouse cerebellum. In: *Cell, Tissue and Organ Culture in Neurobiology*, S. Fedoroff and L. Hertz (Eds.), Academic Press, New York, pp. 539–554.

Hirano, A. and Dembitzer, H. M. (1973) Cerebeller alterations in the Weaver mouse. *J. Cell Biol.*, 56: 478–486.

Kim, S. U. (1971) Electron microscope study of mouse cerebellum in tissue culture. *Exp. Neurol.*, 33: 30–44.

Kornguth, S. E. and Scott, G. (1972) The role of climbing fibers in the formation of Purkinje cell dendrites. *J. comp. Neurol.*, 146: 61–82.

Larramendi, L. M. H. (1969) Analysis of synaptogenesis in the cerebellum of the mouse. In *Neurobiology of Cerebellar Evolution and Development*, R. Llinás (Ed.), Amer. Med. Ass., Chicago, Ill., pp. 803–843.

Llinás, R., Hillman, D. E. and Precht, W. (1973) Neuronal circuit reorganization in mammalian cerebellar cortex. *J. Neurobiol.*, 4: 69–94.

Mallet, J., Pougeois, R., Huchet, M. and Changeux, J.-P. (1976) Anatomical, physiological, and biochemical studies on the cerebellum of mutant mice. III. Protein differences associated with the weaver, staggerer and nervous mutations. *Brain Res.*, 103: 291–312.

McLoon, S. and Hughes, W. F. (1978) Ganglion cell death during retinal development in chick eyes explanted to the chorioallantoic membrane. *Brain Res.*, 150: 398–402.

Messer, A. and Smith, D. M. (1977) In vitro behavior of granule cells from Staggerer and Weaver mutant mice. *Brain Res.*, 130: 13–23.

Murray, M. (1965) Nervous tissues in vitro. In *Cells and Tissues in Culture*, E. N. Willmer (Ed.), Academic Press, New York, pp. 373–455.

Palay, S. L. and Chan-Palay, V. (1974) *Cerebellar Cortex. Cytology and Organization.* Springer, Berlin.

Pearson, D. R., Goodman, R. and Sachs, H. (1975) The fetal guineapig hypothalamo-neurohypophysial complex in organ culture: presence of a stimulatory factor for vasopressin and neurophysin biosynthesis. *Science*, 187: 1081–1082.

Pessac, B., Alliot, F., Girard, A., Combes, P., Guerinot, F., Drian, M. J. and Privat, A. (1978) Properties of mouse cerebellum cells transformed by SV 40. *Neurosci. Lett.*, Suppl. 1: F39.

Pfenninger, K. H. and Bunge, R. (1974) Freeze-fracturing of nerve growth cones and fibers. A study of developing plasma membrane. *J. Cell Biol.*, 63: 180–196.

Pfenninger, K. H. and Rees, R. P. (1975) From the growth cone to the synapse. In *Neuronal Recognition*, S. Barondes (Ed.), Chapman and Hall, London, pp. 131–178.

Privat, A. (1975) Dendritic growth "in vitro". In *Advances in Neurology, Vol. 12*, G. W. Kreutzberg (Ed.), Raven Press, New York, pp. 201–216.

Privat, A. (1976) High resolution radioautographic localization of GABA. A critical study. *J. microsc. Biol. Cell.*, 27: 253–256.

Privat, A. (1978) Dendro-dendritic pentalaminar junctions in the Weaver mouse cerebellum. *Acta neuropath. (Berl.)*, 42: 137–140.

Privat, A. and Drian, M. J. (1976) Postnatal maturation of rat Purkinje cells cultivated in the absence of two afferent systems: an ultrastructural study. *J. comp. Neurol.*, 166: 201–244.

Privat, A., Brian, M. J. and Mandon, P. (1973) The outgrowth of rat cerebellum in organized culture. *Z. Zellforsch.*, 146: 45–67.

Privat, A., Drian, M. J. and Mandon, P. (1974) Synaptogenesis in the outgrowth of rat cerebellum in organized culture. *J. comp. Neurol.*, 153: 291–308.

Puelles, L. and Privat, A. (1977) Do oculomotor neuroblasts migrate across the midline in the fetal rat brain. *Anat. Embryol.*, 150: 187–206.

Rakic, P. (1971) Neuron-glia relationship during granule cell migration in developing cerebellar cortex. A Golgi and electronmicroscopic study in *Macacus rhesus*. *J. comp. Neurol.*, 153: 291–308.

Rees, R. P., Bunge, M. B. and Bunge, R. P. (1976) Morphological changes in the neuritic growth cone and target neuron during synaptic junction development in culture. *J. Cell Biol.*, 68: 240–263.

Sheffield, J. B. and Moscona, A. A. (1970) Electron microscopic analysis of aggregation of embryonic cells: the structure and differentiation of aggregates of neural retina cells. *Develop. Biol.*, 23: 36–61.

Shimada, M. and Langman, J. (1970) Repair of the external granular layer after postnatal treatment with 5-fluorodeoxyuridine. *Amer. J. Anat.*, 129: 247–260.

Silverman, A. J. (1975) The hypothalamic magnocellular neurosecretory system of the guinea pig. II. Immunohistochemical localization of neurophysin and vasopressin in the fetus. *Amer. J. Anat.*, 144: 445–460.

Stefanelli, A., Zacchei, A. M., Caravita, S., Cataldi, A. and Ieradi, L. A. (1967) New forming retinal synapses "in vitro". *Experientia (Basel)*, 23: 199–200.

Sotelo, C. (1975) Synaptic remodeling in mutants and experimental animals. In *Aspects of Neuronal Plasticity*, F. Vital-Durand and M. Jeannerod (Eds.), INSERM, Paris, pp. 167–190.

Sotelo, C. and Changeux, J. P. (1974) Bergmann fibers and granular cell migration in the cerebellum of homozygous weaver mutant mouse. *Brain Res.*, 77: 484–491.

Sotelo, C. and Privat, A. (1978) Synaptic remodeling of cerebellar circuitry in mutant mice and experimental cerebellar malformations. Study "in vivo and in vitro". *Acta neuropath. (Berl.)*, 43: 19–34.

Sotelo, C., Privat, A. and Drian, M. J. (1972) Localization of tritiated GABA in tissue culture of rat cerebellum using electron microscope radioautography. *Brain Res.*, 45: 302–308.

Sotelo, C., Hillman, D. E., Zamora, A. J. and Llinás, R. (1975) Climbing fiber deafferentation: its action on Purkinje cell dendritic spines. *Brain Res.*, 98: 574–581.

Vaughn, J. E., Henrikson, C. R. and Grieshaber, J. A. (1974) A quantitative study of synapses in motor neuron dendrite growth cones in developing spinal cord. *J. Cell Biol.*, 60: 664–672.

Vrensen, G. (1978) Ontogenesis of the visual cortex of rabbits and the effects of visual deprivation. In *Maturation of the Nervous System, Progress in Brain Research, Vol. 48,* M. A. Corner, R. E. Baker, N. E. Van de Poll, D. F. Swaab and H. B. M. Uylings (Eds.), Elsevier, Amsterdam, pp. 231–244.

Wolf, M. K. (1977) Cell and organotypic culture studies of neurological mutations affecting structural development. In *Cell, Tissue and Organ Culture in Neurobiology,* S. Fedoroff and L. Hertz (Eds.), Academic Press, New York, pp. 555–572.

Cerebellum: Certain Features of its Development and Biochemistry

R. BALÁZS

MRC Developmental Neurobiology Unit, Institute of Neurology, 33 John's Mews, London WC1N 2NS (Great Britain)

INTRODUCTION

The cerebellum offers many advantages for studying the biochemical properties of specific neural structures: knowledge of the morphology and physiology of the cerebellum is relatively advanced (Eccles et al., 1967; Palay and Chan-Palay, 1974) and certain characteristics of the cerebellar architecture facilitate the isolation of specific neuronal structures in a pure state. With respect to developmental studies, in addition, important experimental advantages include the great wealth of ontogenetic information and the timing of cerebellar development which takes place to a great extent after birth in many species (e.g., in the rat mainly considered here and also in humans) (for reviews see, e.g., various chapters in Llinás, 1969; Altman, 1969, 1972; Balázs et al., 1978b). This gives a unique opportunity to study the influence of non-genetic factors on neurogenesis and on the establishment of neuronal interconnections under conditions when the powerful mechanisms counteracting metabolic imbalance, functional in the pregnant animal, are not yet fully developed.

CELL ACQUISITION IN THE POSTNATAL RAT CEREBELLUM

At first I will consider certain aspects of cell acquisition in the cerebellum and the influence of metabolic imbalance on this process. I will rely heavily on our own results, and I am indebted to the important contribution of my colleagues, especially to Drs. A. J. Patel from our Unit and P. D. Lewis from Hammersmith Hospital.

Fig. 1 underlines the usefulness of the cerebellum in developmental studies. In the rat, only 3% of the final cell number is present at birth and in man this value is about 17% (Dobbing and Sands, 1973). Since neurones constitute about one-half of the total cell number, extensive neurogenesis must occur in the cerebellum during the postnatal period. This conclusion is also valid for man; it has been shown that the germinal site from which most of the cerebellar interneurones are generated, the external granular layer (EGL), is present till about 1.5 years after birth (Larroche, 1966), and the number of cells in the internal granular layer, which contains a very high density of granule neurones, is very markedly increasing during the first two postnatal years (Gadsdon and Emery, 1976). It will be shown below that the acquisition of cells, including nerve cells, is sensitive to the main-

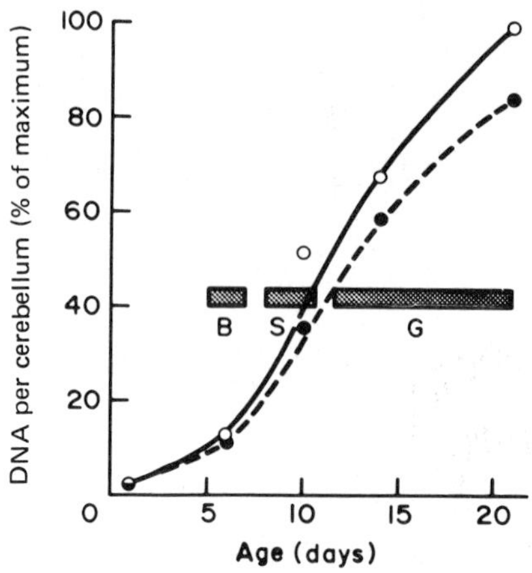

Fig. 1. Effect of undernutrition on postnatal cell acquisition in the cerebellum. The results are expressed as a percentage of the adult DNA content (3.9 μgatom DNA-P). The age curves for controls (○) differ significantly from those for the undernourished rats (●— —●) ($P < 0.01$). The results are taken from Patel et al. (1973). The birthdays of the postnatal cerebellar interneurones are also indicated. The horizontal bars show the period when the formation of basket cells (B) and stellate cells (S) is maximal, and the period when about 50% of the granule cells (G) are formed (Altman, 1969, 1972).

tenance of the metabolic balance, thus the "clumsy" child so well known in paediatric practice may carry the persistent consequences of a metabolic insult of some kind occurring during the postnatal period of cerebellar development.

Postnatally formed cells in the cerebellum are generated either from the EGL (mainly neurones), which is a secondary germinal site or from dispersed glial precursors (e.g. Altman, 1969). In contrast, the Purkinje cells, the only efferent neurones in the cerebellar cortex, the Golgi II cells and the large nerve cells in the deep cerebellar nuclei are formed from the ventricular germinal layer during gestation (or the perinatal period, Golgi II cells). According to present views the EGL is formed from germinal cells at the rhombic lip in the roof of the fourth ventricle before day 17 in the rat embryo and at 60–80 days gestation in man (for references see Balázs et al., 1977). These cells invest the whole surface of the cerebellum where their replication initially results in an increase in the size of the germinal pool. Later some of the daughter cells migrate out from the EGL, the total area of which changes during postnatal development depending on the balance of cells emigrating from and remaining in this layer. In the rat both the total area of the EGL and cell replication, in terms of DNA synthesis rate, reach their maxima at about day 13. After that age, both estimates are sharply decreasing. By about 21 days this germinal zone disappears and extensive DNA synthesis comes to an end, while DNA content reaches the adult level. Replicating cells can also be detected outside the EGL. In the first postnatal week these are numerous in the future internal granular layer and generate astrocytes (Lewis et al., 1977a). The massive proliferation of the oligodendroglia starts later, but, judged from the age curve of the acquisition and synthesis rate of DNA, the extensive proliferation of the glial precursors also terminates at about the same time as that of the neurones. The proliferation kinetics of the neuronal precursors (external granule cells) and astroglial precursors have been found to be similar (Lewis et al., 1977a).

Studies on the effects of metabolic factors have shown that they influence cell acquisition in the cerebellum by interfering either with cell replication directly or with cell migration and differentiation.

Undernutrition during pregnancy, and especially during the suckling period, is a good example of the direct influence on the replicating cells. It has been known for a long time that cell acquisition is depressed under these conditions throughout the brain. The final deficit in cell numbers is somewhat greater in the cerebellum than in the rest of the brain, and under the usual experimental conditions (e.g. halving the normal food given to the dams) is about 20% (for references see Balázs et al., 1979). However, in comparison, the rate of in vivo DNA synthesis is more drastically reduced at its nadir by about 70% (Patel et al., 1973). We have found that the discrepancy between the modest depression of the cell acquisition and the pronounced decrease of DNA synthesis rate results from a derangement of the cell generation cycle in undernutrition (Lewis et al., 1975). Table I shows this effect in the EGL, but similar results have been obtained in the forebrain germinal sites during the neonatal period. It is evident that in undernutrition the DNA synthesis (S) phase is markedly prolonged especially in the first 2 weeks after birth. However, the cell cycle time is much less affected, because of the virtual elimination of the G_1 phase. These changes are consistent with a greater depression in DNA synthesis rate, that is a function of the S phase length, in comparison with cell acquisition rate, which, assuming a growth fraction of 1, is a function of the cell cycle time. Such a perturbation of the generation cycle of the germinal cells is characteristic of the developing brain. In comparison with the S phase, the prolongation of the cell cycle time and of the G_1 phase is about the same or more in other developing organs and in rapidly proliferating cells in various tissues as well as in the cerebral

TABLE I

EFFECT OF UNDERNUTRITION (UN) ON THE LENGTH OF CELL CYCLE PHASES IN THE EXTERNAL GRANULAR LAYER OF THE DEVELOPING CEREBELLUM AND THE FOREBRAIN SUBEPENDYMAL LAYER OF ADULT RATS

Animals were undernourished by halving the normal diet of the mother rats from the 6th day of pregnancy onwards and throughout lactation. At day 26 a group of the undernourished rats was weaned to a restricted amount of normal diet sufficient to hold their body weights at 20–25% of controls (42-day-old experimental group). Estimates are the median values (in hr) obtained by fitting computer generated curves to the data representing the percentage labelled mitoses at 1–32 hr after injection of [^{3}H]thymidine. (We are indebted to Dr. G. G. Steel for the computer analysis.) The results for (a) and (b) are taken from Lewis et al. (1975) and Lewis et al. (1976b), respectively.

		(a) Cerebellar external granular layer				*(b) Forebrain subependymal layer*
Age (days)		*1–2*	*6–7*	*12–13*	*21–22*	*42*
S phase (hr)	Control	9.2	9.6	10.6	9.7	12.3
	UN	14.0	13.7	19.0	12.4	22.8
G_1 phase (hr)	Control	8.3	4.2	3.8	4.8	4.7
	UN	0.7	0.2	0.1	6.2	9.5
Cell cycle	Control	19.0	16.3	16.8	17.3	20.4
time (hr)	UN	20.0	17.0	21.7	21.6	35.4

subependymal layer in adult rats (see Table I) (for refs. see Balázs et al., 1978b). The severe curtailment of the G_1 phase may have important consequences for the progeny of the dividing cells, since processes occurring during a limited period of the G_1 phase may be critical in terms of differentiation (Vonderhaar and Topper, 1974). Besides the distortion of the cell cycle, undernutrition also affects other aspects of cell acquisition in the brain, e.g., especially during the second week, an abnormally great proportion of the postmitotic cells in the germinal zones die (Lewis et al., 1975).

Indirect influences, i.e., interference with cell acquisition through processes other than replication, have been observed when the effects of thyroid state were analysed. Thyroid hormones seem to influence cell acquisition only in those parts of the brain, including the cerebellum, where neurogenesis is extensive in the postnatal period (Patel et al., 1976). In neonatal thyroid deficiency, cell number is reduced in the cerebellum during the second week, but ultimately there is a catch-up, because massive cell proliferation, which under normal conditions ceases by 21 days, persists for about a week longer (Table II). The dissolution of the EGL is correspondingly delayed (Legrand, 1967; Nicholson and Altman, 1972a). The transient reduction of cell acquisition is mainly due to two factors. One is a decrease in the germinal cell population without any apparent alteration in cell proliferation kinetics (Lewis et al., 1976). The other factor is an increased rate of loss of differentiating cells. While the pyknotic index is normal in both the EGL and the molecular layer, it is over 10 times greater in the internal granular layer, which is the major site where cells formed in the EGL differentiate after they have migrated through the molecular layer. It would appear that the effect is primarily due to a retardation of the dendritic arborisation of the Purkinje cells originally described by Legrand (1967). During development the axons of the granule cells are laid down on the surface of the parallel fibres of the earlier cohort of granule cells from the bottom upwards by a stacking process (Altman, 1972). Since the production rate of granule cells is nearly normal, but the Purkinje cell dendritic tree is severely hypoplastic, a proportion of the newly extended parallel fibres has no synaptic partners. In addition, there is also a significant reduction in the number of basket cells in thyroid deficiency (Nicholson

TABLE II

EFFECT OF THYROID STATE ON CELL ACQUISITION IN THE CEREBELLUM

Animals were made thyroid-deficient by feeding daily 50 mg propylthiouracil to mother rats by stomach tube, from the 18th day of gestation throughout the experimental period. Hyperthyroidism was effected by giving daily subcutaneous injection of 3 μg thyroxine. The age curve of DNA acquisition in the normal cerebellum is shown in Fig. 1. Here the results are expressed as a percentage of the control values at the ages indicated. (The results are taken for thyroxine-deficient and hyperthyroid rats from Patel et al., 1976 and 1979, respectively.)

	Percentage of control values (%)						
Age (days)	*1*	*2*	*4*	*6*	*12*	*21*	*35*
Thyroid deficiency	98			94	65*	86*	95
Hyperthyroidism		96	118*	128*	106*	81*	

* Results are significantly different from controls ($P < 0.05$).

and Altman, 1972a; Clos and Legrand, 1973). It is proposed, therefore, that some of the newly formed granule cells die through failure to make adequate synaptic contact. A comparable situation occurs in the cerebellar mutant mouse, the staggerer, and similar events are well documented during embryogenesis (for refs. see Balázs et al., 1977).

Neonatal hyperthyroidism has two major effects on cell acquisition in the cerebellum (Patel et al., 1979). (a) Cell proliferation ceases prematurely throughout the brain (see also Nicholson and Altman, 1972a), and this seems to be consequent to an advancement of cell differentiation under these conditions (for review see Balázs et al., 1975a). (b) Selectively in the cerebellum there is an acceleration of cell acquisition rate during the first postnatal week only (Table II). This is manifested by a greater than normal DNA content (Gourdon et al., 1973), thymidine kinase activity (Weichsel, 1973), incorporation of labelled thymidine into DNA (Patel et al., 1979) and an increase in the area of the EGL (Nicholson and Altman, 1972a). At variance with the claim of Lauder (1977), we have found that cell proliferation kinetics are normal (Patel et al., 1979). Furthermore, the pyknotic index is also normal in the different layers of the cerebellar cortex. Therefore, changes in the rate of cell replication or the loss of newly formed cells cannot account for the effect. Nevertheless, the area of the EGL and thus the germinal cell numbers are greater than in controls during the first week. It is evident that an increase in the number of replicating cells together with an unaltered rate of cell loss, must lead to an elevated rate of cell acquisition.

The transient increase in cell proliferation and its association with an enlarged EGL, which occurs without detectable changes in cell cycle parameters, are effects of treatment with thyroid hormone that are opposite to those seen in thyroid deficiency. Therefore, the major question is, how does thyroid hormone influence the size of the germinal pool in the cerebellum? A lead towards understanding this effect has been provided by the finding of decreased entry of labelled migrating cells into the molecular layer of T_4-treated 4-day-old animals injected with [^{3}H]thymidine 2 days beforehand (Patel et al., 1979). This suggests that in the early postnatal period, when the EGL is expanding, the hormone promotes this process and a higher than normal proportion of the cells are retained in the replicative phase. Since thyroid hormone can only induce an increase in cerebellar thymidine kinase activity and the rate of in vivo DNA synthesis during the first few days after birth the responsive cell population is present in the cerebellum only for a limited period (Patel et al., 1979). From the latter part of the second week onwards, when a progressively increasing proportion of the external granule cells are committed to differentiate, the hormone appears to advance this process, leading to a premature dissolution of the EGL. In contrast to the cerebellum, in the whole forebrain only the advanced termination of cell acquisition is evident. Whether the differences in the effect of neonatal hyperthyroidism in the different brain parts are due to differences in the predominant cell types generated from the EGL (neurones) and the subependymal layer (glia) or to the stage of development of the progenitor cell population would need further experimentation. However, the results obtained in both thyroid deficiency and hyperthyroidism are consistent with the view that the effect of thyroid hormone on cell acquisition in the developing brain is related to changes in either cell migration or differentiation, rather than alterations in the generation cycle of dividing cells.

Recent experiments by our group have indicated further differences in the response of the germinal cells in the forebrain and the cerebellum to metabolic insults of other kinds. It has been found that drugs, such as monoamine depletors and phenothiazines, which interfere with neurotransmitter balance, also affect cell proliferation in the developing brain (Lewis et al., 1977c; Patel et al., 1977, 1979). During the postnatal period the germinal cells in the cerebellum seem to be less sensitive to these drugs than those in the forebrain subependymal layer. In addition, other differences have also emerged in the response, e.g. reserpine treatment results in marked increase in the degeneration of postmitotic cells mainly in the EGL. The mechanisms of the effect of these drugs are currently investigated. The working hypothesis is that neurotransmitters at certain stages of development may also function as neurohumoral agents influencing cell replication and differentiation (see, e.g., Balázs et al., 1977). This is based on the observation that monoaminergic nerve cells are among the earliest differentiating neurones in the developing brain (Loizou, 1972; Lauder and Bloom, 1974, 1975). Furthermore, regulation of cell replication mediated through effects on neurohumoral receptors, is now well documented for various cell types (for review, see Balázs et al., 1977).

There is evidence that the offspring of pregnant animals, which were given certain drugs acting on the CNS, show behavioural anomalies in adulthood (Werboff and Gottlieb, 1963; Barlow and Sullivan, 1975). Interference with cell proliferation in the developing brain may be one of the underlying mechanisms of the behavioural teratological effects of these agents. The functional consequences of exposure to these drugs and to other conditions, discussed above, which result in metabolic imbalance, may also depend on the time of interference with cell proliferation. Because of the chronology of cell formation in the CNS, a transient metabolic insult may interfere with the formation of particular cell types. The cerebellum offers certain advantages to test this hypothesis, since the "birthdays" of the different cell types are now well established (e.g., Altman, 1969). Although powerful compensatory mechanisms are operating to offset the ill effects of various insults, e.g. the persistence of the EGL in thyroid deficiency and the curtailment of the G_1 phase to balance the prolongation of S phase in undernutrition (see above), it has been found that the cellular composition of the cerebellum is indeed altered as a result of neonatal abnormal thyroid state or undernutrition. Under these conditions, the basket cells seem to be most vulnerable, their final number being reduced in abnormal thyroid state and undernutrition to about 50% and 65% of the control values respectively (Nicholson and Altman, 1972a; Clos and Legrand, 1973; Clos et al., 1977). Usually the number of cells, which were generated before the metabolic insult, is unaltered. On the other hand there are marked changes in the glial population, which is reduced in undernutrition (Clos et al., 1977) and increased in thyroid deficiency (Clos and Legrand, 1973).

DIFFERENTIATION OF CELLS IN THE CEREBELLUM

The differentiation of cells in the CNS is manifested in characteristic structural and biochemical changes. Fig. 2 shows some of the parameters that reflect the progress of maturation in the cerebellum. It seems that the biochemical reflections of maturation, such as the development of glucose metabolism and metabolic compartmentation of glutamate (for refs. see Balázs et al., 1975a), precede the morphological manifestations of differentiation (Fig. 2a). However, Fig. 2b and c show that development is not simply a monotonous acquisition of new functions. Transmitter enzymes are good indices of the proliferation of nerve terminals, and, within certain limits, transmitter binding activity of the elaboration of postsynaptic receptor sites. There are marked differences in the age curves for the 3 transmitter systems depicted in the figures. The development of the noradrenergic system is relatively advanced, since at birth the concentrations of both tyrosine hydroxylase and the β-adrenergic receptor are about 50% or more of the adult values. This is consistent with the general developmental

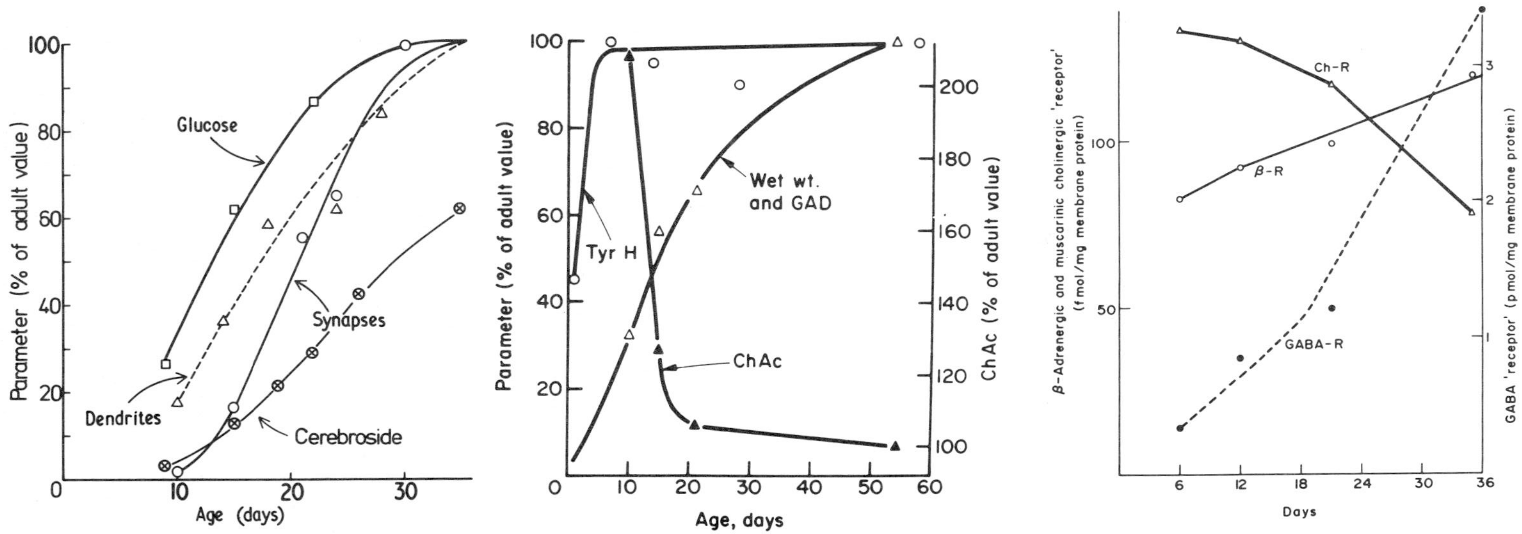

Fig. 2. Structural and biochemical maturation in the rat cerebellum. a: maturation of glucose metabolism (from Patel et al., 1974), □; total number of synapses in the molecular layer of the pyramis (from Nicholson and Altman, 1972b), ○; dendrite arborisation of Purkinje cells in the vermis (from Legrand, 1967), △; cerebroside content (as a marker of myelination; from Balázs et al., 1971), ⊕. b: neurotransmitter enzymes: tyrosine hydroxylase (Tyr H) (from Coyle and Axelrod, 1972), ○; choline acetyltransferase (ChAc), ▲; glutamate decarboxylase (GAD) and wet weight estimates, △ (from Patel et al., 1978). c: neurotransmitter receptor binding capacity. Binding of the musarinic cholinergic ligand, [^{3}H]quinuclidinyl benzylate (QNB) (Ch-R), △, of the β-adrenergic ligand [^{3}H]dihydroalprenelol (β-R), ○, and of the GABA-ergic ligand, [^{3}H]muscimol (GABA-R), ●. I am indebted to Drs. A. J. Patel and R. Smith (CSIRO Division of Human Nutrition, Kintore Avenue, Adelaide, Australia) for their unpublished results.

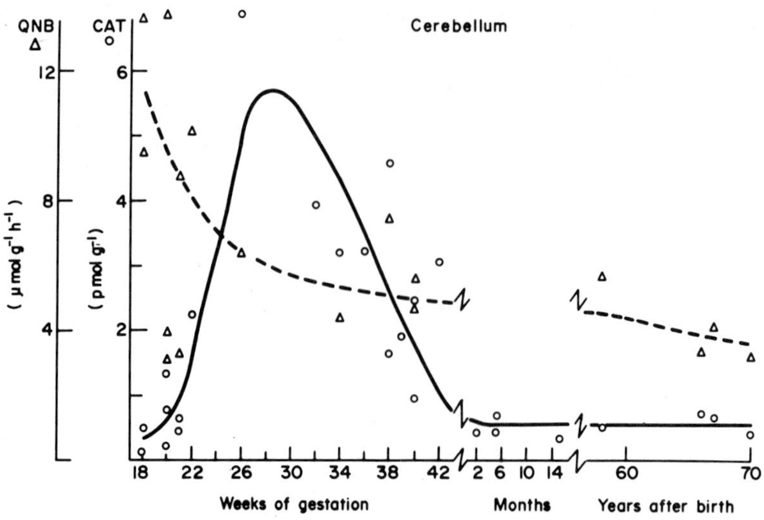

Fig. 3. Development of the cholinergic system in the human cerebellum. The maximal binding capacity of cerebellar membranes for the muscarinic cholinergic ligand (QNB) was estimated from Scatchard plots, △; choline acetyltransferase activity, ○. (From Brooksbank et al., 1979.)

pattern in the CNS and supports the view that the monoaminergic system may have an important regulating role in ontogenesis. On the other hand, the activity of the GABA-ergic system is very low at birth and its development parallels the overall growth of the tissue. The behaviour of markers of the cholinergic system is, however, different from those of either the β-adrenergic or the GABA-ergic systems. The concentration of choline acetyltransferase is maximal during the early postnatal period and it declines sharply afterwards. Although the fall is not as marked, the concentration of the muscarinic cholinergic binding capacity shows the same developmental trend. The sharp decrease in these indices is due to the concentration of cholinergic systems in the rat archicerebellum, which is the earliest developing part of the cerebellum. Thus the concentration of the transmitter enzyme and the receptor decreases with the rapid postnatal growth of the other, principally non-cholinergic parts of the cerebellum, which constitute a very great proportion of the tissue. It is noteworthy that the pattern of development, in terms of these cholinergic markers, is similar in the human cerebellum (Fig. 3, Brooksbank et al., 1979). Because of the great difficulties in collecting sufficient numbers of samples, the exact shape of the choline acetyltransferase curve may be exaggerated but, even with this caveat, Fig. 3 also indicates another important trend, namely that the development of the muscarinic cholinergic receptor (considered here as mainly a postsynaptic marker) precedes that of the transmitter enzyme activity (concentrated in the presynaptic structures). This order of cholinergic development has been reported to occur in the brain of other species, although the relationships with age differ between brain regions (Coyle and Yamamura, 1976; Enna et al., 1976). Postsynaptic neurones often possess at a very early age the capability to respond selectively to the particular transmitter they are destined to receive in maturity, and selective chemosensitivity, or the existence of nucleotide cyclases specifically responsive to certain neurotransmitters, can be demonstrated prior to any major development of synapses or of more than a rudimentary capacity of presynaptic endings to synthesize the appropriate transmitter (see Lanier et al., 1976).

Another putative transmitter receptor and linked second messenger system which has been investigated recently by John Garthwaite in our laboratory is the glutamate-induced increase in cGMP content (Garthwaite and Balázs, 1978). In the adult brain the cerebellum contains the highest levels of cGMP, and these can be altered in vivo by manipulation of excitatory pathways (Biggio and Giudotti, 1976; Rubin and Ferrendelli, 1977), intraventricular injection of glutamate (Mao et al., 1974) and in vitro by certain transmitter candidates including glutamate (Ferrendelli et al., 1974). Fig. 4 shows that the cGMP response to glutamate in cerebellar slices is very low at birth and increases very sharply to reach by day 8 a maximum of about 200-fold stimulation, which is larger than any yet reported for non-tumorous nervous tissue. The degree of stimulation remains high till day 14, but falls precipitously later, so that by day 21 it is only 6-fold. cAMP levels also increase in response to glutamate but the changes are small, about 2-fold, and similar for all ages (inset of Fig. 4). Further studies have shown that the large difference between 21-day-old or adult and 8–14-day-old cerebellar slices in the cGMP response to glutamate does not simply reflect quantitative differences, the potency of acidic amino acids and their analogues being different depending on age (in preparation). We have also been able to narrow down the cell types responsible for the effect (Garthwaite and Balázs, 1978). It seems that in the 8-day-old cerebellum replicating cells, granule cells and cells from the deep cerebellar nuclei are not the major sites involved in the cGMP response to glutamate, and we are currently pursuing these studies using preparations of isolated cell types.

It has been claimed that the cGMP changes in response to excitation and inhibition reside in the Purkinje cells (Biggio and Guidotti, 1976). If so, it is of interest that the period of the maximal response coincides with the restructuring of the climbing fibre–Purkinje cell circuit, namely with the replacement of the multiple innervation on the perikaryon with a single climbing fibre on the dendrites of the Purkinje cells. Thus the magnitude of the observed changes and the confinement of the apparent supersensitivity to this period of

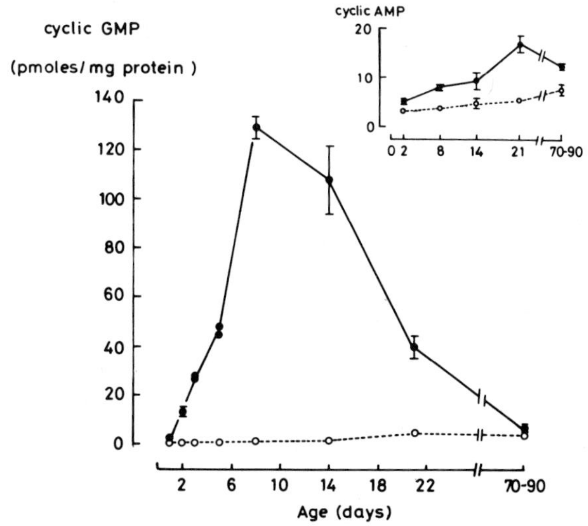

Fig. 4. Age dependence of the effect of glutamate on the level of cGMP and cAMP in cerebellar slices. Unstimulated levels, ○; content of cyclic nucleotides in slices 5 min after the addition of 3 mM glutamate, • (from Garthwaite and Balázs, 1978, by permission of *Nature*).

development might have implications regarding a role of transmitter-induced changes in cGMP in maturing neurones in the cerebellum, e.g., in the stabilisation of synapses (Changeux and Danchin, 1976).

The effects of metabolic factors on the maturation of the cerebellum will not be considered here in detail. In general, the effects are similar to those seen in the rest of the brain and indicate that maturation is advanced after neonatal treatment with thyroid hormone, whereas it is retarded in thyroid deficiency or undernutrition (for reviews see, e.g., Balázs et al., 1975a, 1979). Many, but not all, of the indices of brain maturation are restored to normal after rehabilitation or proper therapy. However, it seems important that metabolic imbalance can also cause distortions in brain development. For example, an immature wiring pattern persists for a long time in the cerebellar cortex of the thyroid deficient animal in terms of the balance between the climbing fibre–Purkinje cell circuit and the mossy fibre–granule cell–Purkinje cell circuit (Hajós et al., 1973; Crepel, 1974). Such changes and delays in attaining adult biochemical constitution and structural organisation may contribute to the persistent behavioural anomalies, e.g. impaired motor coordination, often observed in the adult animals which were exposed to metabolic insults during the period of cerebellar development.

BIOCHEMICAL PROPERTIES OF CHARACTERISTIC SUBCELLULAR STRUCTURES AND CELL TYPES OF THE CEREBELLUM

It would appear that our descriptive knowledge about the effects of metabolic factors in the developing brain is quite extensive. However, our understanding of the underlying mechanisms is limited. To approach these and similar basic questions preparations of well characterised subcellular structures and specific cell types are badly needed. In the last part of my presentation I will describe some of our efforts in this direction.

We have isolated in a pure form large fragments of the cerebellar glomeruli comprising exclusively neuronal processes (Balázs et al., 1975b). This preparation has been used recently for raising antibodies specific to the glomeruli (Goridis et al., 1978). One of our major objectives has been to use the glomerulus particle preparation for testing the hypothesis of selective uptake of transmitters by those nerve terminals which operate with these agents as their transmitter (e.g., Logan and Snyder, 1972). It has been observed that the glomerulus particles have both high and low affinity transport systems for putative transmitter amino acids, including GABA and glycine (Wilson et al., 1976). The uptake of [^{3}H]GABA is competitively inhibited by 2,4-diaminobutyric acid (DABA) (the K_I, about 20 μM, being very near to the K_t of GABA, 10 μM), whereas it is little affected by β-alanine. These results are consistent with the view that the high affinity [^{3}H]GABA transport is selectively inhibited by DABA in neurones and by β-alanine in glia (Schon and Kelly, 1974; however, see below). [^{3}H]GABA uptake is localised to the inhibitory Golgi axon terminals (Wilkin et al., 1974), while the other structures in the preparation, the excitatory mossy fibre terminals and the granule cell dendritic digits show only background labelling. However, in recent studies with Drs. A. Csillag, G. P. Wilkin and J. E. Wilson we have found that [^{3}H]glycine is also selectively taken up by the Golgi terminals, although hitherto this amino acid has not been considered as a transmitter in the cerebellum. Furthermore, since glycine is a weak non-competitive inhibitor of [^{3}H]GABA uptake (K_I about 600 μM) it seems that different sites are involved in the transport of these amino acids. In contrast to a preliminary report (Balázs et al., 1978), it would appear that [^{3}H]glycine and [^{3}H]GABA are taken up by different

Golgi terminals in the glomerulus particles, since the grain counts per terminal are not additive. Currently we are studying the localisation of these two amino acids after their local administration in vivo and in slices.

The other preparations which I want to consider briefly are isolated cell types from the cerebellum. These studies were initiated in collaboration with a team from the Open University (Drs. G. Dutton and N. Currie). We have developed a method which yields ultrastructurally preserved and metabolically competent perikarya from 0–15-day-old postnatal rat cerebella (Wilkin et al., 1976). Depending on age, about 25–50% of the total cells are recovered and the viability of the cells is attested by the high plating efficiency in tissue culture (about 90%; unpublished observations by Rosemary Rodd in our laboratory). The constituent cell types have been separated by unit gravity sedimentation utilising the marked size differences in the perikarya of the various classes of cells. Using ultrastructural, immunocytochemical and combined metabolic and autoradiographic criteria, preparations enriched in the following cell types have been obtained (Cohen et al., 1978) (the dominant cell types as a percentage of the total cell number are given in brackets): large neurones (40%), external granule and primitive granule cells (70%), astroglia-like cells (57%; this fraction is only prominent in preparations from 6–7-day-old cerebella and only few cells show positive reaction with antibody against glial fibrillary acidic protein, GFAP), and a subpopulation of replicating cells in the late S and G_2 phase of the cell cycle (30–40%). Since our group is very much interested in cell proliferation in the CNS, the last fraction is of great importance for our work. DNA synthesis can be detected in this fraction in vitro and the rate is about 6 times greater than that in the mixed cell suspension. Preliminary studies indicate that besides continuing DNA synthesis initiated in vivo, cells also enter the S phase during the first 24 hr in tissue culture. A high proportion of the dividing cells in this fraction are similar to external granule cells, thus raising the possibility of studying replicating neuronal precursors in vitro.

The presence of the replicating cells, however, has also unwanted consequences. Their size changes as they progress through the cell cycle and their heterogeneous sedimentation pattern is one of the major obstacles to the better resolution of the differentiated cells. Improvement of cell separation has been achieved by eliminating the proliferating cells in situ before the fractionation of cells using an inhibitor of cell replication (hydroxy urea, HU) (Cohen et al., 1979). Furthermore, since the "birthdays" of the different cell types in the cerebellum are known, HU treatment at different ages may facilitate the separation of particular cell classes. The schedule hitherto employed involved HU treatment at day 6 and cell separation at day 8 when the numbers of differentiated granule cells and oligodendroglia are relatively low, but in addition to the Purkinje, Golgi and basket cells a great proportion of the astroglia has already been generated (Altman, 1969; Lewis et al., 1977a). This procedure has led to the isolation of fractions remarkably enriched respectively in large neurones, mainly Purkinje cells (80%) and astrocytes (50% of the cells are GFAP positive, but judged by the morphological appearance and metabolic properties the proportion of cells of the same type is markedly greater). These preparations are depicted in Fig. 5, which shows, besides the structural preservation of the cells, the significant enrichment in the particular cell types in terms of the immunological markers GFAP for astrocytes and "Purkinje cell" antigen (we are indebted for the gifts of specific antisera against GFAP and "Purkinje cell" antigen to Drs. A. Bignami (Harvard Medical School, Boston) and J.-P. Changeux and J. Mallet (Pasteur Institute, Paris) respectively). With respect to the specificity of these antisera we have confirmed the observations of Bignami and Dahl (1973) and Ludwin et al. (1976) and found that the GFAP antiserum stained exclusively astroglial elements in the cerebellum. However, the "Purkinje cell" antiserum used in Fig. 5A, although it does not show reaction with neurones

a

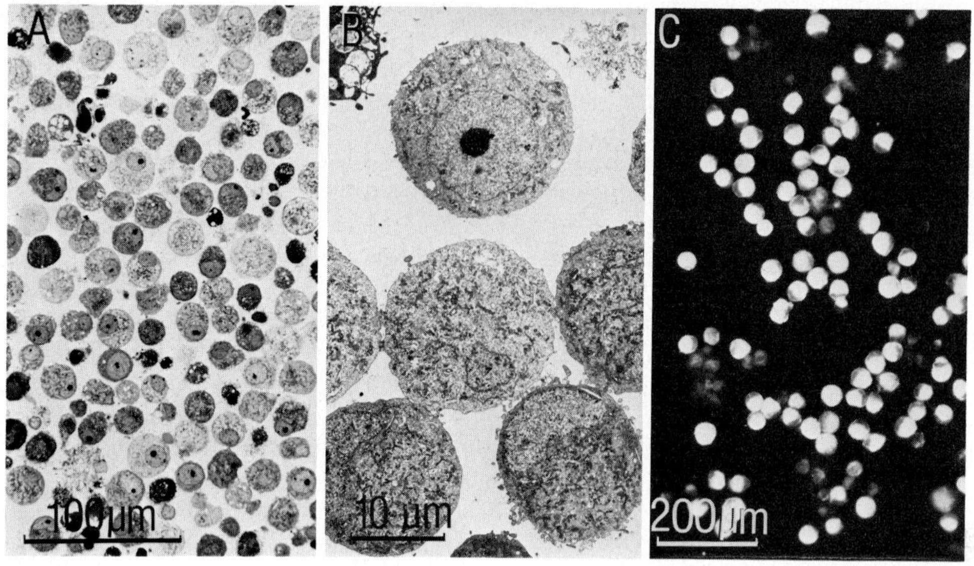

b

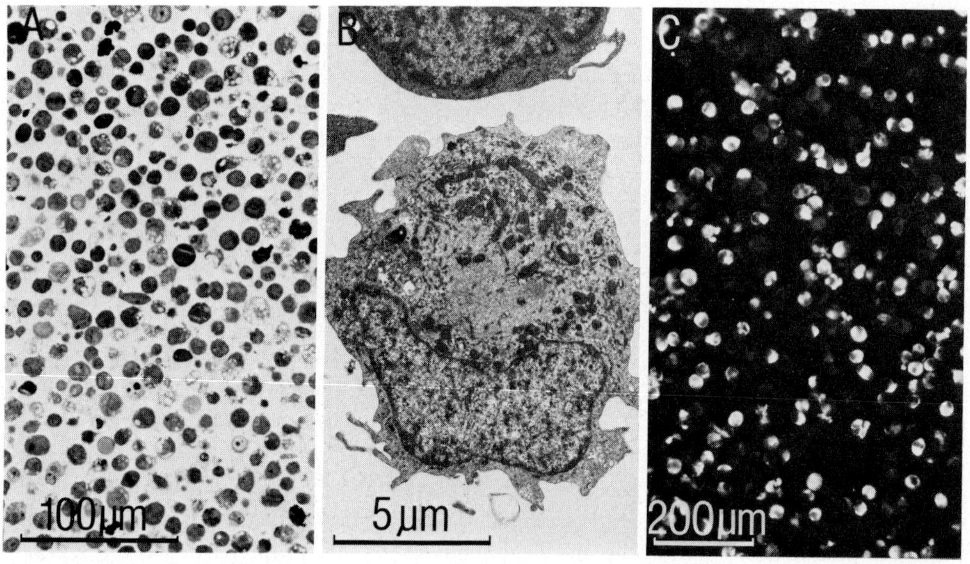

Fig. 5. Morphology of the fraction enriched by Purkinje cells (a, upper panels) or in astrocytes (b, lower panels). The preparations were obtained from the cerebellum of 8-day-old rats treated with hydroxy urea at day 6 as described by Cohen et al. (1979). A: semi-thin sections stained with toluidine blue. B: electron microscopy shows that the structures of the isolated cells are well preserved. C: the enrichment in the dominant cell types is shown by immunofluorescence using antiserum against the "Purkinje cell" antigen (upper panel) and against GFAP (lower panel).

in the forebrain, stains besides the Purkinje cells large nerve cells in the deep cerebellar nuclei and the brain stem. In recent studies, P. Woodhams from our Unit, in collaboration with J. Mallet and J.-P. Changeux from the Pasteur Institute, has further purified the antiserum and obtained a preparation that reacts exclusively with the Purkinje cells.

Thus we have now preparations greatly enriched in two types of neurones (Purkinje and granule cells respectively) and one enriched in astrocytes, and are currently studying the biochemical properties of these classes of cells. Here I want to mention only briefly the investigations with J. Cohen and P. Woodhams on [^{3}H]GABA transport systems using the Purkinje cell and the astrocyte preparations. Although the cells in both preparations exhibit low and high affinity [^{3}H]GABA uptake, they show different structural specificities. β-Alanine (Schon and Kelly, 1974) and cis-1,3-aminocyclohexane carboxylic acid (ACHC) (Bowery et al., 1976) respectively are good competitive inhibitors of the high affinity transport of [^{3}H]GABA in astrocytes and Purkinje cells. (We are grateful to Dr. N. G. Bowery for the gift of ACHC.) However, in contrast to some previous observations (for review see Iversen and Kelly, 1975) DABA inhibits GABA uptake into glial cells as well as into neurones. Autoradiographic studies have extended these observations by showing that the labelling of cells by [^{3}H]GABA is relatively homogeneous and this is reduced markedly in the relevant fractions only by the cell type-specific inhibitors. In spite of the finding that 50% of the cells in the astrocyte preparations are not GFAP positive we could not detect an equivalent proportion of highly labelled cells which are resistant to the inhibitory action of β-alanine. Thus in the astrocyte fraction the properties of the GABA transport system of a much greater fraction of the cells than indicated by GFAP screening are similar.

There are also differences between neurones and astrocytes in the properties of the metabolic processes underlying amino acid transport. Although [^{3}H]GABA transport in both preparations is Na^+-dependent, this process is virtually unaffected in the astrocyte preparation even by 400 μM ouabain that inhibits the activity of the Na^+,K^+-ATPase implicated in the maintenance of the Na^+ gradient. In contrast [^{3}H]GABA uptake in the Purkinje cell fraction is highly sensitive to ouabain (80% inhibition at 50 μM). It has also been found that in comparison with the astrocyte preparation the transport of GABA in the Purkinje cell fraction is much more sensitive to NaF, an inhibitor of glycolysis. The differential effects of NaF and ouabain on the Purkinje cell and astrocyte preparations might reflect underlying differences in the Na^+ permeability of the constituent cells.

Finally, the isolated cells can be cultured after fractionation and they show signs of distinctive differentiation. Under certain conditions granule cells form characteristic aggregates joined by bundles of fibres (Currie et al., 1976). After seeding, astrocytes extend rapidly narrow processes and within a few days the GFAP positive cells cover the whole surface with an elaborate network of processes (Cohen et al., 1979). We have also observed that the cerebellar astrocytes retain the ability, not only to differentiate, but also to replicate in vitro. Furthermore, the cells formed in vitro do express their differentiated function in terms of GFAP production, since after the cultures were exposed to [^{3}H]thymidine during the first day, a great proportion of the GFAP positive cells became labelled by day 7. Even the large neurones of the Purkinje cell preparation plate well initially, although they usually fail to differentiate under these conditions. However, a small proportion of these cells do produce a dendritic tree resembling that of Purkinje cells in vivo, when cultured together with other cells in the mixed cell suspension. It seems therefore that the viability of the cells in the separated fractions is well retained, and thus tissue culture techniques may provide means of studying the factors required for the survival, growth and differentiation of the isolated cells and their interaction in vitro.

REFERENCES

Altman, J. (1969) DNA metabolism and cell proliferation. In *Handbook of Neurochemistry, Vol. 2,* A. Lajtha (Ed.), Plenum Press, New York, pp. 137–182.

Altman, J. (1972) Postnatal development of the cerebellar cortex in the rat. I. The external germinal layer and the transitional molecular layer. *J. comp. Neurol.,* 145: 353–398.

Balázs, R., Brooksbank, B. W. L., Patel, A. J., Johnson, A. L. and Wilson, D. A. (1971) Incorporation of [^{35}S]sulphate into brain constituents during development and the effects of thyroid hormone on myelination. *Brain Res.,* 30: 273–293.

Balázs, R., Lewis, P. D. and Patel, A. J. (1975a) Effects of metabolic factors on brain development. In *Growth and Development of the Brain: Nutritional, Genetic and Environmental Factors, IBRO Monograph Series, Vol. 1,* M. B. Brazier (Ed.), Raven Press, New York, pp. 83–115.

Balázs, R., Hajós, F., Johnson, A. L., Reynierse, G. L. A., Tapia, R. and Wilkin, G. P. (1975b) Subcellular fractionation of rat cerebellum: an electron microscopic and biochemical investigation. III. Isolation of large fragments of the cerebellar glomeruli. *Brain Res.,* 86: 17–30.

Balázs, R., Patel, A. J. and Lewis, P. D. (1977) Metabolic influences on cell proliferation in the brain. In *Biochemical Correlates of Brain Structure and Function,* A. N. Davison (Ed.), Academic Press, New York, pp. 43–83.

Balázs, R., Cohen, J., Garthwaite, J. and Woodhams, P. L. (1978) Isolation and biochemical characterization of morphologically defined structure, including cell types from the cerebellum. In *Amino Acids as Chemical Transmitters,* F. Fonnum (Ed.), Plenum Press, New York, pp. 629–651.

Balázs, R., Lewis, P. D. and Patel, A. J. (1979) Nutritional deficiencies and brain development. In *Human Growth: a Comprehensive Treatise, Vol. 3,* F. Faulkner and J. Tanner (Eds.), Plenum Press, New York, pp. 415–480.

Barlow, S. W. and Sullivan, F. M. (1975) Behavioural teratology. In *Teratology – Trends and Applications,* C. L. Berry and D. E. Poswillo (Eds.), Springer, Berlin, pp. 103–120.

Biggio, G. and Guidotti, A. (1976) Climbing fiber activation and 3′,5′-cyclic guanosine monophosphate content in cortex and deep nuclei of cerebellum. *Brain Res.,* 107: 365–373.

Bignami, A. and Dahl, D. (1973) Differentiation of astrocytes in the cerebellar cortex and the pyramidal tract of the newborn rat. An immunofluorescence study with antibodies to a protein specific to astrocytes. *Brain Res.,* 49: 393–402.

Bowery, N. G., Jones, G. P. and Neal, M. J. (1976) Selective inhibition of neuronal GABA uptake by *cis*-1,3-aminocyclohexane carboxylic acid. *Nature (Lond.),* 264: 281–284.

Brooksbank, B. W. L., Martinez, M., Atkinson, D. J. and Balázs, R. (1979) Biochemical development of the human brain. I. Some parameters of the cholinergic system. *Develop. Neurosci.,* in press.

Changeux, J. P. and Danchin, A. (1976) Selective stabilization of developing synapses as a mechanism for the specification of neuronal networks. *Nature (Lond.),* 264: 705–712.

Clos, J. and Legrand, J. (1973) Effects of thyroid deficiency on the different cell populations of the cerebellum in the young rat. *Brain Res.,* 63: 450–455.

Clos, J., Favre, C., Selme-Matrat, M. and Legrand, J. (1977) Effects of undernutrition on cell formation in the rat brain and specially on cellular composition of the cerebellum. *Brain Res.,* 123: 13–26.

Cohen, J., Balázs, R., Hajós, F., Currie, D. N. and Dutton, G. R. (1978) Separation of cell types from the developing cerebellum. *Brain Res.,* 148: 313–331.

Cohen, J., Woodhams, P. L. and Balázs, R. (1979) Preparations of viable astrocytes from the developing cerebellum. *Brain Res.,* 161: 503–514.

Coyle, J. T. and Axelrod, J. (1972) Tyrosine hydroxylase in rat brain: developmental characteristics. *J. Neurochem.,* 19: 1117–1123.

Coyle, J. T. and Yamamura, H. I. (1976) Neurochemical aspects of the ontogenesis of cholinergic neurons in the rat brain. *Brain Res.,* 118: 429–440.

Crepel, F. (1974) Excitatory and inhibitory processes acting upon the cerebellar Purkinje cells during maturation in the rat: influence of hypothyroidism. *Exp. Brain Res.,* 20: 403–420.

Currie, D. N., Dutton, G. R. and Cohen, J. (1976) Primary cell cultures of separated cell fractions from developing cerebellum. *Neurosci. Lett.,* 3: 86–88.

Dobbing, J. and Sands, J. (1973) The quantitative growth and development of human brain. *Arch. Dis. Childh.,* 48: 757–767.

Eccles, J. C., Ito, M. and Szentágothai, J. (1967) *The Cerebellum as a Neuronal Machine.* Springer, Berlin.

Enna, S. J., Yamamura, H. I. and Snyder, S. H. (1976) Development of muscarinic cholinergic and GABA receptor binding in chick embryo brain. *Brain Res.,* 101: 177–183.

Ferrendelli, J. A., Chang, M. M. and Kinsherf, D. A. (1974) Elevation of cyclic GMP levels in central nervous system by excitatory and inhibitory amino acids. *J. Neurochem.*, 22: 535–540.

Gadsdon, D. R. and Emery, J. L. (1976) Some quantitative morphological aspects of postnatal human cerebellar growth. *J. neurol. Sci.*, 29: 137–148.

Garthwaite, J. and Balázs, R. (1978) Supersensitivity to the cyclic GMP response to glutamate during cerebellar maturation *Nature (Lond.)*, 275: 328–329.

Goridis, C., Martin, J. and Schachner, M. (1978) Characterization of an antiserum to synaptic glomeruli from rat cerebellum. *Brain Res. Bull.*, 3: 45–52.

Gourdon, J., Clos, J., Coste, C., Dainat, J. and Legrand, J. (1973) Comparative effects of hypothyroidism, hyperthyroidism and undernutrition on the protein and nucleic acid contents of the cerebellum in the young rat. *J. Neurochem.*, 21: 861–871.

Hajós, F., Patel, A. J. and Balázs, R. (1973) Effect of thyroid deficiency on the synaptic organization of the rat cerebellar cortex. *Brain Res.*, 50: 387–401.

Iversen, L. L. and Kelly, J. (1975) Uptake and metabolism of gamma-aminobutyric acid by neurones and glial cells. *Biochem. Pharmacol.*, 24: 933–938.

Lanier, L. P., Dunn, A. J. and Van Hartesveldt, C. (1976) Development of neurotransmitters and their function in brain. *Rev. Neurosci.*, 2: 195–256.

Larroche, J.-C. (1966) The development of the central nervous system during intrauterine life. In *Human Development*, F. Falkner (Ed.), Saunders, Philadelphia, Pa., pp. 257–276.

Lauder, J. M. (1977) The effects of early hypo- and hyperthyroidism on the development of rat cerebellar cortex. III. Kinetics of cell proliferation in the external granular layer. *Brain Res.*, 126: 31–51.

Lauder, J. M. and Bloom, F. E. (1974) Ontogeny of monoamine neurones in the locus coeruleus, raphe nuclei and substania nigra of the rat. I. Cell differentiation. *J. comp. Neurol.*, 155: 469–482.

Lauder, J. M. and Bloom, F. E. (1975) Ontogeny of monoamine neurons in the locus coeruleus, raphe nuclei and substantia nigra of the rat. II. Synaptogenesis. *J. comp. Neurol.*, 163: 251–264.

Legrand, J. (1967) Analyse de l'action morphogénétique d'hormones thyroïdiennes sur le cervelet du jeune rat. *Arch. Anat. micr. Morph. exp.*, 56: 205–244.

Lewis, P. D., Balázs, R., Patel, A. J. and Johnson, A. L. (1975) The effect of undernutrition in early life on cell generation in the rat brain. *Brain Res.*, 83: 235–247.

Lewis, P. D., Patel, A. J., Johnson, A. L. and Balázs, R. (1976) Effect of thyroid deficiency on cell acquisition in the postnatal rat brain: a quantitative histological study. *Brain Res.*, 104: 49–62.

Lewis, P. D., Fülöp, Z., Hajós, F., Balázs, R. and Woodhams, P. L. (1977a) Neuroglia in the internal granular layer of the developing rat cerebellar cortex. *Neuropath. appl. Neurobiol.*, 3: 183–190.

Lewis, P. D., Patel, A. J. and Balázs, R. (1977b) Effect of undernutrition on cell generation in the adult rat brain. *Brain Res.*, 138: 511–519.

Lewis, P. D., Patel, A. J., Béndek, G. and Balázs, R. (1977c) Effect of reserpine on cell proliferation in the developing rat brain: a quantitative histological study. *Brain Res.*, 129: 299–308.

Llinás, R. (Ed.) (1969) *Neurobiology of Cerebellar Evolution and Development.* A.M.A. Education and Research Fund, Chicago, Ill.

Logan, W. J. and Snyder, S. H. (1972) High affinity uptake systems for glycine, glutamic and aspartic acids into synaptosomes of rat central nervous tissue. *Brain Res.*, 42: 413–431.

Loizou, L. A. (1972) The postnatal ontogeny of monoamine-containing neurones in the central nervous system of the albino rat. *Brain Res.*, 40: 395–418.

Ludwin, S. K., Kosek, J. C. and Eng, L. F. (1976) The topographical distribution of S-100 and GFA proteins in the adult rat brain: an immunohistochemical study using horseradish peroxidase-labelled antibodies. *J. comp. Neurol.*, 165: 197–208.

Mao, C. C., Guidotti, A. and Costa, E. (1974) The regulations of cyclic guanosine monophosphate in rat cerebellum: possible involvement of putative amino acid transmitters. *Brain Res.*, 79: 510–514.

Nicholson, J. L. and Altman, J. (1972a) The effect of early hypo-and hyperthyroidism on the development of rat cerebellar cortex. I. Cell proliferation and differentiation. *Brain Res.*, 44: 13–23.

Nicholson, J. L. and Altman, J. (1972b) Synaptogenesis in the rat cerebellum. Effects of early hypo- and hyperthyroidism. *Science*, 176: 530–532.

Palay, S. L. and Chan-Palay, V. (1974) *Cerebellar Cortex, Cytology and Organization.* Springer, Berlin.

Patel, A. J., Balázs, R. and Johnson, A. J. (1973) Effect of undernutrition on cell formation in the rat brain. *J. Neurochem.*, 20: 1151–1165.

Patel, A. J., Michaelson, I. A., Cremer, J. E. and Balázs, R. (1974) The metabolism of [^{14}C]glucose by the brains of suckling rats intoxicated with inorganic lead. *J. Neurochem.*, 22: 581–590.

Patel, A. J., Rabié, A., Lewis, P. D. and Balázs, R. (1976) Effect of thyroid deficiency on postnatal cell formation in the rat brain: a biochemical investigation. *Brain Res.*, 104: 33–48.

Patel, A. J., Béndek, G., Balázs, R. and Lewis, P. D. (1977) Effect of reserpine on cell proliferation in the developing rat brain: a biochemical study. *Brain Res.*, 129: 283–297.

Patel, A. J., Del Vecchio, M. and Atkinson, D. J. (1978) Effect of undernutrition on the regional development of transmitter enzymes: glutamate decarboxylase and choline acetyltransferase. *Develop. Neurosci.*, 1: 41–53.

Patel, A. J., Lewis, P. D., Balázs, R., Bailey, P. and Lai, M. (1979) Effect of thyroxine on postnatal cell acquisition in the rat brain. *Brain Res.*, in press.

Rubin, E. H. and Ferrendelli, J. A. (1977) Distribution and regulation of cyclic nucleotide levels in cerebellum in vivo. *J. Neurochem.*, 29: 43–51.

Schon, F. and Kelly, J. S. (1974) The characterisation of [^{3}H]GABA uptake into the satellite glial cells of rat sensory ganglia. *Brain Res.*, 66: 289–300.

Vonderhaar, B. K. and Topper, Y. T. (1974) The role of the cell cycle in hormone-dependent differentiation. *J. Cell Biol.*, 63: 707–712.

Weichsel, Jr., M. E. (1973) Effect of thyroxine on DNA synthesis and thymidine kinase activity during cerebellar development. *Brain Res.*, 78: 455–465.

Werboff, J. and Gottlieb, J. S. (1963) Drugs in pregnancy: behavioural teratology. *Obstet. gynec. Surv.*, 18: 420–423.

Wilkin, G., Wilson, J. E., Balázs, R., Schon, F. and Kelly, J. S. (1974) How selective is high affinity uptake of GABA into inhibitory nerve terminals? *Nature (Lond.)*, 252: 397–399.

Wilkin, G. P., Balázs, R., Wilson, J. E., Cohen, J. and Dutton, G. R. (1976) Preparation of cell bodies from the developing cerebellum: structural and metabolic integrity of the isolated "cells". *Brain Res.*, 115: 181–199.

Wilson, J. E., Wilkin, G. P. and Balázs, R. (1976) Metabolic properties of a purified preparation of large fragments of the cerebellar glomeruli: glucose metabolism and amino acid uptake. *J. Neurochem.*, 26: 957–965.

Quantification of Horizontal Cells in the Domestic Cat Retina

H. WÄSSLE[1], L. PEICHL[1] and B. B. BOYCOTT[2]

[1]*Friedrich-Miescher-Laboratorium der Max-Planck-Gesellschaft, Spemannstr. 37–39, D-74 Tübingen (G.F.R.) and* [2]*MRC Cell Biophysics Unit, King's College, 26–29 Drury Lane, London WC2B 5RL (Great Britain)*

INTRODUCTION

Two morphologically distinct types of horizontal cells have been described from Golgi-stained whole mount preparations (Boycott, 1974; Fisher and Boycott, 1974; Kolb, 1974; Gallego, 1976; Boycott et al., 1978). They differ in their dendritic branching pattern, their overall size and the presence or absence of an axon. The purpose of this paper is to give a qualitative description of the two types, to quantify their receptor contacts and to present a topographical analysis of the network they form in the retina.

MORPHOLOGY OF A- AND B-TYPE HORIZONTAL CELLS

The two types of horizontal cells as observed in whole mount preparations of the cat retina are illustrated in Fig. 1. The A-type cell has 4–6 thick primary dendrites radiating fairly straight out of the perikaryon. The dendrites branch relatively infrequently and adjacent dendritic branches of individual A-type cells hardly ever overlap. The dendritic trees of B-type cells are more densely branched, the primary dendrites are smaller and adjacent branches often overlap. The dendritic field diameter of B-type cells increases from 60 μm in the central area to more than 120 μm in the periphery and is always smaller by a factor of about 0.7 than that of A-type cells. The fine branches of the dendrites of A- and B-type horizontal cells end in characteristic groups of terminals (Figs. 1 and 7). The terminals insert into the cone synapses to form the lateral elements of the triads (Kolb, 1974).

A- and B-type cells can be recognized unequivocally using the above criteria, but a further major difference between the two types is the presence of an axon on each B-type cell. A wide variety of staining methods have never revealed an axon-like process on the A-type cells of cat retina.

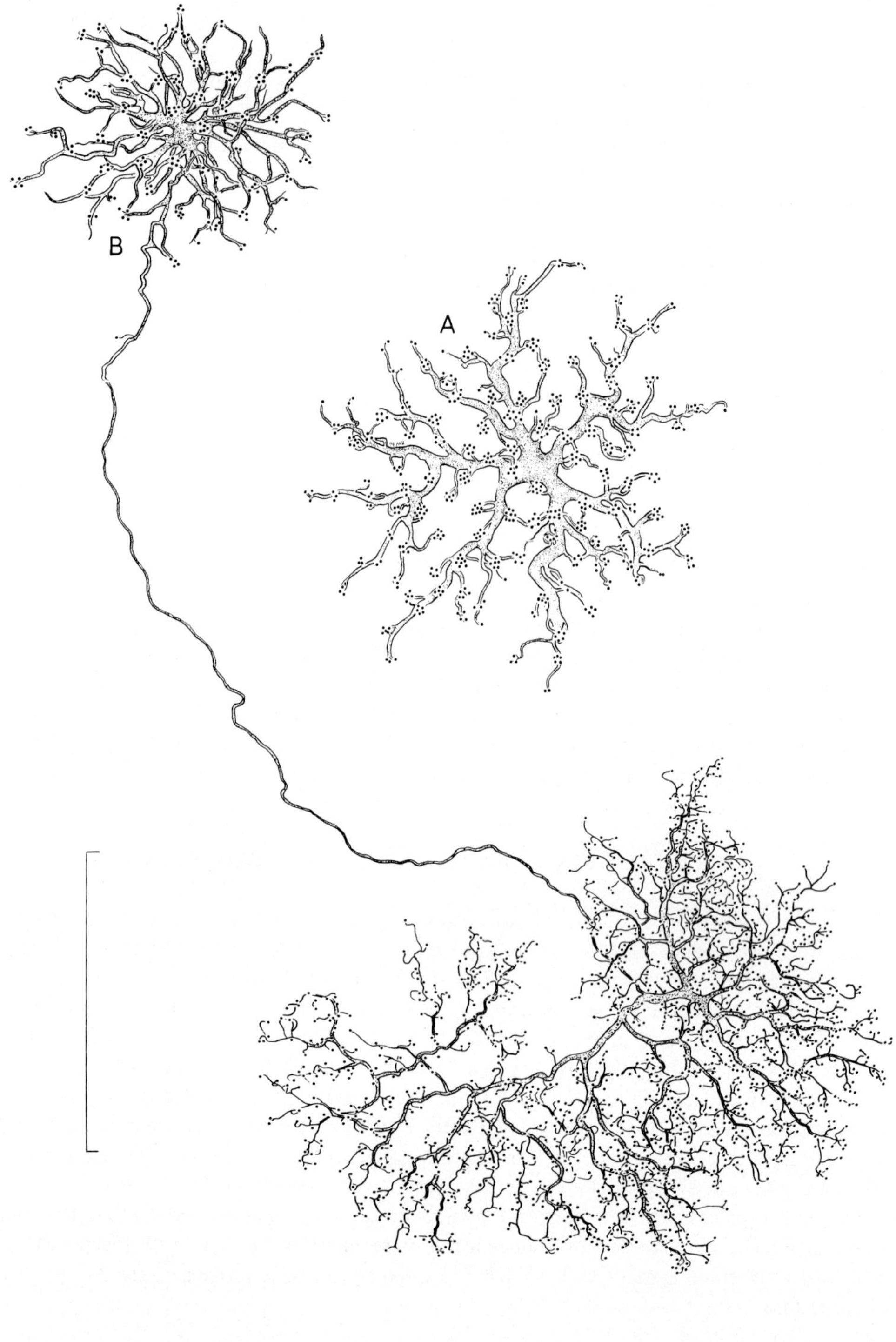

Fig. 1. Drawings of representative A- and B-type horizontal cells from a whole mount of Golgi-Colonnier-stained cat retina (viewed from the receptor side, eccentricity, A = 4.7 mm, B = 7.3 mm). The scale is 100 μm.

THE AXON OF B-TYPE HORIZONTAL CELLS

The axon of B-type horizontal cells always originates from a dendrite (Figs. 4 and 9A). The course of an axon through the outer plexiform layer may be relatively straight or meandering. After a length of approximately 400 μm it always abruptly increases in diameter in a most remarkable manner (Figs. 5 and 6). Successive branches then form the dense plexus of the axon terminal system (Figs. 2 and 3). As shown in Fig. 1 the axon terminal system has a very distinctive morphology which cannot be confused with the branching pattern of A- and B-type cell dendrites. The focus in Fig. 2 illustrates the branching pattern of the axon and that of Fig. 3 its fine terminations. Each terminal forms one of the 3 lateral elements in the single invagination of a rod spherule (Kolb, 1974). Fig. 8 is a micrograph of a vertical section through such an axon terminal system. The terminals are visible as single knobs arrayed at several depths corresponding to the densely packed layers of rod spherules. One axon terminal system could be connected to between 2000 and 3000 rods.

Fig. 9A represents in a small area of retina all the B-type cells that were stained completely through to the axon terminal system. The axons of those cells show no preferred direction with respect to retinal coordinates. To test for directionality on a larger sample of cells we superimposed in Fig. 9B the cell bodies of 70 B-type cells, which were taken along a transect through the retina, and drew just the axons of those cells. The result is a rosette of axons, which go in all directions and show most possible deviations from a straight line. It seems as if, during development, the axons are programmed to synapse with rods, there is a finite length to the axon, and within these constraints it is chance which rods are innervated and which course the axon takes.

CONE CONTACTS OF HORIZONTAL CELLS

Electron microscopy of Golgi-impregnated A- and B-type horizontal cells has shown directly that the terminals of the dendrites form the lateral elements of the cone triads, whereas the axon terminals of the B-type cells form the lateral elements in the rod spherules (Kolb, 1974). However, the horizontal cells of the cat are too large for such a direct demonstration to be made for more than a limited sample of terminal aggregates. For a general demonstration of their connectivity a numerical analysis of Golgi-stained cells by light microscopy is necessary (Wässle et al., 1978a).

Fig. 10A shows an A-type horizontal cell at an eccentricity of 5.4 mm from the central area. In Fig. 10B we have illustrated only the terminals of that cell. Altogether there were 509 terminals. It can immediately be seen that they are not evenly distributed but clustered to form aggregations. Fig. 10D represents a random distribution constructed for the same density of terminals. The difference between the patterns in Fig. 10B and Fig. 10D is obvious to the eye. It has also been shown statistically (Wässle et al., 1978a) that the terminals of horizontal cells are clustered to form separate aggregates. A high power micrograph of an aggregate is illustrated in Fig. 7. A single aggregation in A-type cells contains on the average 5.5 (± 2 S.D.) terminals; in B-type cells the comparable result is 3. The aggregates on peripheral dendrites normally have fewer terminals (often only 1) than those near the cell body (up to 9). In Fig. 10C the terminals are grouped by circles of 5 μm diameter. There are two reasons for choosing a circle of 5 μm diameter to delimit the extent of a single aggregate: (1) In some patches of Golgi-stained retinae several overlapping horizontal cells were stained and contributed terminals to single aggregates, which then were completely filled with termi-

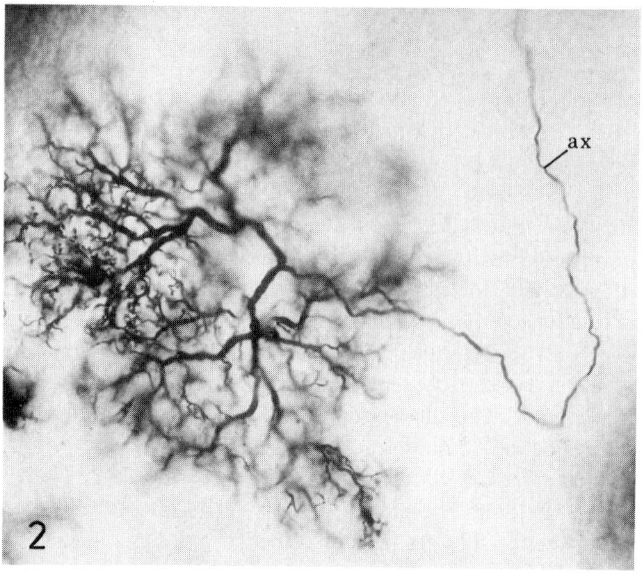
ax
2

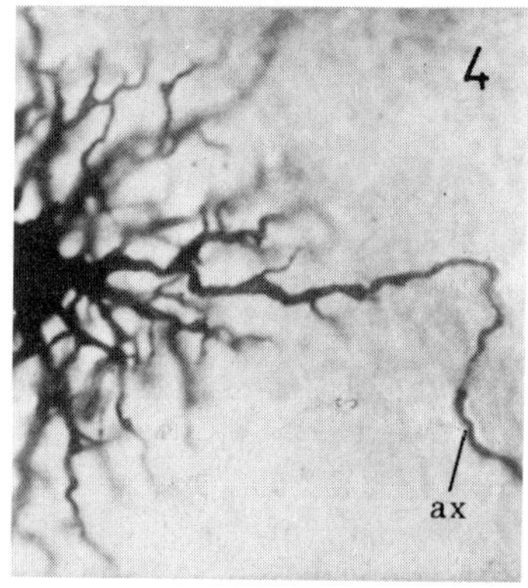
4
ax

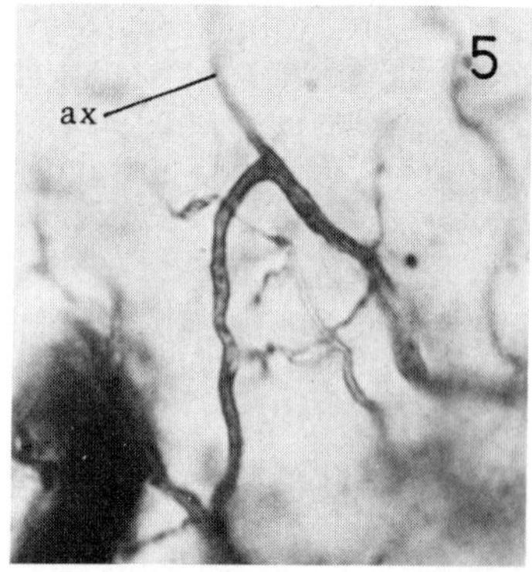
ax
5

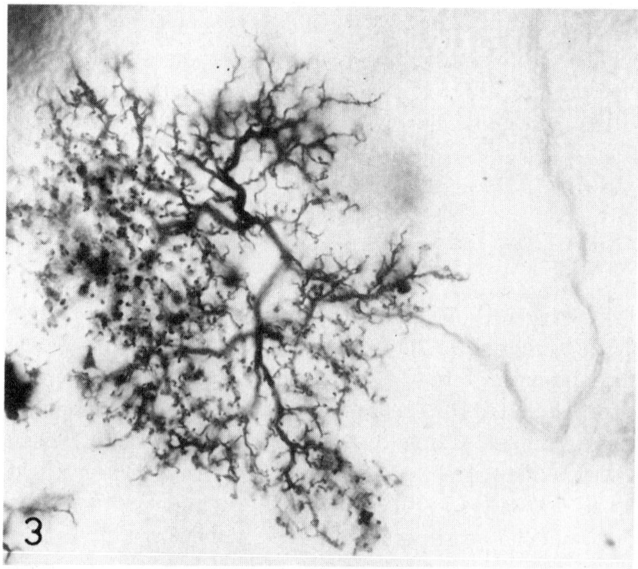
3

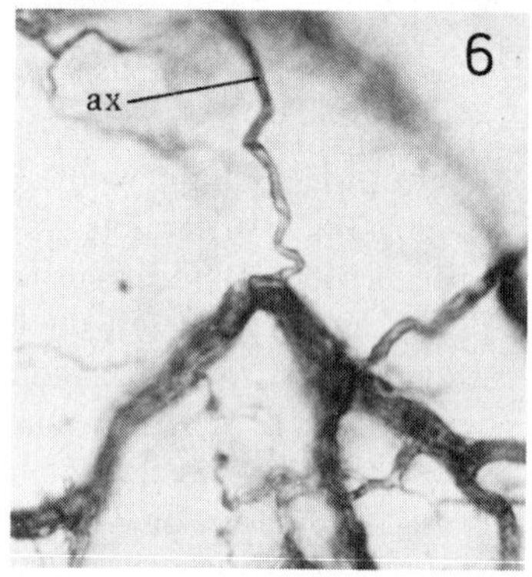
ax
6

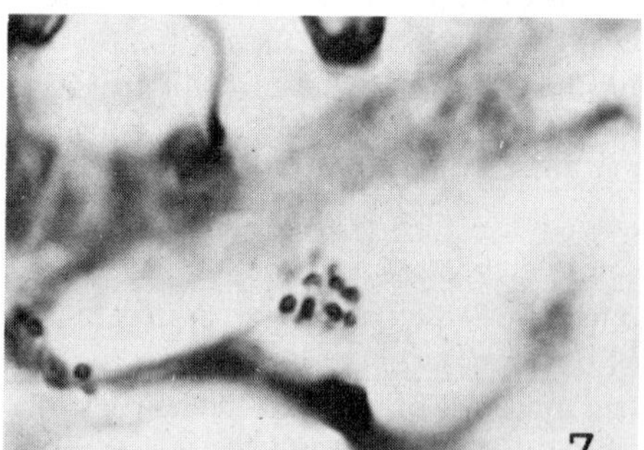
7

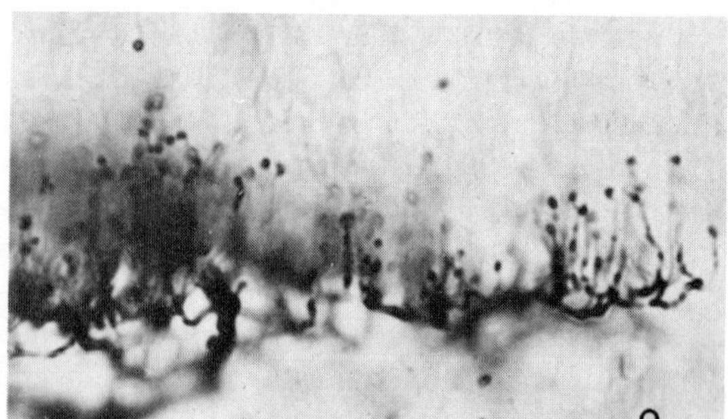
8

nals. Such full aggregates never exceeded 5 μm in diameter. (2) Holländer and Stone (1972) have published electron micrographs of both tangential and vertical sections through cone pedicles of the cat, which were about 5 μm wide.

It has to be demonstrated that each aggregate in Fig. 10C corresponds to one cone pedicle. Unfortunately the cone pattern above the cell in Fig. 10A was not visible and an indirect proof, which can only be outlined briefly here, was necessary. As shown by Wässle and Riemann (1978) the cone pattern in the cat retina is a regular mosaic; the cones are not distributed at random. If the horizontal cell terminal aggregates really are the contact areas with the cones, they must exhibit exactly the same spatial arrangement. The truth of this is given in detail by Wässle et al. (1978a). Fig. 11 illustrates this congruence between cone pattern and terminal aggregation pattern. Fig. 11A shows a B-type cell from the central area. Fig. 11B gives the terminal aggregations of that cell and Fig. 11C the cone pattern of the central area. The density of the dendritic branches and the density of terminal aggregations obviously are adapted for the high cone density in the central area. The same adaptation to the cone pattern can be observed in the B-type cell from the retinal periphery shown in Fig. 11D. The cone density in the periphery is low (Fig. 11F) and this is paralleled by a low density of terminal aggregates (Fig. 11E) and a looser dendritic branching of that cell.

With this analysis we were able to show that A-type horizontal cells contact about 120 cones in the periphery of the retina and up to 170 cones in the central area. B-type cells, correlated with their smaller dendritic fields, contact 60 cones in the periphery and 90 cones in the central area.

◀Figs. 2–8. *The origin and branching of the axon of B-type horizontal cells.* Figs. 2–6 are from retinal whole mounts stained by Golgi-Colonnier and viewed from the receptor side.

Fig. 2. The branching pattern of the main process of the axon of a B-type cell (1 cm = 24 μm).

Fig. 3. The same as Fig. 2 in a focus which shows the terminals that go to rods.

Fig. 4. Part of a B-type cell to show the axon coming off a dendrite (1 cm = 13 μm).

Fig. 5. The initial branch of a B-type axon terminal system (1 cm = 7.7 μm).

Fig. 6. Initial branch of another B-type cell axon terminal system in the same retina and at the same magnification as Fig. 5, showing that the sudden enlargement that occurs differs in magnitude for different cells. In the main these differences are related to retinal eccentricity.

Vertical sections of Golgi rapid stained retinae

Fig. 7. Centre field shows a terminal aggregate on an A-type cell which goes to one cone; to the left is another terminal aggregate just slightly off focus (1 cm = 5 μm).

Fig. 8. Shows the different levels of ending of the terminals of an axon terminal system. Each terminal invaginates into one rod spherule (1 cm = 12.5 μm).

CONE SELECTIVITY OF HORIZONTAL CELLS

Because there are two morphological types of horizontal cell it seemed likely that there might be cone selectivity. For example one kind of horizontal cell might contact only green cones and the other only blue cones. Specific chromatic connections have recently been demonstrated in fish retina (Scholes, 1975; Stell, 1976). In cat we have been unable to identify morphological differences between cones either by light or electron microscopy. Thus assessment of the possible receptor selectivity has to be done numerically.

Fig. 12A shows a B-type cell, Fig. 12B illustrates the terminal aggregations of the cell and Fig. 12C is the cone pattern observed above the dendritic tree. The position of the cell and the extent of the dendritic tree are given by the dotted lines in Fig. 12C. There is a degree of freedom in delineating the boundaries of the dendritic tree and we could only obtain a minimum and maximum estimate of the number of cones this horizontal cell could contact, which was either 99 or 117 cones. The number of terminal aggregations on

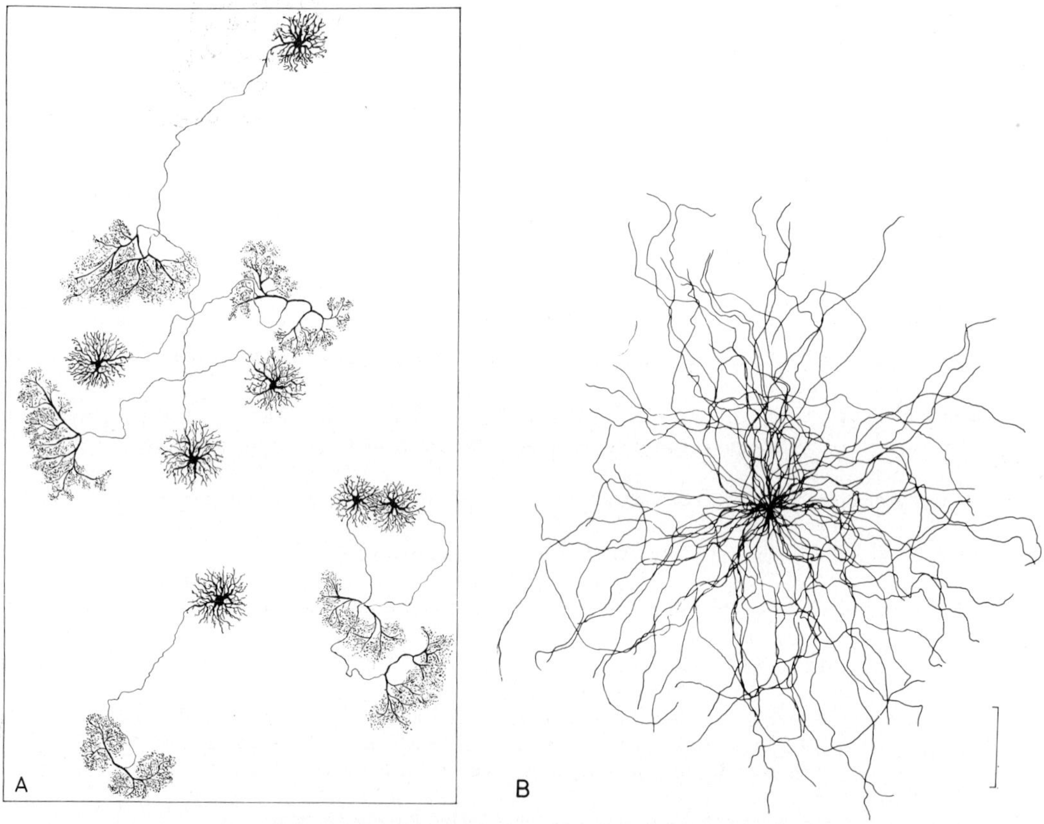

Fig. 9. Course of B-type horizontal cell axons. A: general drawing of 7 B-type horizontal cells which were all that stained at one retinal location by the Golgi-Colonnier method. Frame size 1 mm × 0.6 mm. Central area to the right at approximately 1 mm from the centre of the drawing. The selectivity of the Golgi staining is illustrated by the fact that of the 600 B-type cells which are present in that field only 1% have been stained. B: superposition diagram of 70 B-type horizontal cell axons, sampled from a strip tilted 60° towards the upper nasal retina, scale 100 μm.

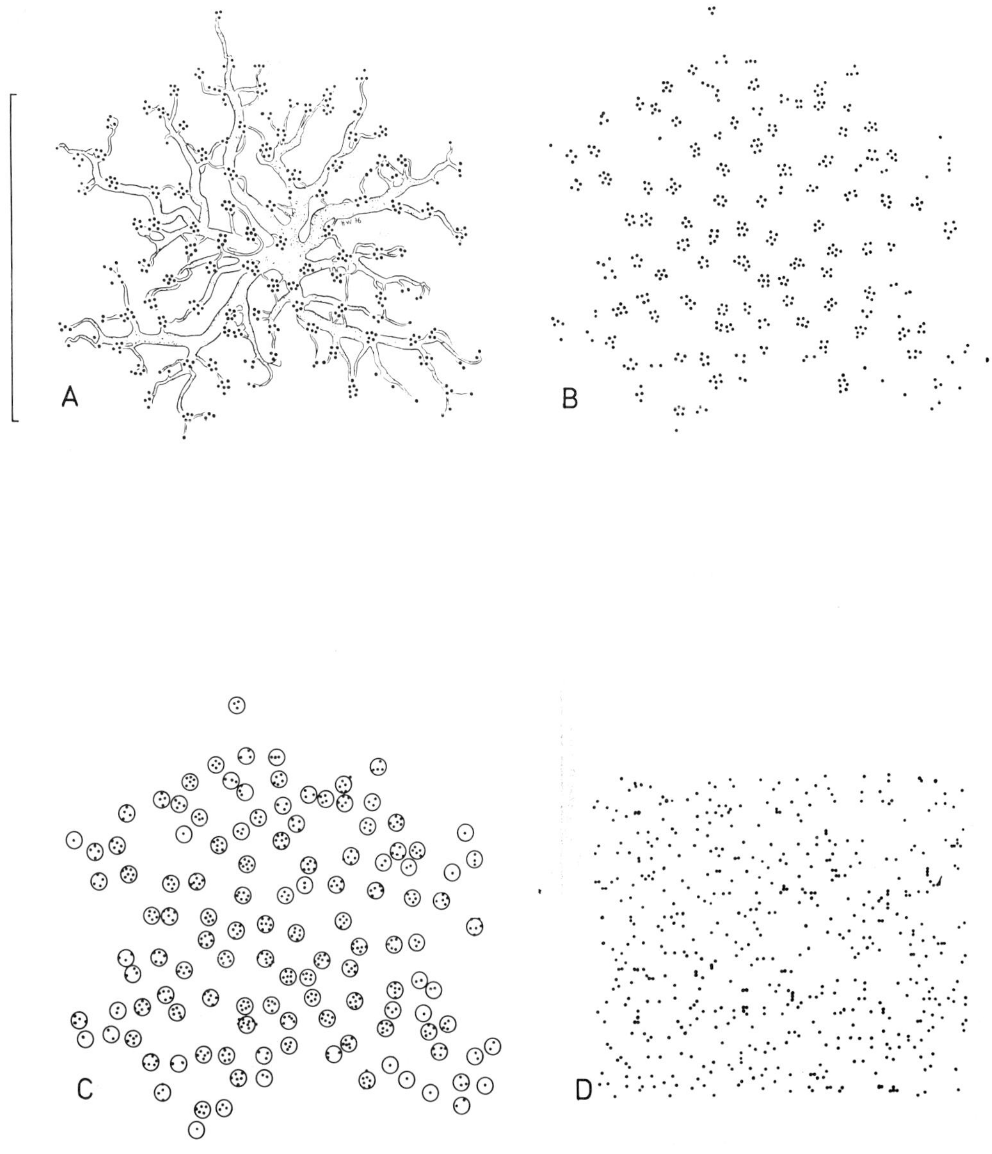

Fig. 10. A: A-type horizontal cell from a Golgi-Colonnier-stained whole mount (scale 100 μm, eccentricity 5.4 mm). B: pattern of the terminals visible above that cell. C: grouping of the terminals into discrete aggregates by 5 μm diameter circles. D: random dot pattern for the same number of terminals as in B.

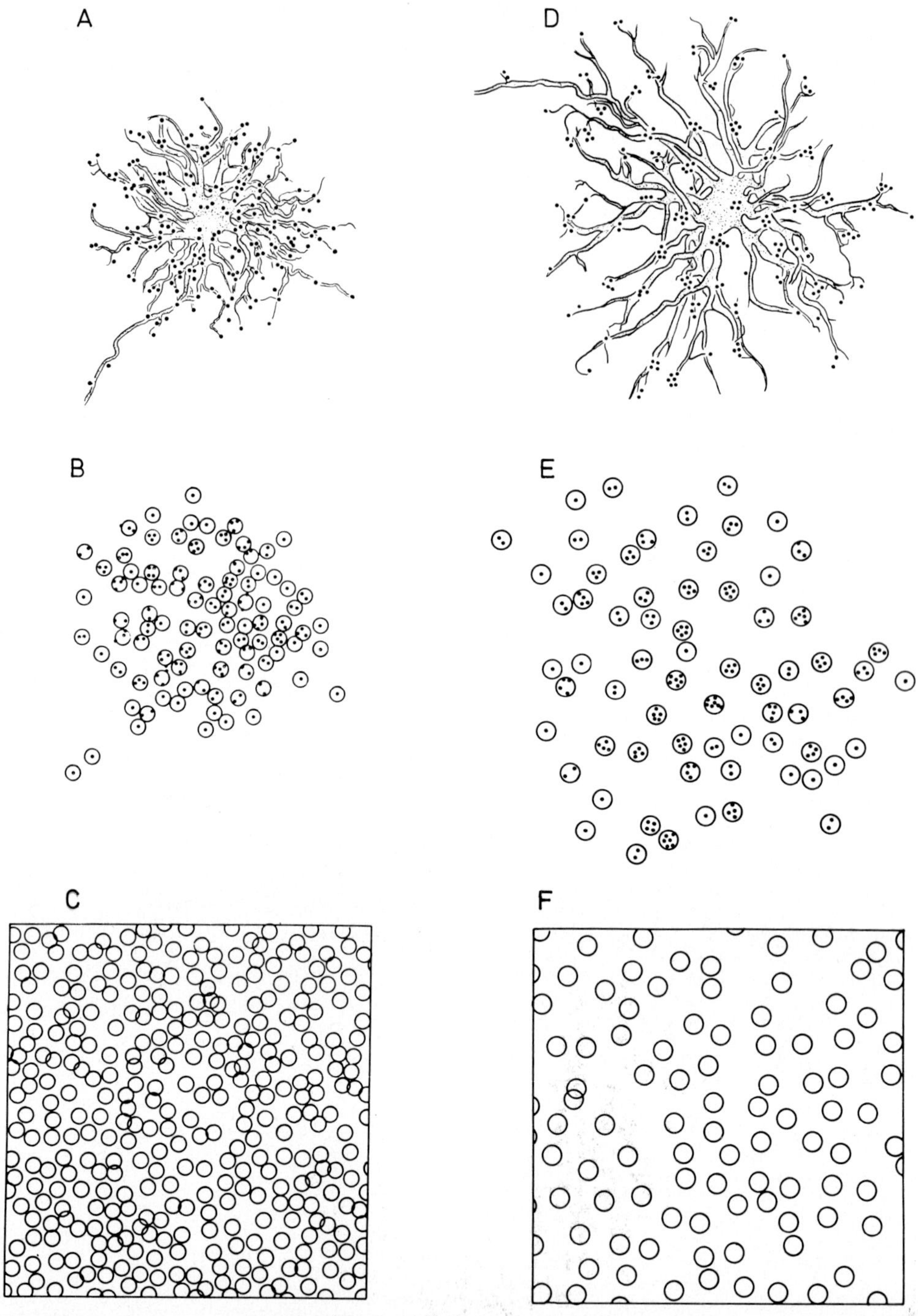

Fig. 11. A: B-type horizontal cell from the central area. B: terminal aggregations of the cell. C: cone pattern in a 100 μm × 100 μm field in the central area drawn from an Azan-stained retinal whole mount. D: B-type cell from an eccentricity of 8.9 mm. E: pattern of terminal aggregations of that cell. F: cone pattern at the same topographical position as E. A–F on same scale, cones and cone pedicles are smaller in the central area and are therefore represented by a 4 μm circle.

the cell was 85. Thus between 72% and 86% of all cones above the cell are contacted by that cell. This percentage was confirmed for many cells of either type (Wässle et al., 1978a). It can be concluded that every horizontal cell makes contact with some 80% of the cones above its dendritic field and that there is no difference in the percentage of cones contacted by either type. For completely overlapping A- and B-type horizontal cells this has the consequence of 60% of the cone input being common to both classes of cell. Thus a strict selectivity, where A-type cells contacted one class of cone and B-type another, is excluded.

TOPOGRAPHICAL ANALYSIS OF HORIZONTAL CELLS IN THE CAT RETINA

In the previous sections the convergence of cones onto horizontal cells has been analyzed. To get information about the divergence of the cone signal, that is to ask how many horizontal cells a cone is connected to, more information is needed. In particular the number of horizontal cells overlapping at each point of the retina has to be determined.

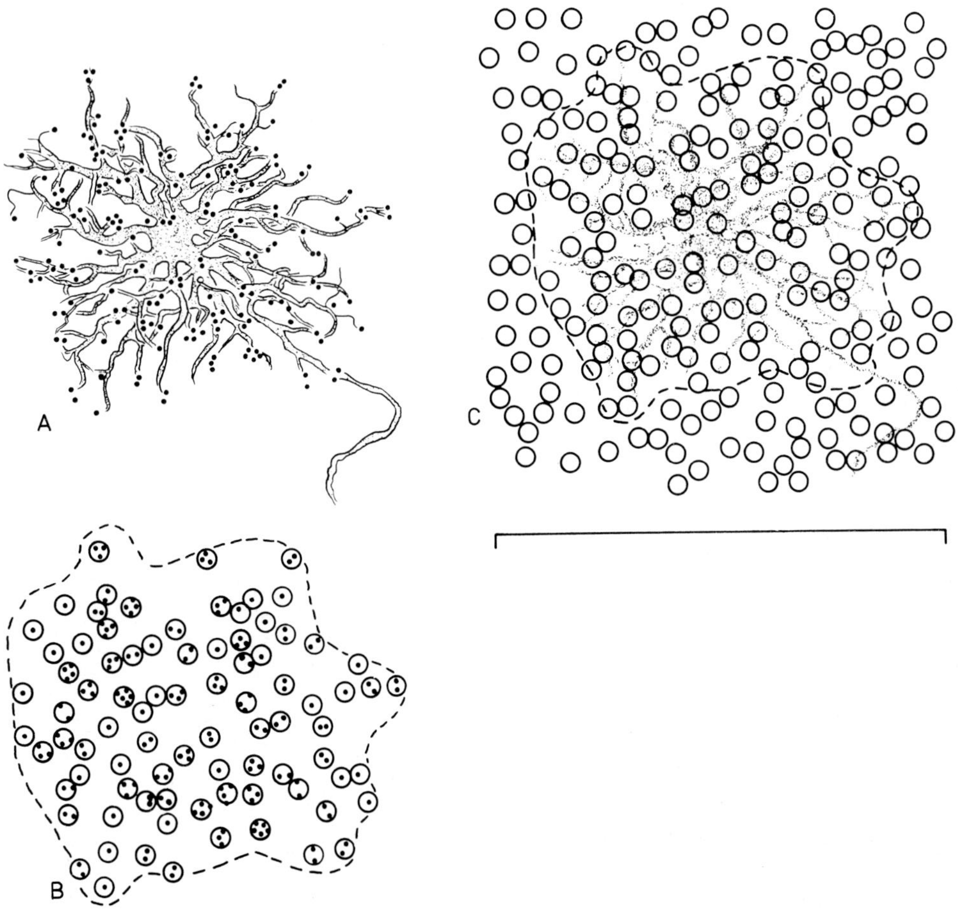

Fig. 12. B-type cell to illustrate the relationship between the terminal aggregations and the cone pattern. Scale 100 μm.

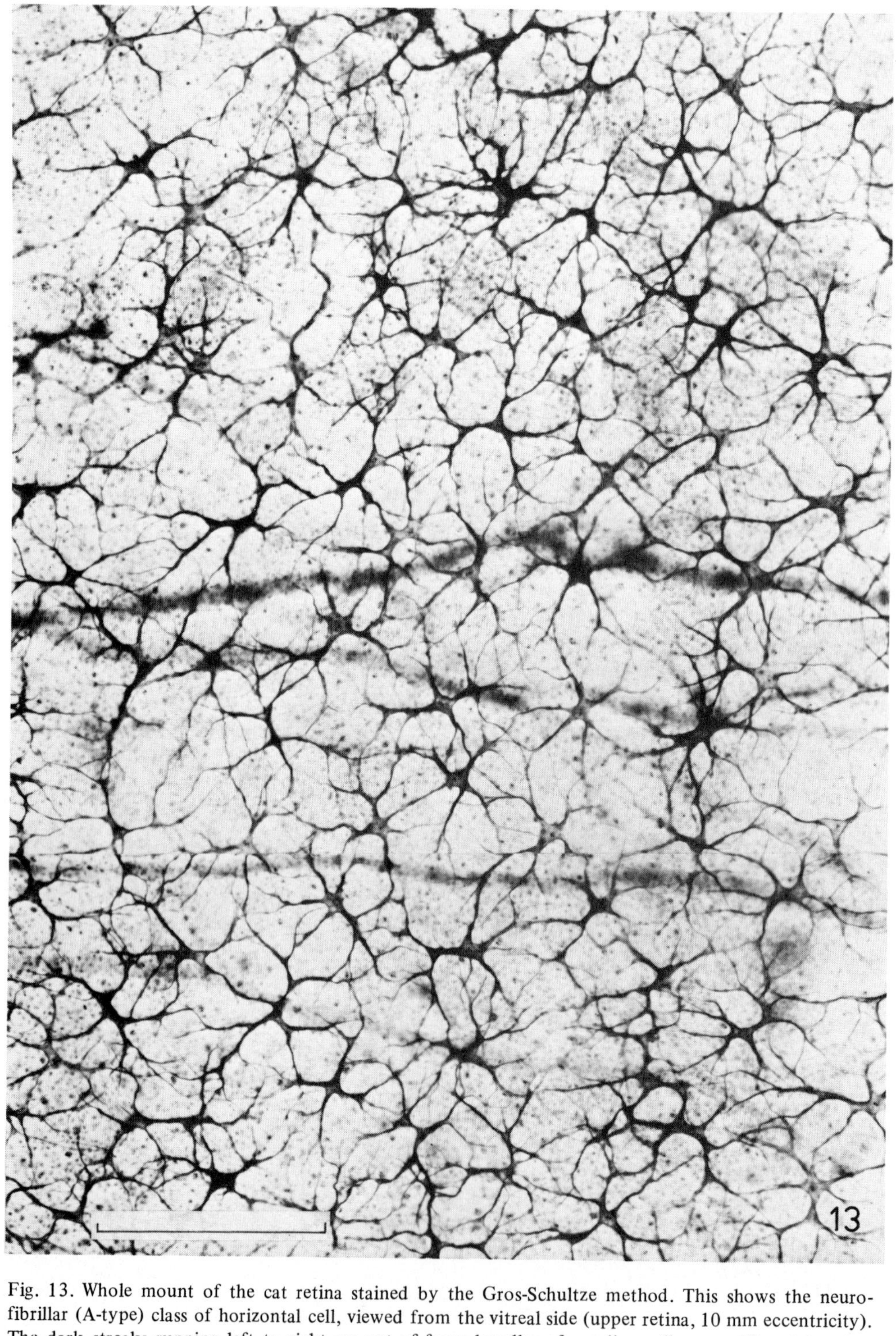

Fig. 13. Whole mount of the cat retina stained by the Gros-Schultze method. This shows the neurofibrillar (A-type) class of horizontal cell, viewed from the vitreal side (upper retina, 10 mm eccentricity). The dark streaks running left to right are out of focus bundles of ganglion cell axons. The picture is a montage of 9 micrographs. Scale 200 μm.

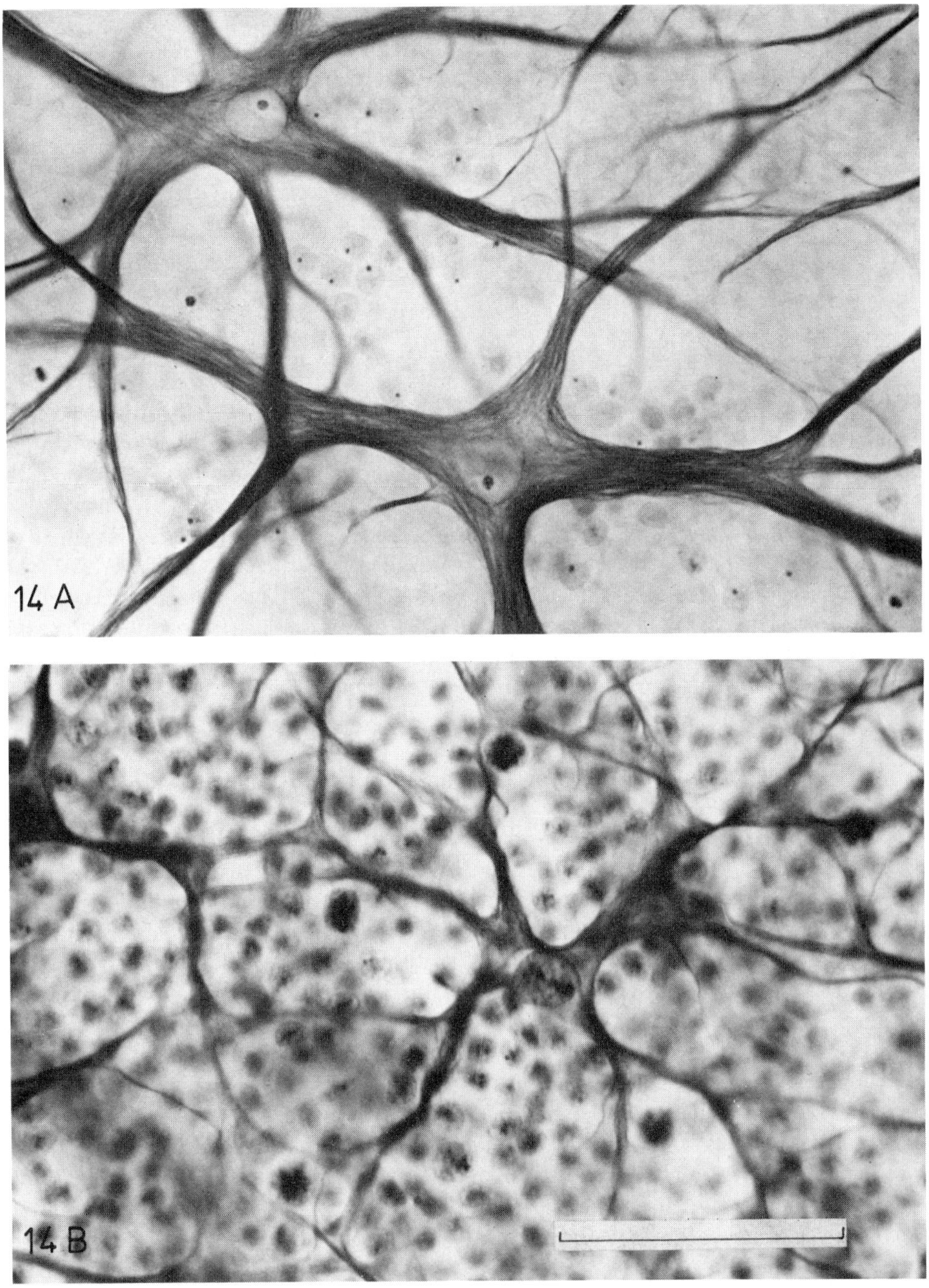

Fig. 14. A: 2 A-type horizontal cells (Richardson's method) to show the fibrillar structure of this class of cell (eccentricity 9.4 mm). B: Gros-Schultze-stained retina to show that the larger and darker staining B-type cell nuclei are clearly identifiable from the numerous small nuclei of bipolar cells. Eccentricity 8 mm, scale 50 μm.

Since the beginning of this century it has been known (Sala, 1904) that neurofibrillar methods stain some of the horizontal cells in the cat retina. Using reduced silver staining methods, such as Bodian, Gros-Schultze and Richardson, we succeeded in staining the total population of one class of the horizontal cells in whole retinae (for details see Wässle et al., 1978b). Fig. 13 illustrates the plexus formed by neurofibrillar horizontal cells. We have shown these horizontal cells to be identical with the A-type horizontal cells of Golgi staining and that B-type cells are not stained by neurofibrillar methods (Wässle et al., 1978b). The reason for this selective staining is the presence of bundles of neurofilaments in the thick processes of A-type cells, which stain with neurofibrillar methods (see Fig. 14A).

DENSITY AND DENDRITIC FIELD DIAMETER OF A-TYPE HORIZONTAL CELLS

The density of A-type horizontal cells measured from a Gros-Schultze-stained whole mount is shown in Fig. 15A. The density decreases from a maximum of 800 cells/mm^2 in the central area to about 100 cells/mm^2 in the far periphery. The isodensity lines show a clear asymmetry along the horizontal meridian. Such a distribution was previously known only for ganglion cell densities, where it is called a streak (Hughes, 1977). A topographical map of the dendritic field diameters was constructed from the same whole mount (Fig. 15B). The dendritic field sizes increase from 80 μm in the central area to 220 μm in the periphery of the retina. The isodendritic field lines are oval and the long axes are also oriented along the horizontal meridian. This shows that the dendritic field size of the cells and their packing density are interdependent parameters.

COVERAGE OF THE RETINA BY A-TYPE HORIZONTAL CELLS

The dendritic fields of neighboring horizontal cells overlap considerably (Figs. 13 and 14A). Each point of the receptor layer is covered by the dendritic tree, not only of a single horizontal cell but by that of several. The number of cells covering each point of the retina is given by the product dendritic field area × density of the cells. This coverage factor was calculated for 3 transects through the retina (Fig. 16). In each graph (Fig. 16A–C) the solid line shows the density of cells, the broken line their dendritic field area. On the chosen logarithmic scale the required product of those data is given by the addition of their ordinates. Fig. 16A–C show very clearly that the two curves, dendritic field area and density, are always a mirror image of each other. This means that, as the density increases the dendritic field area decreases at the same rate. The products of the left hand curves – that is the coverage of the retina – are shown in Fig. 16D–F. Independent of eccentricity (the curves do not show systematic variations), each retinal point is covered by the dendritic fields of 3–4 A-type horizontal cells. It means that a single cone in the periphery and one in the central area will be in contact with the same number of 3–4 A-type horizontal cells, irrespective of the difference in density of the two cell types at these loci. Thus the coverage is an important invariant of retinal construction.

Fig. 15. A: isodensity lines of the A-type horizontal cell distribution in a whole mount of the cat retina. ▶ The map is aligned so that the ridge of higher density extending nasal and temporal from the central area is placed horizontally. The innermost isodensity line indicates 600 cells/mm^2. B: isodendritic field lines of A-type horizontal cells in the same retina as A. The numbers indicate dendritic field diameters in μm. A and B have same scale.

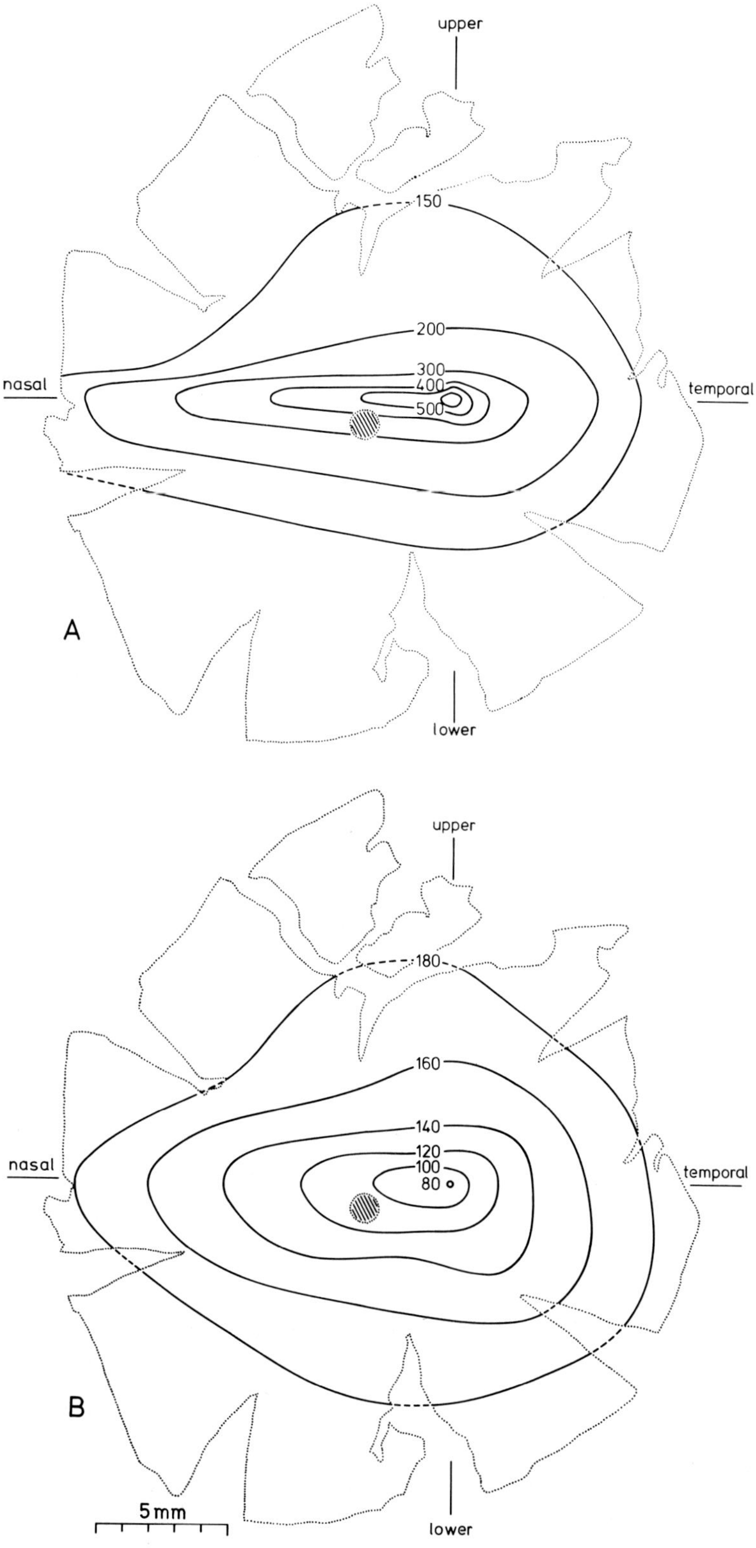
upper
150
200
300
400
500
nasal
temporal
A
lower
upper
180
160
140
120
100
80
nasal
temporal
B
5mm
lower

TOPOGRAPHY OF B-TYPE HORIZONTAL CELLS

B-type horizontal cells do not stain with neurofibrillar methods but their nuclei are recognizable. In Fig. 14B a stained A-type cell is surrounded by several darkly stained nuclei, which are readily distinguished from the smaller nuclei of the bipolar cells of the rest of the inner nuclear layer. We could show that those nuclei belong to B-type horizontal cells and thus were able to determine their density distribution (Wässle et al., 1978b). The B-type density decreases from 2300 cells/mm^2 in the central area to about 300 cells/mm^2 in the periphery. The ratio B-type to A-type horizontal cells is rather constant at a mean of 2.72 (± 0.36 S.D.).

The coverage of the retina by B-type cells can be deduced by combining those density measurements with the dendritic field data derived from measurements of Golgi-stained B-type cells. The coverage assessed in that way is constant over most of the retina at about 4 except for the first 2 mm around the central area, where it is about 7. This shows that the

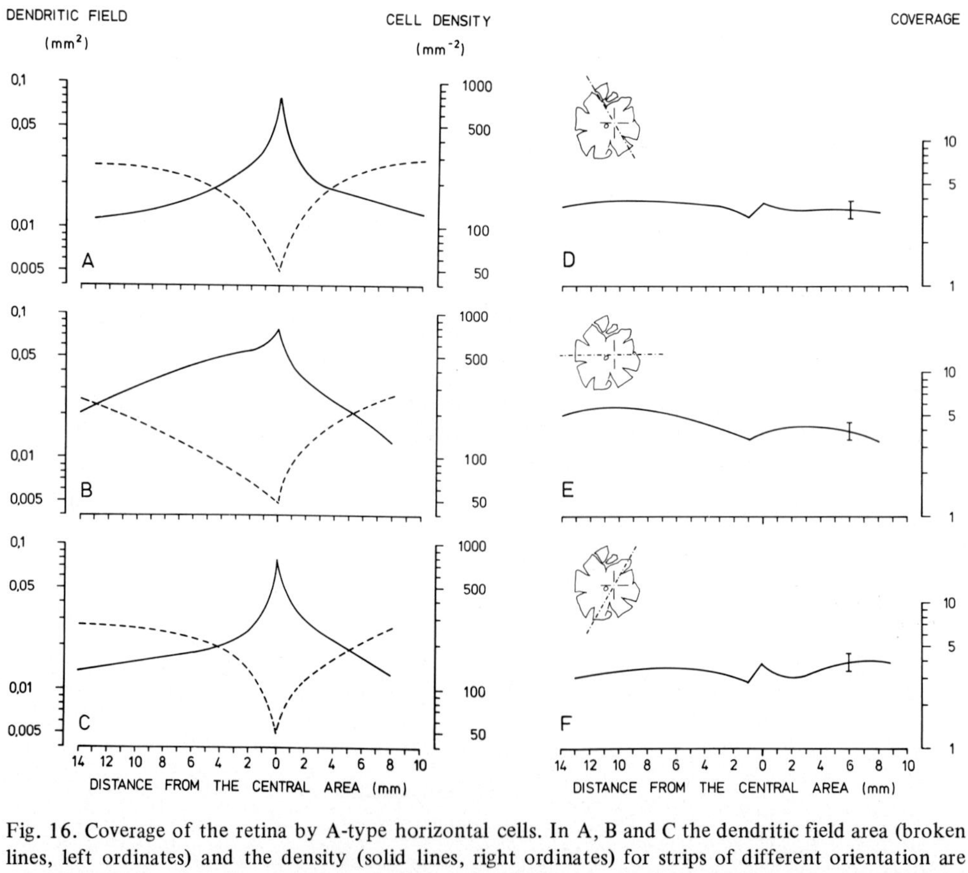

Fig. 16. Coverage of the retina by A-type horizontal cells. In A, B and C the dendritic field area (broken lines, left ordinates) and the density (solid lines, right ordinates) for strips of different orientation are compared. D, E and F show the coverage of the retina with A-type horizontal cells for these 3 strips. The vertical bar in each curve shows the mean scatter of the curves, which results from the scatter of dendritic field dimensions. Because of this scatter the significance of the discontinuity of the curves around the central area is uncertain. The schematic retinal maps indicate the strips whence the samples were taken.

coverage of most of the retina with B-type horizontal cells is of the same order as that of A-type cells. Each retinal point is covered by the dendritic tree of 3–4 A-type horizontal cells and 4 B-type horizontal cells.

NUMBER OF MORPHOLOGICAL TYPES OF HORIZONTAL CELL

From serial sections of cone pedicles of the cat retina (Boycott and Kolb, 1973) it is known that they contain between 9 and 14 triads (mean 11.3 ± 1.4 S.D.) and therefore can accommodate some 23 horizontal cell processes. We have shown a single terminal aggregation of A-type cells to contain an average of 5 terminals and of B-type cells, 3 terminals. No single horizontal cell can fill any particular cone pedicle completely and any cone has to be connected with several horizontal cells. It has been shown above that at each retinal location dendritic trees of 3–4 A-type and 4 B-type horizontal cells overlap. Since every one of those cells must contact at least 80% of all cones in its field, it follows that each cone receives from 3 to 4 A-type horizontal cells with an 80% probability 5 terminals and also from 4 B-type horizontal cells with 80% probability 3 terminals. Summing up we get for each cone from horizontal cells below it $3.5 \times 0.8 \times 5 + 4 \times 0.8 \times 3 = 23.6$ terminals. That number agrees remarkably well with the 23 available sites determined from electron microscopy.

Such agreement makes it highly improbable that there is an as yet unstained and undiscovered type of horizontal cell. We therefore conclude that there are only two basic morphological types of horizontal cell in the cat retina.

SUMMARY

It is shown that there are only two basic morphological types of horizontal cell in the cat retina. Their dendritic patterns differ. One, the A-type, has no axon; the other, the B-type, has an axon ending in a terminal system. There are about 2.5 more B- than A-type cells. The A-type contacts between 120 and 170 cones and the B-type 60–90. The B-type axon connects to between 2000–3000 rods. Both cell types contact at least 80% of the cones in their dendritic field; therefore 60% of the cones that a horizontal cell contacts are common to both classes of horizontal cell, and there is no strict selectivity of cone type. The coverage factor of the retina for the dendrites of both horizontal cell types is about 4, except in the central area where that of the B-type rises to 7.

ACKNOWLEDGEMENTS

All the figures are reproduced, with permission, from our 3 papers in the Proceedings of The Royal Society. We wish also to thank Mr. Z. Gabor and Mr. J. H. Hopkins for their help in the preparation of the paper. The work was done with a grant (Wa 312/5) from the "Deutsche Forschungsgemeinschaft".

REFERENCES

Boycott, B. B. (1974) Aspects of the comparative anatomy and physiology of the vertebrate retina. In: *Essays on the Nervous System; a Festschrift for Professor J. Z. Young,* R. M. Bellairs and E. G. Gray (Eds.), Clarendon Press, Oxford, pp. 223–257.

Boycott, B. B. and Kolb, H. (1973) The connections between the bipolar cells and photoreceptors in the retina of the domestic cat. *J. comp. Neurol.,* 148: 115–139.

Boycott, B. B., Peichl, L. and Wässle, H. (1978) Morphological types of horizontal cell in the retina of the domestic cat. *Proc. roy. Soc. B,* 203: 229–245.

Fisher, S. K. and Boycott, B. B. (1974) Synaptic connections made by horizontal cells within the outer plexiform layer of the retina of the cat and the rabbit. *Proc. roy. Soc. B,* 186: 317–331.

Gallego, A. (1976) Comparative study of the horizontal cells in the vertebrate retina: mammals and birds. In: *Neural Principles in Vision,* F. Zettler and R. Weiler (Eds.), Springer, Berlin, pp. 22–62.

Holländer, H. and Stone, J. (1972) Receptor pedicle density in the cat's retina. *Brain Res.,* 42: 497–502.

Hughes, A. (1977) The topography of vision in mammals of contrasting life style: comparative optics and retinal organisation. In: *Handbook of Sensory Physiology, Vol. VII/5, The Visual System in Vertebrates,* F. Crescitelli (Ed.), Springer, Berlin, pp. 613–756.

Kolb, H. (1974) The connections between horizontal cells and photoreceptors in the retina of the cat: electron microscopy of Golgi preparations. *J. comp. Neurol.,* 155: 1–14.

Sala, G. (1904) Beitrag zum Studium der feineren Struktur der Netzhaut. *Anat. Anz.,* 25: 246–249.

Scholes, J. H. (1975) Colour receptors, and their synaptic connexions, in the retina of cyprinid fish. *Phil. Trans. B,* 270: 61–118.

Stell, W. K. (1976) Functional polarisation of horizontal cell dendrites in goldfish retina. *Invest. Ophthal.,* 15: 895–908.

Wässle, H. and Riemann, H. J. (1978) The mosaic of nerve cells in the mammalian retina. *Proc. roy. Soc. B,* 200: 441–461.

Wässle, H., Boycott, B. B. and Peichl, L. (1978a) Receptor contacts of horizontal cells in the retina of the domestic cat. *Proc. roy. Soc. B,* 203: 247–267.

Wässle, H., Peichl, L. and Boycott, B. B. (1978b) Topography of horizontal cells in the retina of the domestic cat. *Proc. roy. Soc. B,* 203: 269–291.

The Chemical Specificity of Neurones in the Retina

MARY J. VOADEN

Department of Visual Science, Institute of Ophthalmology, Judd Street, London WC1H 9QS (Great Britain)

INTRODUCTION

The vertebrate retina has 5 major classes of neurones (Fig. 1): photoreceptor cells, containing the light sensitive pigments; bipolar and ganglion cells, intermediate neurones on the direct pathway to the brain; and horizontal and amacrine cells that modulate the radial transfer of visual information. In addition, interplexiform neurones, that synaptically link the inner and outer plexiform layers, have recently been described (Dowling et al., 1976; Ehinger, 1976). Each class of cells can be subdivided into several types according to their morphology, synaptic connections and physiological responses (Dowling, 1970; Stell, 1972; Dubin, 1974; Arden, 1976), and superimposed on this, there are species differences, both in the relative sizes and numbers of the various cells.

The results from many studies show that cells within a single class possess different biochemical properties, and that the chemical specificity of neurones of the same class may not be the same between species.

FUNCTIONAL ASPECTS

Ganglion cells, whose axons run in the optic nerve and transmit information from the retina to the brain, fire propagating spikes. Amacrine cells also spike but, as with earlier retinal neurones, are thought to modulate the release of their neurotransmitters by graded hyper- or depolarizing responses. Photoreceptor cells hyperpolarize on light stimulation and indirect physiological evidence suggests that they liberate their neurotransmitter(s) in darkness, the release being curtailed when the cell is stimulated by light (e.g., Dowling and Ripps, 1973; Kaneko and Shimazaki, 1975). This conclusion is supported by EM studies employing horseradish peroxidase and showing a greater turnover of photoreceptor synaptic vesicles in the dark-adapted retina (Ripps et al., 1976; Schacher et al., 1976). Photoreceptor cells synapse with bipolar and horizontal neurones (Fig. 1). The latter generally receive information from more than one photoreceptor, and from other horizontal cells, and hyperpolarize on light stimulation. However, in fish and birds some receive input from various cones whose photopigments absorb maximally at different wave lengths and these shift their membrane potential as a function of wave length. There are not only several morphological

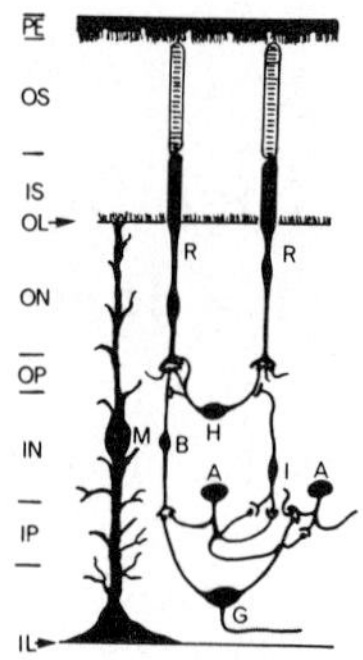

Fig. 1. Schematic diagram of the vertebrate retina. Photoreceptor cells (R) synapse with bipolar (B) and horizontal (H) neurones. Horizontal cells may synapse with bipolar and photoreceptor cells. Bipolars synapse with ganglion (G) and/or amacrine (A) cells, and amacrine cells synapse with ganglion, bipolar and other amacrine cells. Input to interplexiform cells (I) is in the inner plexiform layer from amacrine cells, and output is to amacrine, horizontal and bipolar cells. PE, pigment epithelium; OS, photoreceptor outer segments; IS, photoreceptor inner segments; ON, outer nuclear layer; OP, outer plexiform (synaptic) layer; IN, inner nuclear layer; IP, inner plexiform layer.

varieties of bipolar cells but also two functional ones. "On" bipolars respond to light in the centre of their receptive fields by depolarizing, whereas "off" bipolars hyperpolarize. If one assumes that all photoreceptor cells liberate their transmitter(s) only in the dark then these opposing responses could be caused by the release of inhibitory or excitatory chemicals respectively from the photoreceptors. Alternatively they might result from different membrane responses to the same transmitter. This has been found in carp bipolar cells (Murakami et al., 1975).

Bipolars interact with amacrine and ganglion cells, at a complex terminal known as a dyad. Both depolarizing and, more recently, hyperpolarizing amacrines have been described and the responses may be either transient or sustained. Amacrine cells synapse with other amacrines and with bipolar and ganglion cells.

As might be expected, the complexity of synaptic interconnections increases proximally through the retina and, reflecting this, ganglion cells have a variety of responses. "On-centre" cells increase their firing rate when illuminated in the centres of their receptive fields, whereas "off-centre" cells decrease it. These responses are usually reversed if the spot is replaced by an annulus of light. In both groups, some cells respond in a sustained or tonic fashion, whereas others respond transiently and are said to be phasic. In addition, some are sensitive to motion, with or without directional sensitivity, and some are colour sensitive.

Present evidence suggests that amacrine cells determine such complex ganglion cell responses as tonic versus phasic, and directional sensitivity. In line with this Dowling (1970) and Dubin (1974) have studied the inner plexiform layers of a variety of species and have concluded that retinas with ganglion cells having more complex receptive fields (e.g., amphibia and birds) also have more amacrine synapses.

CHEMICAL SPECIFICITY

The layered arrangement of the neurones of the retina invites tangential sectioning of the tissue, and much can be deduced from the chemical and enzymatic content of the layers

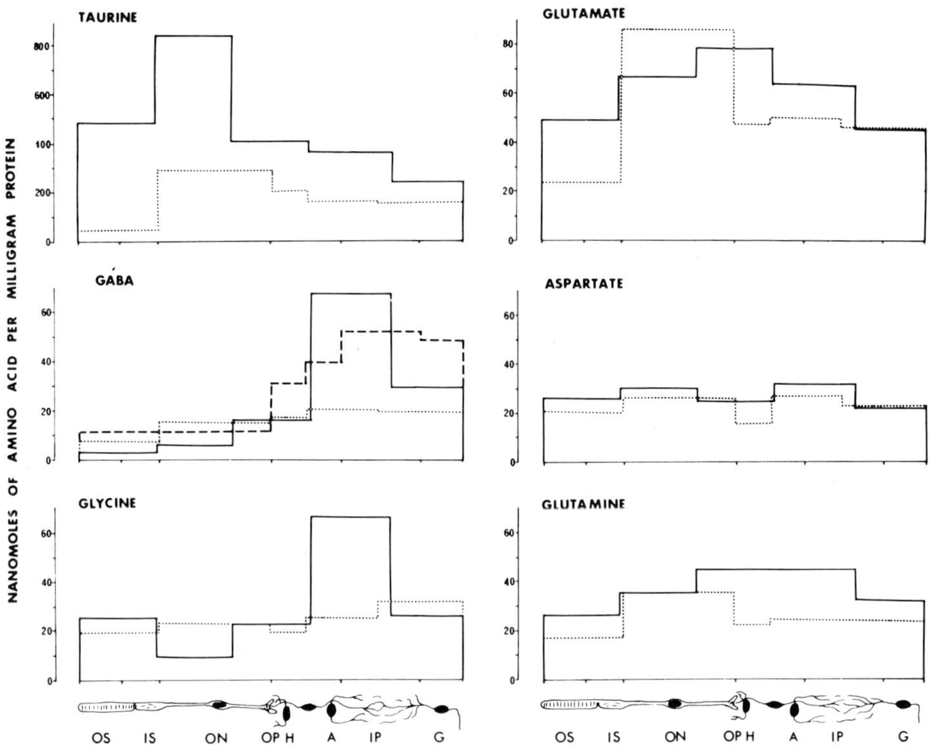

Fig. 2. The distribution of neuroactive amino acids in the rat retina. The values have been obtained from Graham (1974) (– – – – – –), Kennedy et al. (1977) (··········), and Morjaria and Voaden (1979) (————). Recalculations have been based on 12% protein and 83% water contents for the retina. The retinal layers are: OS, photoreceptor outer segments; IS, photoreceptor inner segments; OP, outer plexiform layer; H, horizontal cell rich portion of the inner nuclear layer; A, amacrine cell rich portion of the inner nuclear layer; IP, inner plexiform layer; G, ganglion cell and nerve fibre layer.

(e.g., Lowry et al., 1956). However, the principal glia of the retina, Müller cells, are radially orientated and glial cytoplasm will therefore be present in all fractions from the vitreal surface to the inner segment of the photoreceptor cells (Fig. 1). In the rat retina glial cytoplasm constitutes 100% of the tissue at the vitreal surface, about 10% in the inner plexiform and inner nuclear layers, and only 5% in the nuclear region of the photoreceptor cells (Rasmussen, 1972).

The distribution of neuroactive amino acids through the rat retina has been studied and the results are shown in Fig. 2. The data of Graham (1974) and Kennedy et al. (1977) were obtained by microdissection of freeze-dried, frozen sections of retina; whereas Morjaria and Voaden (1979) have bisected retinas at various depths using the technique of Arden and Ernst (1971) and have obtained their data by differential analysis.

Taurine

It is a consistent finding, in a range of species, that taurine, the predominant free amino acid in retina, with reported levels in the rat of from 11 to 90 μmoles/g wet wt (see Voaden, 1978), has its peak concentration in photoreceptor cells, perhaps in the nuclear layer (Cohen et al., 1973; Orr et al., 1976; Voaden et al., 1977; Cohen, 1978; Voaden, 1978). Allowing for an extracellular space of 30% of the total tissue volume, concentrations here may be in excess of 60 mM. Consistent with the endogenous distribution, autoradiography has shown that endogenously applied [^{3}H]taurine is taken up throughout photoreceptor cells, including the synaptic pedicles (Lake et al., 1978). Its function in these cells is not known, although studies on cats, a species in which taurine is an essential dietary amino acid, show that it is needed for photoreceptor cell viability (Schmidt and Berson, 1978). Taurine entry into the retina is regulated in part by the pigment epithelium (Miller and Steinberg, 1976; Lake et al., 1977, 1978).

Taurine is neuroactive and, in the *Necturus* retina, hyperpolarizes "on" bipolar cells but has no effect on the "off-centre" variety (see Cohen, 1978). It might therefore function as a photoreceptor neurotransmitter. However, its widespread distribution in photoreceptors argues against this, as does its generalized uptake into rods and cones.

Autoradiography (Ehinger, 1973; Pourcho, 1977; Voaden et al., 1977; Lake et al., 1978), the high content of taurine in the inner neuronal layers of various species (Orr et al., 1976; Voaden et al., 1977) and data obtained from degenerate retinae (Lund-Karlsen and Fonnum, 1976) all suggest that there are both glial and neuronal pools of taurine in the inner retina (see Voaden, 1978). However, it may not be evenly distributed as autoradiographs show differential neuronal labelling (Lake et al., 1978). In some species, the particularly prominent uptake of [^{3}H]taurine into select populations of neurones suggests that it might be a transmitter for these cells. In the frog retina, for example, putative bipolars are labelled (Lake et al., 1978). Specificity is not certain as [^{3}H]GABA is taken up by some bipolar cells in this species (Voaden, 1978). However, other neurones are also labelled by [^{3}H]GABA (see later). The association of putative inhibitory transmitters with some bipolar cells is consistent with the observation made on the cat retina that "rod" bipolars may make an inhibitory (sign-inverting) synapse onto rod amacrine cells (Nelson et al., 1976).

Physiological evidence for a transmitter role for taurine is provided by its selective effects both on the b wave of the chicken retina (Mandel et al., 1976) and on ganglion cell activity in the rabbit (Cunningham and Miller, 1976). In addition, prolonged release of preloaded and endogenous taurine from the chicken retina has been observed on light stimulation

TABLE I

TURNOVER OF RADIOACTIVE TAURINE IN THE MOUSE RETINA IN VIVO

Results are expressed as mean ± S.E.M. (n=3). One μCi/g body wt. of [^{35}S]taurine (79 mCi/mmol) was injected into 8-week-old mice. Light-stimulated animals were maintained under a regime of 12 hr dark and 12 hr light (a 40 W tungsten lamp was located 50 cm above the cage). Dark-adapted animals were kept in the dark for 48 hr before use and were injected under a dim, red light. They were then kept in total darkness until sacrifice. Tissue extracts were chromatographed on 20 cm x 20 cm. TLC plastic sheets with layered silica gel (Merck, Darmstadt) using propan-1-ol–ammonia–acetone (7:3:1, v/v/v) as solvent. Carrier amino acids were also plated and the chromatograms developed with ninhydrin in butanol. No labelled metabolites of taurine were detected.

Time after injection (weeks)	*Light-stimulated (dpm/mg wet wt. retina)*	*Dark-adapted (dpm/mg wet wt. retina)*
1	1363 ± 148	1351 ± 263
5	349 ± 27	351 ± 78

(Mandel et al., 1976), perhaps from photoreceptor outer limbs (Salceda et al., 1977), and transient releases of labelled taurine at both the start and cessation of a light stimulus have been found for cat and rat retinas (Schmidt, 1978). Other reports, however, have been negative (Kennedy and Voaden, 1976; Kennedy and Neal, 1978). Endogenous taurine levels do not change on light or dark adaptation in mouse, rat, frog, chicken or goldfish retinas (Cohen et al., 1973; Starr, 1973); although they are higher in dark- as compared with normally reared chickens (Pasantes-Morales et al., 1973). In addition no turnover of preloaded labelled taurine has been observed in frog retinas over a period of 6 weeks (Lake et al., 1977), whereas in chickens there is a decline in the label which is slower in dark-adapted animals (Pasantes-Morales et al., 1973). In mice there is also a steady loss of label (Table I), but no difference between dark-adapted and light-stimulated tissue.

It thus seems that, although taurine is present at high levels in the photoreceptor cells of many species, differences may exist both in its localization and its role(s) in other areas of the retina.

γ-Aminobutyric acid (GABA)

Whereas taurine is most concentrated in photoreceptor cells, GABA, certainly in some species, reaches its greatest levels in the amacrine, inner plexiform and ganglion cell layers of the retina (Fig. 1; rabbit, Kuriyama et al., 1968; frog, Graham, 1974; monkey, Berger et al., 1977). Glutamate decarboxylase has a similar but more localized distribution (Graham, 1974) and evidence from immunohistochemistry suggests that it is present in rat amacrine synaptic terminals (Wood et al., 1976). In addition, GABA, synthesized from glucose or glutamine in the rat retina, is formed predominantly in the amacrine and inner plexiform layers of the tissue (Voaden et al., 1978; Morjaria and Voaden, 1979) and, with species variation, exogenously applied GABA is taken up there, as well as into other cells, e.g., cat, rabbit, guinea pig, frog, goldfish and avian retinas (Bruun and Ehinger, 1974; Lam, 1975; Voaden, 1976; Ehinger, 1977).

In mammalian retinas, there is also uptake by the glial cells of Müller. This predominates in rat and primates to the extent that an initial uptake of GABA into amacrine cells is doubtful (Neal and Iversen, 1972; Bruun and Ehinger, 1974; Voaden, 1976). However, the GABA analogue DABA is taken up, in rat and monkey retinas, by putative amacrine cells, as well as by glia (Bauer and Ehinger, 1978).

The data of Cohen et al. (1973) suggest that GABA levels might be lower in the dark- as compared with the light-adapted mouse retina. This has not been observed in the rat (Starr, 1973) and no difference in in vivo GABA synthesis or turnover from labelled glucose or acetate has been found in this species on light stimulation (Starr, 1975). Preloaded, labelled GABA is released from the rabbit retina on light stimulation (Bauer, 1978), but again this has not been seen in the rat; neither for the preloaded compound (Voaden and Starr, 1972) nor for endogenous GABA (Starr, 1975; Kennedy and Neal, 1978).

Uptake of GABA into Müller cells has also been observed in skate (Lam, 1975), axolotl and salamander retinas (Marshall and Voaden, unpublished). However, there is little or none in goldfish, turtle, frog, pigeon or chicken (Lam, 1975; Voaden, 1976). In these, again with species variation, bipolar and/or horizontal cells, as well as amacrine and/or ganglion cells may be labelled. As regards these differences Lam (1975) has suggested that in lower vertebrates GABA may only be taken up by horizontal cells that are connected solely to cone photoreceptors.

In frog and goldfish retinas the endogenous synthesis and, in goldfish, the uptake of GABA are increased on light stimulation (Starr, 1973, 1975; Lam, 1975), but whereas the horizontal cell layer is responsive in the goldfish, amacrine and ganglion cells may be affected in the frog (Graham et al., 1970; Voaden, 1976). In the skate retina flashing light increases the uptake of GABA by Müller cells (Ripps, personal communication).

As yet we do not know the significance of these many species differences and more studies are needed. However, the evidence suggesting a transmitter role for GABA, certainly in some retinas, is strengthened by the observations of selective effects of the GABA antagonists, picrotoxin and bicuculline on various retinal functions (Kirby and Enroth-Cugell, 1976; Miller et al., 1977; Caldwell and Daw, 1978; Caldwell et al., 1978; see also Graham, 1974; Neal, 1976a). The glycine antagonist strychnine has also been tested in some of the above studies. The overall effects of these drugs, such as increase in the spontaneous and driven activity of ganglion cells, and the removal of specific properties of complex receptive fields, leading to more simple ones, are consistent with the concept that all three are antagonizing specific inhibitory retinal transmitters. In general, bicuculline and picrotoxin have similar effects whereas those of strychnine differ.

Glycine

There is doubt as to the specificity of strychnine in the CNS (Krnjević, 1974) and in the retina it antagonizes taurine as well as glycine actions (Mandel et al., 1976; Miller et al., 1977; Cohen, 1978). However, the effects of strychnine on retinal function are consistent with a role for glycine in synaptic transmission, and the observations of peak levels of this amino acid in the amacrine and inner plexiform layers of rat and monkey retinas (Fig. 1; Berger et al., 1977) must strengthen the possibility that it is a retinal inhibitory neurotransmitter. Particularly as, in a range of species, exogenously applied glycine is taken up by cells in the position of amacrine interneurones (Bruun and Ehinger, 1974; Voaden, 1976). The light-stimulated release of glycine from cat, rabbit and rat retinas has also been observed (Ehinger and Lindberg-Bauer, 1976; Schmidt, 1978) although not consistently in all studies (Voaden, 1974; Kennedy and Neal, 1978), and the time course of the release from rat and cat retinas differs from that found for taurine (Schmidt, 1978). The concentration of endogenous glycine is the same in light- and dark-adapted retinas (Cohen et al., 1973; Starr, 1973).

Glutamic and aspartic acids

Glutamate and aspartate have often been suggested as photoreceptor cell excitatory neurotransmitters (e.g., Dowling and Ripps, 1973; Neal, 1976a; Marshall and Werblin, 1978), but, as in other areas of the CNS, this has been hard to confirm. Conclusions from neurophysiological studies on horizontal cell sensitivity to these amino acids oscillate as to which one is the more likely candidate (e.g., Kleinschmidt and Yazulla, 1978; Wu and Dowling, 1978).

Glutamate is relatively concentrated in photoreceptor cells (Fig. 1; Berger et al., 1977; Voaden, 1978) and the enzymes glutamate dehydrogenase and glutamate-oxaloacetate transaminase are also active there (Lowry et al., 1956). Consistent with this, when radioactively labelled glucose or glutamine are metabolized by the rat retina there is a ready incorporation of label into the photoreceptor pools of both amino acids (Morjaria and Voaden, 1979). Exogenously applied glutamate and aspartate are also, with species variation, taken up by photoreceptor cells, probably by a common carrier mechanism (Neal, 1976a). The uptake is selective and in man, baboon and Cynomolgus monkey retinas in vitro, all of the rods but only some cones are labelled. Others remain unlabelled throughout their length, including the synaptic pedicles (Bruun and Ehinger, 1974; Marshall and Voaden, unpublished). One can speculate as to the possibility of a transmitter function for one or both of these amino acids in the photoreceptors taking them up. However, in goldfish the intravitreal administration of kainic acid specifically destroys the dendrites of second order neurones that penetrate into cone but not rod synaptic terminals, suggesting here that cone photoreceptors are glutamatergic (Yazulla and Kleinschmidt, 1978). Thus species differences may exist.

The principal uptake of exogenously applied glutamate and aspartate is into Müller cells (Bruun and Ehinger, 1974; Neal, 1976a; Voaden, 1978). However, in the rabbit retina, horizontal cells are also labelled (Ehinger, 1977). This has not been observed in other species.

In a survey of amino acid levels in various layers of the rhesus monkey retina, Berger et al. (1977) reported peak concentrations of both glutamate (80–90 μmol/g dry wt) and aspartate (20–30 μmol/g dry wt) in the ganglion cell layer. This is of interest as both amino acids could potentially serve as the transmitter of ganglion cells to the higher visual centres via the optic nerve. However, there is no evidence for a specific uptake of radioactive glutamate or aspartate into ganglion cells in the species studied by autoradiography, including human, monkey and baboon, and such high levels of these amino acids are not present in the ganglion cell nerve fibre layer of the "red spot" area of the pigeon retina (Fig. 3 and Table II), cf. also the values obtained for the combined ganglion cell/inner plexiform fraction of the rat retina (Fig. 2). Nevertheless, Henke et al. (1976) have observed a loss of high-affinity uptake sites for glutamic acid in pigeon optic tectum following retinal ablation and have inferred that glutamate might therefore be a retino-tectal transmitter. Species differences may exist as there was no change in the glutamate transport systems in the rat dorsal lateral geniculate body or in the superior colliculus following enucleation (Lund Karlsen, 1978).

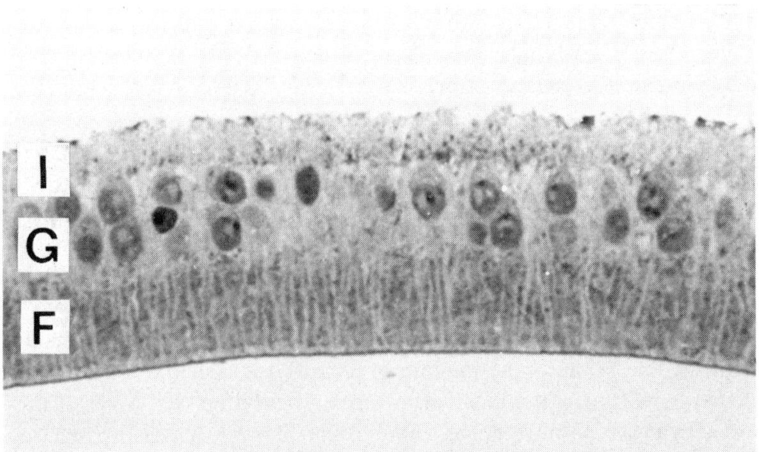

Fig. 3. A section of the ganglion cell layer of the pigeon retina (× 780). The "red spot" area of the pigeon retina was sectioned from the ganglion cell side to a depth of 40 μm, using the technique of Arden and Ernst (1971). The tissue was then fixed in glutaraldehyde followed by osmium tetroxide and processed for light microscopy. I, inner plexiform layer; G, ganglion cells; F, nerve fibre layer.

TABLE II

ENDOGENOUS AMINO ACIDS IN THE "GANGLION CELL LAYER" OF THE PIGEON RETINA

The "red spot" area of the pigeon retina was sectioned from the ganglion cell side to a depth of 40 μm, as described by Morjaria and Voaden (1979) (cf., Fig. 2). The amino acid content of both the ganglion cell layer and the rest of the retina have been measured by double label dansylation (Morjaria and Voaden, 1979) and percentages calculated on the mean total in the tissue. Results are expressed as the mean ± S.E.M. (n=8) and are the levels present in a disc of retina, diameter 3 mm.

	nmol amino acid in the ganglion cell layer		
Amino acid	*per 3 mm disc retina*	*per mg protein*	*% total in the retina*
Taurine	2.15 ± 0.40	72.6	7.6
GABA	0.72 ± 0.15	24.3	7.6
Glycine	0.40 ± 0.07	13.5	6.8
Glutamate	0.84 ± 0.18	28.4	8.3
Aspartate	0.21 ± 0.04	7.1	7.7
Glutamine	1.71 ± 0.21	57.8	16.0
Protein (μg)	29.60 ± 3.40		16.0

When radioactive glutamine is metabolized by the pigeon retina, the principal retention of label is in glutamic acid and, in autoradiographs, exposed grains are seen over perikarya in a position characteristic of bipolar cells (Voaden et al., 1978). A population of these may, therefore, use glutamate as a transmitter. This was not observed in rat, cat or frog retinas.

Acetylcholine (ACh)

It has been known for many years that the retina is a rich source of choline acetyl transferase (ChAc), perhaps the richest in the CNS, with values in the inner plexiform layer of the goldfish reaching 318 mmol/ kg dry wt/hr (Ross and McDougal, 1976). Retinas also show the largest species variation, however, and activity in the inner plexiform layer of the cat is only about 4 mmol/kg dry wt/hr (Ross and McDougal, 1976; see also Graham, 1974; Neal, 1976b). With the exception of the mudpuppy retina, it is a general finding that the enzyme is concentrated in the amacrine, inner plexiform and ganglion cell layers of the tissue, with only minor activity in photoreceptor and horizontal cells. Levels appear to correspond quantitatively with the distribution of amacrine cells (Ross and McDougal, 1976) but the species differences in enzyme activity are generally greater than the variation in numbers of amacrine cell synapses, and, in addition, some bipolar cells may be cholinergic (see below). Optic nerves possess little or no ChAc activity. The pigeon optic nerve is an exception, but here the activity may be associated with centrifugal fibres (Graham, 1974).

As with ChAc, acetyl cholinesterase activity is also concentrated in the inner plexiform layer and, in many species, is reported to be localized in the bodies and processes of amacrine cells (see Graham, 1974; and Neal, 1976b, for refs.). In some species minor activity has also been detected in cell processes in the outer plexiform layer.

When [^{3}H]choline is used as a precursor of acetylcholine in the chicken retina, soluble compound autoradiography reveals label in both the outer and inner plexiform layers (Baughman and Bader, 1977). Cell bodies in positions characteristic of bipolar, amacrine and ganglion cells are discernible; the latter may be displaced amacrine cells.

α-Bungarotoxin (α-bgt) binds to both plexiform layers in avian, goldfish, turtle and rabbit retinas (Vogel and Nirenberg, 1976; Yazulla and Schmidt, 1976, 1977). However, binding in the outer plexiform layer may not always reflect a typical nicotinic synapse as, in the pigeon, it is not readily inhibited by nicotine (Yazulla and Schmidt, 1977), although, in the goldfish, it is (Schwartz and Bok, 1978). Corresponding with the sites of synthesis of radioactive ACh from [^{3}H]choline in the chicken retina, α-bgt also binds to select populations of dendrites postsynaptic to both bipolar and amacrine cells (Vogel et al., 1977). However, sometimes only one postsynaptic terminal in a bipolar dyad reacts, suggesting that both muscarinic and nicotinic receptors are present in the same terminal (see also Sugiyama et al., 1977). In mouse and rat retinas only terminals postsynaptic to amacrine cells are labelled by α-bgt, and in these species there is no binding in the outer plexiform layer (Vogel and Nirenberg, 1976; Pourcho, 1978).

The results from neurophysiological studies are consistent with the conclusion that, with species variation, ACh may be an excitatory neurotransmitter of select populations of amacrine and bipolar cells (see Graham, 1974; and Neal, 1976b, for refs.). In particular, the responses of ganglion cells in the rabbit retina to ACh, anticholinesterase and cholinergic antagonists suggest that "on-centre" bipolar cells may be cholinergic (Masland and Ames, 1976). ACh, synthesized from exogenous [^{14}C]choline is released from the rabbit retina on light stimulation (Masland and Livingstone, 1976).

The function(s) of the cholinergic system in the outer plexiform layer of the retina are not known. The observation by Lam (1975) that isolated cones of the turtle are able to synthesize ACh has led to the speculation that it might be an excitatory photoreceptor neurotransmitter. However, the generally low level of ChAc in the photoreceptor and outer plexiform layers of retinas argues against this, as does the observation that ACh application to horizontal cells has no appreciable effect (e.g., Murakami et al., 1972; carp and guecko retinas). Nevertheless, in the turtle, agents known to block ACh muscarinic receptors, block preferentially transmission from cones to horizontal cells, but not to hyperpolarizing bipolar cells (Gerschenfeld and Piccolino, 1977), and in the goldfish retina α-bgt may bind selectively to bipolar dendrites (Schwartz and Bok, 1978). In the tiger salamander, ACh appears to interrupt synaptic input into horizontal cells from neighbouring horizontal cells (Marshall and Werblin, 1978). Thus there may be species differences.

The biogenic monoamines

Of the biogenic monoamines (adrenaline, noradrenaline, dopamine and 5-hydroxy-tryptamine [5-HT]) dopamine is the strongest transmitter candidate in the retina. However, the presence of small numbers of adrenergic and noradrenergic neurones cannot be excluded, e.g., adrenaline is present in frog and toad retinas (see Ehinger, 1976). The evidence as regards 5-HT as a retinal transmitter can best be described as intriguing.

A detailed survey of the results obtained from application of the Falck-Hillarp technique to retinas has been given by Ehinger (1976) and little purpose would be served by reproducing the data here. In summary it can be said that cells exhibiting dopamine fluorescence have been observed in all vertebrate retinas processed by this procedure, and these most commonly form 5–10% of the innermost cell row of the inner nuclear layer – a position characteristic of amacrine cells. A few are also seen among ganglion cells (probably displaced amacrines as no catecholamine-containing axons have been found in optic nerves) and occasionally a fluorescent cell is positioned in the middle of the inner plexiform layer. These have been observed in all species so far examined. There is no obvious evolutionary pattern to the differences that exist (Ehinger, 1976). In mammals complex nerve fibre arrangements are seen in rabbits, dogs and some New World monkeys, whereas simple ones occur in mouse, rat, cat, some Old World monkeys and man.

In two groups of animals, teleost fish and New World monkeys, dopamine-containing interplexiform cells extend processes widely in both plexiform layers. However, in other species (e.g., cat and rhesus and squirrel monkeys) these cells are non-fluorescent, and remain so even when treated with monoamine oxidase inhibitors and with both indole and catecholamine analogues (Dowling et al., 1976; Ehinger, 1976). These observations again emphasize that morphologically similar cells may use different transmitters in different species.

Direct electrophysiological studies on the effects of dopamine on retinal neurones are scarce. In general, inhibitory effects on ganglion cells have been observed and, correlating with this, systemic and intraocular administration of reserpine, which depletes catecholamine stores, makes animals photophobic (Ehinger, 1976; Kramer, 1976). Release of preloaded, labelled dopamine from cat retinas has been reported (Kramer, 1976) and the rate of release plus the amount released per light flash increases with increasing flash frequency. In light-adapted animals a high rate of dopamine release is observed regardless of flash frequency.

With the exception of tissue from chicks (Hauschild and Laties, 1973), no indoleamine-containing neurones have been observed in retinas processed by the Falck-Hillarp method. However, significant amounts of 5-HT and its metabolic enzymes have been detected in many species (Ehinger, 1976; Ehinger and Florén, 1976). In addition, indoleamine-accumulating neurones, clearly distinguishable from the dopaminergic ones, are present in rabbit, cat and goldfish retinas (Ehinger and Florén, 1976, 1978). Again, the location of the cell bodies suggests a subpopulation of amacrine cells.

The significance of these observations is not clear, it may be that the endogenous level of 5-HT is normally low, or alternatively that this is the precursor, or an analogue of the precursor, of a different, non-fluorescing amine in these cells. A candidate is melatonin. However, although hydroxy-indole-*O*-methyl transferase (which forms melatonin from 5-acetyl-5-hydroxytryptamine) is present in retinas from fish, amphibians, a turtle and leghorn chickens, little or none was found in other reptiles, birds, rats or monkeys (see Ehinger, 1976). In addition melatonin is not actively taken up by the rabbit retina (Ehinger and Florén, 1978). Thus more studies are needed.

Neuroactive peptides

Very little is known of neuroactive peptides in the retina. Thyrotropin-releasing hormone-like material has been detected in the rat retina, and is low during the night and higher during the day (Schaeffer et al., 1977). In addition, substance P-like activity has been reported and this may be influenced by the level of retinal illumination (see Stern, 1963). However, Winder and Patsalos (1974) have shown that activity in the bovine retina is essentially limited to the optic nerve stump.

Conclusions

Many of the compounds discussed here are good candidates as retinal neurotransmitters. Some of the evidence supporting this, such as the kinetics of transport systems and the effects of high external potassium concentrations and electrical stimulation on their retention by the retina, has not been dealt with. For this information the reader is referred to Neal (1976a, amino acids), Neal (1976b, acetylcholine) and Ehinger and Florén (1978, dopamine and indoleamines).

Considering the layered structure of the retina and the meticulous work that is being done to define the retinal circuits (e.g., Nelson et al., 1976), it is clear that the application of many of the histological techniques now available will enable us to locate putative transmitters at the EM level, and to correlate these with the neurophysiology and morphology. However, it will require a great deal of patience, especially as it may have to be done a species at a time.

SUMMARY

Present evidence suggests considerable chemical as well as morphological specialization of retinal neurones. Analysis of tangential sections of the retina has shown peaks of, e.g., choline acetyltransferase, GABA and glutamate decarboxylase in the amacrine cell and inner plexiform layers, and α-bungarotoxin binding and immunohistochemistry respectively have been used to locate these systems at the EM level. Endogenous pools of monoamines have been detected by fluorescent histochemistry and autoradiography has localised the uptake of radiolabelled putative neurotransmitters to specific neuronal populations.

Where many transmitters have been associated with subpopulations of one cell type, it is not always clear whether single cells are e.g. accumulating more than one transmitter. However, effects of antagonists do imply specificity in the neuronal circuits.

REFERENCES

Arden, G. B. (1976) The retina – neurophysiology. In: *The Eye, 2nd ed., Vol. 2A, Visual Function in Man,* H. Davson (Ed.), Academic Press, New York, pp. 229–356.

Arden, G. B. and Ernst, W. (1971) A method of determining photoreceptor ion contents. *J. Physiol. (Lond.),* 216: 5P-7P.

Bauer, B. (1978) Photic release of radioactivity from rabbit retina preloaded with [^{3}H]GABA. *Acta ophthal. (Kbh.),* 56: 270–283.

Bauer, B. and Ehinger, B. (1978) Retinal uptake and release of [^{3}H]DABA. *Exp. Eye Res.,* 26: 275–290.

Baughman, R. W. and Bader, C. R. (1977) Biochemical characterization and cellular localization of the cholinergic system in the chicken retina. *Brain Res.,* 138: 469–485.

Berger, S. J., McDaniel, M. L., Carter, J. G. and Lowry, O. H. (1977) Distribution of four potential transmitter amino acids in monkey retina. *J. Neurochem.,* 28: 159–163.

Bruun, A. and Ehinger, B. (1974) Uptake of certain possible neurotransmitters into retinal neurons of some mammals. *Exp. Eye Res.,* 19: 435–447.

Caldwell, J. H. and Daw, N. W. (1978) Effects of picrotoxin and strychnine on rabbit retinal ganglion cells: changes in centre surround receptive fields. *J. Physiol. (Lond.),* 276: 299–310.

Caldwell, J. H., Daw, N. W. and Wyatt, H. J. (1978) Effects of picrotoxin and strychnine on rabbit retinal ganglion cells: lateral interactions for cells with more complex receptive fields. *J. Physiol. (Lond.),* 276: 277–298.

Cohen, A. I. (1978) Retinal organization and function: possible roles for taurine. In: *Taurine and Neurological Disorders,* A. Barbeau and R. J. Huxtable (Eds.), Raven Press, New York, pp. 249–264.

Cohen, A. I., McDaniel, M. and Orr, H. (1973) Absolute levels of some free amino acids in normal and biologically fractionated retinas. *Invest. Ophthal.,* 12: 686–693.

Cunningham, R. and Miller, R. F. (1976) Taurine: its selective action on neuronal pathways in the rabbit retina. *Brain Res.,* 117: 341–345.

Dowling, J. E. (1970) Organization of vertebrate retinas. *Invest. Ophthal.,* 9: 655–680.

Dowling, J. E. and Ripps, H. (1973) Effects of magnesium on horizontal cell activity in skate retina. *Nature (Lond.),* 242: 101–103.

Dowling, J. E., Ehinger, B. and Hedden, W. L. (1976) The interplexiform cell: a new type of retinal neuron. *Invest. Ophthal.,* 15: 916–926.

Dubin, M. W. (1974) Anatomy of the vertebrate retina. In: *The Eye, Vol. 6, Comparative Physiology,* H. Davson and L. T. Graham, Jr. (Eds.), Academic Press, New York, pp. 227–256.

Ehinger, B. (1973) Glial uptake of taurine in the rabbit retina. *Brain Res.,* 60: 512–516.

Ehinger, B. (1976) Biogenic monoamines as transmitters in the retina. In: *Transmitters in the Visual Process,* S. L. Bonting (Ed.), Pergamon Press, Oxford, pp. 145–163.

Ehinger, B. (1977) Glial and neuronal uptake of GABA, glutamic acid, glutamine and glutathione in the rabbit retina. *Exp. Eye Res.,* 25: 221–234.

Ehinger, B. and Florén, I. (1976) Indoleamine-accumulating neurons in the retina of rabbit, cat and goldfish. *Cell Tiss. Res.,* 175: 37–48.

Ehinger, B. and Florén, I. (1978) Quantitation of the uptake of indoleamines and dopamine in the rabbit retina. *Exp. Eye Res.,* 26: 1–11.

Ehinger, B. and Lindberg-Bauer, B. (1976) Light-evoked release of glycine from cat and rabbit retina. *Brain Res.,* 113: 535–549.

Gerschenfeld, H. M. and Piccolino, M. (1977) Muscarinic antagonists block cone to horizontal cell transmission in turtle retina. *Nature (Lond.),* 268: 257–259.

Graham, Jr., L. T. (1974) Comparative aspects of neurotransmitters in the retina. In: *The Eye, Vol. 6, Comparative Physiology,* H. Davson and L. T. Graham, Jr. (Eds.), Academic Press, New York, pp. 283–342.

Graham, L. T., Baxter, C. F. and Lolley, R. N. (1970) In vivo influence of light or darkness on the GABA system in the retina of the frog *(Rana pipiens). Brain Res.,* 20: 379–388.

Hauschild, D. and Laties, A. M. (1973) An indoleamine-containing cell in chick retina. *Invest. Ophthal.,* 12: 537–540.

Henke, T. E., Schenker, T. M. and Cuénod, M. (1976) Effects of retinal ablation on uptake of glutamate, glycine, GABA, proline and choline in pigeon tectum. *J. Neurochem.,* 26: 131–134.

Kaneko, A. and Shimazaki, H. (1975) Effects of external ions on the synaptic transmission from photoreceptors to horizontal cells in the carp retina. *J. Physiol. (Lond.),* 252: 509–522.

Kennedy, A. J. and Neal, M. J. (1978) The effect of light and potassium depolarization on the release of endogenous amino acids from the isolated rat retina. *Exp. Eye Res.,* 26: 71–75.

Kennedy, A. J. and Voaden, M. J. (1976) Studies on the uptake and release of radioactive taurine by the frog retina. *J. Neurochem.,* 27: 131–137.

Kennedy, A. J., Neal, M. J. and Lolley, R. N. (1977) The distribution of amino acids within the rat retina. *J. Neurochem.,* 29: 157–159.

Kirby, A. W. and Enroth-Cugell, C. (1976) The involvement of gamma-aminobutyric acid in the organization of cat retinal ganglion cell receptive fields. A study with picrotoxin and bicuculline. *J. gen. Physiol.,* 68: 465–484.

Kleinschmidt, J. and Yazulla, S. (1978) Effects of glutamate agonists and antagonists on goldfish horizontal cells (ARVO Abstr.). *Invest. Ophthal. Vis. Sci.,* 18 (Suppl.): 284.

Kramer, S. G. (1976) Dopamine in retinal neurotransmission. In: *Transmitters in the Visual Process,* S. L. Bonting (Ed.), Pergamon Press, Oxford, pp. 165–198.

Krnjević, K. (1974) Chemical nature of synaptic transmission in vertebrates. *Physiol. Rev.,* 54: 418–540.

Kuriyama, K. E., Sisken, B., Haber, B. and Roberts, E. (1968) The γ-aminobutyric acid system in rabbit retina. *Brain Res.,* 9: 165–168.

Lake, N., Marshall, J. and Voaden, M. J. (1977) The entry of taurine into the neural retina and pigment epithelium of the frog. *Brain Res.,* 128: 497–503.

Lake, N., Marshall, J. and Voaden, M. J. (1978) High affinity uptake sites for taurine in the retina. *Exp. Eye Res.,* 27: 713–718.

Lam, D. M. K. (1975) Synaptic chemistry of identified cells in the vertebrate retina. *Cold Spr. Harb. Symp. quant. Biol.*, 40: 571–579.

Lowry, O. H., Roberts, N. R. and Lewis, C. (1956) The quantitative histochemistry of the retina. *J. biol. Chem.*, 220: 879–892.

Lund Karlsen, R. (1978) The mammalian visual system. In: *Amino Acids as Neurotransmitters*, F. Fonnum (Ed.), Plenum Press, New York, pp. 241–256.

Lund Karlsen, R. and Fonnum, F. (1976) The toxic effect of sodium glutamate on rat retina: changes in putative transmitters and their corresponding enzymes. *J. Neurochem.*, 27: 1437–1441.

Mandel, P., Pasantes-Morales, H. and Urban, P. F. (1976) Taurine, a putative transmitter in retina. In: *Transmitters in the Visual Process*, S. L. Bonting (Ed.), Pergamon Press, Oxford, pp. 89–105.

Marshall, L. M. and Werblin, F. S. (1978) Synaptic transmission to the horizontal cells in the retina of the larval tiger salamander. *J. Physiol. (Lond.)*, 279: 321–346.

Masland, R. H. and Ames, III, A. (1976) Responses to acetylcholine of ganglion cells in an isolated mammalian retina. *J. Neurophysiol.*, 39: 1220–1235.

Masland, R. H. and Livingstone, C. J. (1976) Effect of stimulation with light on synthesis and release of acetylcholine by an isolated mammalian retina. *J. Neurophysiol.*, 39: 1210–1219.

Miller, R. F., Dacheux, R. F. and Frumkes, T. E. (1977) Amacrine cells in *Necturus* retina: evidence for independent γ-aminobutyric acid- and glycine-releasing neurons. *Science*, 198: 748–750.

Miller, S. and Steinberg, R. H. (1976) Transport of taurine, L-methionine and 3-*O*-methyl-D-glucose across frog retinal pigment epithelium. *Exp. Eye Res.*, 23: 177–190.

Morjaria, B. and Voaden, M. J. (1979) The formation of glutamate, aspartate and GABA in the rat retina; glucose and glutamine as precursors. *J. Neurochem.*, in press.

Murakami, M., Ohtsu, K. and Ohtsuka, T. (1972) Effects of chemicals on receptors and horizontal cells in the retina. *J. Physiol. (Lond.)*, 227: 899–913.

Murakami, M., Ohtsuka, T. and Shimazaki, H. (1975) Effects of aspartate and glutamate on the bipolar cells in the carp retina. *Vision Res.*, 15: 456–458.

Neal, M. J. (1976a) Amino acid transmitter substances in the vertebrate retina. *Gen. Pharmacol.*, 7: 321–332.

Neal, M. J. (1976b) Acetyl choline as a retinal transmitter substance. In: *Transmitters in the Visual Process*, S. L. Bonting (Ed.), Pergamon Press, Oxford, pp. 127–143.

Neal, M. J. and Iversen, L. L. (1972) Autoradiographic localisation of ^{3}H-GABA in rat retina. *Nature New Biol.*, 235: 217–218.

Nelson, R., Kolb, H., Famiglietti, Jr., E. V. and Gouras, P. (1976) Neural responses in the rod and cone systems of the cat retina: intracellular records and Procion stains. *Invest. Ophthal.*, 15: 946–953.

Orr, H. T., Cohen, A. I. and Lowry, O. H. (1976) The distribution of taurine in the vertebrate retina. *J. Neurochem.*, 26: 609–611.

Pasantes-Morales, H., Klethi, J., Ledig, M. and Mandel, P. (1973) Influence of light and dark on the free amino acid pattern of the developing chick retina. *Brain Res.*, 57: 59–65.

Pourcho, R. G. (1977) Distribution of ^{35}S taurine in mouse retina after intravitreal and intravascular injection. *Exp. Eye Res.*, 25: 119–127.

Pourcho, R. G. (1978) Localization of nicotinic acetyl choline receptors in the retina (ARVO Abstr.). *Invest. Ophthal. Vis. Sci.*, 18 (Suppl.): 285.

Rasmussen, K.-E. (1972) A morphometric study of the Müller cell cytoplasm in the rat retina. *J. Ultrastruct. Res.*, 39: 413–429.

Ripps, H., Shakib, M. and MacDonald, E. D. (1976) Peroxidase uptake by photoreceptor terminals of the skate retina. *J. Cell Biol.*, 70: 86–96.

Ross, C. D. and McDougal, Jr., D. B. (1976) The distribution of choline acetyl transferase activity in the vertebrate retina. *J. Neurochem.*, 26: 521–526.

Salceda, R. López-Colomé, A. M. and Pasantes-Morales, H. (1977) Light-stimulated release of [^{35}S]taurine from frog retinal rod outer segments. *Brain Res.*, 135: 186–191.

Schaeffer, J. M., Brownstein, M. J. and Axelrod, J. (1977) Thyrotropin-releasing hormone-like material in the rat retina: changes due to environmental lighting. *Proc. nat. Acad. Sci. (Wash.)*, 74: 3579–3581.

Schacher, S., Holtzman, E. and Hood, D. C. (1976) Synaptic activity of frog retinal photoreceptors. A peroxidase uptake study. *J. Cell Biol.*, 70: 178–192.

Schmidt, S. Y. (1978) Taurine fluxes in isolated cat and rat retinas: effects of illumination. *Exp. Eye Res.*, 26: 529–535.

Schmidt, S. Y. and Berson, E. L. (1978) Taurine in retinal degenerations. In: *Taurine and Neurological Disorders,* A. Barbeau and R. J. Huxtable (Eds.), Raven Press, New York, pp. 281–287.

Schwartz, I. R. and Bok, D. (1978) Autoradiographic localization of ^{125}I-α bungarotoxin binding sites in the outer plexiform layer of the goldfish retina (ARVO Abstr.). *Invest. Ophthal. Vis. Sci.,* 18 (Suppl.): 115–116.

Starr, M. S. (1973) Effect of dark adaptation on the GABA system in retina. *Brain Res.,* 59: 331–338.

Starr, M. S. (1975) Effect of light stimulation on the synthesis and release of GABA in rat and frog retinae. *Brain Res.,* 100: 343–353.

Stell, W. K. (1972) The morphological organization of the vertebrate retina. In: *Handbook of Sensory Physiology, Vol. VII/2, Physiology of Photoreceptor Organs,* M. G. F. Fuortes (Ed.), Springer, Berlin, pp. 111–213.

Stern, P. (1963) Substance P as a sensory transmitter and its other central effects. *Ann. N.Y. Acad. Sci.,* 104: 403–414.

Sugiyama, H., Daniels, M. P. and Nirenberg, M. (1977) Muscarinic acetyl choline receptors of the developing retina. *Proc. nat. Acad. Sci. (Wash.),* 74: 5524–5528.

Voaden, M. J. (1974) Light and the spontaneous efflux of radioactive glycine from the frog retina. *Exp. Eye Res.,* 18: 467–475.

Voaden, M. J. (1976) γ-Aminobutyric acid and glycine as retinal neurotransmitters. In: *Transmitters in the Visual Process,* S. L. Bonting (Ed.), Pergamon Press, Oxford, pp. 107–125.

Voaden, M. J. (1978) The localization and metabolism of neuroactive amino acids in the retina. In: *Amino Acids as Neurotransmitters,* F. Fonnum (Ed.), Plenum Press, New York, pp. 257–274.

Voaden, M. J. and Starr, M. S. (1972) The efflux of radioactive GABA from rat retina in vitro. *Vision Res.,* 12: 559–566.

Voaden, M. J., Lake, N., Marshall, J. and Morjaria, B. (1977) Studies on the distribution of taurine and other neuroactive amino acids in the retina. *Exp. Eye Res.,* 25: 249–257.

Voaden, M. J., Lake, N., Marshall, J. and Morjaria, B. (1978) The utilization of glutamine by the retina: an autoradiographic and metabolic study. *J. Neurochem.,* 31: 1069–1076.

Vogel, Z. and Nirenberg, M. (1976) Localization of acetyl choline receptors during synaptogenesis in retina. *Proc. nat. Acad. Sci. (Wash.),* 73: 1806–1810.

Vogel, Z., Maloney, G. J., Ling, A. and Daniel, M. P. (1977) Identification of synaptic acetyl choline receptor sites in retina with peroxidase-labelled α-bungarotoxin. *Proc. nat. Acad. Sci. (Wash.),* 74: 3268–3272.

Winder, A. F. and Patsalos, P. N. (1974) Substance P and retinal neurotransmission. *Biochem. Soc. Trans.,* 2: 1260–1261.

Wood, J. G., McLaughlin, B. J. and Vaughn, J. E. (1976) Immunocytochemical localization of GAD in electron microscopic preparations of rodent CNS. In: *GABA in Nervous System Function,* E. Roberts, T. Chase and D. B. Tower (Eds.), Raven Press, New York, pp. 133–148.

Wu, S. M. and Dowling, J. E. (1978) A re-examination of putative photoreceptor transmitters (ARVO Abstr.). *Invest. Ophthal. Vis. Sci.,* 18 (Suppl.): 284.

Yazulla, S. and Kleinschmidt, J. (1978) Kainic acid differentially affects rod and cone synaptic connections in goldfish retina (ARVO Abstr.). *Invest. Ophthal. Vis. Sci.* 18 (Suppl): 284.

Yazulla, S. and Schmidt, J. (1976) Radioautographic localization of [^{125}I]α-bungarotoxin binding sites in the retinas of goldfish and turtle. *Vision Res.,* 16: 878–880.

Yazulla, S. and Schmidt, J. (1977) Two types of receptors for α-bungarotoxin in the synaptic layers of the pigeon retina. *Brain Res.,* 138: 45–57.

A Speculative Essay on Geniculate Lamination and its Development

R. W. GUILLERY*

Department of Pharmacological and Physiological Sciences, University of Chicago, 947 East 58th Street, Chicago, Ill. 60637 (U.S.A.)

INTRODUCTION

The dorsal lateral geniculate nucleus shows clear signs of lamination in many mammals. The laminar arrangement varies considerably from one order to another and in some instances it even shows marked differences between sub- or infra-orders. Many different laminar patterns have been described (see e.g. Minkowski, 1920; Nichterlein and Goldby, 1944; Walls, 1953; Polyak, 1957; Hassler, 1964; Giolli and Tigges, 1970; Kaas et al., 1972, 1978; Sanderson, 1974) and a number of suggestions have been made for schematizing the various laminar patterns. Two quite different approaches can be used for an analysis of these laminar patterns. The laminae can be considered from a functional point of view by asking whether different laminae or laminar groupings subserve different functions, and this approach has made some significant advances recently; or they can be looked at from a developmental point of view by enquiring about the mechanisms that produce the adult laminated structure. These two approaches are complementary and in this paper I will discuss the functional analysis first, and then consider the developmental mechanisms. I will try to show briefly how these approaches relate to each other and where each can help us to understand the laminar structure. The review will focus especially upon problems that are as yet unsolved.

(1) THE TWO INDEPENDENT RETINO-GENICULO-CORTICAL PATHWAYS

The simplest and most obvious functional interpretation of geniculate lamination is that this is a device for segregating two independent ocular inputs, one from each eye. Each retina is represented as a topographically organized map within one set of geniculate layers, and the two pathways are independent of each other in the lateral geniculate nucleus. Binocular interactions, on this view, first occur in the visual cortex.

This interpretation presents an adequate explanation for two geniculate layers, but it can provide no functional basis for more than two layers; and most mammals have more than two geniculate layers. Further, if the lateral geniculate nucleus is, indeed, a nucleus within which the pathways from the two eyes are kept clearly segregated, then it is difficult to

* Supported by Grants NS 14283 and EY 02374 from the NIH.

understand why the two representations of the visual field, one coming from each eye, should be accurately in register within the nucleus. In all mammalian species that have been studied from this point of view one finds that each geniculate layer carries a map of the contralateral visual field and that these maps are in precise alignment (see Walls, 1953; Polyak, 1957; Kaas et al., 1972). I shall return to this point, but note here that the developmental mechanisms that could produce such an alignment are not simple, for within the geniculate layers, axons arising from homonymous retinal points (i.e. points viewing the same position in the visual field) terminate in precise alignment. These homonymous retinal points have no known common morphological feature, nor do they have a shared developmental history. Thus, a complex developmental problem is solved with remarkable accuracy and it is reasonable to look for the functional significance of such a developmental achievement.

(2) FUNCTIONALLY DISTINCT RETINO-GENICULATE PATHWAYS

(A) The X, Y, W systems

The view that there are separate, functionally distinct retino-geniculate pathways and that the geniculate layers represent separate relays for these pathways is not new (e.g. LeGros Clark, 1942; Walls, 1953) but it has recently received strong support from observations on cats and monkeys. In the cat, 3 functionally distinct retino-geniculate systems have been identified as X, Y and W systems (see e.g. Cleland et al., 1976; Wilson et al., 1976) and each appears to have a relatively independent relay to the cortex (Stone and Dreher, 1973; Wilson and Stone, 1975). The functional characteristics of these systems do not concern us at present; the Y system has the thickest, most rapidly conducting axons, the W system the finest. In the laminar part of the lateral geniculate nucleus the X and Y systems have a largely overlapping distribution within the dorsal layers (layers A, A1 and C of Hickey and Guillery, 1974) while the W system terminates mainly further ventrally among the smaller cells of layers C1 and C2 (Cleland et al., 1976; Wilson et al., 1976; Mitzdorf and Singer, 1977).

In the monkey (owl monkey and macaque monkey) it has been possible to recognize that an X-like system, with color opponent cells responding in a sustained manner to stationary stimuli and having slowly conducting axons, relays in the parvocellular layers, while a Y-like system, with broadly tuned cells that have transient responses and rapidly conducting axons, relays in the magnocellular layers (Dreher et al., 1976; Sherman et al., 1976; Schiller and Malpeli, 1978). No system that might correspond to the W system of cats has yet been described, but it should be noted that there are very thin layers of extremely small cells on either side of the magnocellular layers (Guillery and Colonnier, 1970; Hubel and Wiesel, 1977), and the functional properties of these small cells remain to be defined, as do, of course, the detailed parallels between the cat and the monkey "X" and "Y" systems. Schiller and Malpeli (1978) have further found that cells within the dorsal two parvocellular layers (layers 5 and 6) are mainly "on center", while cells in the ventral parvocellular layers (3 and 4) are mainly "off center."

Other species have not been studied in detail from the point of view of the laminar segregation of cell types. Although Sherman et al. (1975a) were able to distinguish X-like and Y-like cells within the lateral geniculate nucleus of tree shrews, they were not able to localize functionally distinct cell types within individual layers. Possibly, however, the reason for this is a technical difficulty and not the absence of such a segregation, since the layers in the tree shrew are extremely thin. Certainly, there is good evidence that in the tree shrew the different geniculate layers send axon terminals to different cortical laminae (Harting et al., 1973) and this in itself suggests some functional segregation.

The view that the geniculate layers represent sets of functionally distinct pathways, one set coming from each eye, may account for many of the features of geniculate structure in many mammalian forms. Clearly, the precise correspondence between laminar structure and the functionally distinct pathways needs to be studied in more species. Further, it will be of interest to determine whether the separate layers merely represent topographically separate relays, each performing a similar function for each of its several pathways, or whether the layers may represent relays each of which imposes its own characteristic transfer functions upon its pathway.

There is, at present, very little evidence on this last point. It is recognized that perikaryal size differs within the several geniculate laminae of many species, and where evidence is available it appears that cell size relates to axon diameter and thus to conduction velocity within the visual pathways (e.g. Stone and Fukuda, 1974; Wässle et al., 1975). However, the significance of conduction velocity to the performance of the several pathways remains somewhat obscure. A potentially more interesting possibility has been raised recently by the suggestion that in the cat, geniculate X and Y cells may be distinguishable on the basis of their dendritic branching patterns (LeVay and Ferster, 1977), the X cells being the class 2 cells and the Y cells the class 1 cells that are recognizable in Golgi preparations (see Guillery, 1966). Since there is reason to believe that retino-geniculate axons synapse with class 2 cells at specialized grape-like appendages clustered around primary dendritic branch points (Szentágothai, 1963, 1964; Guillery, 1967a, 1969a), whereas these axons synapse with class 1 cells upon dendritic stems nearer the perikaryon (Guillery, 1971a; Guillery and Scott, 1971), one can be led by an, as yet, rather tenuous argument to conclude that in the cat the geniculate transfer characteristics of the X and Y systems may differ significantly. Here, again, however, we need more information about how the specific retino-geniculate synapses are related to other synapses or to the membrane properties of geniculate cells for each of the two cell types.

In the cat, the X and Y systems share layers A, A1 and C and, thus, particular differences between these cell types cannot be regarded as representative of laminar differences. In the monkey the X-like and Y-like systems show a laminar segregation, but we do not know yet whether the magnocellular and parvocellular cells are distinguishable in terms of features such as those that distinguish class 1 from class 2 cells in cats.

(B) Varying degrees of functional segregation: a comparison of cat and monkey

The conclusion that functionally distinct pathways tend to be kept separate within the lateral geniculate nucleus seems reasonable on the basis of currently available information, and the laminar arrangements that characterize the nucleus would appear to represent this segregation of functional systems to some extent. However, the degree to which any two systems may be separated varies between species, and it does not seem possible to suggest any single schema that might account for mammalian geniculate patterns in general. A comparison of cat and monkey illustrates this point quite strikingly and also suggests that individual laminar patterns occurring in any one species may represent varying degrees of segregation of functionally different pathways.

One striking feature of the monkey's lateral geniculate nucleus, which is also seen in the nucleus of other primates but is absent in the cat and in most other mammals, is a feature that can be called "binocular balance". In a geniculate nucleus having binocular balance there is, for the binocular part of the visual field, one lamina innervated by the ipsilateral eye corresponding to every lamina innervated by the contralateral eye*. Most non-primate nuclei are unbalanced; the contralaterally innervated layers outnumber those that receive an ipsilateral input, and this is the situation in the cat.

Of the layers receiving X and Y inputs in the cat, layers A and C are contralaterally innervated while layer A1, lying between them, is ipsilaterally innervated. Mitzdorf and Singer (1977) have presented evidence from current source density studies that laminae A and C together are equivalent to lamina A1, with most of the crossed Y input going to lamina C, and A1 receiving uncrossed X and Y inputs. There is a tendency for those Y inputs that terminate in layers A and A1 to end ventral to the X inputs (that is, closer to lamina C). This distribution suggests a system that is partially split, with the Y relays moving ventrally, the X relays dorsally, and the split for the crossed system being more nearly complete than the split for the uncrossed system. This is an appealing interpretation and there is some support for it from the pattern of geniculo-cortical projections described by Holländer and Vanegas (1977). However, others have not consistently confirmed such a geniculo-cortical pattern (Garey and Blakemore, 1977; Geisert, 1978) and electrophysiological studies of single geniculate cells have not shown the distribution of X and Y systems described by Mitzdorf and Singer (1977).

An organization similar to that proposed by Mitzdorf and Singer for the X and Y systems can also be suggested for the fine fibered (W) input that goes to the ventral C layers of the cat and the mink (see Guillery and Oberdorfer (1977) for details regarding the mink and for the comparison with the cat; see Sanderson (1974) for a description of the general carnivore pattern of geniculate lamination including specifically the cat and mink). There are 3 C layers in receipt of retinal inputs: C, C1 and C2. C and C2 receive crossed inputs while C1 receives an uncrossed input. The dorsal part of C is large celled and receives the coarse afferents discussed above, but the cells become smaller as the border of lamina C1 is approached and there is evidence for a W input to this ventral part of layer C (Wilson et al., 1976). The afferents to layer C1 are fine axons (Guillery, 1970) identifiable as belonging to the W system (Cleland et al., 1976; Wilson et al., 1976) and there are reasons for thinking that the afferents to layer C2 are even finer than those to C1 (Guillery and Oberdorfer, 1977). Thus, the crossed W system may have a relatively coarse fibered dorsal component going to the ventral part of layer C and a very fine fibered component going to layer C2. The uncrossed inputs show no clear separation, all go to C1 and the average of the fiber diameters would appear to lie between those of the C and C2 afferents.

In the monkey, then, the X-like and Y-like systems are clearly separated, whereas in the cat they are partially separated, and the separation is more advanced for the crossed than for the uncrossed pathways. There is evidence for inhibitory interactions between X and Y systems in the lateral geniculate nucleus of the cat (Singer and Bedworth, 1973; Dubin and Cleland, 1977) and the occurrence of these interactions may be related to the incomplete anatomical separation of the two systems. It is not known whether the interactions are more

---

* The S layer which receives primarily an ipsilateral input (see Giolli and Tigges, 1970; Kaas et al., 1972, 1978) is excluded from this argument since it may represent a folding of one of the other ipsilateral layers and probably represents only a part of the visual field (Kaas et al., 1972, 1978; Casagrande, 1978). Clearly, including layer S in the following argument would accentuate the difference between the primate nucleus and others.

marked for the crossed than for the uncrossed pathways in the cat, nor is it known whether comparable interactions occur in the monkey. It is possible that such interactions tend to take place in the cortex to a greater extent in species in which the geniculate pathways are separated.

(3) OTHER ASPECTS OF GENICULATE ORGANIZATION

Several problems remain that cannot be accounted for by the view that lamination is a means of segregating functionally distinct pathways. One is that some layers represent only a small part of the contralateral visual hemifield; another is that there are well defined interlaminar zones and these do not easily fit into such a schema; a third, which has been mentioned already is that it is difficult to see why the several visual field representations should be in register. Naturally, there are others, but these are the three that will concern us in the following paragraphs.

(A) Laminae that represent small segments of the visual field

The partial layers that do not represent a complete hemifield are well seen in the parvocellular layers of Old World monkeys and have been discussed previously by Kaas et al. (1972). There are 4 parvocellular layers for central vision, but only two for peripheral vision (Malpeli and Baker, 1975). One could regard this as representing a morphological basis for some system that is present for central vision but not for peripheral vision. However, at present there is no evidence for such a view. Schiller and Mapeli (1978) have some evidence that where the 4 parvocellular layers fuse to form two, the segregation of functional types is maintained, and one cell type tends to concentrate in the dorsal parts of a single layer while another concentrates in the ventral parts. This is reminiscent of the suggestions made by Mitzdorf and Singer (1977) regarding a partial segregation of cell types in cats and suggests that the segregation is more advanced for central than it is for peripheral vision. Since it is not unusual to find that the laminar structure is better defined in the parts of the nucleus representing central vision (e.g. Guillery (1970) for the cat), this may prove to be a rather general gradient of segregation.

In some primate nuclei, particularly in the human nucleus (Hickey and Guillery, 1978) one finds geniculate segments that contain 6 rather than 4 parvocellular laminae. At first sight it is tempting to treat these segments as representing a further stage in the segregation of functional types. However, in the human nucleus the occurrence of the 6-layered parvocellular segment is very variable and this segment does not lie in the zone that represents central vision. Instead, it lies at various locations along the plane where the two parvocellular layers split into four, and commonly lies close to the representation of the optic disc. Further, in the human nucleus the dorsal layer (6) shows a tendency to form small spurs that look like abortive attempts at the formation of yet another lamina, and these spurs also occur along the plane where two parvocellular layers split to form four (see Hickey and Guillery (1978) for details). Thus, it is possible to consider this reduplication of parvocellular layers as a developmental aberration, reflecting an intrageniculate mechanism that produces a laminar splitting along a reasonably well defined plane. In some nuclei this mechanism appears to go beyond the simple production of four layers out of two; the reasons for this developmental aberration are not known.

(B) The interlaminar zones

The interlaminar zones were long regarded as being myelinated leaflets that serve merely to separate cell layers (Walls, 1953). Some interlaminar zones may represent a functionally quite neutral myelinated zone of this type (see e.g. Fig. 14 of Hassler, 1964), but in most nuclei the interlaminar zones are a synaptically rich, relatively cell free zone into which one can trace the peripheral segments of dendrites from adjacent cellular laminae (Guillery (1966, 1969a) for the cat; Casagrande et al. (1978b) for the tree shrew). The interlaminar zones are further characterized by being relatively free of retinal input and rich in corticofugal and tecto-geniculate inputs. The lack of retinal input is evident especially in autoradiographs that label retino-geniculate axons (see Hickey and Guillery (1974), Casagrande et al. (1978) and Hubel and Wiesel (1977) for the cat, tree shrew and monkey respectively), and is most striking where adjacent layers are innervated by the same eye, as for example, between layers 2 and 3 of the Old World monkey or layers 2, 3, and 4 of the tree shrew. In a normal cat adjacent layers are not innervated by the same eye, but in mink, a carnivore whose nucleus resembles that of the cat, layers A and A1 both split into two leaflets, and these leaflets are separated by a well defined interlaminar zone which is clearly not in receipt of a significant retinal input (Guillery and Oberdorfer, 1977; Fig. 2). The A/A1 interlaminar zone can be seen to be similarly free of retinal input in an albino mink, in which layers A and A1 both receive crossed inputs (Sanderson et al., 1974; Guillery et al., 1978).

The cortical input to the interlaminar zones is shown clearly by fiber degeneration or autoradiographic methods (e.g., Guillery, 1967b; Holländer, 1972; Updyke, 1976, for the cat; Sanderson and Kaas, 1974, for the mink; Casagrande et al., 1978b, for the tree shrew; Holländer and Martinez Millán, 1975, for the Old World monkey). Generally, the corticogeniculate projection from area 17 distributes equally to the laminae and to the interlaminar zones. However, in the tree shrew there is a preponderance of inputs to the interlaminar regions (Casagrande et al., 1978b). In the cat, the corticofugal pathway from area 18 shows a similar tendency to concentrate within the interlaminar zones (Updyke, 1976).

In addition to the cortico-geniculate afferents to the interlaminar zones there are also tecto-geniculate afferents which terminate predominantly within the interlaminar zones in the squirrel monkey (Harting et al., 1978) and tree shrew (Casagrande et al., 1978b). However, it is possible that in some species this input is particularly concentrated around the smallest geniculate cells (Graham, 1977).

It is, thus, necessary to regard the interlaminar zones as specialized synaptic regions, where cortico-geniculate systems impinge upon dendritic segments that are free of retinal inputs. Regions showing a similar organization can also be seen in the main laminae (the interstitial zones; Guillery, 1969a) and so long as one considers the nerve cell as the functional unit one cannot easily regard the interlaminar zones as representing a functionally discrete region comparable to a lamina or to a nucleus. However, by the localized absence of retinal inputs, by the concentration of some cortical inputs and by the orientation of corticofugal axons, which tend to run in the plane of the laminae in the interlaminar zones but perpendicular to this in the laminae (Guillery, 1967b), it is possible to distinguish the interlaminar zones as regions that are in some way specialized for the receipt of cortical inputs. There is a difference between the interstitial zones and the interlaminar zones, but at present the functional significance of this difference is undefined.

Not only are the interlaminar zones receptor zones for cortical inputs, but there is reason to believe that each of the different cortical areas (17, 18, 19, etc.) relates to the several interlaminar zones in a characteristic patterned manner (see Updyke, 1976). Thus it is possible to look at laminar splits in a new light. These splits may arise not only to produce a clearer segregation of the functionally distinct retino-geniculate pathways discussed in section A, but perhaps some of the splits occur because a new interlaminar zone, receptive to a particular pattern of cortical inputs, has been developed. The fact that some interlaminar zones represent only a limited part of the visual field may well be related to the observation that some cortical areas only represent a part of the visual field (e.g. Palmer et al., 1978). However, the precise relationship between the several cortical areas and the interlaminar zones in different mammalian species remains to be worked out.

(C) The alignment of the several visual field representations

To account for the alignment of the visual field representations it is necessary to look for interactions between the laminae. We have seen that there is some evidence for interactions between functionally distinct pathways (X pathways and Y pathways, see above) but there is no clear evidence yet that this involves interlaminar interactions. For understanding the alignment it may be more important to consider binocular interactions of the type that have been described by Sanderson et al. (1971) and that probably involve either translaminar interneurons (see Tömböl, 1969) or translaminar dendrites (Guillery, 1966) or both. Perhaps the most significant feature that may account for the alignment is the cortico-geniculate fiber system. The axons of this system pass through the geniculate layers roughly along the lines of projection (Beresford, 1962; Guillery, 1967b) and they can often be traced across laminar borders. Almost half of the axon terminals identifiable within layers A and A1 have the morphological characteristics of cortico-geniculate axons (Guillery, 1969b) and one can reasonably conclude that there is a large cortical input to the lateral geniculate nucleus. Mitzdorf and Singer (1977) found that cortical stimulation produces activity comparable in intensity to that produced by retinal stimulation. Curiously, even though this is an impressive system in terms of the number of its axons, in terms of their orientation and translaminar organization, and in terms of their widespread cortical origin (Updyke, 1976), very little is known regarding its functions. From the point of view of the present discussion, we can regard it as a major system that may well demand a precise interlaminar alignment of visual field representations, but a system whose function is reluctantly left as beyond the scope of the present review.

(4) THE DEVELOPMENT OF THE LATERAL GENICULATE LAMINAE

The account I have given so far indicates some of the problems that an analysis of geniculate development can usefully address. A mechanism for generating the differentiation of laminae must be related to ingrowth of the axons from the two eyes, and must also be related to the ingrowth of functionally distinct fiber types, which show varying degrees of laminar segregation, depending upon the species. Where two different systems overlap within a single lamina, as do the X and Y systems in layers A and A1 of cats, each system may need to establish connections with a particular cell type. The maps from the two eyes must be in register within the whole set of the geniculate laminae and these maps themselves must be in register with the visual field maps that are carried in the cortico-geniculate systems. The axons of the several corticofugal systems must develop their characteristic laminar distributions and the terminal segments of these axons must distribute appropriately along the lines of projection, or perpendicular to these. As the laminae develop, so the regions between them must differentiate their characteristic synaptic organization.

A simple summary of some of the known features of geniculate organization such as the above stresses the complexity of the developmental problems and draws attention to the limited knowledge that is available about developmental mechanisms for any complex neural center. The same general problems, of matching several separate maps, of segregating functionally distinct inputs, and of connecting morphologically different cell types to specific sets of inputs, occur over and again in the developing brain. Geniculate development may prove of particular interest because the complexities of the adult structure are beginning to be reasonably well understood and because many of the developmental problems one can define have a clear topographic component. So far, 3 approaches have been used to study geniculate development. The first is to study normal development, the second is to study the changes produced by removal of one input, and the third is to study congenitally abnormal development. Here we are concerned only with the laminated nucleus and will therefore confine the discussion to cat, monkey, mink and ferret.

(A) Normal developmental sequences

Knowledge of the normal time sequence will clearly provide the basis for an eventual understanding of geniculate development. So far very few details are known. Anker (1977) has shown that the retino-geniculate axons of the cat reach the lateral geniculate nucleus by embryonic day 37, and that cortico-geniculate afferents have entered the nucleus by embryonic day 48. In contrast to this, Cragg (1975) has shown that within layers A and A1 of the cat most synaptic development occurs postnatally. Lamination is recognizable in a newborn kitten (Kalil, 1978) but the first appearance of lamination has not been defined for cats. Preliminary observations of ferrets, in which the young are born very early, show that in this species the characteristic carnivore pattern of lamination appears during the first 10 postnatal days; at birth the major retinal input to the lateral geniculate nucleus is crossed, and there is no clear segregation of the small ipsilateral input until about the time at which lamination appears (Card-Linden, 1978). Rakic's (1976, 1977a, b) studies of the rhesus monkey show that the inputs from the two eyes appear to overlap at early stages of geniculate development and that the cytoarchitectonic differentiation of laminae appears at about the same time as the two inputs segregate during intrauterine life. Rakic (1977b) has shown that the cells of the magnocellular layers are generated somewhat earlier than those of the parvocellular layers, although there is considerable overlap. Further, Rakic has suggested that neurons grouped around a single line of projection in the adult, that is, viewing the same point in visual space, may have a common origin from a limited cell group of the early germinal epithelium. It is possible that such a common "clonal" origin may serve as a marker during later development (Stryker, 1977) but there is no evidence yet to suggest how the two populations of ingrowing axons, one from each eye, may use such a marker.

(B) Congenitally abnormal geniculate development

The relatively normal geniculate development that has been described by Kaiserman-Abramoff et al. (1975) in anophthalmic mice is a striking illustration of the degree to which a considerable part of geniculate development must be independent of retinal input. However, the nucleus of the mouse does not show the laminar organization that is the main topic of this review, and no comparable anophthalmic strains have been studied in carnivores or primates, so that we do not know the extent to which the laminated nucleus may depend upon retinal inputs. Early enucleations, however, do provide some clues, and these are discussed in the next section.

In cats, mink and ferrets it has been possible to study congenital abnormalities of the retino-geniculate pathways that do provide some clues about the development of laminar structures (see Guillery, 1969c, 1971b; Guillery and Kaas, 1971; Hubel and Wiesel, 1971; Sanderson et al., 1974; Shatz, 1977a, b; Guillery et al., 1979). The abnormal animals show an abnormality of retinal development which produces a misrouting of retino-geniculate axons; fibers from the temporal retina cross in the optic chiasm instead of staying on their own side. The size of the abnormal contingent varies in different abnormal genotypes, so that in some individuals there are only a few misrouted axons while in others almost all of the retino-geniculate axons are crossed (see Sanderson et al., 1974; Guillery et al., 1979; for details about abnormal mink, in which the greatest variety of abnormalities can be seen).

It has been possible to find several modifications of geniculate structure that are relevant to understanding how the laminar development may be related to the binocular input. These modifications affect layers A and A1 quite clearly, and the following discussion will be limited to these layers. Because the C layers are less clearly differentiated, abnormalities in these layers are more difficult to evaluate, and they will not be considered further.

When some of the retinofugal axons are abnormally crossed, as for example in Siamese cats, one finds a normal complement of geniculate layers, but there is a marked tendency for any two layers which are innervated by the same eye, to fuse. Further, one finds that where a single layer has two parts, one innervated normally by the ipsilateral eye, and the other receiving an abnormal crossed input, these two parts are separated by a region resembling an interlaminar zone (Guillery and Kaas, 1971; Shatz, 1977a, b). That is, the retinal input appears to be capable of modifying the perikaryal distribution in the nucleus so that regions receiving from the same eye tend to form a continuous cell group, while regions receiving from different eyes form cytoarchitectonically separate groups. It should be noted, however, that this retinal "control" of geniculate structure is never complete. Athough two geniculate segments receiving from different eyes seem always to be separated by a narrow, cell-free zone*, it is not uncommon to find two adjacent cell groups that are innervated by the same eye and that are nonetheless not fused (Guillery and Kaas, 1971; Shatz, 1977a, b; Montero and Guillery, 1978; for the Siamese cat; Guillery et al., 1979; for the mink). Thus, in many Siamese cats the part of lamina A1 receiving a crossed input fuses with lamina A in the medial, but fuses less or not at all in the lateral parts of the nucleus (Shatz, 1977a). Similarly in albino mink, most of the nucleus receives a crossed input, there are only tiny patches receiving ipsilateral afferents, yet the normal complement of laminae is clearly recognizable in most of the nucleus. The abnormal fusions only occur in some parts, mostly medially (Guillery et al., 1979).

One can argue that this lack of complete fusion of the abnormally innervated layers shows that the retinal input only has a partial control of the cellular arrangements in the nucleus and that other factors, some of which may be intrinsic geniculate factors, or factors

* This statement applies to layers A and A1 of the congenitally abnormal mink and cats, and it also applies to normal carnivores and Old World primates (see Hickey and Guillery, 1978). However, it does not apply to New World monkeys, in which parvocellular laminae innervated by different eyes are cytoarchitectonically completely fused.

dependent upon the cortical afferents, also tend to produce the laminar separations and to control the differentiation of the interlaminar zones. The alternative is to argue that the abnormal pathways develop rather late, after the normal laminar arrangements of the nucleus have already been established under the control of a relatively normal retino-geniculate input, which is lost at later developmental stages. The first interpretation is more attractive for a number of reasons, but the second clearly needs to be ruled out by a close study of the abnormal developmental sequence, which is currently being undertaken. Preliminary observations show that abnormal pathways are established prior to laminar differentiation. There are two further reasons for favoring the first interpretation. One is that the pathway abnormality is closely related to specific developmental abnormalities of the retinal pigment epithelium, which occur very early in intrauterine life, at a time when retinofugal pathways are first being established. Thus, it is more likely that the initial development of the pathways is abnormal. The second reason is that in some abnormal mink which are described in the next paragraph, the laminar structure of the normally innervated layers is modified in a manner strongly suggestive of some non-retinal control of laminar development.

These abnormal mink have been described by Guillery et al. (1979). They show a reduced ipsilateral input to layer A1; this leads to a reduced size of layer A1 and also, in many instances, to an interruption in the layer. Opposite such interruptions one sees reduplications of the normally innervated layer A. These reduplications can often be clearly identified as belonging to layer A rather than A1 because in the mink, layers A and A1 both consist of paired adjacent leaflets. Where there is a hiatus in one or both leaflets of layer A1 there is in many instances a reduplication of the anterior leaflet of layer A, with no involvement of the posterior leaflet. In contrast to this, where layer A1 is involved in fusions with A, the posterior leaflet of A, nearest A1, is modified.

There are some reasons, then, for thinking that there may be two mechanisms interacting to produce the normal complement of geniculate layers. One is an intrinsic geniculate mechanism, or one depending upon cortico-geniculate inputs, which tends to produce the number of laminae appropriate for the particular species, and the other is a mechanism that depends upon the characteristics of the ingrowing retinal afferents. In normal development these two mechanisms would reinforce each other to produce the same outcome. In the abnormal mink and the Siamese cat they tend to act against each other, and one sees a compromise outcome, of partial fusions and partial reduplication of layers, which are difficult to explain in terms of a single mechanism.

It is possible to regard the variable reduplication of parvocellular layers in the human nucleus described above (p. 407), as an expression of the non-retinal mechanism. It is more difficult to understand this as a result produced by a sorting of functionally distinct inputs coming from the eyes.

(C) Experimental manipulations

The considerable amount of work that has been done on postnatal development of the geniculo-cortical system, particularly as this relates to visual deprivation by lid suture, dark-rearing, or more subtle means, is beyond the scope of this brief review, since the known geniculate changes do not affect the general arrangement of the laminae or their afferents. However, it should be pointed out that there is evidence that in cats and tree shrews the Y system is more severely affected by postnatal deprivation than is the X system (Sherman et al., 1972, 1975b; Norton et al., 1977) and there is clearly a possibility that this involves a switch in the specific geniculate connectivity patterns established by each system during development. Interestingly, there is no evidence that the two systems are differentially affected in monkeys (Von Noorden and Middleditch, 1975) where the X-like and Y-like pathways appear to be more clearly segregated within individual layers. Perhaps the modification of the Y system that is seen in cats depends upon interactions between X and Y systems that are possible in cats but are excluded in monkeys by the clear laminar segregation. The possibility that in the cat one of the two systems may develop at the expense of the other has also recently been considered by LeVay and Ferster (1977).

Monocular enucleation has a more dramatic effect upon geniculate development than does monocular deprivation. Removing one eye in an adult itself produces quite dramatic cell shrinkage in the deafferented geniculate layers (Minkowski, 1920; LeGros Clark and Penman, 1934; Cook et al., 1951) and some cell death may also occur (Goldby, 1957; Matthews et al., 1960). When one eye is removed in an infant the change is more marked (Guillery, 1973 for the cat), and in cats there may be up to 35% cell death (Guillery, unpublished observations of enucleations done on the 7th postnatal day). Within the lateral geniculate nucleus of an adult cat, which had had one eye removed at the 3rd–20th postnatal day, it is possible to see that the deafferented layers are extremely shrunken and contain very small cells; and the earlier enucleations appear to produce the more severe changes. In addition to these atrophic changes one sees that parts of the deafferented layers adjacent to a normally innervated layer are invaded by translaminar axonal sprouts, and in the region of these sprouts geniculate cells develop an apparently normal size (Guillery, 1971c, 1972; Kalil, 1972; Hickey, 1975; Robson et al., 1978). Further, in the region of the translaminar invasion the interlaminar zone often becomes obscured and this is seen especially after the earliest enucleations. This translaminar invasion only occurs in young kittens enucleated during the first 3 weeks of postnatal life (Guillery, 1972). It does not occur at all in adults.

When a kitten is born the geniculate layers are differentiated (Kalil, 1978) and appropriately innervated (Richards and Kalil, 1974). Thus, the enucleation experiments show that when one set of retino-geniculate axons is destroyed the other set can invade some of the territory in the vacated layers, can successfully reinnervate the denervated cells (Robson et al., 1978) and can save them from the shrinkage (and possible death) they would presumably have suffered had they not been reinnervated. Individual axons can have some terminal branches in their original layers and others in the foreign, originally deafferented layers (Robson et al., 1978) so that one must conclude that in normal development each set of retino-geniculate axons may be kept out of inappropriate territory by the presence of another set, rather than by specific properties of geniculate cells.

When one set of retino-geniculate axons is removed two concurrent changes thus occur: some deafferented cells atrophy, and others are reinnervated by axons whose main termination is in the supposedly unaffected layers. We do not know how the balance between these two changes is maintained nor do we know exactly how this balance changes with age. It is probable that the cell death and shrinkage produced by deafferentation is most rapid at the earliest stages and that axonal growth also slows down with increasing age. Thus, the cells that are "saved" may be the ones that can be reached within a certain critical time period (which, too, is probably related to age) by the most rapidly growing axons.

In macaque monkeys, Hubel and Wiesel (1977) found very severe transneuronal atrophy when one eye was removed at 2 weeks after birth and the animal was examined about 18 months later. There was no evidence for any significant translaminar sprouting; their figure shows clear interlaminar borders and a reasonably good survival of interlaminar zones. Rakic (1977c) has done unilateral enucleations on younger monkeys. He finds that after an enucleation at embryonic day 63 the nucleus in the 3 month postnatal monkey has developed without any evidence of lamination. When the enucleation is done at a later intrauterine stage (91 days) some lamination is recognizable in the nucleus at 3 months postnatally, and this is comparable to the stage of laminar development attained at the time of the enucleation.

It is possible that there is no stage at which the monkey's system shows the type of translaminar growth of axons found in cats. However, it will clearly be of interest to look at intermediate stages from this point of view and to determine the extent to which the alaminar nucleus produced by an early enucleation results from a complete failure of laminar development, a complete new innervation of the deafferented cells, or a complete atrophy of the deafferented cells.

A comparison of normal development, congenitally abnormal development, and experimentally modified development shows that each can provide clues about the mechanisms by which the adult laminar patterns are produced and that the necessary studies of these developmental process in each area are only just beginning. The sequence demonstrable in normal development will offer useful limitations to the number of different mechanisms that can reasonably be postulated; abnormal development can offer some illuminating clues regarding the capacities of the system, and experimental manipulation can provide some planned attacks upon the mechanisms themselves. However, at present the manipulations that are possible are extremely limited and even such an apparently simple maneuver as removing one eye has complex effects. There is an important difference between, on the one hand, producing a monocular input by enucleation, which reduces the input to each geniculate nucleus and which may lead to cellular atrophy and abnormal axonal growth, and on the other hand, producing a monocular input by a rerouting of axons in the optic chiasm. Of course, the latter is more difficult. So far, a complete decussation of all retinofugal axons has not been reported in any mammalian form, but the albino mink has an almost completely decussated retino-geniculate system. The structure of this system suggests that the laminar differentiation possible with a truly monocular input may be quite different from that produced in a nucleus receiving from only one hemiretina.

GENERAL CONCLUSIONS

Clearly the lateral geniculate nucleus is a rather special case amongst central relays, and the functional demands and developmental forces producing this nucleus may be of limited relevance to understanding other nuclei, even other thalamic relays. Perhaps the occurrence of the binocular input itself has initiated a tendency to lamination that is less evident in other comparable relays such as the ventrobasal nucleus or the medial geniculate nucleus. However, many of the developmental problems that have had to be solved in the production of a functionally adequate lateral geniculate relay are general problems for many other relays. Topographic order is commonly maintained, two or more maps must often be made congruent, and functionally distinct pathways must be kept apart while yet being allowed some degree of interaction. Clearer knowledge about the geniculate relay and its development will help us to understand visual mechanisms, it may also illuminate some more general developmental problems, and will perhaps prove useful for understanding a number of other central relays, particularly thalamic relays, which must to some extent have a shared developmental history.

REFERENCES

Anker, R. L. (1977) The prenatal development of some of the visual pathways in the cat. *J. comp. Neurol.*, 173: 185–204.

Beresford, W. A. (1962) A Nauta and gallocyanin study of the corticolateral geniculate projection in the cat and monkey. *J. Hirnforsch.*, 5: 210–228.

Card-Linden, D. (1978) Unpublished observations.

Casagrande, V. A. (1978) Unpublished observations.

Casagrande, V. A., Guillery, R. W. and Harting, J. K. (1978a) Differential effects of monocular deprivation seen in different layers of the lateral geniculate nucleus. *J. comp. Neurol.*, 179: 469–486.

Casagrande, V. A., Guillery, R. W. and Scott, G. L. (1978b) Unpublished observations.

Cleland, B. G., Levick, W. R., Morstyn, R. and Wagner, H. G. (1976) Lateral geniculate relay of slowly conducting retinal afferents to cat visual cortex. *J. Physiol. (Lond.)*, 255: 299.

Cook, W. H., Walker, J. H. and Barr, M. L. (1951) A cytological study of transneuronal atrophy in the cat and the rabbit. *J. comp. Neurol.*, 94: 267–292.

Cragg, B. G. (1975) The development of synapses in the visual system of the cat. *J. comp. Neurol.*, 160: 147–166.

Dreher, B., Fukada, Y. and Rodieck, R. W. (1976) Identification, classification, and anatomical segregation of cells with X-like and Y-like properties in the lateral geniculate nucleus of Old World primates. *J. Physiol. (Lond.)*, 258: 432–452.

Dubin, M. W. and Cleland, B. G. (1977) Organization of visual inputs to interneurons of lateral geniculate nucleus of the cat. *J. Neurophysiol.*, 40: 390–427.

Garey, L. J. and Blakemore, C. (1977) The effects of monocular deprivation on different neuronal classes in the lateral geniculate nucleus of the cat. *Exp. Brain Res.*, 28: 259–278.

Geisert, Jr., E. E. (1978) *The Cortical Projections of the Lateral Geniculate Nucleus in the Cat.* Ph.D. Thesis. University of Wisconsin, Madison.

Giolli, R. A. and Tigges, J. (1970) The primary optic pathways and nuclei of primates. In: *The Primate Brain. Advances in Primatology, Vol. 1*, C. R. Noback and W. Montagna (Eds.), Appleton-Century-Crofts, New York, pp. 29–54.

Goldby, F. (1957) A note on transneuronal atrophy in the human lateral geniculate body. *J. Neurol. Neurosurg. Psychiat.*, 20: 202–207.

Graham, J. (1977) An autoradiographic study of the efferent connections of the superior colliculus in the cat. *J. comp. Neurol.*, 173: 629–654.

Guillery, R. W. (1966) A study of Golgi preparations from the dorsal lateral geniculate nucleus of the cat. *J. comp. Neurol.*, 128: 21–50.

Guillery, R. W. (1967a) A light and electron microscopical study of neurofibrils and neurofilaments at neuro-neuronal junctions in the dorsal lateral geniculate nucleus of the cat. *Amer. J. Anat.*, 120: 583–604.

Guillery, R. W. (1967b) Patterns of fiber degeneration in the dorsal lateral geniculate nucleus of the cat following lesions in the visual cortex. *J. comp. Neurol.*, 130: 197–222.

Guillery, R. W. (1969a) The organization of synaptic interconnections in the laminae of the dorsal lateral geniculate nucleus of the cat. *Z. Zellforsch.*, 96: 1–38.

Guillery, R. W. (1969b) A quantitative study of synaptic interconnections in the dorsal lateral geniculate nucleus of the cat. *Z. Zellforsch.*, 96: 39–48.

Guillery, R. W. (1969c) An abnormal retino-geniculate projection in Siamese cats. *Brain Res.*, 14: 739–741.

Guillery, R. W. (1970) The laminar distribution of retinal fibers in the dorsal lateral geniculate nucleus of the cat: a new interpretation. *J. comp. Neurol.*, 138: 339–368.

Guillery, R. W. (1971a) Patterns of synaptic interconnections in the dorsal lateral geniculate nucleus of cat and monkey: a brief review. *Vision Res.*, 3 (Suppl.): 211–227.

Guillery, R. W. (1971b) An abnormal retino-geniculate projection in the albino ferret *(Mustela furo)*. *Brain Res.*, 33: 482–485.

Guillery, R. W. (1971c) Survival of large cells in the dorsal lateral geniculate laminae after interruption of retinogeniculate afferents. *Brain Res.*, 28: 541–544.

Guillery, R. W. (1972) Experiments to determine whether retino-geniculate axons can form translaminar collateral sprouts in the lateral geniculate nucleus of the cat. *J. comp. Neurol.*, 146: 407–420.

Guillery, R. W. (1973) Quantitative studies of transneuronal atrophy in the dorsal lateral geniculate nucleus of cats and kittens. *J. comp. Neurol.*, 149: 423–438.

Guillery, R. W. and Colonnier, M. (1970) Synaptic patterns in the dorsal lateral geniculate nucleus of the monkey. *Z. Zellforsch.*, 103: 90–108.

Guillery, R. W. and Kaas, J. H. (1971) A study of normal and congenitally abnormal retino-geniculate projections in cats. *J. comp. Neurol.*, 143: 73–100.

Guillery, R. W. and Oberdorfer, M. D. (1977) A study of fine and coarse retino-fugal axons terminating in the geniculate C laminae and in the medial interlaminar nucleus of the mink. *J. comp. Neurol.*, 176: 515–526.

Guillery, R. W. and Scott, G. L. (1971) Observations on synaptic patterns in the dorsal lateral geniculate nucleus of the cat: the C laminae and the perikaryal synapses. *Exp. Brain Res.*, 12: 184–203.

Guillery, R. W., Oberdorfer, M. D. and Murphy, E. H. (1979) Abnormal retino-geniculate and geniculo-cortical pathways in several genetically distinct color phases of the mink *(Mustela vison)*. *J. comp. Neurol.*, in press.

Harting, J. K., Diamond, I. T. and Hall, W. C. (1973) Anterograde degeneration study of the cortical projection of the lateral geniculate and pulvinar nuclei in the tree shrew *(Tupaia glis)*. *J. comp. Neurol.*, 150: 393–439.

Harting, J. K., Casagrande, V. A. and Weber, J. T. (1978) The projection of the primate superior colliculus upon the dorsal lateral geniculate nucleus: autoradiographic demonstration of interlaminar distribution of tectogeniculate axons. *Brain Res.*, 150: 593–599.

Hassler, R. (1964) Die zentralen Systeme des Sehens. In: *Bericht über den 66te Zusammenkunft der Deutschen Ophthalmol. Gesellsch., Heidelberg.* J. F. Bergmann, Munich, pp. 229–251.

Hickey, T. L. (1975) Translaminar growth of axons in the kitten dorsal lateral geniculate nucleus following removal of one eye. *J. comp. Neurol.*, 161: 359–382.

Hickey, T. L. and Guillery, R. W. (1974) An autoradiographic study of retino-geniculate pathways in the cat and the fox. *J. comp. Neurol.*, 156: 239–254.

Hickey, T. L. and Guillery, R. W. (1978) Variability of laminar patterns in the human lateral geniculate nucleus. *J. comp. Neurol.*, 183: 221–246.

Holländer, H. (1972) Autoradiographic evidence for a projection from the striate cortex to the dorsal part of the lateral geniculate nucleus in the cat. *Brain Res.*, 41: 464–466.

Holländer, H. and Martinez-Millán, L. (1975) Autoradiographic evidence for a topographically organized projection from the striate cortex to the lateral geniculate nucleus in the rhesus monkey *(Macaca mulatta)*. *Brain Res.*, 100: 407–411.

Holländer, H. and Vanegas, H. (1977) The projection from the lateral geniculate nucleus onto the visual cortex in the cat: a quantitative study with horseradish peroxidase. *J. comp. Neurol.*, 173: 519–536.

Hubel, D. H. and Wiesel, T. N. (1971) Aberrant visual projections in the Siamese cat. *J. Physiol. (Lond.)*, 218: 33–62.

Hubel, D. H. and Wiesel, T. N. (1977) Functional architecture of macaque visual cortex. *Proc. roy. Soc. B*, 198: 1–59.

Kaas, J. H., Guillery, R. W. and Allman, J. M. (1972) Some principles of organization in the dorsal lateral geniculate nucleus. *Brain Behav. Evol.*, 6: 253–299.

Kaas, J. H., Huerta, M. F., Weber, J. T. and Harting, J. K. (1978) Patterns of retinal terminations and laminar organization of the lateral geniculate nucleus of primates. *J. comp. Neurol.*, 182: 517–554.

Kaiserman-Abramoff, I. R., Graybiel, A. M. and Nauta, W. J. H. (1975) Neural connections of area 17 in anophthalmic mouse strain. *Neurosci. Abstr.*, 1: 102.

Kalil, R. E. (1972) Formation of new retino-geniculate projections in kittens after removal of one eye. *Anat. Rec.*, 172: 339–340.

Kalil, R. E. (1978) Development of the dorsal lateral geniculate nucleus in the cat. *J. comp. Neurol.*, 182: 265–291.

LeGros Clark, W. E. (1942) The visual centers of the brain and their connections. *Physiol. Rev.*, 22: 205–232.

LeGros Clark, W. E. and Penman, G. G. (1934) The projection of the retina on the lateral geniculate body. *Proc. roy. Soc. B*, 114: 291–311.

LeVay, S. and Ferster, D. (1977) Relay cell classes in the lateral geniculate nucleus of the cat and the effects of visual deprivation. *J. comp. Neurol.*, 172: 563–584.

Malpeli, J. G. and Baker, F. H. (1975) The representation of the visual field in the lateral geniculate nucleus of *Macaca mulatta*. *J. comp. Neurol.*, 161: 569–594.

Matthews, M. R., Cowan, W. M. and Powell, T. P. S. (1960) Transneuronal degeneration in the lateral geniculate nucleus of the macaque monkey. *J. Anat. (Lond.)*, 94: 146–169.

Minkowski, M. (1920) Über den Verlauf, die Endigung, und die zentrale Repräsentation von gekreuzten und ungekreuzten Sehnervenfasern bei einigen Säugethieren und beim Menschen. *Schweiz. Arch. Neurol. Psychiat.*, 6: 201–252.

Mitzdorf, U. and Singer, W. (1977) Laminar segregation of afferents to lateral geniculate nucleus of the cat: an analysis of current source density. *J. Neurophysiol.*, 40: 1227–1244.

Montero, V. M. and Guillery, R. W. (1978) Abnormalities of the cortico-geniculate pathway in Siamese cats. *J. comp. Neurol.*, 179: 1–12.

Nichterlein, O. E. and Goldby, F. (1944) An experimental study of optic connections in the sheep. *J. Anat. (Lond.)*, 78: 59–67.

Norton, T. T., Casagrande, V. A. and Sherman, S. M. (1977) Loss of Y-cells in the lateral geniculate nucleus of monocularly deprived tree shrews. *Science*, 197: 784–786.

Palmer, L. A., Rosenquist, A. C. and Tusa, R. J. (1978) The retinotopic organization of lateral suprasylvian areas in the cat. *J. comp. Neurol.*, 177: 237–256.

Polyak, S. (1957) *The Vertebrate Visual System.* University of Chicago Press, Chicago, Ill.

Rakic, P. (1976) Prenatal genesis of connections subserving ocular dominance in the rhesus monkey. *Nature (Lond.)*, 261: 467–471.

Rakic, P. (1977a) Prenatal development of the visual system in the rhesus monkey. *Phil. Trans. B*, 278: 245–326.

Rakic, P. (1977b) Genesis of the dorsal lateral geniculate nucleus in the rhesus monkey: site and time of origin, kinetics of proliferation, routes of migration and pattern of distribution of neurons. *J. comp. Neurol.*, 176: 23–52.

Rakic, P. (1977c) Effect of prenatal unilateral eye enucleation on the formation of layers and retinal connections in the dorsal lateral geniculate nucleus (LGd) of the rhesus monkey. *Neurosci. Abstr.*, 3: 573.

Richard, W. and Kalil, R. E. (1974) Dissociation of retinal fibers by degeneration rate. *Brain Res.*, 72: 288–293.

Robson, J. A., Mason, C. A. and Guillery, R. W. (1978) Terminal arbors of axons that have formed abnormal connections. *Science*, 201: 635–637.

Sanderson, K. J. (1974) Lamination of the dorsal lateral geniculate nucleus of carnivores of the weasel *(Mustelidae)*, raccoon *(Procyonidae)* and fox *(Canidae)* families. *J. comp. Neurol.*, 153: 239–266.

Sanderson, K. J., Bishop, P. O. and Darian Smith, I. (1971) The properties of the binocular receptive fields of lateral geniculate neurons. *Exp. Brain Res.*, 13: 178–207.

Sanderson, R. J. and Kaas, J. H. (1974) Thalamocortical interconnections of the visual system of the mink. *Brain Res.*, 70: 139–143.

Sanderson, R. J., Guillery, R. W. and Shackelford, R. M. (1974) Congenitally abnormal visual pathways in mink *(Mustela vison)* with reduced retinal pigment. *J. comp. Neurol.*, 154: 225–248.

Schiller, P. H. and Malpeli, J. G. (1978) Functional specificity of lateral geniculate nucleus laminae of the rhesus monkey. *J. Neurophysiol.*, 41: 788–797.

Shatz, C. J. (1977a) A comparison of visual pathways in Boston and Midwestern Siamese cats. *J. comp. Neurol.*, 171: 205–228.

Shatz, C. J. (1977b) Abnormal interhemispheric connections in the visual system of Boston Siamese cats: a physiological study. *J. comp. Neurol.*, 171: 229–246.

Sherman, S. M., Hoffman, K. P. and Stone, J. (1972) Loss of a specific cell type from the dorsal lateral geniculate nucleus in visually deprived cats. *J. Neurophysiol.*, 35: 532–541.

Sherman, S. M., Norton, T. T. and Casagrande, V. A. (1975a) X- and Y-cells in the dorsal lateral geniculate nucleus of the tree shrew *(Tupaia glis)*. *Brain Res.*, 93: 152–157.

Sherman, S. M., Wilson, J. R. and Guillery, R. W. (1975b) Evidence that binocular competition affects the post-natal development of Y-cells in the cat's lateral geniculate nucleus. *Brain Res.*, 100: 441–444.

Sherman, S. M., Wilson, J. R., Kaas, J. H. and Webb, S. V. (1976) X- and Y-cells in the dorsal lateral geniculate nucleus of the owl monkey *(Aotus trivirgatus)*. *Science*, 192: 475–477.

Singer, W. and Bedworth, N. (1973) Inhibitory interaction between X and Y units in the cat lateral geniculate nucleus. *Brain Res.*, 49: 291–307.

Stone, J. and Dreher, B. (1973) Projections of X- and Y-cells of the cat's lateral geniculate nucleus to area 17 and 18 of visual cortex. *J. Neurophysiol.*, 36: 551–567.

Stone, J. and Fukuda, Y. (1974) The naso-temporal division of the cat's retina re-examined in terms of Y-, X- and W-cells. *J. comp. Neurol.*, 155: 377–394.

Stryker, M. P. (1977) Abnormal neural development. In: *Function and Formation of Neural Systems*, G. S. Stent (Ed.), Dahlem Konferenzen, Berlin, pp. 285–308.

Szentágothai, J. (1963) The structure of the synapse in the lateral geniculate body. *Acta anat. (Basel)*, 55: 166–185.

Szentágothai, J. (1964) The use of degeneration methods in the investigation of short neuronal connections. In: *Progress in Brain Research, Vol. 14, Degeneration Patterns in the Nervous System*, M. Singer and J. P. Schadé (Eds.), Elsevier, Amsterdam, pp. 1–32.

Tömböl, T. (1969) Two types of short axon (Golgi 2nd) interneurons in the specific thalamic nuclei. *Acta morph. Acad. Sci. hung.*, 17: 285–297.

Updyke, B. V. (1976) The patterns of projection of cortical areas 17, 18 and 19 onto the laminae of the dorsal lateral geniculate nucleus in the cat. *J. comp. Neurol.*, 163: 377–396.

Von Noorden, G. K. and Middleditch, P. R. (1975) Histology of the monkey's lateral geniculate nucleus after unilateral lid closure and experimental strabismus: further observations. *Invest. Ophthal.* 14: 674–683.

Walls, G. L. (1953) The lateral geniculate nucleus and visual histophysiology. *Univ. Calif. Publ. Physiol.*, 9: 1–100.

Wässle, H., Levick, W. R. and Cleland, B. G. (1975) The distribution of the alpha type of ganglion cells in the cat's retina. *J. comp. Neurol.*, 159: 419–437.

Wilson, P. D. and Stone, J. (1975) Evidence of W-cell input to the cat's visual cortex via the C-laminae of the lateral geniculate nucleus. *Brain Res.*, 92: 472–478.

Wilson, P. D., Rowe, M. H. and Stone, J. (1976) Properties of relay cells in cat's lateral geniculate nucleus: a comparison of W-cells with X- and Y-cells. *J. Neurophysiol.*, 39: 1193–1209.

Specific Thalamo-cortical Afferents and their Presumptive Targets in the Visual Cortex. A Golgi Study

A. FAIRÉN and F. VALVERDE

Sección de Neuroanatomía Comparada, Instituto Cajal, CSIC, Velázquez 144, Madrid 6 (Spain)

INTRODUCTION

In the present paper, two questions relating to the circuitry of the visual cortex are discussed on the basis of Golgi observations. The first is: What types of neurons with intracortical axons can be contacted by geniculo-cortical fibres? the second: How are these fibres three-dimensionally arranged in layer IV of the primary visual cortex? Clearly, although the answers that the Golgi method offers to the first question are not conclusive, they nevertheless provide the necessary background for the interpretation of experimental data. To this end, a classification of presumptive recipient non-pyramidal cells is introduced, which takes into account dendritic, as well as axonal, characteristics.

Some preliminary results on the geometrical arrangement of geniculo-cortical fibres are also discussed and some possible consequences of geometry on connectivity are considered.

The observations were made on a large collection of brains of mice, cats and monkeys stained during the last 12 years by the rapid Golgi method, as described elsewhere (Valverde, 1970, 1978). Details of interest were recorded on camera lucida drawings or photographed to be later assembled as mosaic reconstructions. Selected examples of individual cortical afferent fibres were tracked for storage on magnetic tape, to be later displayed on an X-Y plotter in various spatial orientations, using a micro-computer based system (Valverde, 1976, 1978).

RECEPTIVE CELLS IN THE INTERNAL GRANULAR LAYER: AN ESSAY ON CLASSIFICATION

Despite considerable efforts during recent years, identification of the diverse types of neurones receiving thalamo-cortical synapses is not yet complete. Recent approaches like anterograde degeneration combined with a new Golgi-EM technique (Fairén et al., 1977; Peters et al., 1977) or intracellular labelling of physiologically identified cells (Kelly and Van Essen, 1974; Christensen and Ebner, 1978) offer new possibilities. For obvious reasons, however, these techniques have to deal with a rather limited number of cells. To facilitate interpretation of the experimental data, then, a detailed catalogue of the types of presumptive recipient cells is wanting. In spite of many recent attempts to define neuronal types in the sensory areas of a number of species (Garey, 1971; Shkol'nik-Yarros, 1971; Valverde, 1971, 1976; Lund, 1973; Szentágothai, 1973; Jones, 1975b; Parnavelas et al., 1977; Feldman and Peters, 1978; Tömböl, 1978) some clarification is needed, for the results are not completely concordant, owing to differences in cataloguing criteria, and are not applicable to all animal species.

For this reason, a classification is proposed of non-pyramidal cell types in the primary visual cortex, specially of those present in layer IV. These cells possess, with a few exceptions, intracortical axons. The main criteria used are morphology of dendritic surfaces and axonal arborization patterns. In no way is it intended to cover all cell types exhaustively, but rather to characterize some clear groups which are well represented in our material, and to follow possible homologies between different animal species. Two major categories are distinguished on the basis of the presence or absence of dendritic spines, because this is relevant in interpreting EM results on anterograde degeneration.

In area 17 of rats, cats and monkeys, 14–15% of the degenerating terminals resulting from lateral geniculate lesions contact dendritic shafts; 2–3% contact neuronal somata and the remainder, 83–84%, dendritic spines (Garey and Powell, 1971; Peters and Feldman, 1976). These cell somata and dendritic shafts have been interpreted as belonging to stellate cells (Colonnier and Rossignol, 1969; Garey and Powell, 1971; Peters et al., 1976) of the type which either lacks spines or is poor in them (sparsely spined stellate cells). This has been confirmed in Golgi-electron microscopic (EM) studies of the rat visual cortex (Peters, 1978). These cells, however, do not constitute a uniform group: Peters et al. (1976) have pointed out, on EM grounds, that two different cell types might be involved and Feldman and Peters (1978), basing their observations on dendritic morphology in Golgi material, have described various types of spineless neurones.

On the other hand, the spines which receive geniculo-cortical afferents belong to dendrites of small diameter (Garey and Powell, 1971; Peters and Feldman, 1976, 1977), which show different morphologies, indicating that they belong to different cell types (Peters and Feldman, 1977). Golgi-EM studies in both rat visual and mouse somatosensory cortex have indicated that they are in fact diverse parts of pyramidal cells (Peters et al., 1977; Peters, 1978; Somogyi, 1978; White, 1978). Stellate cells with spiny dendrites are also involved (Peters et al., 1977; Peters, 1978; White, 1978). These results indeed agree with those obtained through dye injections in the cat visual cortex (Kelly and Van Essen, 1974). Interestingly enough, many of these connections have previously been suggested by Golgi studies (Valverde, 1968, 1971; Valverde and Ruiz-Marcos, 1969; Ruiz-Marcos and Valverde, 1970).

Besides the presence or absence of dendritic spines, neuronal types are considered as having either *generalized* or *specialized* axonal arborization patterns. Generalized axons are defined by exclusion, for their lack of specific preterminal arborizations, being common in rats (Feldman and Peters, 1978; Peters and Fairén, 1978) and mice.

Neurones with smooth and sparsely spined dendrites and generalized intracortical axons

In the mouse, spineless or sparsely spined neurones have axons that can be included in classes I, II and III of the Valverde (1976) classification. Class I and III axons bear certain similarities, whereas those of class II constitute a quite different entity.

Another group recently described in rats as bipolar cells (Feldman and Peters, 1978) does not show well impregnated axonal plexuses in our mouse material and is not dealt with here, but, undoubtedly, its frankly interesting features deserve further study.

(a) Cells with recurving axonal arcades (classes I and III). Axons of classes I and III belong to cells stellate in form, whose dendrites are smooth or bear a very small number of spines. They are present in all cortical layers of the mouse area 17, with the exception of layer I. An example of a layer II–III cell bearing a class III axon is shown in Fig. 1,b.

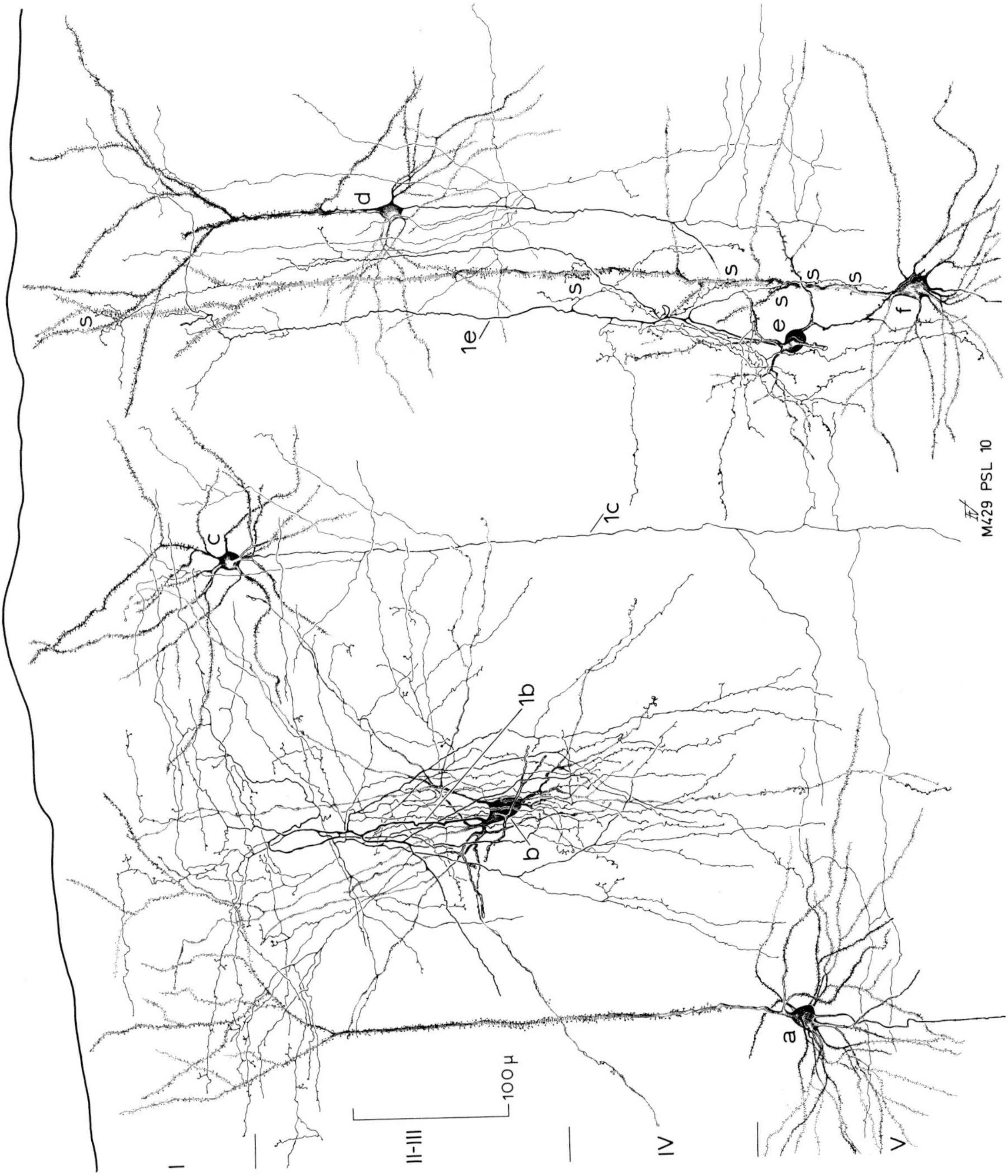

Fig. 1. Frontal section through the visual cortex of the mouse. Varieties of cells with intracortical axons (b, e) and pyramidal cells (a, c, d, f) can be observed. The figure shows the contrasting difference between the extension of the axonal plexus of cell b (labelled 1b) and the ascending axon (labelled 1e) of cell e. In the latter, the possible sites of synaptic contacts with dendrites of pyramidal cells are labelled s. Golgi method, camera lucida drawing. Mouse, 21 days old.

Typically, the axon emerges from the upper pole of the cell body or from the base of a dendrite, ascends vertically and after the first bifurcation forms thick recurving arcades giving rise to horizontal or oblique branches. These form a plexus of variable density, within or in the vicinity of the dendritic field. On occasion (Fig. 1,b) there is a dense local plexus forming a curtain around the central portion of the neurone, while some branches form looser plexuses which in this case invade layer I.

Class I axons ramify exclusively above the cell body, whereas class III do so above and below; these distinct axonal patterns result in different connection possibilities. An interesting fact, also observed in rats (Peters and Fairén, 1978) is that the axon is not exclusively confined to the vicinity of the cell body, for a descending branch may sometimes be followed over considerable distances.

In a recent study, the structural characteristics of spine-free stellate cells were studied in rat (Peters and Fairén, 1978). Some cells (numbered 1, 2, 3 and 6) are entirely comparable to those bearing class I/III axons in the mouse. By their cytological features they correspond to one of the cell types shown to receive geniculo-cortical input (Peters et al., 1976). After an electron microscopic analysis of their axonal plexuses it became feasible to define the role played by these cells in the intracortical circuits.

Entirely comparable neurones are present in monkey (Lund, 1973) visual and somatosensory (Jones, 1975b, type 2) cortices and have been described as large stellate cells in several electron microscopic studies (see Tigges et al., 1977, for a review).

(b) Cells with ascending axons (class II). Neurones possessing class II axonal arborizations (Valverde, 1976) are rather frequently observed in mice. They are stellate cells whose dendrites range from smooth (spine-free) to sparsely spinous (Fig. 1,e). In some instances, even in adult animals, the dendrites are so richly endowed with spines that their classification as sparsely spinous would seem inadequate, although the number of spines never reaches the level typical of true spiny stellate cells (Figs. 2–5); however, it is clear that only quantification can lead to conclusive criteria.

The axon (Fig. 1,1e) emerges from the upper pole of the cell body and forms a straight ascending stem which reaches layer I, where it arborizes. According to the localization of the cell bodies, two subtypes may be recognized. Neurones located in layer II–III send the ascending axon towards layer I, where it bends and follows horizontal courses for variable distances. Collaterals originate from the main stem throughout its course in the form of long, thin descending branches, but thick arcades are never present. On the other hand, cells located in lower layer IV or in layer V originate a more conspicuous ascending axon; a main group of thin, descending collaterals originates from the initial portion of the axonal trunk and forms a relatively dense local arborization (Fig. 1). A second group of axonal branches derives from the upper part of the axonal stem and distributes within layer I. These deeply located cells correspond to the type described by Cajal (1911) as Martinotti cells. On the basis of Golgi observations, Ruiz-Marcos and Valverde (1970) considered these cells to be recipient of thalamo-cortical synapses.

No data on the types of terminals formed by these neurones are available. Golgi observations in mice suggest that the axon might synapse with apical dendritic shafts (s-s on cells f and d), but also other postsynaptic elements may well be involved.

Neurones with specialized axonal arborizations

Several neurone types of the non-spiny variety have been described whose axonal terminal branches adopt very specific arborization patterns. These include pericellular baskets (Cajal,

1911; Marín-Padilla, 1969; Szentágothai, 1973; Tömböl, 1978), horse-tail arborizations (Cajal, 1899, 1911; Colonnier, 1966; Szentágothai, 1973; Jones, 1975b), vertical axonal bundles provided with grape-like knobs (Valverde, 1978), and candlesticks (Szentágothai and Arbib, 1974). In a broader sense, clewed cells (Valverde, 1971; Jones, 1975b) which show very elaborate, strictly local arborizations might also be included in this group.

Although the versatility of the Golgi procedure can create false quantitative impressions, the information gathered from the study of our own Golgi material seems to support the idea that cells with specialized axons are more frequently present in higher species. If this were true, it could be that in lower species, generalized types assume the same roles in cortical circuitry as specialized ones do in higher species. In rat, cells with generalized axons have shown the same connections as those presumed, on the basis of Golgi studies, to have at least two different types of neurones with well organized axonal formations (Peters and Fairén, 1978). However, generalized and specialized axons have been found to coexist in the cerebral cortex of a given animal species.

It is evident that more precise data on connectivity patterns of specialized neurones are needed to clarify this problem. To date, there is a single instance (Somogyi, 1977; Szentágothai, 1978) in which a type of neurone, in rat visual cortex, has been shown to produce a unique type of synaptic contact, in relation to axon initial segments of pyramidal cells. Work in progress in this laboratory shows, in cat visual cortex, the presence of such a type of specific synaptic relationship.

Some types of neurones with specialized axons are not well enough represented in our Golgi material and consequently, our review is restricted to 3 categories only: clewed cells, chandelier cells and neurones with vertical axonal bundles.

(a) Clewed cells. In layer IVc of monkey area 17, Valverde (1971) described short axon cells which were named "clewed cells" on account of the complex, twisted disposition of their dendritic and axonal branches. An example is shown in Fig. 3g. They are small cells with a low number of smooth, beaded dendrites. The axon (1g) may issue from any point around the cell body and soon resolves into numerous collaterals which are densely interwoven with the dendrites of the same cell, forming a plexus strictly local in nature. On the basis of Golgi observations, it was suggested that clewed cells were contacted by specific afferents (Valverde, 1971).

This cell type corresponds to Jones' (1975b) type 5; a comparable granular cell is present in monkey area 18 (Valverde, 1978) but here, axonal plexuses are not so dense and the dendritic fields are vertically elongated.

In layer IV of cat area 17, a type of short axon cell is observed (Fig. 2,e) which bears resemblance to primate clewed cells. In cat, the cells are larger and the axonal arborizations looser. Clewed cells are not present in rodents but, interestingly, some class III axonal arborizations are reminiscent of clewed cell axons.

(b) Chandelier cells. These cells, described by Szentágothai and Arbib (1974), Szentágothai (1975) and Tömböl (1978) are similar to type 4 cells of Jones (1975b). They are considered ubiquitous cells in the cortex but to our knowledge, no examples of such cells have been described in monkey visual cortex. In area 17 of cats we have recently found some examples which agree in almost every detail with previous descriptions (Fig. 2,a). Usually, dendrites are sparsely spinous. The terminal axonal formations (candlesticks) are apparent (2a). One major point of discrepancy is that, almost invariably, a thick axonal trunk (1a) leaves the principal area of axonal arborization and descends to lower layers where it arborizes again, though never so richly as in superficial levels, or even enters the white matter.

No data showing that chandelier cells could be targets of the geniculo-cortical input are available. In cat visual cortex they are frequently present in layer IV but no evidence for these connections has been found so far.

(c) Cells with vertical axonal bundles and grape-like terminal knobs. These cells have been described by Valverde (1978) in layer II and upper III of area 18 in monkeys, but no examples have been found in area 17. They are considered here only because their axons bear certain similarities with class I/III axons in mice (see Figs. 3,a and 5,b, in Valverde, 1978).

The dendrites of these neurones are smooth and beaded. The axon, originating from the upper or lower pole of the cell body, forms arcades from which several long, thin collaterals arise. These descend to lower levels, emitting characteristic grape-like terminal knobs, specially abundant in layer IV, and group together constituting compact bundles.

Non-pyramidal neurones with spinous dendrites

In cats and monkeys, spinous non-pyramidal neurones are frequent in all subdivisions of layer IV. They are multipolar cells whose dendrites are almost as densely studded with spines as pyramidal cells (see Jones, 1975b). However, a typical apical dendrite is lacking. Density of spines is, then, a criterion which serves to differentiate true spiny stellate cells from other neuronal types whose dendrites bear *some* spines. Although the term *spiny stellate cell* is not entirely adequate, it is retained here for the sake of simplicity. It is clear that they do not constitute a uniform group (Figs. 2–5); subgroups can be defined according to cell size, dendritic orientation and axonal distribution. In all cases axons can be considered generalized, as defined above, for they lack specific terminal arborizations. However, their overall distributions follow rather definite patterns, which can also help to fully define spiny stellate cells as a special neurone category.

In layer IV of cat visual cortex (Fig. 2,b, c, d) cell bodies are large (up to 18 μm in diameter) and sometimes show cilia (Fig. 4A). Dendrites are richly supplied with drumstick-like spines and span a very large field. The axon (Figs. $2_{1b,\ 1c,\ 1d}$ and Fig. $4A_1$) originates from the lower pole and soon gives rise to collaterals, either horizontal or recurrent. Horizontal collaterals (Figs. $2_{2b,\ 3b,\ 2c,\ 2d}$ and Fig. $4A_4$) are thick and extend for long distances; less frequently, they ascend and ramify poorly in upper layers (Fig. 2_{3b}). Recurrent collaterals form loops (Fig. $4A_{2,\ 3}$) and ascend obliquely or in some cases, vertically (Figs. 2 and $4A_5$). It has been possible to observe these ascending branches in intimate contact with the spines of apical dendrites (Figs. $2_{s\ on\ ap2}$ and Fig. $4B_b$) in a way suggesting functional contacts.

The main descending branch of the axon (Figs. 2_{4b} and $4A_6$) descends vertically and sometimes enters the white matter.

These spiny stellate cells clearly correspond to the giant stellate cells described by Cajal (1899, 1911, 1921) and should be considered presumptive targets of thalamic afferent fibres (Szentágothai, 1975).

In monkey area 17, spiny stellate cells vary in morphology according to the sublayer where they are located.

In layer IVa (which receives input from the parvocellular geniculate laminae), stellate cells (Fig. 3,b, c) are medium sized and in some cases their dendrites adopt horizontal courses. The axon (1b, 1c) leaves the lower pole of the perikaryon and descends vertically for variable distances, sending off recurrent collaterals which ascend more or less vertically (2b).

Layer IVb contains a group of clearly multipolar stellate cells (Fig. 3,d, e), which resemble

Fig. 2 (see following page). Frontal section through the visual cortex of the cat. The figure is a composite drawing recording varieties of cells from several adjacent sections and one specific afferent fibre (in red) which has been traced in 3 consecutive sections. Large stellate cells with markedly spinous dendrites are labelled b, c, d. One cell (e) with smooth dendrites and localized axonal field (1e) and one "chandelier" cell (a) with characteristic terminal formations (2a) complete a pattern of cell varieties most frequently stained in kittens. Golgi method, camera lucida drawing. Cat, 1 month old.

Fig. 3 (see following right-hand page). Frontal section through the visual cortex of the monkey. The drawing is a composite illustration of varieties of cells recorded in adjacent sections corresponding to the central part of the thickness of the cortex and showing also specific afferent fibres (*1, 2,* in red). Medium sized conventional pyramidal cells can be observed in layer III (a) as well as in the middle of sublayer IVb (f). Small stellate cells with spinous dendrites (h, i, j) and recurrent axons (in blue) ascend to develop localized axonal plexuses in sublayer IVa. Here another variety of stellate cell with spinous dendrites (b, c) have dendrites running horizontally probably in relation to the disposition of specific afferent cortical terminal fibres of sublayer IVa. This level might also be affected by recurrent axon terminals (in yellow) of small pyramidal cells (k, l, m) located in the upper part of layer V. Two stellate cells with spinous dendrites (d, e) and one clewed cell (g) can also be observed. Golgi method, camera lucida drawing. Adult monkey *(Macaca rhesus)*.

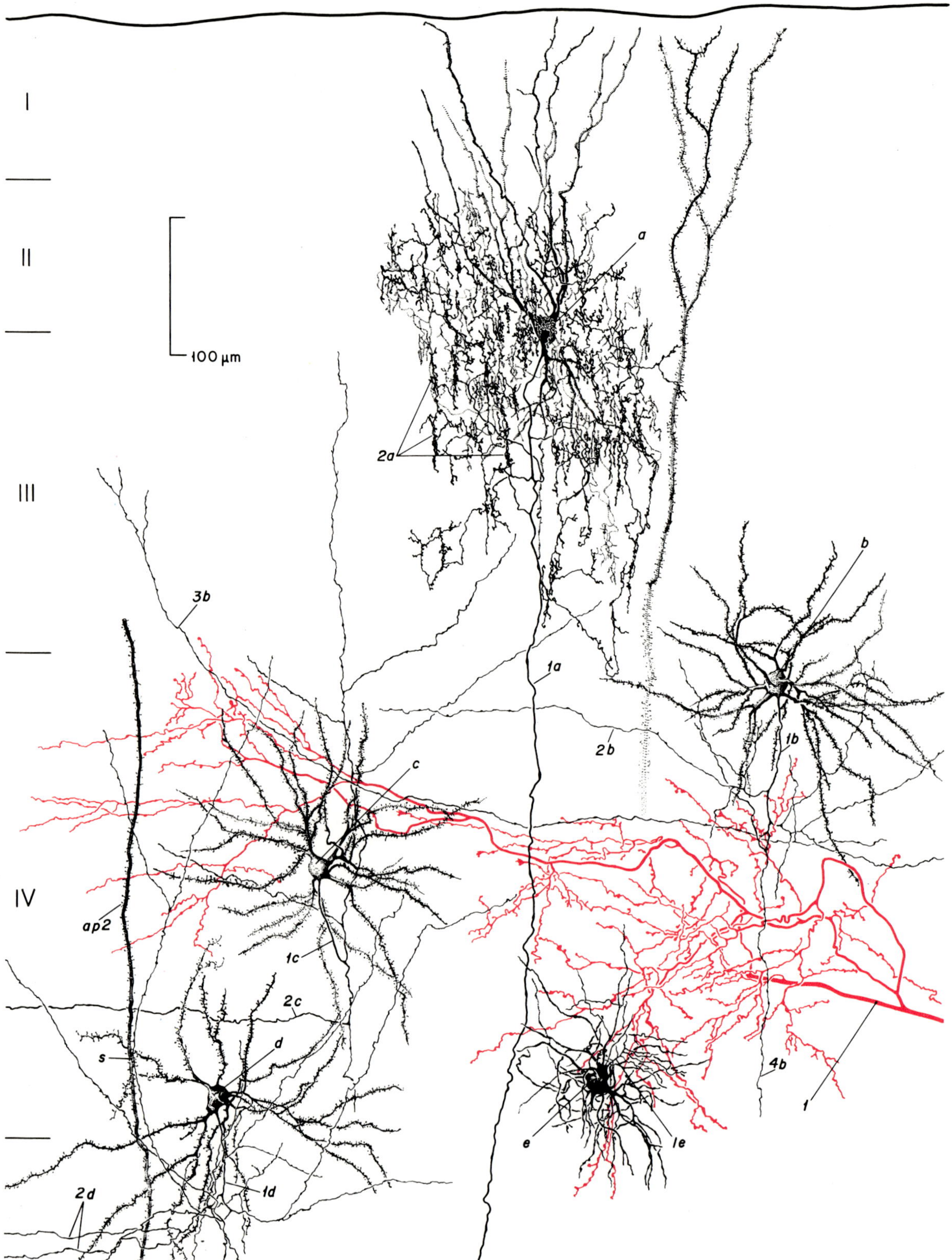

I
II
III
IV
V
100 µm
a
2a
b
1a
3b
1b
2b
c
ap2
1c
2c
d
s
4b
1
e
1e
1d
2d

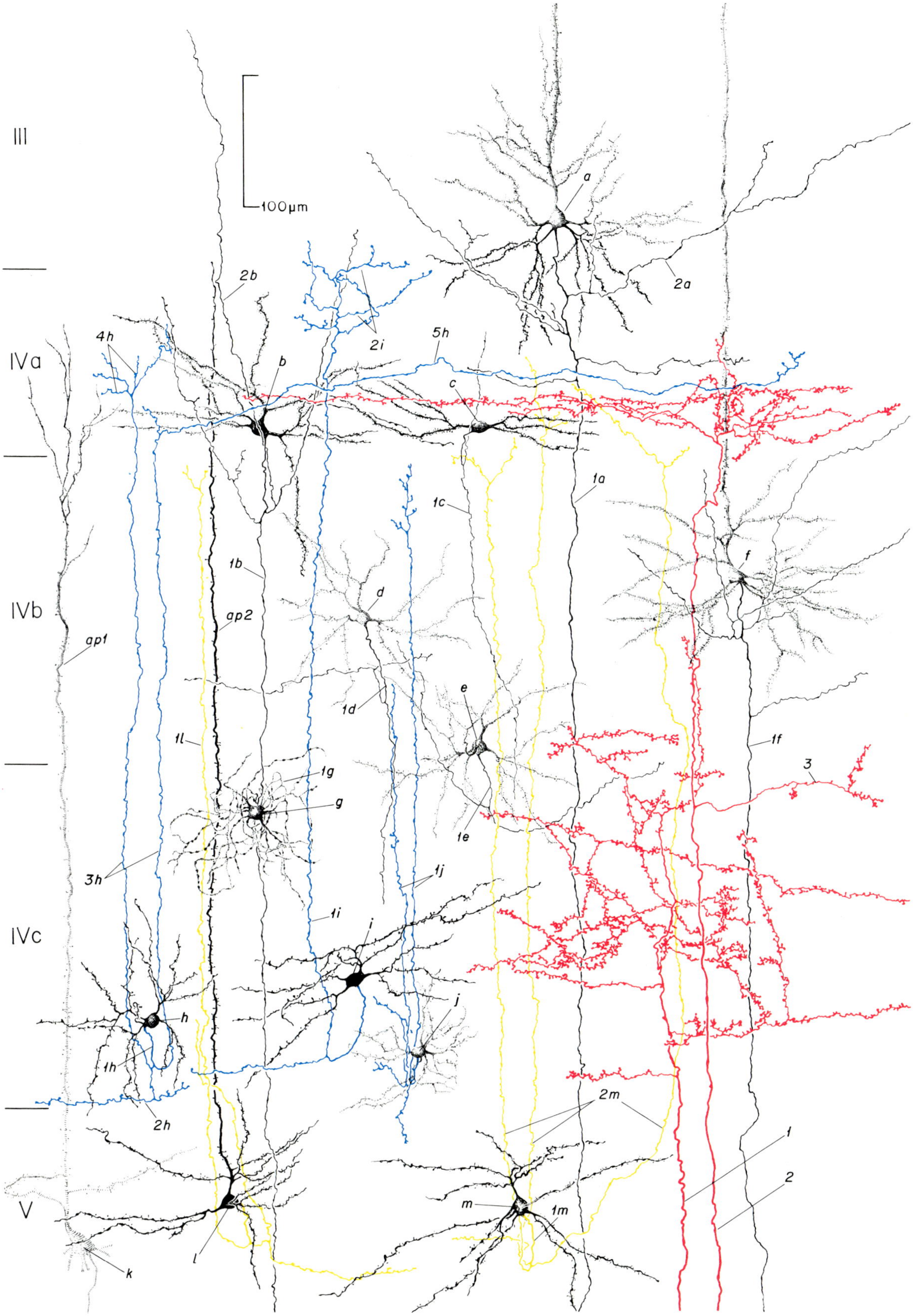

III
IVa
IVb
IVc
V
100µm
a
b
c
d
e
f
g
h
i
j
k
l
m
1
2
3
1a
1b
1c
1d
1e
1f
1g
1h
1i
1j
1l
1m
2a
2b
2h
2i
2m
3h
4h
5h
ap1
ap2

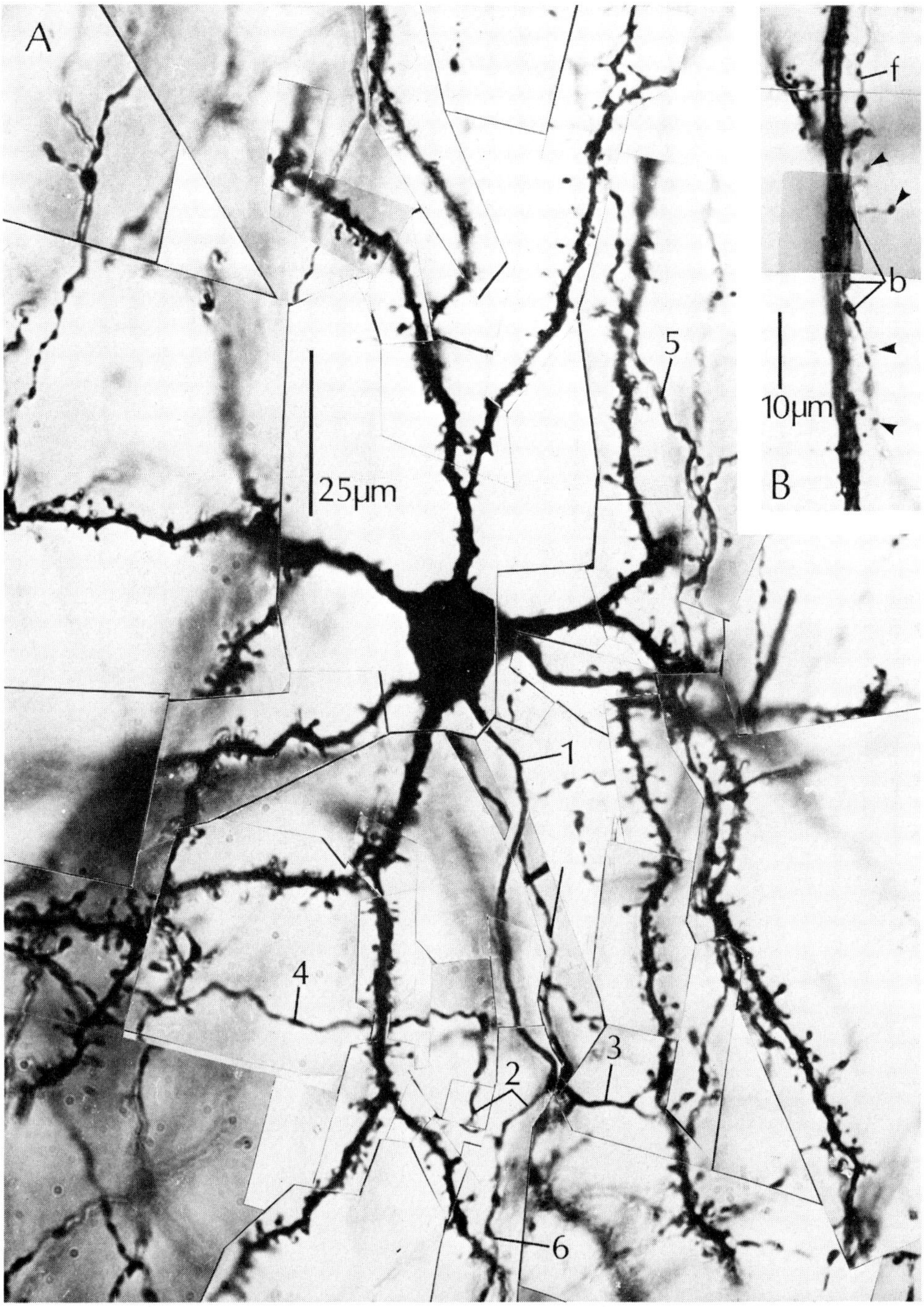

Fig. 4A: mosaic photomicrographic reconstruction of one large stellate cell with spinous dendrites in layer IV of the visual cortex of the cat. The main axonal trunk *(1)* splits into several collateral branches *(2–5)* coursing in various directions. Inset B shows a series of parallel contacts (b) of a fibre f which is a continuation outside the field of the collateral *4* in A, along a portion of one apical dendrite. Note spine heads (arrowheads) at the end of long stalks attached to the dendrite. Golgi method. Cat, 1 month old.

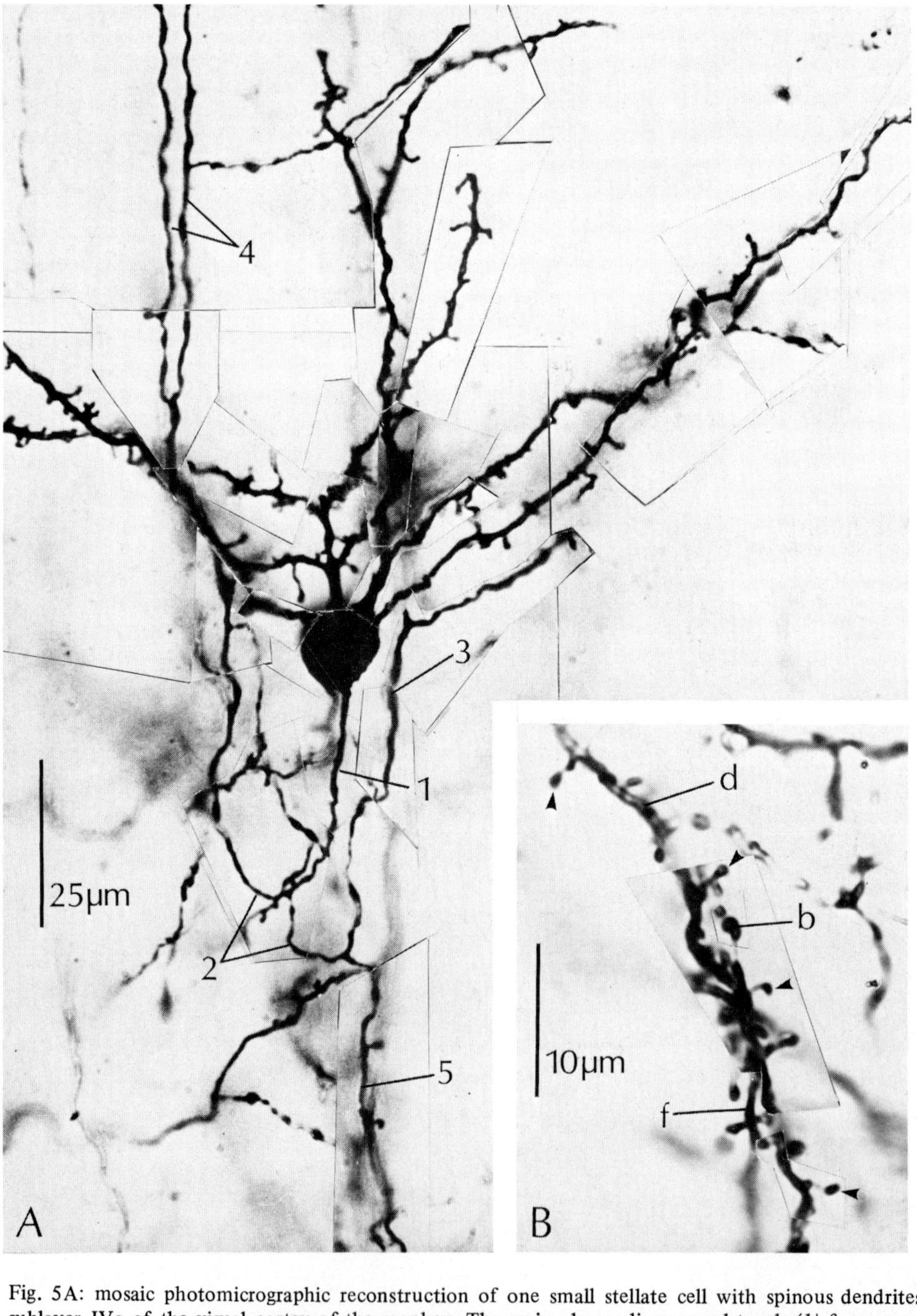

Fig. 5A: mosaic photomicrographic reconstruction of one small stellate cell with spinous dendrites in sublayer IVc of the visual cortex of the monkey. The main, descending axonal trunk *(1)* forms several loops *(2)* which emit recurrent *(3, 4)* and descending *(5)* collaterals. In comparison with the cell in Fig. 4, this cell shows dendrites with fewer, but larger long-stalked spines. Both reconstructions were made to the same final magnification to facilitate comparison. Inset B shows one portion of a dendrite (d) belonging to a similar stellate cell enveloped by a fibre (f) which is a collateral of one specific afferent fibre. Notice spines marked by arrowheads and enlargements of fibre f, notably b, which might be sites of synaptic contact. Golgi method, adult monkey *(Macaca rhesus)*.

the large stellate cells of Cajal. They are clearly smaller than in the cat, however (compare with Fig. 2), and cannot receive direct thalamic input, except if located at the borders of IVb; those located in lower IVb (e) do not differ from spiny stellate cells in upper layer IVc.

The lower part of layer IVc, which also receives parvocellular geniculate input, contains a very typical group of spiny stellate cells (Figs. 3,h, i, j and 5A). The cell bodies are some 12 μm in diameter, while dendrites are less densely covered with spines and some are long stalked. As in other spiny stellate cells, the axon goes down initially but soon forms recurving loops (Fig. $5A_{1,2}$) which are followed by vertically ascending collaterals (Figs. $3_{3h, 1i, 1j}$ and Fig. $5_{3,4}$), strictly columnar in distribution, that reach sublayer IVa where they form terminal arborizations (4h, 2i) or follow horizontal courses (5h). Other collaterals are horizontal (2h) and, sometimes, the main axonal trunk continues as a descending fibre (Fig. 5_5).

These layer IVc stellate cells are likely to receive fibres of geniculate origin. In Fig. 5B, a fibre (f) identified as a specific afferent apparently makes contact with a dendritic spine of one such stellate cell.

In layer V there is a group of pyramidal cells with recurrent axons (Cajal, 1911, 1921) which have a quite similar pattern of axonal distribution (Fig. $3_{l,m}$); they have also been described in monkey area 18 (Valverde, 1978).

In seeking for cell types in mice that might be considered homologous of the spiny stellate cells, it became evident that they were not as abundant as in higher species or, alternatively, that they were not so easily stainable by the Golgi method. However, typical examples are present and a very clear one has been illustrated previously (Valverde, 1968, Fig. 7). The axonal distribution of these stellate cells follows the pattern described as class V by Valverde (1976). This arborization pattern does not differ from the one shown by some pyramidal cells with intracortical axons in mouse, and by star pyramids (Lorente de Nó, 1949; Jones, 1975b).

GEOMETRY OF THE SPECIFIC AFFERENT FIBRES

Presumed specific, geniculo-cortical fibres have been studied in layer IV. In young mice, as well as in cat and monkey, the criteria for identification of geniculo-cortical fibres in Golgi preparations are based entirely on consideration of the following points: (a) the parent branch can be traced to the white matter, (b) the intracortical trajectories correspond to those shown by degeneration studies, and (c) the level of termination and extension of their final branches agrees with degeneration and autoradiography results (cf., Valverde, 1971; Lund, 1973; Jones, 1975a).

The mouse

In young mice, specific afferents can be recognized as the thickest fibres entering the visual cortex from the white matter. As they ascend in the cortex, they follow oblique ascending, wavy courses (see Fig. 2 in Valverde and Ruiz-Marcos, 1969, and Fig. 1 in Ruiz-Marcos and Valverde, 1970). In layer V, or sometimes even below in layer VI, they may divide dichotomously, giving rise to secondary fibres generally unequal in thickness.

In layer IV, these secondary fibres give origin to preterminal branches provided with both en passant and terminal dilations of presumably synaptic character (cf., Peters and Fairén, 1978). The fibres form a plexus which distributes mainly in layer IV but also in the deepest part of layer III; isolated fibres can be followed up to layer I. In Golgi preparations, preterminal fibres occur in elongated clouds possessing an oblique major axis 300–400 μm in length (Ruiz-Marcos and Valverde, 1970). Within the domain of these clouds, repeated branching at acute angles is observed. In their spatial distribution, preterminal fibres tend to follow oblique courses, as has previously been shown (Cajal, 1911; Lorente de Nó, 1949) and sometimes they are vertical. Except for these characteristics, it seems that mice show rather unspecific patterns of terminal distribution when compared to cats or monkeys.

Successful staining of the specific afferent fibres can only be attained in young mice and, therefore, it is not infrequent to observe enlarged growing tips. During postnatal development the thick fibres myelinate and thus become refractory to Golgi staining. However, in adult animals it is frequent to observe plexuses of fine horizontal or oblique fibres in layers IV and lower III, corresponding in part to specific axons.

Fig. 6A shows, in a frontal view, a computer reconstructed afferent cortical fibre as it enters the visual cortex from the white matter. This fibre was digitized from a 220 μm thick Golgi section of a mouse 10 days old. Although the fibre shows a principal bifurcation in a lower level corresponding to the bottom of layer VI, most branches originate at the level of layer IV and lower II–III. Some long collaterals ascend unbranched to higher levels. Fig. 7A shows the same fibre after computer rotation of 90° around the horizontal OX axis; the fibre thus appears as if it were seen from the surface of the brain. No definite preferential orientation is observed, so that any possible direction of its collaterals seems to be equally probable (cf., Fig. 9 in Valverde, 1976).

The cat

Golgi impregnations of specific fibres have been particularly successful in 1-month-old kittens; by this age, most neurones exhibit adult features even though myelination is not complete. As has been shown by LeVay et al. (1978), segregation of ocular dominance columns is completed between the 33rd and 39th postnatal days.

Fig. 2 is a composite drawing synthetising information from several adjacent Golgi-stained sections. In red, a reputed geniculo-cortical fibre is depicted; it has been traced in 3 consecutive sections and can be considered quite complete. It stems from a thick fibre *(1)* which has been partially impregnated, as if it were an unmyelinated segment of a myelinated fibre. The thick parent fibre follows an oblique, almost horizontal course in the bottom of layer IV. Whenever it has been possible to trace the specific fibres down to the white matter, specially in younger animals, it has been found that the parent fibres are thick (up to 3 μm) and sometimes divide into diverging fibres before entering the cortex, in such a way that the span of a single afferent fibre may be quite large.

Fibre *1* in Fig. 2 gives rise to a thick ascending branch which soon subdivides dichotomously into slightly thinner secondary branches, which follow long, wavy trajectories inside layer IV. Preterminal branches originate from the secondary branches and, on occasions, even from the primary trunk. They follow oblique ascending or descending, but not vertical, courses and originate, by repeated subdivisions, interlacing bouquet-like plexuses which are denser than the ones present in mice. The fine fibres show synaptic enlargements along their lengths and short appendages ending in dilations also occur. It is worth noting, however, that the thick secondary branches (which presumably acquire myelin sheaths later in development) also give rise to synaptic contacts (unpublished Golgi-EM observations). This fact agrees with the observation by Garey and Powell (1971) of degenerating geniculo-cortical axons making synapses immediately after the loss of a myelin sheath.

Fig. 6B shows a computer display of the same specific fibre shown in Fig. 2_1 in the same

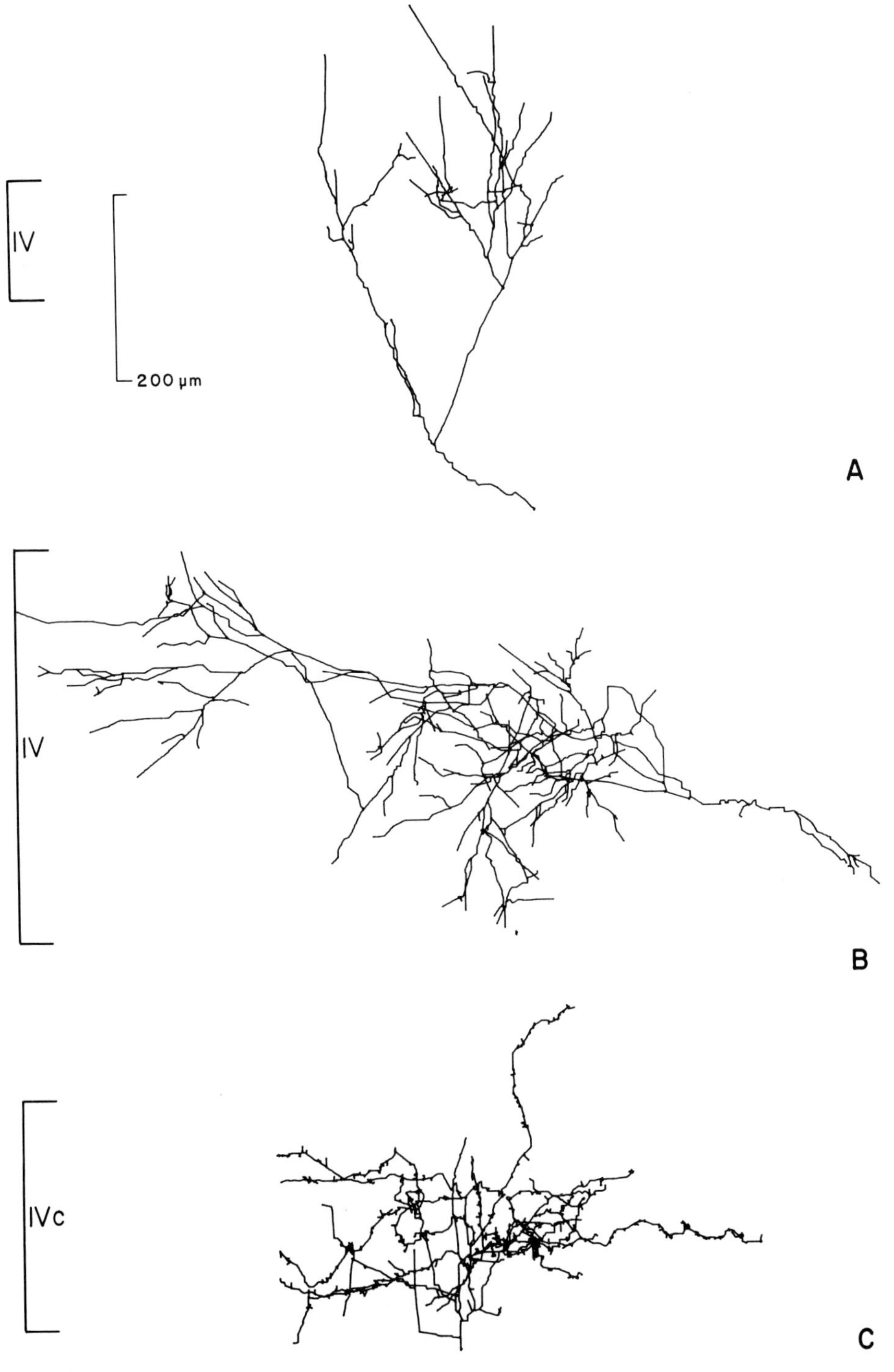

Fig. 6. Computer display of specific afferent fibres in the visual cortex. A: mouse, 10 days old. B: cat, 1 month old. C: adult monkey. From Golgi material.

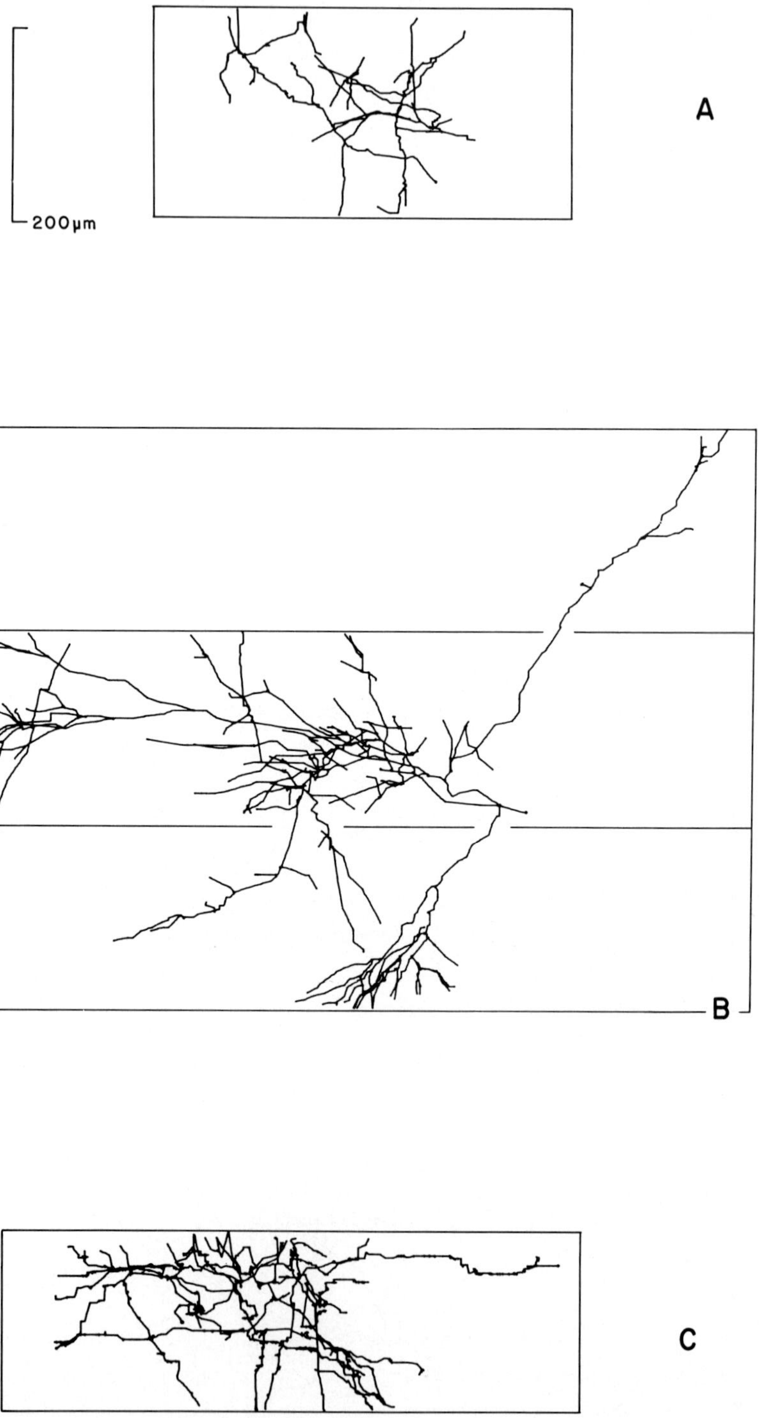

Fig. 7. Computer display of the same fibres shown in Fig. 6 after rotation of 90° on the horizontal OX axis.

position. The fibre is here represented as seen in a frontal section. As the figure shows, the total tangential spread of the fibre is in the order of 700 μm. A dense preterminal plexus is visible in the centre of the picture and a less profuse one appears on the left.

After a 90° computer rotation on the OX axis (Fig. 7B), the tangential distribution of the fibre becomes visible, as if it were seen perpendicularly from the pial surface. Horizontal lines indicate the limits of the 3 Golgi-stained sections used to reconstruct the fibre. One of the salient features revealed by the rotation is that the dense plexus shown in the centre of Fig. 6B is resolved into distinct plexuses coming out from main collaterals extending in a slightly oblique anteroposterior direction. Another interesting feature observed in computer rotations like this is that the plexuses of preterminal fibres occur as discrete entities, roughly 100–150 μm in diameter, separated by clear fields of the same size. From Golgi observations, it is impossible to know whether or not other incoming fibres overlap and then obscure such a pattern, but in support of the suggestion that the pattern does exist, there is the observation that, after geniculate lesions, degeneration occurs in clusters with a periodicity of about 100 μm (Garey and Powell, 1971).

The monkey

As seen in Golgi preparations of the visual cortex in adult monkeys, presumed geniculo-cortical fibres entering from the white matter, ascend vertically through layers VI and V. Immediately above the well marked boundary between IVc and V, the parent fibres begin to arborize by sending out at right angles a number of collateral branches which extend for variable distances in sublayer IVc. These collaterals are provided with numerous tightly packed short-side appendages and dilations giving a most characteristic image in well impregnated Golgi preparations (Fig. 3, red fibre 1). These collateral branches pierce through groups of stained small stellate cells with spinous dendrites and clewed cells (cf., Fig. 6 in Valverde, 1971), where it is not infrequent to observe close approximations to spinous dendritic segments in a way suggesting functional relationships (Fig. 5B). There is a second and thinner stratum of terminal fibres in sublayer IVa. Here parent fibres (Fig. 3, red fibre 2) can be traced ascending vertically from the white matter to end in this plexus of sublayer IVa; collaterals from the same parent fibre are also seen in sublayer IVc (Fig. 3, fibre 3), so that dual innervation of both levels from an identical origin can be presumed to exist.

Fig. 6C is a computer display of the terminal arborization of a single afferent fibre entering sublayer IVc in which all short-sided appendages and terminal dilations were recorded. The computed total number of terminal end bulbs in this fibre is 366; these are distributed in a volume of tissue of 32.7×10^6 μm^3. The high concentration of presumed synaptic sites in a given space is notorious. This fibre can be seen in Fig. 7C after 90° rotation around the horizontal OX axis. In this view it seems evident that the plexus of terminal fibres extends in a more or less elongated field with predominant transverse orientation, though no definite patterns are visible.

General considerations

Despite some common characteristics, which served for identification purposes, the patterns of distribution of specific fibres in the 3 animal species studied are rather diverse, probably in correlation with the progressive complication of the mammalian brain during evolution.

In mouse, the distribution of preterminal fibres on the tangential plane appears to be unspecific and does not seem to bear any correspondence with the cellular composition of layer IV, and in the rat visual cortex, Peters and Feldman (1976) found that degenerating axon terminals were no more densely grouped around apical dendritic clusters (Peters and Walsh, 1972) than elsewhere. Afferent fibres in cat (Fig. 7B) form distinct groupings of preterminal fibres. Whether this pattern as seen in Golgi preparations reflects a discreteness in the distribution of terminals is not clear. However, Garey and Powell (1971) found that such discreteness bears no relation to any morphological feature in layer IV.

The situation in the motor cortex appears to be different. In monkey (Sloper, 1973), a denser aggregation of degenerating terminals of thalamic origin occurs around apical dendrites. It seems that this different grouping of terminals reflects the fact that in the motor cortex, thalamo-cortical synapses on apical dendritic spines are apparently frequent; they have moreover been reported in EM degeneration studies (Strick and Sterling, 1974). In the primary visual cortex no such synapses have been seen by using this technique, suggesting that they do not exist or perhaps are less frequent.

In Golgi preparations of cat and monkey visual cortex, the majority of preterminal fibres follow horizontal or oblique courses (Fig. 6B, C). The probability for these fibres to establish synaptic contacts with apical dendritic spines is therefore less than if they followed vertical trajectories (cf., Szentágothai, 1975). If this were true, preterminal thalamo-cortical fibres in the motor cortex would be expected to course vertically. From the data shown by Jones (1975a, Fig. 15), it is clear that this is indeed the case. In mouse, preterminal fibres distribute in a more perpendicular fashion, much as they do in monkey motor cortex; our mouse material, however, is probably immature. Unfortunately, no EM degeneration data are available on mouse to decide whether or not apical dendrites are involved. In the closely related rat, a case of such contact has been found by the Golgi-EM technique (Peters, 1978), but the distribution of geniculo-cortical fibres in rat visual cortex is still unknown.

In fact, one major unsolved question remains behind these considerations: are axonal arborizations specific, in terms of the postsynaptic elements they contact? To approach this problem, a much more detailed knowledge of the connectivity of diverse types of axons, extrinsic or intrinsic, must be attained.

SUMMARY

The Golgi method is used to study the forms of non-pyramidal cells in the primary visual cortex in 3 animal species; neuronal types that could be recipients of the geniculo-cortical input are sought. These neurones are classed according to dendritic and axonal characteristics, into several distinct groups: spine-free (or sparsely spinous) neurones with either generalized or specialized axons, and spiny neurones always bearing axons of the generalized type.

Specific afferent fibres are identified in Golgi preparations and their geometrical properties analysed by means of computer rotations. The morphology differs in the animal species studied, but some basic properties are maintained. Except for laminar distribution, no definite patterns of arborization are found in mouse and monkey, whereas, in cat, afferent fibres form discrete preterminal arborizations.

ACKNOWLEDGEMENTS

We wish to thank Miss Laura López for her excellent technical assistance. The work was supported in part by a grant from Fundación E. Rodriguez Pascual to A.F. and by Fondo Nacional para el Desarrollo de la Investigación Científica.

REFERENCES

Cajal, S. Ramón y (1899) Comparative study of the sensory areas of the human cortex. In: *Centennial Volume,* Clark University, Worcester, Mass., pp. 311–382.

Cajal, S. Ramón y (1911) *Histologie du Système Nerveux de l'Homme et des Vertébrés, Tome II,* Maloine, Paris (Reimpress., Consejo Superior de Investigaciones Científicas, Instituto Cajal, Madrid, 1955).

Cajal, S. Ramón y (1921) Textura de la corteza visual del gato. *Trab. Lab. Invest. biol. Univ. Madrid,* 19: 113–144.

Christensen, B. N. and Ebner, F. F. (1978) The synaptic architecture of neurons in opossum somatic sensory-motor cortex: a combined anatomical and physiological study. *J. Neurocytol.,* 7: 61–70.

Colonnier, M. (1966) The structural design of the neocortex. In: *Brain and Conscious Experience,* J. C. Eccles (Ed.), Springer, Berlin, pp. 1–23.

Colonnier, M. and Rossignol, S. (1969) Discussion: heterogeneity of the cerebral cortex. In: *Basic Mechanisms of the Epilepsies,* H. H. Jasper, A. A. Ward and A. Pope (Eds.), Little, Brown and Co., Boston, Mass., pp. 29–40.

Fairén, A., Peters, A. and Saldanha, J. (1977) A new procedure for examining Golgi impregnated neurons by light and electron microscopy. *J. Neurocytol.,* 6: 311–337.

Feldman, M. L. and Peters, A. (1978) The forms of non-pyramidal neurons in the visual cortex of the rat. *J. comp. Neurol.,* 179: 761–794.

Garey, L. J. (1971) A light and electron microscopic study of the visual cortex of the cat and monkey. *Proc. roy. Soc. B,* 179: 21–40.

Garey, L. J. and Powell, T. P. S. (1971) An experimental study of the termination of the lateral geniculo-cortical pathway in the cat and monkey. *Proc. roy. Soc. B,* 179: 41–63.

Jones, E. G. (1975a) Lamination and differential distribution of thalamic afferents within the sensory-motor cortex of the squirrel monkey. *J. comp. Neurol.,* 160: 167–204.

Jones, E. G. (1975b) Varieties and distribution of non-pyramidal cells in the somatic sensory cortex of the squirrel monkey. *J. comp. Neurol.,* 160: 205–268.

Kelly, J. P. and Van Essen, D. C. (1974) Cell structure and function in the visual cortex of the cat. *J. Physiol. (Lond.),* 238: 515–547.

LeVay, S., Stryker, M. P. and Shatz, C. J. (1978) Ocular dominance columns and their development in layer IV of the cat's visual cortex: a quantitative study. *J. comp. Neurol.,* 179: 223–244.

Lorente de Nó, R. (1949) Cerebral cortex: architecture, intracortical connections, motor projections. In: *Physiology of the Nervous System,* J. F. Fulton (Ed.), Oxford University Press, London, pp. 288–330.

Lund, J. S. (1973) Organization of neurons in the visual cortex, area 17, of the monkey *(Macaca mulatta). J. comp. Neurol.,* 147: 455–496.

Marín-Padilla, M. (1969) Origin of the pericellular baskets of the pyramidal cells of the human motor cortex: a Golgi study. *Brain Res.,* 14: 633–646.

Parnavelas, J. G., Lieberman, A. R. and Webster, K. E. (1977) Organization of neurons in the visual cortex, area 17, of the rat. *J. Anat. (Lond.),* 124: 305–322.

Peters, A. (1978) Personal communication.

Peters, A. and Fairén, A. (1978) Smooth and sparsely-spined stellate cells in the visual cortex of the rat: a study using a combined Golgi-electron microscope technique. *J. comp. Neurol.,* 181: 129–172.

Peters, A. and Feldman, M. L. (1976) The projection of the lateral geniculate nucleus to area 17 of the rat cerebral cortex. I. General description. *J. Neurocytol.,* 5: 63–84.

Peters, A. and Feldman, M. L. (1977) The projection of the lateral geniculate nucleus to area 17 of the rat cerebral cortex. IV. Terminations upon spiny dendrites. *J. Neurocytol.,* 6: 669–689.

Peters, A. and Walsh, T. M. (1972) A study of the organization of apical dendrites in the somatic sensory cortex of the rat. *J. comp. Neurol.,* 144: 253–268.

Peters, A., Feldman, M. and Saldanha, J. (1976) The projection of the lateral geniculate nucleus to area 17 of the rat cerebral cortex. II. Terminations upon neuronal perikarya and dendritic shafts. *J. Neurocytol.,* 5: 85–107.

Peters, A., White, E. L. and Fairén, A. (1977) Synapses between identified neuronal elements. An electron microscopic demonstration of degenerating axon terminals synapsing with Golgi impregnated neurons. *Neurosci. Lett.*, 6: 171–175.

Ruiz-Marcos, A. and Valverde, F. (1970) Dynamic architecture of the visual cortex. *Brain Res.*, 19: 25–39.

Shkol'nik-Yarros, E. G. (1971) *Neurons and Interneuronal Connections of the Central Visual System.* Plenum Press, New York.

Sloper, J. J. (1973) An electron microscope study of the termination of afferent connections to the primate motor cortex. *J. Neurocytol.*, 2: 361–368.

Somogyi, P. (1977) A specific "axo-axonal" interneuron in the visual cortex of the rat. *Brain Res.*, 136: 345–350.

Somogyi, P. (1978) The study of Golgi stained cells and of experimental degeneration under the electron microscope: a direct method for the identification in the visual cortex of three successive links in a neuron chain. *Neuroscience*, 3: 167–180.

Strick, P. L. and Sterling, P. (1974) Synaptic termination of afferents from the ventrolateral nucleus of the thalamus in the cat motor cortex. A light and electron microscope study. *J. comp. Neurol.*, 153: 77–106.

Szentágothai, J. (1973) Synaptology of the visual cortex. In: *Handbook of Sensory Physiology, Vol. VII/3, Central Processing of Visual Information, Part B, Visual Centers in the Brain,* R. Jung (Ed.), Springer, Berlin, pp. 269–324.

Szentágothai, J. (1975) The "module-concept" in cerebral cortex architecture. *Brain Res.*, 95: 475–496.

Szentágothai, J. (1978) The neuron network of the cerebral cortex: a functional interpretation. *Proc. roy. Soc. B*, 201: 219–248.

Szentágothai, J. and Arbib, M. A. (1974) Conceptual models of neural organization. *Neurosci. Res. Progr. Bull.*, 12: 307–510.

Tigges, M., Bos, J., Tigges, J. and Bridges, E. (1977) Ultrastructural characteristics of layer IV neuropil in area 17 of monkeys. *Cell Tiss. Res.*, 182: 39–59.

Tömböl, T. (1978) Comparative data on the Golgi architecture of interneurons of different cortical areas in cat and rabbit. In: *Architectonics of the Cerebral Cortex,* M. A. B. Brazier and H. Petsche (Eds.), Raven Press, New York, pp. 59–76.

Valverde, F. (1968) Structural changes in the area striata of the mouse after enucleation. *Exp. Brain Res.*, 5: 274–292.

Valverde, F. (1970) The Golgi method. A tool for comparative structural analyses. In: *Contemporary Research Methods in Neuroanatomy,* W. J. H. Nauta and S. O. E. Ebbesson (Eds.), Springer, Berlin, pp. 12–31.

Valverde, F. (1971) Short axon neuronal subsystems in the visual cortex of the monkey. *Int. J. Neurosci.*, 1: 181–197.

Valverde, F. (1976) Aspects of cortical organization related to the geometry of neurons with intra-cortical axons. *J. Neurocytol.*, 5: 509–529.

Valverde, F. (1978) The organization of area 18 in the monkey. *Anat. Embryol.*, 154: 305–334.

Valverde, F. and Ruiz-Marcos, A. (1969) Dendritic spines in the visual cortex of the mouse: introduction to a mathematical model. *Exp. Brain Res.*, 8: 269–283.

White, E. L. (1978) Identified neurons in mouse SmI cortex which are postsynaptic to thalamocortical axon terminals: a combined Golgi-electron microscopic and degeneration study. *J. comp. Neurol.*, 181: 627–662.

Systems-Matching by Degeneration in the Developing Retino-tectal Projection of the Chicken

G. RAGER and U. RAGER

Department of Neurobiology, Max Planck Institute for Biophysical Chemistry, Am Fassberg, 3400 Göttingen (G.F.R.)

INTRODUCTION

The increase of fibre diameters in the optic nerve of the developing chicken has been described previously (Rager, 1976a). The results were shown to fit a model which is based on the assumption that the increase of fibre diameter is a function of the increase of the axonal flow. The axonal flow has been assumed to depend linearly on the axonal arborization.

This model implies that the final maturation and the survival of a retinal ganglion cell depend on the axonal branching process. Thus, in the special case of the formation of the retino-tectal connection in the chicken, if there is an abundance of retinal ganglion cell axons over termination sites in the tectum, the matching together of these two systems will be accompanied by death of the supernumerary cells. This should be considered in the more widespread phenomenon of cell death seen during ontogenesis which has been reviewed elsewhere (Rager and Rager, 1978).

THE TOTAL NUMBER OF OPTIC NERVE FIBRES

We have tested the hypothesis introduced above quantitatively by determining the total number of ganglion cell axons in the optic nerve from incubation day 5 to 100 days after hatching. The optic nerves of 50 animals were fixed for electron microscopy and embedded in Epon-Araldite. Cross-sections of nerves were obtained from the region where the nerves leave the orbita and enter the skull cavity. Since fibre density was measured on micrographs obtained from ultrathin sections, it had to be multiplied by the area of the same section. We measured this area by following the pial border of the nerve, by drawing out the circumference of the nerve with a plotter connected linearly to the stage control of the electron microscope, by recording the x-y coordinates of 30–40 points on the circumference, and by computing a polygon from these points. The cross-sectional area of the ultrathin section measured in this way turned out to be up to 20% smaller than the area of the semithin section. This is of some importance since the area of the semithin section is usually used for fibre counts.

In addition, a rectangle was drawn around the nerve so that each side made a tangent with the nerve's circumference. The rectangle was subdivided into small fields each of which had the size of an electron micrograph. This was the set of adjoining fields, from which samples were selected pseudorandomly. We found that no less than 60 electron micrographs had to be taken per nerve to get a sufficiently good approximation to the fibre density of the population (percentage error of the mean $\leqslant$ 5%). Thus, on average, 10,000 fibres were counted per nerve.

Fig. 1 shows the results. The total number of fibres is plotted in millions against the logarithm of the developmental age in days. Each of the 50 points represents one nerve. The total number of fibres is approximately 4400 on incubation day 5. It increases nearly exponentially during the following days with a maximal increment on incubation day 8. On days 10 and 11 a maximum of 4 million fibres is reached. Only 1 day later, the number of axons has already decreased. By incubation day 18 the final value is reached which is about 2.4 million. This is a reduction of 40% from the maximum.

It could be argued that the number of axons in the optic nerve is not equal to the number of ganglion cells because of the formation of collaterals. However, we were unable to detect axon collaterals in the retina or in the optic nerve (either in Golgi whole mounts of the developing retina or in longitudinal sections of Golgi impregnated nerves or in our electron micrographs). This is supported by the observations of Goldberg (1974). We, therefore, extend our findings from ganglion cell axons to ganglion cell perikarya.

Incubation day 18 is the time when an electroretinogram and a visual evoked response in the optic tectum can first be recorded (Rager, 1979). Thus, both the formation and the degeneration of retinal ganglion cells end before the visual system begins to transmit light signals.

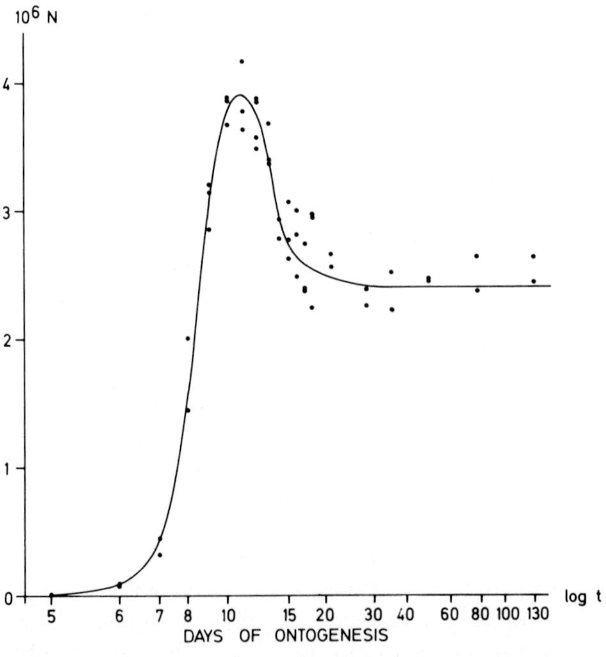

Fig. 1. The total number of ganglion cell axons at 20 subsequent developmental stages is plotted against the logarithm of days of ontogenesis. The curve was obtained from the model; it was fitted to the measured values with the Gauss-Newton method. (From G. and U. Rager (1978), with permission of Springer Verlag.)

DEGENERATING CELLS IN THE RETINA

With the extensive degeneration of retinal axons found by counting nerve fibres, it should be expected that degenerating cells are also visible in the retina. We examined the ganglion cell layer of the retina at various developmental stages with the electron microscope. We sometimes found a few perikarya showing initial signs of degeneration on incubation day 8. From incubation day 9 onwards we saw a considerable number of cells at various stages of degeneration. Thus cell death can be detected in the retina 2–3 days earlier than in the optic nerve (i.e. from counting the total number of axons). This is mainly because generation and degeneration of ganglion cells overlap for a while so that degeneration cannot be recognized from the total counts before incubation day 12.

INTRARETINAL SPREAD OF DEGENERATION

Electron microscopy provides information about the size and the time of appearance of degenerating cells. This in turn enables us to localize these cells with the light microscope. In an additional series of preparations, eyes were cut perpendicularly to the pecten. Sections whose plane was near the lens centre were examined under oil immersion. The position of each degenerating cell was recorded with a plotter which was connected to the stage control of the microscope via linear potentiometers. With this procedure we see that on incubation day 9 degenerating cells are concentrated in the region around the papilla. Three days later they are distributed over the whole retina, but are slightly less concentrated in the central area. On incubation day 15 degenerating cells are found mainly in more peripheral zones. Thus, a wave of degeneration spreads from the centre of the retina to its periphery. It reflects the mode of innervation of the optic tectum by retinal fibres.

A MATHEMATICAL MODEL

Our results show that the number of retinal ganglion cells does not initially match the number of tectal termination sites. Obviously the two systems, retina and optic tectum, are matched in size by degeneration. Our quantitative data serve as a basis to interpret this phenomenon with a mathematical model, which will now be outlined (for details see Rager, 1978).

First, the formation of retinal ganglion cells and of tectal termination domains is described with differential equations based on the mechanism of mitosis. Then the idea of a competent cell is introduced. From our Golgi studies we know that ganglion cell axons of the central retina already start to branch and to invade the central tectal area on incubation day 8 (Rager and von Oeynhausen, 1978). One day later we find a great number of degenerating cells in the retina for the first time. From these two findings, the invasion of the optic tectum on day 8 and the onset of degeneration on day 9, we conclude that ganglion cells do not degenerate before their axons have arrived at the optic tectum and started branching. Apparently a new stage in the maturation of ganglion cells begins when axons start to branch and to form contacts. We propose, therefore, that ganglion cells become competent to continue to develop or to die only after they have arrived at their termination sites. Now, to find the actual number of competent cells, the extension of the fibre pathway between the retina and the optic tectum had to be measured and introduced into the model.

The central proposition of the model is that retinal axons compete for an adequate termination domain and that the total number of supernumerary axons at any given time decreases with a certain time constant.

By this model the mathematical function was determined. The unknown parameter values of this function were optimized with the Gauss-Newton method. The good fit which was obtained between the theoretical and measured values (Fig. 1) allows us to conclude that, to a first approximation, the model is satisfactory.

COMPETITION AND SYNAPTOGENESIS

The mechanisms underlying competition are still unknown. Therefore, we use the term competition in an operationally defined sense. We say that a minimum number of target sites are required for the survival of a neurone. Fibres compete for this subsistence minimum. Those fibres which do not succeed have to die.

Degeneration starts earlier than synaptogenesis as judged from morphological as well as electrophysiological criteria (Rager, 1976b). However, from our Golgi preparations, there is some evidence that the growing tips of retinal axons come into close proximity of tectal dendrites from incubation day 8 onward (Rager and von Oeynhausen, 1979). Thus it might be possible that there is some kind of molecular interaction between afferent fibres and tectal target cells already at this stage leading to some sort of selective stabilization (Changeux et al., 1973) of the surviving ganglion cells. Non-stabilized cells will die. This is expressed in our concept of a competent cell introduced above.

CONCLUSION

Competition for adequate targets and degeneration of supernumerary cells seem to be simple and powerful mechanisms influencing the formation of connections in the brain. They adapt the sizes of the two systems (retina and optic tectum) which are obviously not matched in their Anlage.

SUMMARY

We have used quantitative methods to show that 40% of retinal ganglion cells of the chick embryo degenerate. The degeneration of these cells starts shortly after their axons have reached their termination domains in the optic tectum. It is postulated, therefore, that ganglion cell axons compete for a minimum number of termination sites. If more retinal fibres arrive than tectal termination sites are available, supernumerary fibres may degenerate. The two systems, retina and optic tectum, are finally matched in size after degeneration. This process is interpreted in terms of a mathematical model.

REFERENCES

Changeux, J. P., Courrège, Ph. and Danchin, A. (1973) A theory of the epigenesis of neuronal networks by selective stabilization of synapses. *Proc. nat. Acad. Sci. (Wash.)*, 70: 2974–2978.

Goldberg, S. (1974) Studies on the mechanics of development of the visual pathways in the chick embryo. *Develop. Biol.*, 36: 24–43.

Rager, G. (1976a) Morphogenesis and physiogenesis of the retino-tectal connection in the chicken. I. The retinal ganglion cells and their axons. *Proc. roy. Soc. B*, 192: 331–352.

Rager, G. (1976b) Morphogenesis and physiogenesis of the retino-tectal connection in the chicken. II. The retino-tectal synapses. *Proc. roy. Soc. B*, 192: 353–370.

Rager, G. (1978) Systems-matching by degeneration. II. Interpretation of the generation and degeneration of retinal ganglion cells by a mathematical model. *Exp. Brain Res.*, 33: 79–90.

Rager, G. (1979) The cellular origin of the b-wave in the electroretinogram. A developmental approach. In preparation.

Rager, G. and von Oeynhausen, B. (1978) Ingrowth and ramification of retinal fibres in the developing optic tectum of the chick embryo. *Exp. Brain Res.*, 35: 213–227.

Rager, G. and Rager, U. (1978) Systems-matching by degeneration. I. A quantitative electron microscopic study of the generation and degeneration of retinal ganglion cells in the chicken. *Exp. Brain Res.*, 33: 65–78.

Visual Deprivation in Monkeys: its Effects and its Reversal

L. J. GAREY*, COLIN BLAKEMORE** and F. VITAL-DURAND

Institut d'Anatomie, University of Lausanne, Rue du Bugnon 9, CH-1011 Lausanne (Switzerland), The Physiological Laboratory, Cambridge CB2 3EG (Great Britain) and Laboratoire de Neuropsychologie Expérimentale, INSERM U.94, 16, Avenue du Doyen-Lépine, 69500 Bron (France)

INTRODUCTION

At first sight the highly complex and specialized mammalian central nervous system would seem to be an unlikely place to try to study the theme of this meeting, the problems of chemical specificity of neurons. Many of these proceedings are concerned with simple neural systems and models, provided by isolated cell populations and tissue culture, and it is from such studies that advances at the "molecular" level are likely to come. However, the more global approach of studying the intact or experimentally altered nervous system gives a different set of data which will, hopefully, contribute to our understanding of underlying mechanisms.

The visual system has been the object of intense study for very long. Like other systems its complexity and inherent precision strikes one as soon as one begins to look at it in detail, either from the point of view of its exquisite functional efficiency or its anatomical intricacy. Although the structure and performance of the normal adult visual system are far from understood, some of the principles underlying visual perception, and indeed neural mechanisms more generally, can be investigated by looking at developmental stages, either in the normal brain or in the context of experimental intervention. The stages of development of the primate visual system up to birth have been investigated in a series of studies by Rakic (see Rakic, 1977, for a review), but it is with the very important period just after birth that we shall concern ourselves at present.

The technique of sensory deprivation of experimental animals is not new. Probably the first to exploit these techniques in a systematic way was Gudden (1870). He sutured the eyelids of young rabbits in order to investigate the effects of visual deprivation, without the explicit trauma of actual physical lesions, on the development of the brain. The suturing technique was taken up by Berger (1900) in cats and dogs and he was able to show actual reduction in size and cellular content of the visual cortex when the animal matured after such visual deprivation.

---

* Correspondence to: L. J. Garey, Institut d'Anatomie, Université de Lausanne, Rue du Bugnon 9, CH-1011 Lausanne-CHUV, Switzerland.

** Royal Society Locke Research Fellow.

After many years of eclipse, the lid-suture method was reintroduced by Hubel and Wiesel at the beginning of a series of innovative experiments which they, and many others, still continue. They (Wiesel and Hubel, 1963a, b; Hubel and Wiesel, 1970) formulated several important concepts which provide the basis for most similar work at present. Their findings were that if one eye of a kitten was sutured closed soon after birth, then certain features of the normal mature visual system were radically altered when the deprived animal was investigated several weeks later. The first of these changes was that the neurons of the visual cortex, recorded by extracellular microelectrodes, almost exclusively responded to the eye which had remained open, functional connections with the deprived eye being effectively lost. This contrasted with normal cats of the same age in which at least three-quarters of visual cortical cells were influenced by both eyes (Hubel and Wiesel, 1963). The second big effect of monocular lid suture was that in the lateral geniculate nucleus (LGN), the thalamic relay of fibres from the retina to the cortex, the neurons innervated by the deprived eye failed to grow normally and, when examined histologically, were markedly smaller than normally innervated cells. Furthermore, they defined a "critical" or "sensitive" period from about 3 weeks to 3 months postnatally during which these effects could be elicited, and beyond which the brain seemed mature and exempt from such abuse.

The principal findings concerning the physiology of the cortex mentioned above have been confirmed and extended (see, for example, Pettigrew, 1974; Blakemore and Van Sluyters, 1975), as have the morphological effects (e.g., Guillery and Stelzner, 1970; Garey et al., 1973).

More recently the primate visual system has come under study using similar experimental paradigms. The monkey's visual system is in many ways more convenient than that of the cat, for its cortex is more distinctly laminated and the only cortical projection of the LGN is probably to the primary visual cortex, area 17, whereas in the cat the LGN projects to secondary areas (e.g., Wilson and Cragg, 1967; Garey and Powell, 1967, 1971). The neonatal monkey cortex is more mature than that of the cat (Wiesel and Hubel, 1974; Hubel and Wiesel, 1977) but monocular deprivation is effective in reducing cortical binocularity (Baker et al., 1974; Crawford et al., 1975; Hubel et al., 1977; Blakemore et al., 1978) and in preventing normal LGN growth (Headon and Powell, 1973; Von Noorden, 1973; Hubel et al., 1977; Vital-Durand et al., 1978).

If monocular deprivation is so effective in changing physiological and morphological parameters in the visual pathways, to what extent can the changes be reversed? In cats this question has been partially answered using the technique of "reverse suture". The animal is monocularly deprived for a time calculated to assure a marked effect in both cortex and thalamus, and then the closed eye is re-opened and the other closed. When done before about 6 weeks of age the procedure leads to "recapture" of cortical units by the initially deprived eye and, if left for two weeks or so, to a total reversal of ocular dominance (Blakemore and Van Sluyters, 1974; Movshon, 1976).

At the same time the LGN cells, having undergone a growth failure (or "shrinkage", to use a convenient, if not strictly accurate, term) of about 30–40% in terms of cross-sectional area in histological sections, recover their size, so that within 3 days after reverse suturing they are as big as normal cells, and within a couple of weeks they are 30% larger than the newly deprived cells (Dürsteler et al., 1976).

In view of the dramatic results from these reverse-suturing experiments in cats, and as no similar work had been reported in the primate, we undertook the experiments described below to extend our observations to the monkey.

EXPERIMENTAL METHODS

A total of 35 monkeys of both sexes was used. All were Old World monkeys, and all but four were patas *(Erythrocebus patas).* Infants, born in captivity of wild mothers, were reared by hand from the day of birth. In 31 of these, eyelid suture was performed under ketamine anesthesia at ages ranging from a few hours to about 4 years. In 11, reverse suture was done under ketamine anesthesia. For the electrophysiological experiments, 16 monkeys were anesthetized, paralyzed and maintained during recording by intravenous infusion of Nembutal and Flaxedil, with artificial ventilation. Single units were recorded in area 17 with glass-coated tungsten microelectrodes (Merrill and Ainsworth, 1972; Fig. 1) and visual stimuli were back-projected on a screen 70 cm from the eyes.

At the end of the physiological experiment, or after the required survival time, animals were perfused with physiological saline followed by 10% formalin or 1% paraformaldehyde plus 1.25% glutaraldehyde in 0.1 M phosphate buffer. Cortical electrode tracks were reconstructed from frozen sections stained with cresyl violet. A block containing the thalamus was embedded in paraffin and coronal sections were cut and stained with cresyl violet. Neurons in the LGN were selected and measured using the following technique. The sections were examined with a microscope whose stage was driven by stepping motors. Drawings were made through a drawing tube on a digital graphics tablet interfaced to a computer. The central axis of each LGN layer was drawn at low magnification and the computer selected 5 sampling points spaced equally along the layer. At each sampling point the outlines of 10 neurons with clear nucleoli were drawn on the graphics tablet at × 1000 magnification, and the computer calculated the cross-sectional area of each cell. 600 or 1200 cells were measured in each brain.

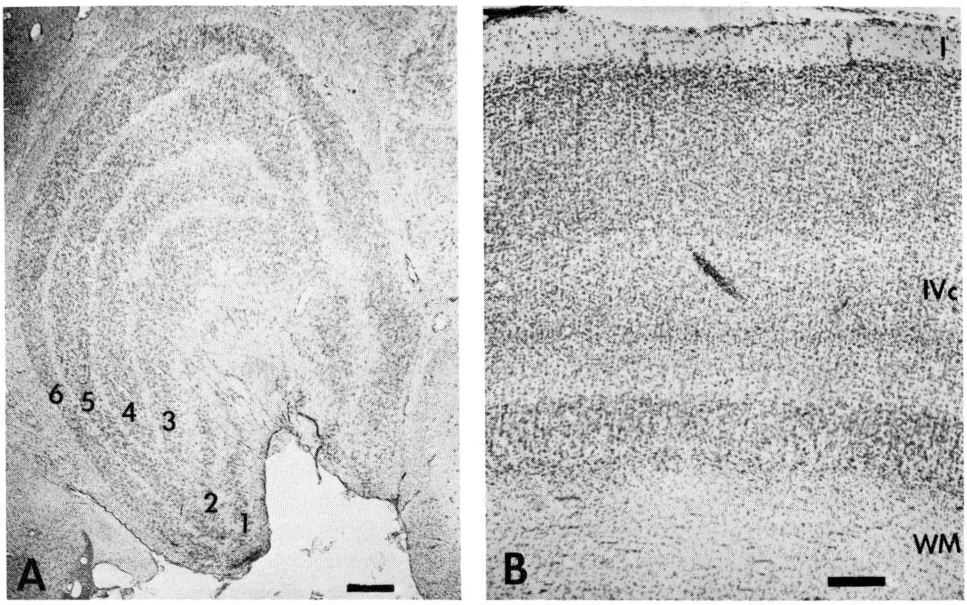

Fig. 1. A: coronal section, stained with cresyl violet, of the LGN of a monkey. Note the 2 magnocellular laminae (1 and 2) and the 4 parvocellular laminae (3–6). Scale bar, 500 μm. B: cresyl violet section of area 17 of a monkey. The white matter (WM) and layers I and IVc (in which an oblique electrode track is visible) are indicated. Scale bar, 250 μm.

EXPERIMENTAL RESULTS

Normal animals

In the visual cortex of a normal 8-month-old monkey (Fig. 2) most cells above and below layer IVc were orientation-selective and binocularly driven, but in layer IVc units were not orientation-selective and almost all were monocular. Cells occurred in alternating patches dominated first by one eye then by the other, reflecting the anatomical distribution of afferent axons in left-eye and right-eye "stripes" (Hubel et al., 1977). The preferred stimulus orientation from one cell to the next progressed in a regular, ordered manner (cf., Hubel and Wiesel, 1977). Fig. 4A shows ocular dominance histograms for all cells recorded in this normal animal.

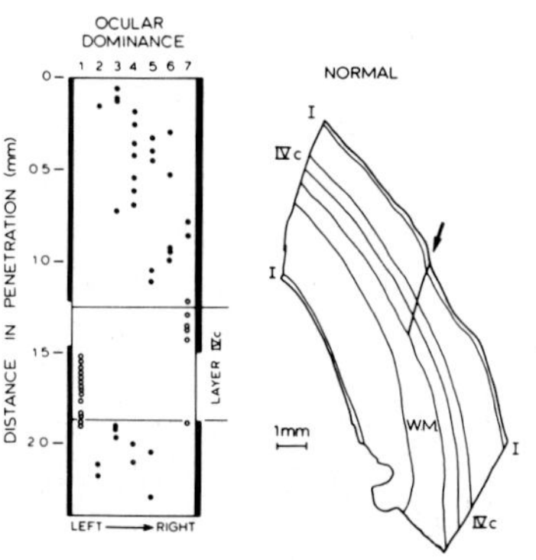

Fig. 2. Diagrams of an electrode penetration in the right area 17 of a normal, 8-month-old, monkey. On the right is a reconstruction of the oblique electrode track (arrowed), with the positions of the white matter (WM) and of layers I and IVc indicated. On the left, the distribution of the ocular dominance of units encountered is expressed with relation to the distance along the penetration (layer IVc, determined from histology, is marked). Ocular dominance groups 1–7 refer to monocular cells driven by, respectively, the contralateral and ipsilateral eye; group 4 cells are totally binocular, while groups 2 and 3, 5 and 6 are binocular but dominated by, respectively, the contralateral and the ipsilateral eye. Filled circles indicate orientation-specific units; open circles are non-oriented units. The thick vertical lines mark areas where the background activity was influenced by the left or right eye.

Monocular deprivation

We recorded from the visual cortex of 4 animals monocularly deprived by closure of the right eye. In 2 of them, deprived within the first 2 months of life, the shift in ocular dominance was very marked. Fig. 3A shows the distribution of ocular dominance for cells recorded in a penetration in the left hemisphere of a vervet monkey *(Cercopithecus aethiops)* monocularly deprived from 2 to 5.5 weeks of age. Most cells were only excitable by the non-deprived left eye, although background activity could be elicited through the deprived eye in small areas occurring at intervals along the track. Another animal, deprived from birth to 24 days of age, confirmed this strong dominance by the non-deprived eye (cf., Hubel et al., 1977). In both, the proportion of layer IVc dominated by the non-deprived eye was almost 3 times larger than that dominated by the deprived eye. Hubel et al. (1977) also

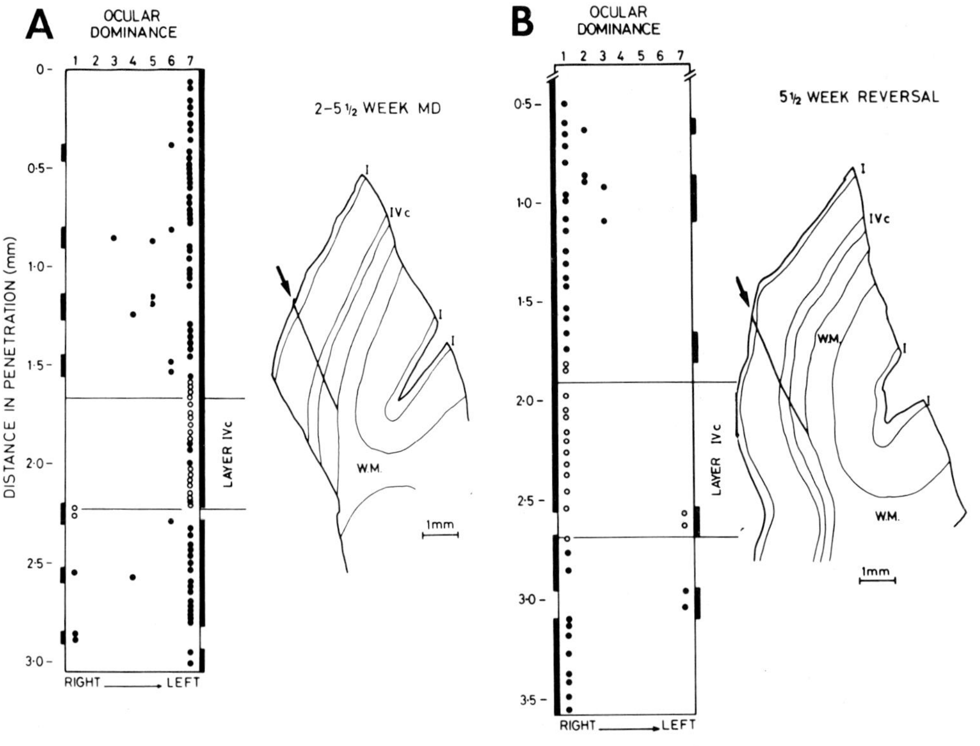

Fig. 3. A: ocular dominance distribution, as in Fig. 2, for a penetration in the left area 17 of a monkey monocularly deprived (MD) in the right eye from 2 to 5.5 weeks of age. B: a similar penetration in a monkey monocularly deprived until 5.5 weeks and then reverse-sutured for 4 months. An almost mirror-image shift in ocular dominance is seen, compared with the experiment in A.

observed that in early monocularly deprived monkeys the "stripes" from the non-deprived eye were up to 3 times wider than those from the deprived eye.

We examined 2 late deprived animals; one was a cynomolgus *(Macaca fascicularis)* monocularly deprived from 11 to 16 months of age and the other a normal adult of about 4 years of age monocularly deprived for more than 6 months. In neither was there any evidence of a shift in ocular dominance within layer IVc. However, in the animal deprived at around the age of a year, there was some change in ocular dominance outside layer IVc, as shown in Fig. 4C. Thus, monocular deprivation late in the first year seems to modify the ocular dominance of cells in the monkey's visual cortex, except for those in layer IVc. The sensitive period is probably different for cells in layer IVc and those outside IVc, and the sensitive period for the latter is longer than that in the cat.

Our measurements of the cross-sectional areas of LGN cells in 16 monocularly deprived monkeys confirm previous studies (Headon and Powell, 1973; Von Noorden, 1973; Hubel et al., 1977) in that after monocular deprivation during the first 6 weeks of life, cells in both magnocellular and parvocellular layers innervated by the deprived eye are smaller, on average, than the corresponding cells with input from the non-deprived eye (Fig. 5). However, we found that the effects were less pronounced than in the kitten, where deprived cells are typically 30–40% smaller than non-deprived (Guillery and Stelzner, 1970; Garey et al., 1973). In the monkey the size difference after early deprivation averaged about 15–20%

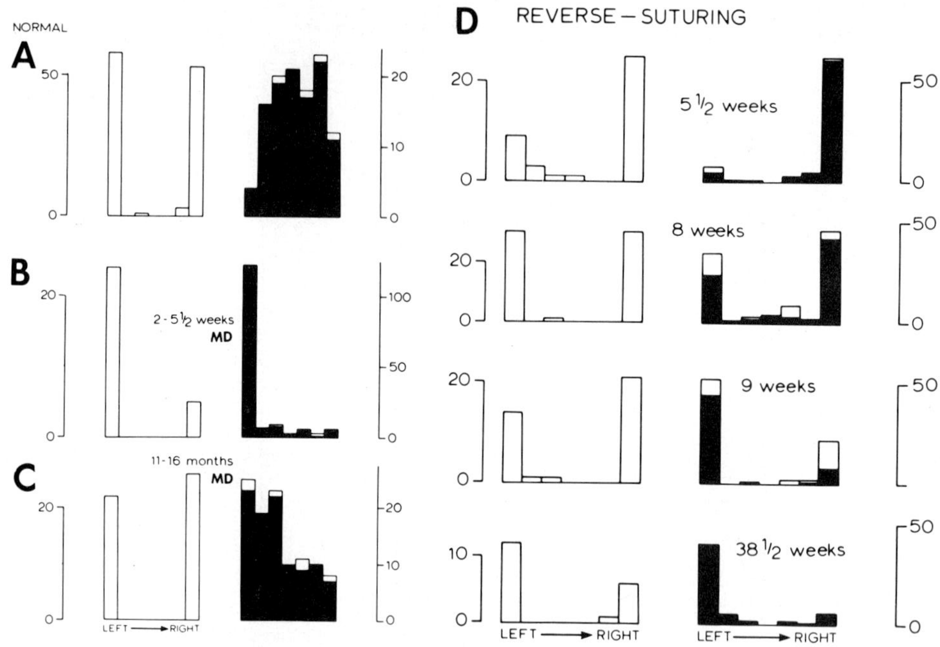

Fig. 4. A series of histograms to show the changes in ocular dominance found in the present study. In all cases, on the left are non-oriented cells recorded in layer IVc (open columns), while on the right are oriented cells (filled columns) and non-oriented cells (open columns) outside layer IVc. Samples from both hemispheres are combined for each experiment as if all were from the right. The ocular dominance groups are then standardized so that the left column represents monocular units dominated by the left eye, and so on. A: normal, 8 months old. B: monocularly deprived from 2 to 5.5 weeks. C: monocularly deprived from 11 to 16 months. D: reverse-sutured for 4 months or more at the ages indicated.

(Fig. 6A). Deprivation as brief as a few days, even starting on the day of birth, can cause a significant change in the size of LGN cells. In the 2 animals deprived at about 1 year and 4 years of age respectively, there was, however, no significant difference between right-eye and left-eye laminae of the LGN.

These results suggest that the sensitive period for effects on LGN cell growth is similar to that for modification of ocular dominance stripes in layer IVc of the cortex, as might be expected if perikaryal size is correlated with the extent of the cell's axonal arborization (Guillery, 1972).

We measured LGN cells in several normal monkeys: in an 8-month-old adolescent, in a mature adult, in a term fetus and in a cynomolgus monkey born about a week prematurely and perfused 4 days postnatally.

In all these animals, cells in the LGN laminae connected to the right eye were no different in size from those in the left-eye laminae, although cells in the magnocellular laminae (1 and 2) were, of course, larger than those in the parvocellular (3–6). From these data, and from cell sizes in non-deprived LGN layers in deprived animals, we can draw some conclusions about the normal growth of LGN cells. This is complicated by the variability in average cell size from animal to animal, which is at least partly accounted for by generally larger cells in male monkeys. Growth in both magnocellular and parvocellular laminae continues after birth and may be complete at about 1 month of age.

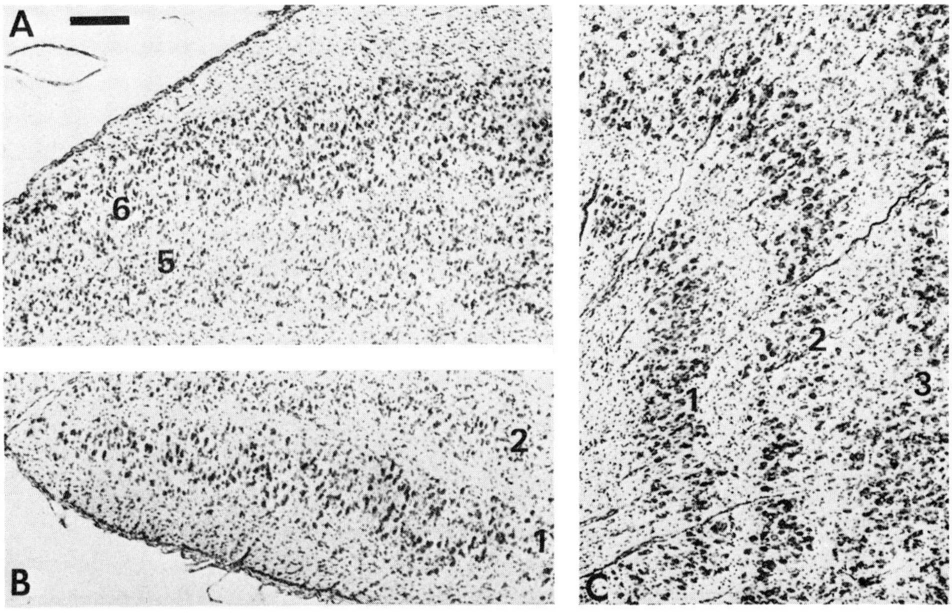

Fig. 5. Coronal cresyl violet sections from the LGN. Scale bar, 250 μm. A: parvocellular laminae 5 and 6 in the right LGN after ipsilateral monocular deprivation from 2 to 5.5 weeks, to show the reduced size of cells in layer 5. B: the magnocellular laminae (1 and 2) of the same animal; lamina 2 cells are small. C: laminae 1, 2 and 3 in the left LGN after early contralateral monocular deprivation. Cells in lamina 1 are smaller than in 2 and 3.

Two animals were *binocularly* deprived on the day of birth, one until 3 weeks, the other until 8 months. Cell growth appears to have been arrested at the neonatal value in both (cf., Headon and Powell, 1978). We conclude that both monocular and binocular deprivation may simply arrest cell growth at the size achieved at the time of eye closure; we have no evidence of hypertrophy of non-deprived cells, unlike the situation in the kitten (Guillery, 1972; Garey et al., 1973).

Reversal of the effects of monocular deprivation

In 8 monkeys, initially deprived in the right eye, the closed eye was re-opened and the other eye closed at ages between 4 and 38.5 weeks. First we shall describe 4 animals that were reverse-sutured at 5.5, 8, 9 and 38.5 weeks and then allowed more than 4 months in which to use the newly opened eye.

In one, deprived in the right eye until 5.5 weeks and then reverse-sutured, the ocular dominance distribution of cortical cells was a mirror image of the monkey monocularly deprived until 5.5 weeks: most cells were monocularly driven by the originally deprived right eye (Fig. 3B). The ordered sequences of preferred orientation were re-established. Later reverse-suture leads to less effective recapture of the cortex by the newly opened eye. Animals deprived until 8 or 9 weeks and then reverse-sutured for more than 4 months had alternating groups of cells dominated by each eye, and the original deprivation effect had not been cancelled. Very late reverse suturing (at 38.5 weeks in a cynomolgus) had no apparent effect on ocular dominance distribution. The ocular dominance histograms in Fig. 4 summarize the results in these 4 reverse-sutured animals compared with normal and monocularly deprived animals.

By comparing the relative dimensions of regions of layer IVc dominated by left and right eyes we calculated that the right-eye regions were roughly the same width as the left-eye stripes in animals reverse-sutured at 9 weeks or before. This contrasts with a ratio of about 1:3 after initial monocular deprivation. Our determination of the boundaries of ocular dominance stripes is purely physiological, of course, and we are now looking at the actual distribution of afferent axons to layer IVc, using the method of transneuronal transport of radioactive label injected into the eye (Hubel et al., 1977).

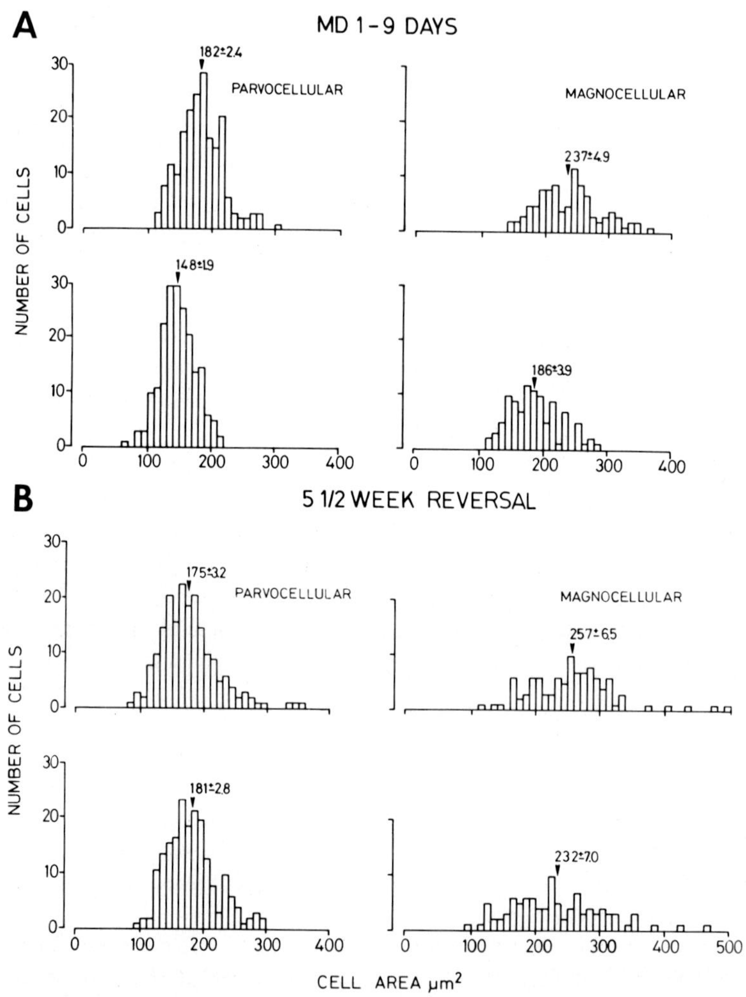

Fig. 6. A: histograms of the areas of 600 LGN cells in an animal monocularly deprived (MD) from 1 to 9 days. Data from the parvocellular laminae are pooled, as are those from the magnocellular laminae. Arrowheads mark the mean cross-sectional area, ± S.E. Mean cell area in the deprived laminae is reduced by about 20% . B: similar histograms for a monkey reverse-sutured at 5.5 weeks. The lower histograms represent the originally deprived laminae. There is no significant difference in cell size in the parvocellular laminae, while in the magnocellular the size difference is less than in a non-reversed monocular deprivation.

The other 4 reverse-sutured monkeys were initially deprived in the right eye until 4 weeks of age and then reversed for between 3 days and 18 weeks. The shift in ocular dominance and the physiological re-expansion of ocular dominance stripes in layer IVc was already detectable after 3 days and virtually complete in 2 weeks.

LGN cell size was measured in the 8 reverse-sutured monkeys described above, and in 3 others reverse-sutured at ages between 1 and 12 weeks. When reverse suture took place before 12 weeks the difference in cell size between LGN laminae was reduced or even slightly reversed (Fig. 6B). The later the age at reverse suturing the less marked was the effect on LGN cell size. In the monkey reverse-sutured at 38.5 weeks, whose cortical physiology was unaffected by the procedure, the LGN showed no sign of reversal. As with the cortical physiology, LGN cell sizes showed a recovery after only 3 days with complete recovery within 2 weeks. We conclude that the sizes of cells in the LGN correlate well with the widths of functional ocular dominance stripes in layer IVc of the visual cortex. Early reverse suturing restores right-eye and left-eye stripes to approximately equal width, and cancels cell size differences in the LGN. In 2 control animals, the closed eye was simply re-opened after 4 weeks of monocular deprivation: in neither case, one for 2 weeks, the other for 14 weeks, was there recovery, either in cortex or LGN.

From our physiological measurement of the widths of ocular dominance stripes in IVc we calculated the ratio ($\bar{L}/\bar{R}$) of the average width of left-eye to right-eye stripes. It had a maximum of 2.85 after monocular deprivation from 2 to 5.5 weeks. The normal control animal had a ratio very close to unity (1.03), as did the animal monocularly deprived at the end of the first year ($\bar{L}/\bar{R}$ = 1.06). The abscissa of Fig. 7 expresses the ratio of average cell size in left-eye laminae of the LGN to that in right-eye laminae. The normal and the late-

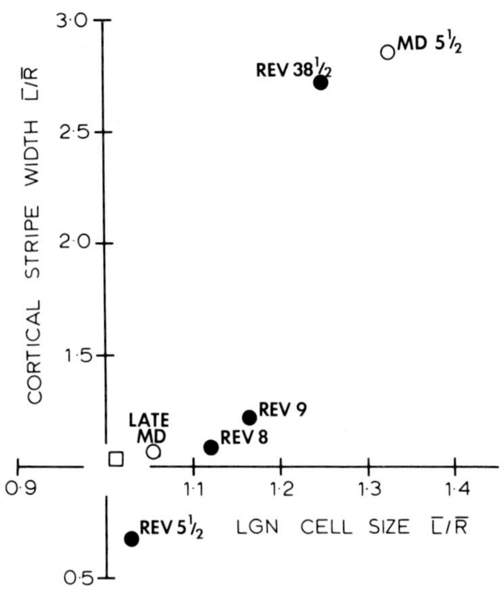

Fig. 7. A comparison of the ratios ($\bar{L}/\bar{R}$) of the left-eye and right-eye stripe widths in layer IVc (ordinate) and of the area of LGN cells innervated by the left eye and the right eye. The square refers to a normal animal, the open circles are monocular deprivations, one until 5.5 weeks (MD 5½), the other from 11 to 16 months (LATE MD). The filled circles were reverse-sutured for at least 4 months at ages 5.5 weeks (REV 5½), 8 weeks (REV 8), 9 weeks (REV 9) and 38.5 weeks (REV 38½).

deprived animals again have values close to unity, but the animal monocularly deprived from 2 to 5.5 weeks has a marked cell size difference ($\overline{L}/\overline{R}$ = 1.33). The filled circles in Fig. 7 describe data for reverse-sutured monkeys. The reversal at 5.5 weeks produced an LGN cell size ratio close to one (1.02) and the right eye cortical stripes were actually slightly wider on average than those for the left eye (cortical $\overline{L}/\overline{R}$ = 0.67). The 2 animals reverse-sutured at 8 and 9 weeks had small differences in cortical stripe widths and LGN cell sizes, just in favour of the original deprivation. The animal reverse-sutured at 38.5 weeks showed no recovery in either cortical stripes or LGN cells.

DISCUSSION

This study has shown that the well-established anatomical and physiological sequelae of monocular visual deprivation in the primate brain can be reversed by forced usage of the deprived eye, although it seems that the good eye must be occluded for this to be effective in the relatively simple paradigm used here. The possible reversal of an experimental deprivation condition is obviously of considerable importance in the clinical treatment of childhood amblyopia (Awaya et al., 1973).

It is not easy to determine the exact limits of the sensitive period, either to monocular deprivation or to reverse suture, but the main effects for LGN and cortical layer IVc seem to be terminated within about the first 2 months of life, rather as in the cat (Hubel and Wiesel, 1970), although cortical ocular dominance outside layer IVc can be modified for up to a year or so. The morphological changes in the LGN seem entirely parallel to the cortical effects and support the concept of a relation between soma size and axonal arborization (cf., Guillery, 1972).

Several problems remain. To what extent are genetically determined factors responsible for the functional properties of the mature visual system and to what extent environmental factors? Can the idea of competition for cortical neurons between the axon terminals of each eye (Guillery and Stelzner, 1970) be confirmed? Certainly, with regard to competition, we know that almost all cells in layer IVc, the main site of termination of thalamo-cortical afferents, are monocularly driven at the times of reverse suture studied here. It is, therefore, unlikely that a straightforward competitive factor is involved. It should be remembered that in the monkey the effect on LGN cells of monocular deprivation is to cause a 15–20% "shrinkage", rather than the 30–40% in the cat, and that, again, unlike the cat, where reverse suture leads to a 30% overshoot in the opposite direction (Dürsteler et al., 1976), in the monkey reversal causes little more than a shift to equality of cell size in all layers. Thus, in the cat we may be seeing an effect of deprivation plus competition, whereas in the monkey an effect dependent on pure deprivation may be operating.

What is actually happening to synapses that become silent after monocular deprivation and are reactivated by reverse suture? Are they withdrawing anatomically and regrowing, or are they simply being suppressed, at least for a limited time, during which reversal can recall them quickly to activity? Although it is not possible to be sure, the rapid re-establishment of cortical response properties, including orientation specificity, after reversal suggests that actual physical removal of axons has not taken place. The results of autoradiography after experiments to label monocular terminals in layer IVc transneuronally, as mentioned above, should help to elucidate the problem, and initial results do suggest that not all terminals are, in fact, lost in deprived ocular dominance columns at an age when reverse suturing is effective in causing re-expansion of the ocular dominance stripes.

SUMMARY

Unilateral eyelid closure in kittens or baby monkeys causes most visual cortical neurons to become unresponsive to the deprived eye (Hubel and Wiesel, 1970). In kittens, "reverse suture" (opening the deprived eye and closing the other) leads to "recapture" of cortical cells by the initially deprived eye, if done sufficiently early (Blakemore and Van Sluyters, 1974). In the monkey also, reverse suture causes total recapture if done early (up to about 6 weeks) with expansion of the ocular dominance "columns" in layer IVc of area 17 related to the newly opened eye. Late reversal is ineffective and intermediate reversal (8–9 weeks) causes partial recapture.

Monocular deprivation also affects normal cell growth in the lateral geniculate nucleus (LGN) of monkeys (Headon and Powell, 1973; Von Noorden, 1973), such that the neurons innervated by the deprived retina are smaller than normal. Reverse suture in kittens leads to a recovery of cell size in the initially deprived LGN laminae and to a shrinkage in the others (Dürsteler et al., 1976). In the monkey, monocular deprivation leads to less effect on LGN cells than in the cat; reverse suture results in recovery of LGN cell size.

ACKNOWLEDGEMENTS

The monkeys in this study were kindly donated by Institut Mérieux and IFFA Merieux, Lyon, to whom we are very grateful. We thank M. C. Cruz, C. Frenois and M. Gaillard for technical help.

The work was supported by INSERM, by the European Training Programme in Brain and Behaviour Research and by grants from the Swiss National Science Foundation (No. 3.2460.74) and the Medical Research Council (No. G972/463/B).

REFERENCES

Awaya, S., Miyake, Y., Imaizumi, Y., Shiose, Y., Kanda, T. and Komuro, K. (1973) Amblyopia in man, suggestive of stimulus deprivation amblyopia. *Jap. J. Ophthalmol.*, 17: 69–82.

Baker, F. H., Grigg, P. and Von Noorden, G. K. (1974) Effects of visual deprivation and strabismus on the response of neurons in the visual cortex of the monkey, including studies on the striate and prestriate cortex in the normal animal. *Brain Res.*, 66: 185–208.

Berger, H. (1900) Experimentell-anatomische Studien über die durch den Mangel optischer Reize veranlassten Entwicklungshemmungen im Occipitallappen des Hundes und der Katze. *Arch. Psychiat. Nervenkr.*, 33: 521–567.

Blakemore, C. and Van Sluyters, R. C. (1974) Reversal of the physiological effects of monocular deprivation in kittens: further evidence for a sensitive period. *J. Physiol. (Lond.)*, 237: 195–216.

Blakemore, C. and Van Sluyters, R. C. (1975) Innate and environmental factors in the development of the kitten's visual cortex. *J. Physiol. (Lond.)*, 248: 663–716.

Blakemore, C., Garey, L. J. and Vital-Durand, F. (1978) The physiological effects of monocular deprivation and their reversal in the monkey's visual cortex. *J. Physiol. (Lond.)*, 283: 223–262.

Crawford, M. L. J., Blake, R., Cool, S. J. and Von Noorden, G. K. (1975) Physiological consequences of unilateral and bilateral eye closure in macaque monkeys: some further observations. *Brain Res.*, 84: 150–154.

Dürsteler, M. R., Garey, L. J. and Movshon, J. A. (1976) Reversal of the morphological effects of monocular deprivation in the kitten's lateral geniculate nucleus. *J. Physiol. (Lond.)*, 261: 189–210.

Garey, L. J. and Powell, T. P. S. (1967) The projection of the lateral geniculate nucleus upon the cortex in the cat. *Proc. roy. Soc. B*, 169: 107–126.

Garey, L. J. and Powell, T. P. S. (1971) An experimental study of the termination of the lateral geniculo-cortical pathway in the cat and monkey. *Proc. roy. Soc. B*, 179: 41–63.

Garey, L. J., Fisken, R. A. and Powell, T. P. S. (1973) Effects of experimental deafferentation on cells in the lateral geniculate nucleus of the cat. *Brain Res.*, 52: 363–369.

Gudden, B. A. (1870) Experimentaluntersuchungen über das periphere und centrale Nervensystem. *Arch. Psychiat. Nervenkr.*, 2: 693–723.

Guillery, R. W. (1972) Binocular competition in the control of geniculate cell growth, *J. comp. Neurol.*, 144: 117–130.

Guillery, R. W. and Stelzner, D. J. (1970) The differential effects of unilateral lid closure upon the monocular and binocular segments of the dorsal lateral geniculate nucleus in the cat. *J. comp. Neurol.*, 139: 413–422.

Headon, M. P. and Powell, T. P. S. (1973) Cellular changes in the lateral geniculate nucleus of infant monkeys after suture of the eyelids. *J. Anat. (Lond.)*, 116: 135–145.

Headon, M. P. and Powell, T. P. S. (1978) The effect of bilateral eye closure upon the lateral geniculate nucleus in infant monkeys. *Brain Res.*, 143: 147–154.

Hubel, D. H. and Wiesel, T. N. (1963) Receptive fields on cells in striate cortex of very young, visually inexperienced kittens. *J. Neurophysiol.*, 26: 994–1002.

Hubel, D. H. and Wiesel, T. N. (1970) The period of susceptibility to the physiological effects of unilateral eye closure in kittens. *J. Physiol. (Lond.)*, 206: 419–436.

Hubel, D. H. and Wiesel, T. N. (1977) Functional architecture of macaque monkey visual cortex. *Proc. roy. Soc. B*, 198: 1–59.

Hubel, D. H., Wiesel, T. N. and LeVay, S. (1977) Plasticity of ocular dominance columns in monkey striate cortex. *Phil. Trans. B*, 278: 377–409.

Merrill, E. G. and Ainsworth, A. (1972) Glass-coated platinum-plated tungsten microelectrodes. *Med. Biol. Engng*, 10: 662–672.

Movshon, J. A. (1976) Reversal of the physiological effects of monocular deprivation in the kitten's visual cortex. *J. Physiol. (Lond.)*, 261: 125–174.

Pettigrew, J. D. (1974) The effect of visual experience on the development of stimulus specificity by kitten cortical neurones. *J. Physiol. (Lond.)*, 237: 49–74.

Rakic, P. (1977) Prenatal development of the visual system in rhesus monkey. *Phil. Trans. B*, 278: 245–260.

Vital-Durand, F., Garey, L. J. and Blakemore, C. (1978) Monocular and binocular deprivation in the monkey: morphological effects and reversibility. *Brain Res.*, 158: 45–64.

Von Noorden, G. K. (1973) Histological studies of the visual system in monkeys with experimental amblyopia. *Invest. Ophthal.*, 12: 727–738.

Wiesel, T. N. and Hubel, D. H. (1963a) Effects of visual deprivation on morphology and physiology of cells in the cat's lateral geniculate body. *J. Neurophysiol.*, 26: 978–993.

Wiesel, T. N. and Hubel, D. H. (1963b) Single-cell responses in striate cortex of kittens deprived of vision in one eye. *J. Neurophysiol.*, 26: 1003–1017.

Wiesel, T. N. and Hubel, D. H. (1974) Ordered arrangement of orientation columns in monkeys lacking visual experience. *J. comp. Neurol.*, 158: 307–318.

Wilson, M. E. and Cragg, B. G. (1967) Projections from the lateral geniculate nucleus in the cat and monkey. *J. Anat. (Lond.)*, 101: 677–692.

Neuronal Mechanisms in Experience Dependent Modification of Visual Cortex Function

W. SINGER

Max-Planck-Institut für Psychiatrie, Kraepelinstr. 2, 8000 Munich 40 (G.F.R.)

INTRODUCTION

In mammals the development of brain functions depends to a substantial degree on epigenetic factors, in particular during early postnatal life. The maturation of numerous sensory and motor functions requires practice and active interaction with the environment (e.g., Held and Bossom, 1961; Held and Bauer, 1974). Severe and often irreversible impairment of sensorimotor performance can be the result of restricted postnatal experience. In search for neuronal correlates of such experience dependent changes in the brain the visual system of mammals has served as the substrate for most of the pioneering studies. Monocular (Wiesel and Hubel, 1963a, b, 1965; Hubel and Wiesel, 1970; Blakemore and Van Sluyters, 1974; Peck and Blakemore, 1975; Maffei and Fiorentini, 1976a; Hoffmann and Sireteanu, 1977) and binocular deprivation (Wiesel and Hubel, 1965; Imbert and Buisseret, 1975; Singer and Tretter, 1976b) of contour vision but also interference with eye position (Hubel and Wiesel, 1965; Ikeda and Wright, 1976; Ikeda et al., 1978) and motility (Maffei and Fiorentini, 1976b) and restriction of the range of visible features (Blakemore and Cooper, 1970; Hirsch and Spinelli, 1970; Pettigrew, 1974; Tretter et al., 1975b) have all been shown to lead to rather specific morphological and/or functional changes in visual centers.

These important observations can be interpreted in two ways: It is conceivable that the functional organization of the visual system is specified in detail right from birth and that adequate visual experience is merely required to maintain the initial functional state. Alternatively it has to be considered that genetic and other intrinsic factors allow only for incomplete development of the visual system, and that further maturation processes require additional information that is only available from visual experience. It is evident from several studies that certain features of the functional organization of the visual system develop independently of experience; if they require sensory practice then only for their consolidation and maintenance. Among such inborn experience independent properties are the basic pattern of connectivity in the retino-cortical pathway (Singer and Tretter, 1976b), some features of the functional architecture of striate cortex such as orientation and ocular dominance columns (Hubel and Wiesel, 1963; Stryker and Sherk, 1975) and the orientation and direction selectivity of a certain class of cortical neurons (Imbert and Buisseret, 1975; Singer and Tretter, 1976b). But there are other properties that seem to develop only when visual experience is available. Such experience dependent acquisitions seem to be the high selectivity for stimulus orientation of most cells outside layer IV (Barlow and Pettigrew, 1971; Imbert and Buisseret, 1975), the shrinkage and sharp delineation of their receptive fields (Singer and Tretter, 1976a), and the increase in the safety factor of synaptic transmission along the retino-cortical pathway (Singer and Tretter, 1976b).

This experience dependent specification of neuronal response properties could be accounted for either by increased efficiency and selectivity of inhibitory pathways or by differential weighting of pre-existing excitatory connections. The experiments described in this paper were designed to test these hypotheses and to further delineate the neuronal mechanisms through which experience, i.e. structured retinal activity, can induce changes in cortical circuitry. Monocular deprivation was chosen as paradigm since it leads to clear and reproducible changes of neuronal response properties.

CAUSES AND SITES OF TRANSMISSION FAILURE IN MONOCULAR DEPRIVATION

After monocular deprivation (MD) the large majority of neurons in striate cortex become dominated by the normal eye and only a small fraction remains excitable by the deprived eye. A number of published observations suggest that this inability of cortical cells to respond to the deprived eye is due to disconnection of deprived afferents from cortical target cells: the cortical territories occupied by afferents from the deprived eye show a marked shrinkage (Hubel et al., 1977) and this retraction of terminal arborizations is associated in turn with shrinkage of relay cells in those layers of the lateral geniculate nucleus (LGN) that are connected to the deprived eye (Wiesel and Hubel, 1963a; Guillery, 1972; Garey and Blakemore, 1976; LeVay and Ferster, 1977; Hoffmann and Hollaender, 1978). Since these drastic morphological changes are not observed in the monocular segment of the LGN nor with binocular deprivation, it has been proposed that they result from competitive interactions between the afferents from the two eyes at their common cortical target cells (Wiesel and Hubel, 1965; Guillery, 1972). In support of a disconnection of thalamo-cortical afferents is also the finding that a particular cell type in the LGN, the transient cells, are less frequently recorded in the deprived laminae (Sherman et al., 1972).

Also the investigation of surface potentials over striate cortex (A17) as well as extra- and intracellularly recorded single unit responses to electrical stimulation of the two optic nerves had suggested that the failure of afferents from the deprived eye to drive cortical neurons was due to decreased excitatory synaptic activity at cortical target cells (Singer, 1977).

The hypothesis of impaired excitatory transmission in the deprived pathways has, however, been challenged by the recent finding that responsiveness to the deprived eye increases instantaneously when activity from the normal eye is blocked (Kratz et al., 1976). It was concluded from this observation that the inability of cortical cells to respond to the deprived eye was to a large extent due to tonic inhibition exerted by the normal eye and not caused by selective inactivation of excitatory connections between deprived afferents and cortical target cells.

For further clarification of this problem we attempted a methodological approach which is complementary to single unit analysis. As shown previously, the current source density analysis of electrically evoked field potentials provides a valuable tool for the investigation of synaptic activity in striate and particularly in parastriate cortex (Mitzdorf and Singer, 1978). It allows to assess the site and amplitude of inward currents generated at excitatory synapses and, thus, reveals the basic pattern of synaptic activity in the various cortical layers as it is induced by synchronous volleys in the specific afferents. Unfortunately, analysis of responses to electrical stimulation of the optic nerves is difficult in cat striate cortex. Reasons are the inhomogeneity in conduction velocity of afferents to striate cortex and the low safety factor of transmission in the slow conducting fibers (Singer and Bedworth, 1973; Singer et al., 1975; Mitzdorf and Singer, 1978). These problems can, however, be overcome in cat parastriate cortex. As shown previously this cortical area is organized in parallel to area 17 (Singer et al., 1975; Tretter et al., 1975b; Singer, 1976a) and its retinal input comes mainly, if not exclusively, from ganglion cells of the transient type (Stone and Dreher, 1973; Tretter et al., 1975a); their axons are homogeneously fast conducting, and synchronous volleys are reliably transmitted through the LGN to A18 (Tretter et al., 1975a; Mitzdorf and Singer, 1978). Because of this methodological advantage we have extended the investigation of monocular deprivation to parastriate cortex. Previous single unit analysis had revealed that also parastriate cortex was susceptible to monocular deprivation (Singer, 1978). With the exception that deprivation effects were less severe in the hemisphere contralateral to the deprived eye, the results were rather similar to those obtained in area 17. It was thus possible to investigate the causes and the site of transmission failure in a substrate providing more favorable conditions for the electrophysiological approach than area 17.

The results obtained from this analysis indicated clearly that monocular deprivation leads to a marked reduction of excitatory synaptic activity in the deprived pathway (Mitzdorf and Singer, 1979b). As exemplified in Fig. 1 already the activity generated by the synapses between thalamic afferents and the monosynaptically driven cortical target cells is substantially reduced. No further impairment of transmission seems to occur beyond this stage along the intracortical pathways. The amplitude reduction of polysynaptic intracortical activity is proportionally the same as the reduction of monosynaptic activity. From previous studies in normal cortex it can be excluded that this reduction of synaptic currents is due to shunting effects caused by concomitant IPSPs (Mitzdorf and Singer, 1978). It can thus be concluded that (1) transmission failure in the deprived pathway occurs at, or prior to, the thalamo-cortical synapses and (2) the decreased responsiveness of cortical neurons is primarily due to a reduction of excitatory input to the monosynaptically driven cortex cells and not caused by tonic inhibition. In the latter case one would expect unimpaired excitatory synaptic activity at the monosynaptically driven cells but reduced polysynaptic responses. These conclusions are in good agreement with results obtained from electrically elicited single unit responses: among the cells still responding to the deprived eye the proportions of mono- and polysynaptic responses to geniculate afferents were the same as for the neurons driven from the open eye (Singer, 1978). This indicates that once thalamic activity from the deprived eye has reached threshold in the cortical target cells it is relayed along polysynaptic pathways without further impairment.

Field potentials recorded from the cortical surface (Singer, 1977) and in particular those recorded from white matter below visual cortex (Mitzdorf and Singer, 1979b) have suggested that transmission failure in the deprived pathway is not restricted to the thalamo-cortical synapses: as shown in Fig. 2 already the earliest potential reflecting activity in the optic radiation is strongly reduced in amplitude when the deprived nerve is stimulated. This is further substantiated by current source density analysis of synaptic activity in the LGN. Among other abnormalities, the synaptic currents produced by the afferents from the deprived eye were consistently smaller than those produced by afferents from the experienced eye (Mitzdorf and Singer, 1979a). These findings led to the unexpected conclusion that monocular deprivation causes impaired synaptic transmission even prior to the sites where afferents from the two eyes converge onto common target cells and are capable of direct

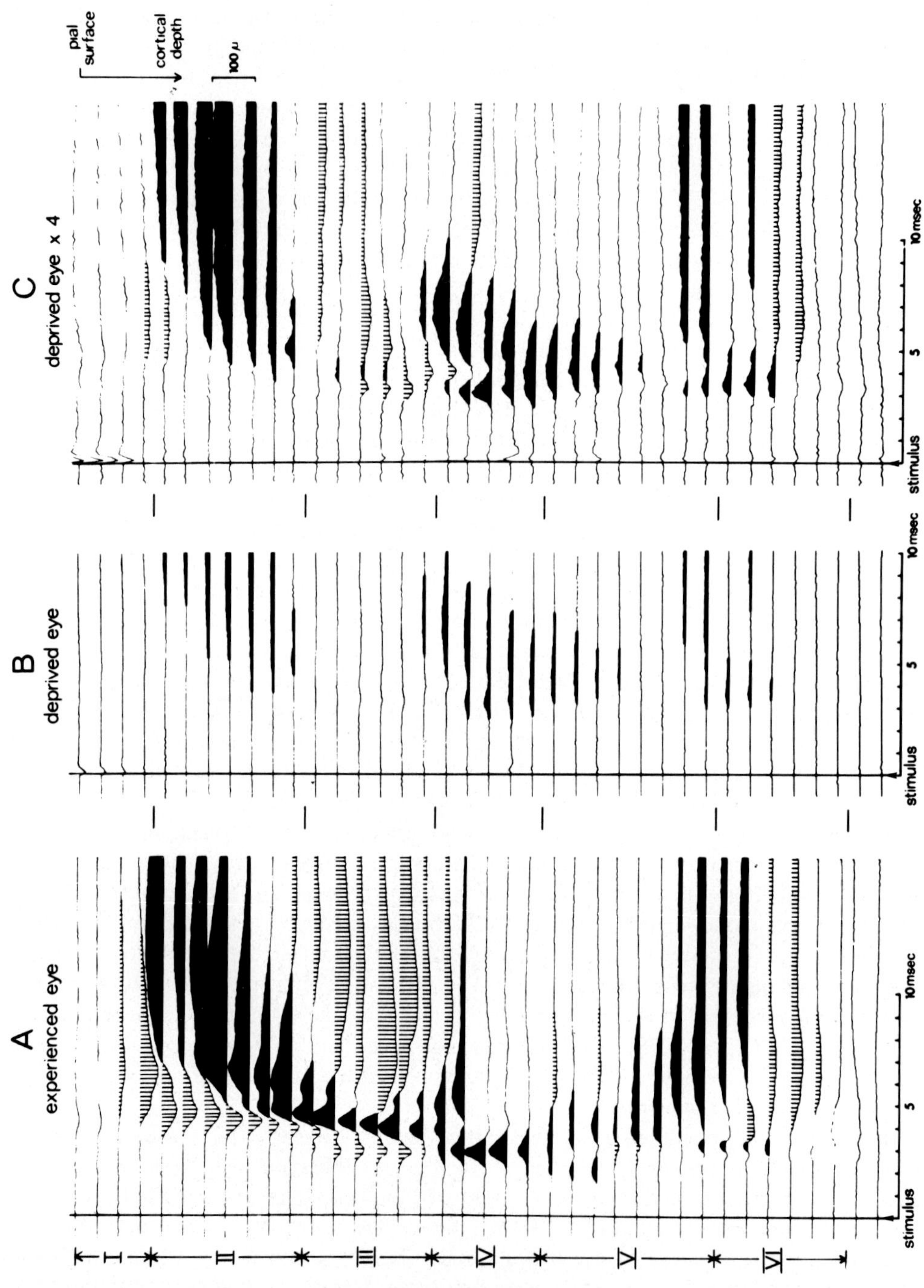

Fig. 1. Current source density (CSD) profiles from parastriate cortex of a monocularly deprived cat. The responses elicited by stimulation of the optic nerves of the normal eye (A) and the deprived eye (B, C). The CSD profiles are calculated from field potentials recorded every 50 μm along penetrations directed orthogonal to the cortical lamination. The respective cortical layers are indicated by numbers I–VI at the left-hand margin. Upward deflections of the CSD traces (sinks) correspond to inward currents at active

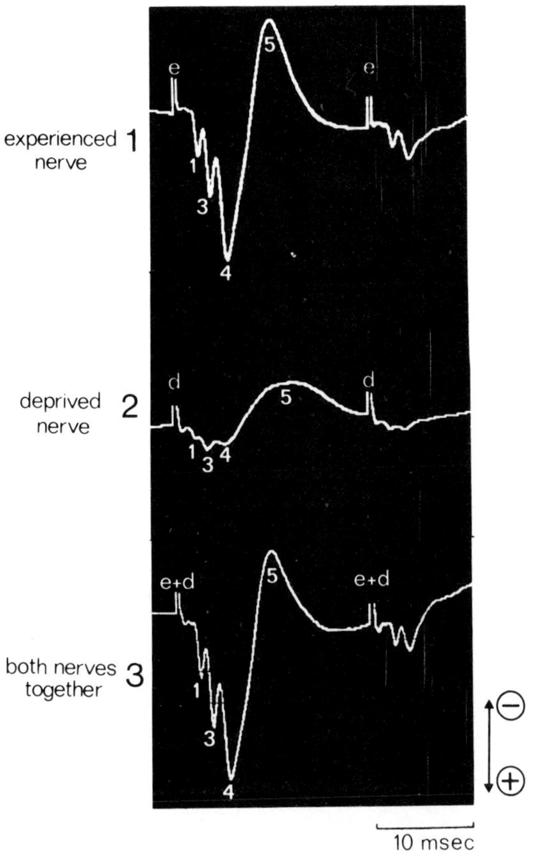

Fig. 2. Evoked potentials recorded from the surface of striate cortex of a monocularly deprived cat after double shock stimulation of the normal nerve (1), the deprived nerve (2) and both nerves together (3). Deflection 1 corresponds to the presynaptic volley in thalamic afferents, deflection 3 to the monosynaptic responses in layer IV, deflection 4 to the disynaptic responses in layer III and the deflection 5 with inverted polarity to trisynaptic activity in supragranular layers. In the response to the deprived nerve, all deflections are markedly reduced in amplitude indicating that already the presynaptic volley in thalamo-cortical afferents is reduced. Deprivation has thus affected transmission of excitatory activity already at the subcortical level.

---

excitatory synapses; the hatched downward deflections (sources) result mainly from loop-closing passive currents. The short latency sinks in layers IV and VI originate from monosynaptic EPSPs, the later sinks in layers IV, III and V are from disynaptic responses and the broad peaks in layer II reflect mainly subthreshold trisynaptic activity. The activity profile induced from the deprived eye (B) was recorded in the same track as the responses in A and has a similar spatio-temporal sink-source distribution but the amplitudes of all sinks, including the monosynaptic responses are considerably smaller. In C the responses to the deprived eye are magnified by a factor of 4: with the exception of the disynaptic sink in layer III, the amplitude relations between the various sinks are identical to those in A. This indicates that intracortical transmission is only little impaired by deprivation. Transmission failure must have occurred at, or prior to, the thalamo-cortical synapses.

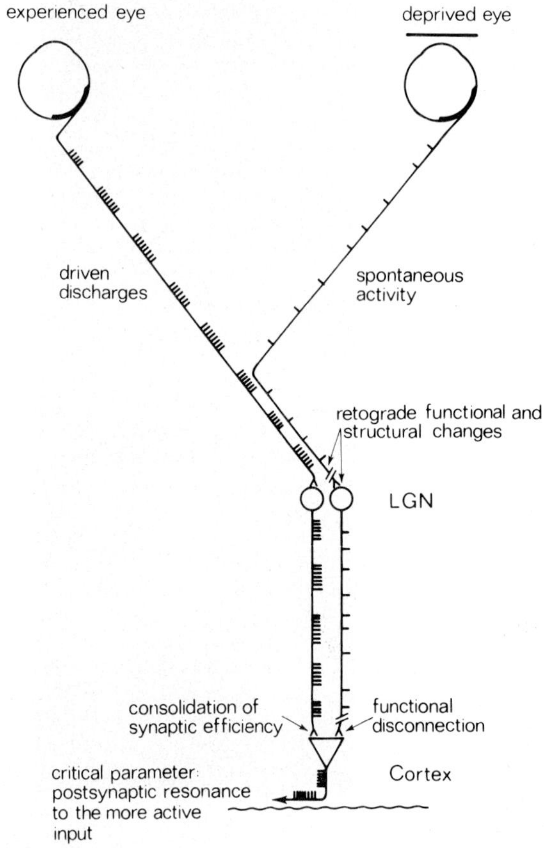

Fig. 3. Schematic representation of afferent pathways and target cells that are involved in circuit changes as they occur with monocular deprivation. Competitive interaction at common cortical target cells leads to functional disconnection of afferents from the deprived eye and to impaired thalamic transmission.

competitive interactions. In Fig. 3 these conditions are summarized in diagrammatic form; they serve as a basis for the following experiments which were designed in search for the mechanisms that gate such activity dependent changes in excitatory transmission.

THE ROLE OF POSTSYNAPTIC RESPONSES FOR INPUT SELECTION AT THALAMO-CORTICAL SYNAPSES

The conclusions reached above provide support for the working hypothesis that experience dependent changes in neuronal response properties are brought about by differential weighting of excitatory connections rather than by modification of inhibitory interactions. If, however, such activity dependent selection among pre-existing excitatory connections was to account also for the specification of functional properties as it occurs during normal postnatal development, a number of predictions can be made about the mechanisms involved. A necessary prerequisite for such selection processes is mechanisms that gate the consolidation and disruption of circuits with respect to the functional adequacy of transmitted activity; this, in turn, requires matching operations between signals in various converging pathways.

This implies that selection among pre-existing circuits must not depend solely on the amount of activity in a particular afferent pathway. The consolidation and disruption of connections should rather be gated by comparison between the presynaptic activity patterns and the respective response properties of the postsynaptic target cells.

An appropriate paradigm in search for such matching operations is again monocular deprivation. By manipulating the activity pattern in afferents from the open eye, it can be determined whether it is a sufficient condition for the suppression of input from the deprived eye that the activities in the afferents from the two eyes differ in amplitude or whether it is required in addition that the activity in the afferents from the open eye matches the response properties of the cortical target cell.

Even in visually inexperienced animals cortical cells respond only little if at all to diffuse brightness changes. In particular the target cells of the thalamic afferents in layer IV show a marked preference for oriented contours already prior to visual experience (unpublished observations). Thus, by monocular stimulation with diffuse light the activity levels in the afferent pathways from the two eyes can be made highly asymmetric but none of the competing afferents will convey activity that matches the response properties of the cortical target cells. As reported recently (Singer et al., 1977) such asymmetry of activity in presynaptic pathways is apparently not sufficient to induce selection among converging afferents. The ocular dominance distribution of cortical cells remains normal even when this asymmetric stimulation is maintained over 200 hr; under conditions of conventional monocular deprivation, by contrast, much shorter exposure has been shown to lead to a complete shift in ocular dominance (Peck and Blakemore, 1975). It thus appears as if postsynaptic responses to one of the converging pathways were required in order to induce suppression of the other.

This result predicted that competitive disconnection of afferents from the deprived eye should occur selectively only at neurons with particular receptive field properties when vision in the open eye is restricted to a narrow range of features: neurons with receptive field properties that match the experienced environment should become dominated by the open eye, whereas neurons with non-corresponding response properties should remain connected to both eyes.

This prediction was tested in two different experiments. In a first series two dark-reared kittens were exposed monocularly to vertically oriented contours. This was achieved by restraining the kittens in the center of a slowly rotating drum whose inner walls were painted with vertically oriented stripes (Singer, 1976b). Total exposure time amounted to at least 60 hr. The results from these two kittens were similar and supporting the notion that afferent activity patterns have to match the neuronal response properties in order to induce circuit changes. Neurons with vertically oriented receptive fields were dominated by the experienced eye; cells with different response properties remained equally well excitable from both eyes or were dominated by the deprived eye. Consequently the orientation preferences of neurons, dominated from either of the two eyes, were complementary (Singer, 1976b, 1979a).

The most likely interpretation of these results is that input selection is gated by a matching operation between inborn response properties and actually available sensory activity. But it is also conceivable that sensory activity has instructed the corresponding response properties in that fraction of cortical cells that happened to be dominated already from birth by the open eye. A prerequisite for such an instruction process would be that numerous target cells of thalamic afferents had still unselective and specifiable receptive field properties when exposure was started. To overcome this ambiguity we have designed a two-stage exposure paradigm which assured that cortical target cells had acquired mature feature selectivity before the afferents from one eye were given competitive advantage. Detailed

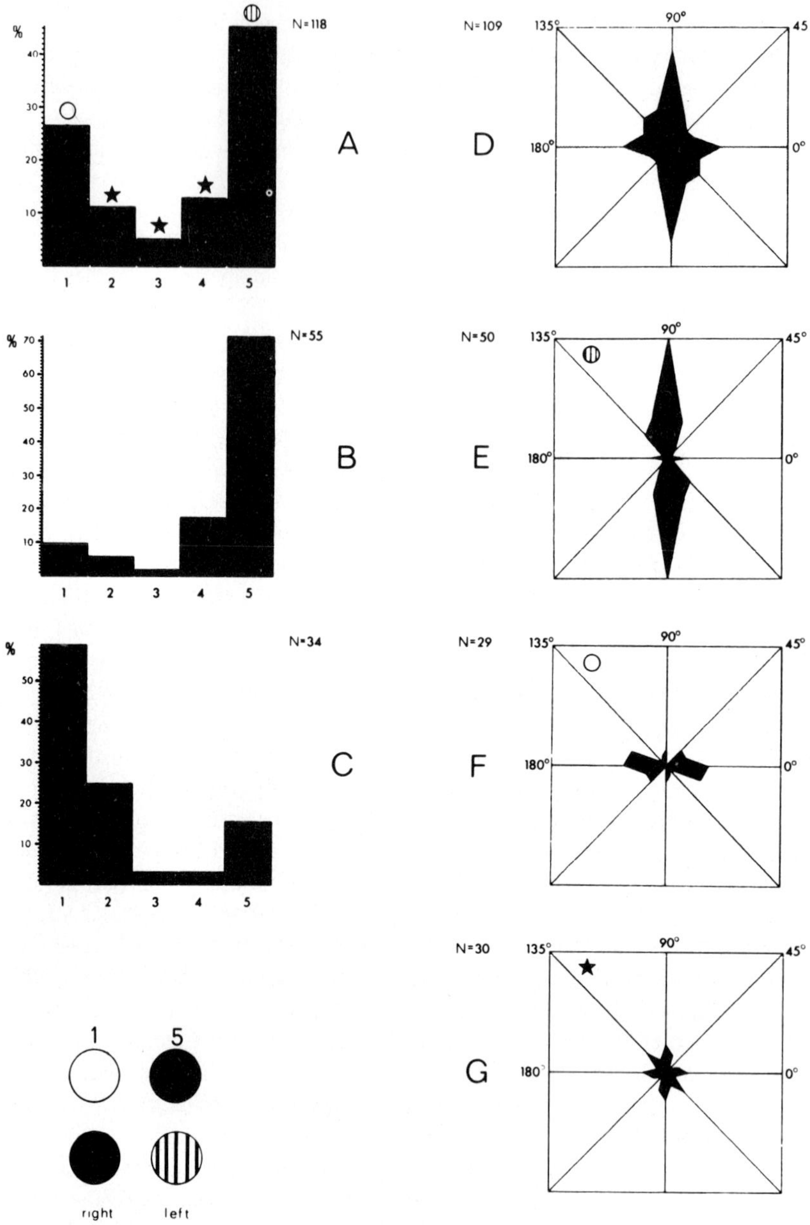

Fig. 4. Ocular dominance distributions (A–C) and polar diagrams of receptive field orientations (D–G) of striate cortex cells in cats with restricted visual experience. The exposure paradigm is indicated schematically below the ocular dominance histograms. The cats were first exposed to normal visual environment for 10 days with the right eye (1) open and the left eye (5) closed. Subsequently the right eye was closed and the left eye exposed selectively to vertically oriented contours. The ocular dominance (OD) histogram in A shows the OD distribution of all cells recorded; the fraction of binocular cells (classes 2–4) is reduced and more cells are driven monocularly by the eye that was open last (class 5) than by the eye that previously had normal experience (class 1). The OD histograms B and C comprise only cells whose receptive field orientation is vertical (± 22°) (B) or horizontal (± 22°) (C). Cells, whose orientation preference matches the orientations experienced during the second stage of exposure (vertical) are dominated by the eye that

description of this experiment is given by Rauschecker and Singer (1979).

Three kittens were dark reared until the age of 38 days and subsequently exposed with one eye closed to a normal environment during 9 consecutive days. Our own control experiments as well as previous studies (Blakemore and Van Sluyters, 1974; Peck and Blakemore, 1975) have shown that by this time most cortical cells have become dominated by the open eye and have acquired normal orientation selectivity. At this age the animals are still within the critical period; thus, the initial shift in ocular dominance can be reversed completely when the previously open eye is closed and the deprived eye opened (Blakemore and Van Sluyters, 1974).

To restrict the range of visible orientations during this second exposure period, a cylindrical lens of –25 dpt was mounted in a polyurethane helmet and this ensemble was fitted on the kitten's head so that the initially deprived eye viewed through the lens. The other, previously open, eye was occluded. Through the cylindrical lens only orientations within $\pm 10°$ off the zero-axis remain visible. Wearing these helmets, the kittens were allowed to freely explore an enriched environment containing contours of high contrast and all orientations. After 10 days of 10 hr exposure daily – during the night the kittens were returned to the dark room – the kittens were again permanently kept in the dark until the experiment.

There was remarkably little interindividual variability in the results obtained from the 3 kittens. As expected after sequential monocular occlusion, the large majority of neurons were monocular and the eye that was open last was slightly more effective. In full agreement with our hypothesis, this eye had regained dominance selectively over those cells whose receptive field properties matched the visible spectrum of orientations. Afferents from the closed eye, in turn, had become ineffective in these cells; they remained, however, efficient in neurons whose orientation preference corresponded to the range of orientations that was invisible during the second stage of exposure. This is exemplified in Fig. 4 with data from a kitten which had experienced only vertical contours during the second stage of exposure. Thus, circuit changes had occurred only for those neurons whose functional predisposition had enabled them to react to the activity from the open eye. As in the one-stage experiment this feature dependent reversal of ocular dominance leads of course to different but complementary distributions of the orientation preferences of cells in different ocular dominance classes.

In conclusion, the results from these two experiments provide strong support for the hypothesis that it is a necessary condition both for the consolidation and the inactivation of converging complementary circuits that the postsynaptic targets are able to get in resonance with the pattern of afferent activity. As shown most clearly in the experiment with reversed occlusion, excitatory transmission cannot only be reduced but also enhanced by appropriate sensory signals. Both processes do, however, require postsynaptic responses as mediators.

---

was open last (5) while cells with preference for orthogonal orientations (C) have remained connected to the eye that was open previously and had experienced normal environment (1). The polar diagram in D shows the distribution of orientation preferences in all recorded cells. It reveals a bias for the restricted range of orientations visible during the second stage of exposure. The polar plots in E, F and G show the orientation distribution as a function of ocular dominance. E comprises only cells driven monocularly from the eye that was open last (OD class 5), F contains cells driven monocularly from the other eye (OD class 1), and G comprises all binocular cells (OD classes 2–4). As expected, the orientation distributions of cells dominated by either the right (1) or the left (5) eye are complementary. These results indicate that the left eye, which was open during the second stage of exposure, had reconnected again only to those cells whose response properties matched the available visual experience (with courtesy of J. Rauschecker).

According to Hebb's (1949) postulate only those connections become facilitated and eventually consolidated that convey activity which matches the response properties of the postsynaptic target cells. Similarly, pathways conveying activity that cannot be matched successfully become disconnected only when the postsynaptic target cells are activated by other converging afferents. When none of the subsets of converging afferents conveys adequate activity, as is the case with diffuse light stimulation and binocular deprivation, there is neither consolidation of certain connections nor selective disruption of others. The only consequence in this case seems to be global impairment of transmission in all converging pathways (Wiesel and Hubel, 1965; Singer and Tretter, 1976b).

The finding that experience dependent modifications in circuitry are obviously gated by matching operations between pre- and postsynaptic activity defines the limits within which experience can be expected to alter functional properties. It is not to be expected that visual experience can instruct functional properties that are not at least in a rudimentary form anticipated by the inborn organization. Sensory signals which are inadequate with respect to the response characteristics of cortical cells will not be able to alter cortical circuits; their effect will be as unspecific as that of complete deprivation. Thus, the role of experience has to be considered as selective rather than instructive.

ARE ADAPTIVE CHANGES IN CIRCUITRY GATED BY CENTRAL EVALUATION OF STIMULUS ADEQUACY?

The conclusions reached above raise the question whether it is a sufficient or only a necessary condition for the induction of circuit changes that the pattern of afferent activity matches the response properties of cortical cells. It is conceivable that it is required in addition that the afferent sensory signals are adequate also with respect to more integral sensorimotor processes. To answer this question dark-reared kittens were monocularly deprived by unilateral lid suture. At the same time the other, open, eye was surgically rotated within the orbit. This intervention leaves the spatio-temporal pattern of retinal responses to contours unaffected and consequently should not interfere with the ability of cortical cells to respond to afferent activity. But eye rotation disturbs the correspondence between retinal coordinates and other sensory and motor maps which leads to severe conflicts in visuomotor integration. In this preparation it is thus possible to determine whether experience dependent changes in cortical circuitry are gated only by matching operations between presynaptic activity and the response properties of the respective postsynaptic target cells or whether the adequacy of sensory signals is evaluated in a more complex behavioral context before sensory activity is enabled to alter local circuitry.

In 5 dark-reared kittens one eye was rotated and the other was closed by lid suture at age 28 days. Subsequently the kittens lived together with their mothers in a normal animal house environment. For the surgical rotation of the eye the conjunctiva was dissected around the eyeball and the extraocular muscles were severed at their insertion to the bulbus. The eyes were then rotated and fixed in the new position by attaching one of the severed distal muscle tendons to the intraorbital conjunctive tissue. This operation resulted in a transient immobilization of the rotated eye. But after a few weeks the eye muscles had apparently reattached and small eye movements reappeared. The degree of rotation was determined from the orientation of retinal vessels on fundus pictures taken before and after the operation and immediately before the neurophysiological experiment. Three of the 5 kittens had their open eyes rotated by 180° and two by 90°. They were recorded from when 6 months old. A number of controls were made to determine whether eye rotation had caused damage to the retina or the optic nerve but none of them provided evidence that such might have occurred (for details see Singer et al., 1979a).

In all kittens visually guided behavior was highly abnormal. During the first weeks after rotation they displayed partially vigorous head nystagmus and circling behavior. As more time elapsed, these behavioral patterns disappeared and a number of tests (forced jumping, obstacle avoidance, visual tracking, visually guided reaching and placing) revealed that the kittens no longer used their open eye for visual orientation. Nevertheless, when alert they kept the rotated eye open. This behavioral abnormality is reflected in the response properties of

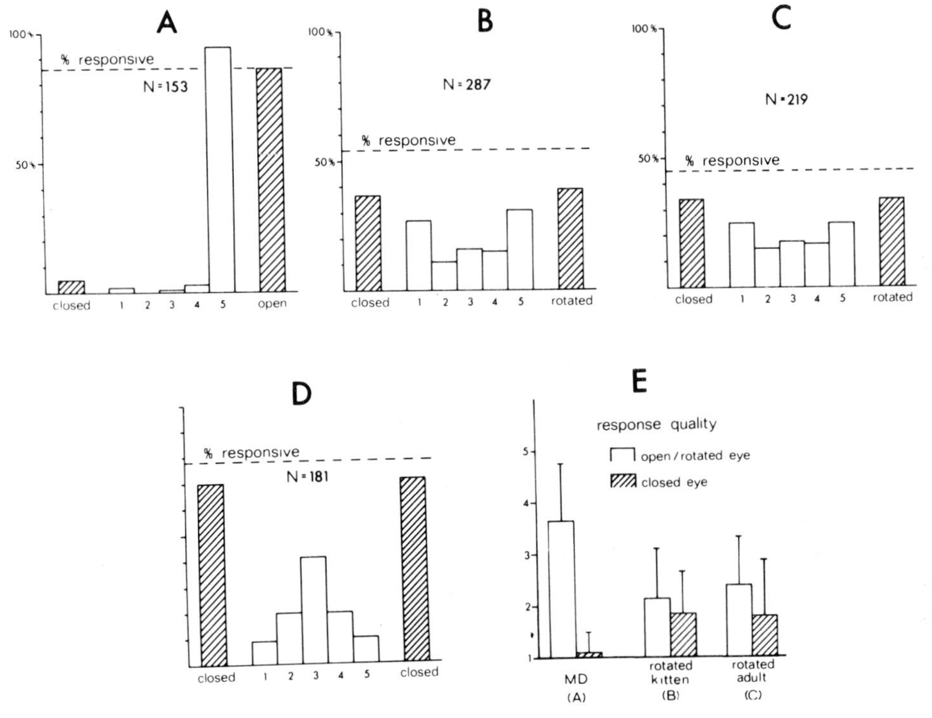

Fig. 5. Ocular dominance (OD) distributions (blank columns), percentages of light reactive cells (interrupted horizontal lines) and percentages of neurons excitable from the right or the left eye (hatched columns) from striate cortex of monocularly deprived animals (A), experimental groups with one eye rotated (B+C) and binocularly deprived cats (D). The OD distributions are calculated in per cent of the light responsive cells; the percentages of cells excitable from either of the two eyes (hatched columns) are calculated from the sum of OD classes 1–4 and 2–5 and refer to the total sample of analyzed cells corresponding to the respective "N" in the graphs. A: data from 2 MDs (6 months old) that were dark-reared till lid closure at age 28 days. B: pooled data from 5 kittens (6 months old) that were dark-reared till age 28 days and then had one eye closed and the other rotated. C: pooled data from 3 adult cats with previously normal vision that were recorded 6 months after lid closure and eye rotation. D: pooled data from 3 binocularly deprived (lid suture) kittens (age 3 months). E: mean response quality of neurons in the experimental groups A, B and C after stimulation of the open or rotated eye (blank columns) and the closed eye (hatched columns). Response quality is estimated from the vigorousness of the responses and rated in classes 1–5 (ordinate), "1" corresponding to a barely detectable response and "5" to the most vigorous reactions encountered in normal cats. The vertical bars indicate the standard deviation. (From Singer et al., 1979a.)

cortical neurons which differed markedly from cats that had undergone normal monocular deprivation (MD). The percentage of cells responding to light stimulation of either eye had markedly decreased. Of the 287 analyzed cells only 54% could be driven with light stimuli. For comparison, in MD cats of similar age (Fig. 5A), clear and vigorous responses could be obtained with hand-held light stimuli in 87% of the recorded neurons. Furthermore, the average quality of light responses of cells still responding was considerably worse than in cats with conventional monocular deprivation (Fig. 5E). The most striking finding was that the open eye had failed to induce the shift in ocular dominance that usually occurs with monocular deprivation (cf., Fig. 5A and B). Of the 156 responsive cells the open rotated eye drove 114 neurons and the deprived eye 108 cells. On average the quality of responses elicitable from the open rotated and the deprived eye was equally poor (Fig. 5E). Although the percentage of binocular cells is markedly reduced when compared to normal cats, it is still surprisingly high (42%) with respect to the fact that these cats had only monocular visual experience.

A significant correlation was found between the neurons' ocular dominance and the vigorousness of their responses. Cells with weak responses had remained binocular or were still dominated by the closed eye. The few neurons (19% of responsive cells) with vigorous reactions to light (quality classes 4 and 5) were predominantly monocular (65%) and 75% of these cells were dominated by the open rotated eye (OD classes 4 and 5).

The symmetrical impairment of the pathways from both eyes and the lack of a clear shift in ocular dominance towards the open eye is also in good agreement with LGN morphology.

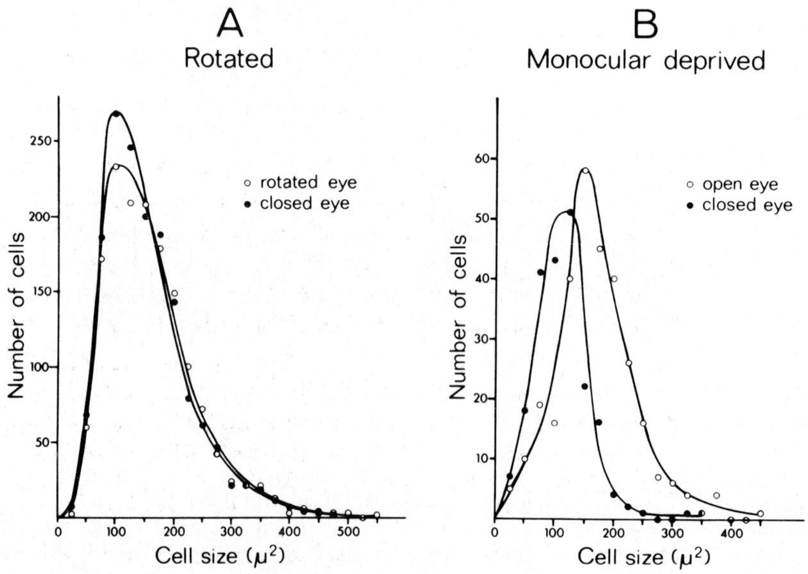

Fig. 6. Distribution of cell size in the lateral geniculate of 3 kittens raised with one eye closed and the open eye rotated (A) and in a kitten raised with conventional monocular deprivation (B). To account for the normal difference in cell size between layers A and A1, the cells from layers A and A1 which are connected to the deprived eye were added together (filled circles) and compared to the sum of cells in layers A and A1 connected to the open rotated eye (open circles). In contrast to the marked difference in cell size between deprived and non-deprived layers in a conventional MD cat (B), there is no significant difference between deprived and non-deprived laminae in cats with the open eye rotated. (From Singer et al., 1979a.)

In contrast to monocularly deprived cats, it proved impossible to tell from inspection of Nissl-stained LGN sections which laminae were connected to the deprived and the rotated eye. Cell shrinkage, if it had occurred at all, must have been similar in the layers connected to the rotated and the closed eye. To substantiate this finding the diameters of LGN cells were measured in Nissl-stained sections according to the method described by Hollaender and Vanegas (1977). Neither the individual data from the two LGNs of the 3 cats analyzed so far nor the pooled data shown in Fig. 6A revealed a significant difference between the cell size in the respective laminae. By contrast, a clear difference in cell diameter was found with identical methods in monocularly deprived control cats (Fig. 6B).

These results clearly indicate that local correspondence between retinal signals and response properties of cortical target cells is not sufficient to induce consolidation and disruption of afferent connections, such as occurs with conventional monocular deprivation. The inadequacy of retinal signals with respect to more integral sensorimotor processes has apparently prevented selective consolidation of afferents from the open eye and competitive suppression of input from the closed eye. Since the normal, non-rotated eye was permanently closed, the inadequacy of afferent retinal signals is detectable only through comparison of retinal signals with other sensory maps or motor commands. This leads to postulate additional gating signals that control consolidation and disruption of local circuits as a function of a more integral evaluation of stimulus adequacy. At present, origin and nature of these postulated gating signals are entirely unknown. The results presented in the next paragraph provide evidence that they might play an important role also in determining the functional state of the mature brain.

INADEQUATE SENSORY SIGNALS DISTORT FUNCTIONS IN THE MATURE NERVOUS SYSTEM

Five cats that had normal visual experience from birth were operated on in the same way as the kittens but only after they were at least 2 years old. One eye was sutured closed and the open eye was rotated by 180° (n = 2) or 90° (n = 3). Survival time between eye rotation and recording was at least 6 months.

The behavioral and electrophysiological investigation of these cats revealed that inverted vision impairs the functional state of visual cortex also beyond the classical critical period. After an initial period of head nystagmus and false orienting responses, the adult cats no longer relied on their open rotated eye for visual orientation. As in the kittens the responsiveness of cortical units to light stimulation was markedly reduced. The percentage of light reactive units and the score of response quality were even lower than in the kittens operated on at the beginning of the critical period (Fig. 5B and C). On average the decrease in responsiveness was equally severe for both eyes (Fig. 5D, hatched columns), although in individual animals either the closed (n = 2) or the rotated eye (n = 3) could be slightly dominant. This is further support for the notion that the decrease in responsiveness cannot be attributed to damage of the rotated nerve; in that case responsiveness to stimulation of the merely closed eye should have remained normal since the lids were only closed well beyond the critical period. Comparison with corresponding data from binocularly deprived animals (Fig. 5E) shows that the reduction of cortical responsiveness is more severe after eye rotation than after complete deprivation of contour vision.

A number of observations suggest that this decrease in responsiveness is not general but selective for cells with particular properties. In the cats operated on as adults there was a

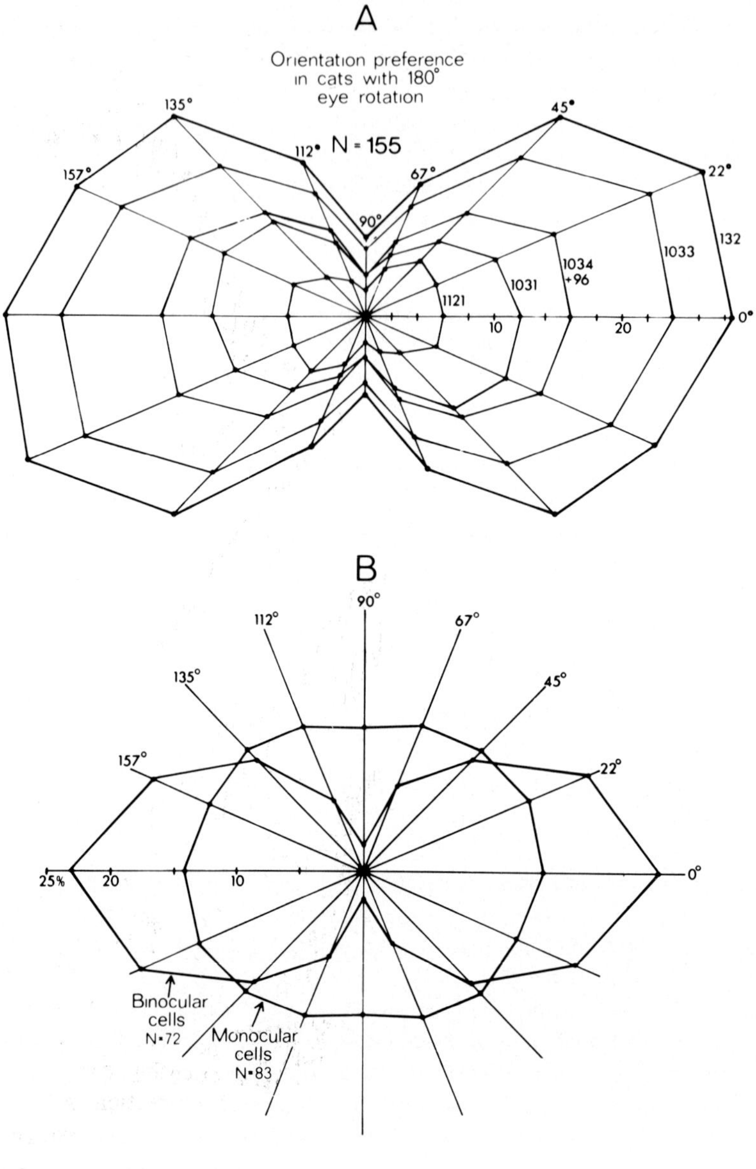

Fig. 7. Polar plots of orientation preferences in cats with inverted (180° rotation of the eye) monocular vision. The polar plots in A are cumulative and calculated from 6 different animals. The 0° radius corresponds to horizontally and the 90° radius to vertically oriented receptive fields. The number of cells with a particular orientation preference is plotted along the 8 different meridians (scale on the 0° meridian). In all animals, cells with orientation preferences close to vertical are markedly underrepresented. The polar plots in B were calculated separately for cells driven from both eyes and for cells driven monocularly from either eye. These distributions indicate that the distortion in the orientation distribution is apparent only in the population of binocular cells. (From Singer et al., 1976b.)

significant reduction of binocular cells; the ocular dominance distributions were flat and clearly different from those in normal cats. As described in detail elsewhere (Singer et al., 1979b) the most surprising observation was, that in cats with 180° eye rotation, both in kittens and adults, cells with vertically oriented receptive fields were remarkably underrepresented. Fig. 7 indicates that this bias in the orientation distribution is seen only in cells receiving binocular input and is absent in the population of cells that are excitable only from either the rotated or the closed eye. In addition to this distortion in the orientation domain also direction selectivity was influenced in the sense that neurons were underrepresented that encode movements towards the vertical meridian. These rather selective effects of inverted vision are further evidence that the observed changes are not due to damage of the rotated nerve. This would have resulted in binocular deprivation and, since it started only well beyond the critical period, should not have influenced cortical functions.

The hypothetical gating signals that have prevented the shift in ocular dominance towards the open rotated eye in the kittens have thus also led to severe alteration in the functional state of previously normal, mature cortex.

DISCUSSION AND CONCLUSIONS

The present results are compatible with the hypothesis that experience dependent changes in neuronal circuitry are based on a selection process among pre-existing excitatory connections. The safety factor of transmission in excitatory pathways can both increase and decrease and these changes in the efficiency of synaptic transmission are gated by a matching operation between presynaptic activity and postsynaptic response properties. Criterion for successful matching seems to be the contingency of pre- and postsynaptic activity.

Nothing is known to date about the mechanisms that could mediate such a comparison between pre- and postsynaptic activity; nor do we know which processes alter the efficiency of synaptic transmission. Nevertheless, the present data allow to define some of the requirements that have to be fulfilled. They are summarized schematically in Fig. 8. The postsynaptic target cell must generate a signal R whenever it is excited and transmitting activity to other cells. This signal must then be made available for a brief period of time to all afferent synaptic contacts. It is then required that those synapses become facilitated which are active while signal R is available while those should become weakened which are inactive while signal R is present. In the absence of signal R the efficiency of all synapses should remain unchanged or perhaps decrease slowly regardless of the state of activity of the respective afferents. We ignore the duration of the time span within which synaptic activity is interpreted as contingent with the postsynaptic response. It cannot be inferred, therefore, whether signal R has to be a fast electrical signal or whether it could be a slower chemical signal as well. The marked changes in cell morphology (Wiesel and Hubel, 1963a; Guillery, 1972; Garey and Blakemore, 1976; LeVay and Ferster, 1977; Hoffmann and Hollaender, 1978) and synaptic transmission (Wiesel and Hubel, 1963a; Mitzdorf and Singer, 1979a) at the level of the LGN suggest, furthermore, that signals are conveyed back to the LGN relay cells about the functional state of their synapses with cortical target cells: functional disconnection at the cortical level leads to shrinkage of the thalamic cells and in turn to reduced synaptic transmission from retinal afferents onto the LGN cells. Again, it is unknown through which communication system these signals are conveyed back to the thalamic relay cells. It could be chemical signals mediated by the retrograde axonal flow. But the message about the functional state of thalamo-cortical synapses could also be transmitted by neuronal activity in the cortico-thalamic feedback loops. Irrespective of the pathways involved in this retrograde signaling it is of interest – in particular for the following consideration – that functional disconnection at the cortical level leads to secondary changes at an earlier stage of the transmission chain.

Most of the phenomena observed in the cats with inverted vision could be accounted for by such retrograde disconnection. As indicated by the schematical drawing in Fig. 9, inverted vision is likely to lead to a mismatch between converging signals in centers that integrate visual information together with other sensory signals and motor commands. Due to eye rotation retinal signals about the direction of image motion will always be in conflict with proprioceptive or corollary signals about eye, head and body movement. It is unlikely that

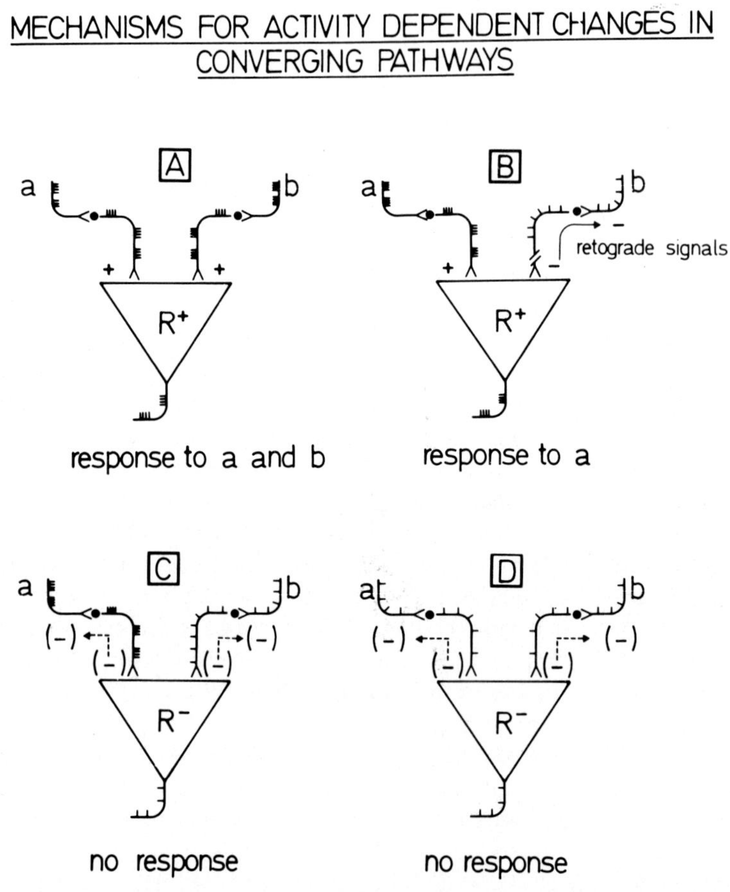

Fig. 8. Summary diagram of local matching operations that gate competitive changes in circuitry as a function of postsynaptic responses (R). In A, both afferents (a and b) are active simultaneously and trigger postsynaptic responses (R). Both converging pathways are consolidated (+). In B only pathway a is successfully driving the postsynaptic target cell: pathway a is consolidated (+) and pathway b disconnected (–). The functional disconnection of pathway b from the target cell results in impaired synaptic transmission also at the preceding synaptic relay. In C, neither pathway triggers postsynaptic responses. In spite of the fact that pathway a is more active than pathway b, both fail to become consolidated. But impairment of synaptic transmission is less severe than in case B. In D, activity levels in pathways a and b are similar and neither is driving the postsynaptic cell. The result is identical to that in D.

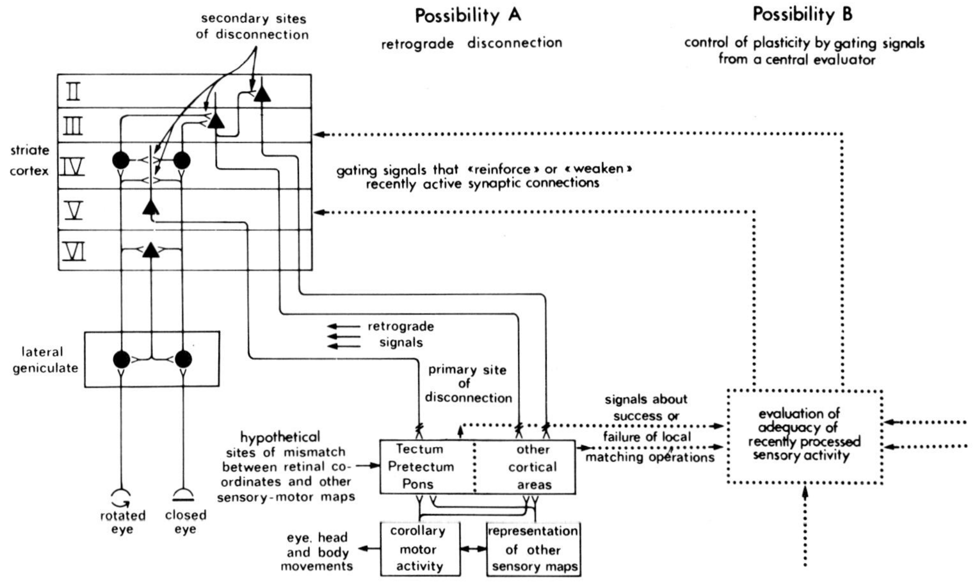

Fig. 9. Schematic representation of the two mechanisms (retrograde disconnection or central gating of neuronal plasticity) that could account for the changes in functional properties as they are induced by inadequate sensory signals. For further details see text.

such polymodal integration occurs at the level of striate cortex, but it can be assumed with great confidence that striate cortex cells convey signals about the localization and the movement of retinal images to such polysensory centers as, e.g., the suprasylvian cortex or subcortical structures in the di- and mesencephalon. In these structures, the conflicting activity conveyed by afferents from striate cortex could lead to functional disconnection of the corticofugal fibers. This disruption could be induced by the same selection through matching operation as that described for the disconnection of thalamo-cortical afferents in the case of monocular deprivation. If such were the case the changes at the level of striate cortex would have to be considered as secondary to the disconnection of cortico-fugal pathways; such a retrograde process would in turn be analogous to changes in the geniculate after disconnection of thalamo-cortical afferents.

This hypothesis predicts that the functional changes at the cortical level should be particularly severe in cells which possess cortico-fugal axons and convey signals about retinal image movements. Although we have not yet identified these projection cells in cats with inverted vision, a number of observations do indeed suggest that these cells are affected most. In the cats operated on as adults it was mainly the cells with symmetrical binocular input that had become unresponsive. Similarly, in both kittens and adults with 180° eye rotation, the distortion in the distribution of orientation and direction preferences were present only in binocular cells. Thus, inadequate retinal signals had affected binocular cells more than monocular cells. There is a trend for cortical output cells, in particular for those projecting to the tectum, to receive symmetrical binocular input while cells at the cortical input stage in layer IV are more often monocular (Palmer and Rosenquist, 1974; Gilbert, 1977). Thus, there is at least some indirect evidence for preferential disconnection of efferent cells.

The hypothesis of activity dependent disconnection of efferent cells could also account for the selective loss of cells with vertically oriented receptive fields in cats with 180° eye rotation. These cells encode retinal image movements along the horizontal plane. With respect to visuomotor coordination image displacements in this plane are distinguished among all others: horizontal eye and head movements are the most frequent and special reflex loops are reserved for horizontal optokinetic and vestibulo-ocular nystagmus. Finally, vergence movements are exclusively performed in the horizontal plane. Although inverted vision leads to mismatch along all meridians, it is conceivable that the most pronounced effects are observed in those subsystems which serve as substrate for the most frequent and most important visuomotor performances. This preponderance of systems involved in the guidance of horizontal eye movements could explain the preferential disconnection of cells which convey signals about horizontal displacements of retinal images.

Retrograde disconnection could account also for the unexpected finding that inverted monocular vision prevents the induction of functional and morphological changes as they normally occur with monocular deprivation. It is conceivable that the retrograde disruptive process, which propagates back to striate cortex, counteracts the facilitation and consolidation of the connections with afferents from the open rotated eye and thereby reduces their competitive advantage over the afferents from the deprived eye. This could explain the low safety factor of transmission in the pathways from either eye and the failure of the afferents from the open eye to inactivate the connections with the deprived eye. The lack of differential cell shrinkage in the LGN would thus be fully accounted for by the absence of competitive disconnection at the cortical level.

The fact that inverted vision in adult cats led to deterioration of previously normal cortical functions, that was at least as severe as the impairment seen after binocular deprivation in kittens, suggests that plasticity of neuronal connections persists well beyond the classical critical period. Within the framework of the hypothesis formulated above this implies (1) that the synapses of corticofugal pathways remain susceptible to competitive disconnection also in adult brains, and (2) that also the retrograde disruptive processes can propagate along previously normal pathways and cause substantial impairment of synaptic transmission. If such were the case the adaptive changes seen with monocular deprivation and squint would have to be considered as a special form of a much more general principle of neuronal plasticity; especially, because it occurs already at a rather peripheral site of sensory processing and because it is restricted to a critical period in early development. This idea does in fact receive some experimental support from recent studies which showed adaptive changes in those brain stem structures of adult cats which control optokinetic and vestibulo-ocular reflexes (Ito et al., 1974; Miles and Fuller, 1974; Melvill Jones, 1977).

Thus, most of the findings reported can be accommodated by assuming (1) local selection processes that are gated by matching operations between converging activity, and (2) retrograde changes that propagate backwards from the site of primary disconnection and impair transmission along the whole chain of afferent neurons. The existence of local matching operations between pre- and postsynaptic activity and the persistence of neuronal plasticity at higher levels of sensorimotor integration in the adult brain are supported rather well by the present experiments. Furthermore, retrograde transneuronal disconnection processes are known to occur quite commonly after lesion in the central nervous system even in adult animals (e.g. Cowey, 1974).

Nevertheless, an alternative to retrograde disconnection should be discussed briefly that could also account at least for some of the results obtained in the cats with inverted vision. It is conceivable that the activity dependent selection processes are in turn controlled by a superimposed gating system. This "master system" would have to have access to information about the adequacy of activity that is or has just been processed. When this activity is identified as adequate and behaviorally relevant the gating system should enable selection of circuits according to the rules of the above described matching operation; if, however, afferent signals are "judged" as inadequate in the context of more integral sensorimotor processing, local activity should be disabled to induce changes in circuitry. Such a superimposed gating system could thus alternatively account for the absence of circuit changes in the kittens with inverted vision. Moreover, such gating could also explain why no selection among converging excitatory pathways occurs when none of these afferents is capable of inducing postsynaptic responses. In that case adequacy of afferent activity cannot be evaluated and consequently the gating system cannot emit the signals that enable circuit changes. The hypothesis that such efferent signals might be required in addition to local activity is supported also by other recent results.

As described elsewhere, we were unable to induce a shift in ocular dominance in anesthetized kittens (Singer, 1979b), although the stimuli applied are known to induce postsynaptic responses. This suggests, that in addition to matching of local activity further requirements have to be fulfilled for the alteration of neuronal connections. Along the same lines are the results obtained by Buisseret et al. (1978); these authors found that contour vision leads to maturation of normal cortical receptive field properties only when the kittens are able to move their eyes. When the kittens are curarized, visual stimulation remains ineffective even though the EEG indicates that the kittens were awake during exposure to visual stimulation. These findings could be accounted for by assuming that neuronal plasticity is gated by intrinsic signals which are only available when the animal is alert and actually "interested" in the afferent sensory activity. Pettigrew and Kasamatsu (1978) have reported that a certain level of extracellular norepinephrine is required to enable activity dependent circuit changes as they occur with monocular deprivation. Although it remains to be seen to which extent this reflects a specific role of norepinephrine in gating neuronal plasticity, this finding indicates that connectivity changes are not solely controlled by local activity.

To account for the findings in the adult cats with inverted vision, one would have to assume, however, that such a superimposed gating system is not only capable of preventing activity dependent changes in circuitry; it would have to have the additional ability to actually disrupt previously consolidated pathways and this disruption would have to be selective for particular pathways. At the present stage it is premature to continue speculation along these lines. Both mechanisms, the retrograde transneuronal disconnection and a supervisor system gating local changes in circuitry, could account for numerous phenomena related to neuronal plasticity in the developing and mature visual system. So far there is no evidence against either of the two concepts and it is very well conceivable that both mechanisms coexist, but the answer to this question requires further experimentation.

REFERENCES

Barlow, H. B. and Pettigrew, J. D. (1971) Lack of specificity of neurones in the visual cortex of young kittens. *J. Physiol. (Lond.)*, 218: 98–100.

Blakemore, C. and Cooper, G. F. (1970) Development of the brain depends on the visual environment. *Nature (Lond.)*, 228: 477–478.

Blakemore, C. and Van Sluyters, R. C. (1974) Reversal of the physiological effects of monocular deprivation in kittens: further evidence for a sensitive period. *J. Physiol. (Lond.)*, 237: 195–216.

Buisseret, P., Gary-Bobo, E. and Imbert, M. (1978) Ocular motility and recovery of orientational properties of visual cortical neurones in dark-reared kittens. *Nature (Lond.)*, 272: 816–817.

Cowey, A. (1974) Atrophy of retinal ganglion cells after removal of striate cortex in a rhesus monkey. *Perception,* 3: 257–260.

Garey, L. J. and Blakemore, C. (1976) Monocular deprivation: morphological effects on different classes of neurons in the lateral geniculate nucleus. *Science,* 195: 414–416.

Gilbert, Ch. D. (1977) Laminar differences in receptive field properties of cells in cat primary visual cortex. *J. Physiol. (Lond.),* 268: 391–421.

Guillery, R. W. (1972) Binocular competition in the control of geniculate cell growth. *J. comp. Neurol.,* 144: 117–127.

Hebb, D. O. (1949) *The Organization of Behaviour.* Wiley, New York.

Held, R. and Bauer, Jr., J. A. (1974) Development of sensorially guided reaching in infant monkeys. *Brain Res.,* 71: 265.

Held, R. and Bossom, J. (1961) Neonatal deprivation and adult rearrangement: complementary techniques for analyzing plastic sensory-motor coordinations. *J. comp. physiol. Psychol.,* 54: 33–37.

Hirsch, H. V. B. and Spinelli, D. N. (1970) Visual experience modifies distribution of horizontally and vertically oriented receptive fields in cats. *Science,* 168: 869–871.

Hoffmann, K. P. and Hollaender, H. (1978) Physiological and morphological changes in cells of the lateral geniculate nucleus of monocularly deprived and reverse-sutured cats. *J. comp. Neurol.,* 177: 145–157.

Hoffmann, K. P. and Sireteanu, R. (1977) Interlaminar differences in the effects of early and late monocular deprivation on the visual acuity of cells in the lateral geniculate nucleus of the cat. *Neurosci. Lett.,* 5: 171–175.

Hollaender, H. and Vanegas, H. (1977) The projection from the lateral geniculate nucleus onto the visual cortex in the cat. A quantitative study with horseradish peroxidase. *J. comp. Neurol.,* 173: 519–536.

Hubel, D. H. and Wiesel, T. N. (1963) Receptive fields of cells in striate cortex of very young, visually inexperienced kittens. *J. Neurophysiol.,* 26: 994–1002.

Hubel, D. H. and Wiesel, T. N. (1965) Binocular interaction in striate cortex of kittens reared with artificial squint. *J. Neurophysiol.,* 28: 1041–1059.

Hubel, D. H. and Wiesel, T. N. (1970) The period of susceptibility to the physiological effects of unilateral eye closure in kittens. *J. Physiol. (Lond.),* 206: 419–436.

Hubel, D. H., Wiesel, T. N. and LeVay, S. (1977) Plasticity of ocular dominance columns in monkey striate cortex. *Phil. Trans. B,* 278: 377–409.

Ikeda, H. and Wright, M. J. (1976) Properties of LGN cells in kittens reared with convergent squint: a neurophysiological demonstration of amblyopia. *Exp. Brain Res.,* 25: 63–77.

Ikeda, H., Tremain, K. E. and Einon, G. (1978) Loss of spatial resolution of lateral geniculate nucleus neurones in kittens raised with convergent squint at different stages in development. *Exp. Brain Res.,* 31: 207–220.

Imbert, M. and Buisseret, P. (1975) Receptive field characteristics and plastic properties of visual cortical cells in kittens reared with or without visual experience. *Exp. Brain Res.,* 22: 25–36.

Ito, M., Shida, T., Yagi, N. and Yamamoto, M. (1974) The cerebellar modification of rabbit's horizontal vestibulo-ocular reflex induced by sustained head rotation combined with visual stimulation. *Proc. Jap. Acad.,* 50: 85–89.

Kratz, K. E., Spear, P. D. and Smith, D. C. (1976) Postcritical period reversal of effects of monocular deprivation on striate cortex cells in the cat. *J. Neurophysiol.,* 39: 501–511.

LeVay, S. and Ferster, D. (1977) Relay cell classes in the lateral geniculate nucleus of the cat and the effects of visual deprivation. *J. comp. Neurol.,* 172: 563–584.

Maffei, L. and Fiorentini, A. (1976a) Monocular deprivation in kittens impairs the spatial resolution of geniculate neurons. *Nature (Lond.),* 264: 754–755.

Maffei, L. and Fiorentini, A. (1976b) Asymmetry of motility of the eyes and change of binocular properties of cortical cells in adult cats. *Brain Res.,* 105: 73–78.

Melvill Jones, G. (1977) Plasticity in the adult vestibulo-ocular reflex arc. *Phil. Trans. B,* 278: 319–334.

Miles, F. A. and Fuller, J. H. (1974) Adaptive plasticity in the vestibulo-ocular responses of the rhesus monkey. *Brain Res.,* 80: 512–516.

Mitzdorf, U. and Singer, W. (1978) Prominent excitatory pathways in the cat visual cortex (A17 and A18): a current source density analysis of electrically evoked potentials. *Exp. Brain Res.,* 33: 371–394.

Mitzdorf, U. and Singer, W. (1979a) Effects of monocular deprivation in the lateral geniculate nucleus of the cat. *J. Physiol. (Lond.),* in press.

Mitzdorf, U. and Singer, W. (1979b) Monocular activation of visual cortex (A17 and A18) in normal and monocularly deprived cats. *J. Physiol. (Lond.)*, in press.

Palmer, L. A. and Rosenquist, A. C. (1974) Visual receptive fields of single striate cortical units projecting to the superior colliculus in the cat. *Brain Res.*, 67: 27–42.

Peck, C. K. and Blakemore, C. (1975) Modification of single neurons in the kitten's visual cortex after brief periods of monocular visual experience. *Exp. Brain Res.*, 22: 57–68.

Pettigrew, J. D. (1974) The effect of visual experience on the development of stimulus specificity by kitten cortical neurons. *J. Physiol. (Lond.)*, 237: 49–74.

Pettigrew, J. D. and Kasamatsu, T. (1978) Local perfusion of norepinephrine maintains visual cortical plasticity. *Nature (Lond.)*, 271: 761.

Rauschecker, J. and Singer, W. (1979) Changes in the circuitry of the kitten visual cortex are gated by postsynaptic activity. *Nature (Lond.)*, in press.

Sherman, S. M., Hoffmann, K. P. and Stone, J. (1972) Loss of a specific cell type from the dorsal lateral geniculate nucleus in visually deprived cats. *J. Neurophysiol.*, 35: 532–541.

Singer, W. (1976a) The functional organization of the cat striate and parastriate cortex: a correlation between receptive field structure and synaptic connectivity. *Exp. Brain Res.*, Suppl. I: 374–379.

Singer, W. (1976b) Modification of orientation and direction selectivity of cortical cells in kittens with monocular vision. *Brain Res.*, 118: 460–468.

Singer, W. (1977) Effects of monocular deprivation on excitatory and inhibitory pathways in cat striate cortex. *Exp. Brain Res.*, 30: 25–41.

Singer, W. (1978) The effect of monocular deprivation on cat parastriate cortex: asymmetry between crossed and uncrossed pathways. *Brain Res.*, 157: 351–355.

Singer, W. (1979a) The role of matching operations between pre- and postsynaptic activity in experience dependent modification of striate cortex functions. In press.

Singer, W. (1979b) Central core control of visual cortex functions. In: *IV. Intensive Study Program.* MIT Press, Cambridge, Mass., in press.

Singer, W. and Bedworth, N. (1973) Inhibitory interaction between x and y units in the cat lateral geniculate nucleus. *Brain Res.*, 49: 291–307.

Singer, W. and Tretter, F. (1976a) Unusually large receptive fields in cats with restricted visual experience. *Exp. Brain Res.*, 26: 171–184.

Singer, W. and Tretter, F. (1976b) Receptive field properties and neuronal connectivity in striate and parastriate cortex of contour-deprived cats. *J. Neurophysiol.*, 39: 613–630.

Singer, W., Cynader, M. and Tretter, F. (1975) On the organization of cat striate cortex: a correlation of receptive field properties with afferent and efferent connections. *J. Neurophysiol.*, 38: 1080–1098.

Singer, W., Rauschecker, J. and Werth, R. (1977) The effect of monocular exposure to temporal contrasts on ocular dominance in kittens. *Brain Res.*, 134: 568–572.

Singer, W., Yinon, U. and Tretter, F. (1979a) Inverted monocular vision prevents ocular dominance shift in kittens and impairs the functional state of visual cortex in adult cats. *Brain Res.*, 164: 294–299.

Singer, W., Tretter, F. and Yinon, K. (1979b) Inverted vision causes selective loss of striate cortex neurons with binocular, vertically oriented receptive fields. *Brain Res.*, in press.

Stone, J. and Dreher, B. (1973) Projection of x- and y-cells of the cat's lateral geniculate nucleus to areas 17 and 18 of visual cortex. *J. Neurophysiol.*, 36: 551–567.

Stryker, M. P. and Sherk, H. (1975) Modification of cortical orientation selectivity in the cat by restricted visual experience: a reexamination. *Science*, 190: 904–905.

Tretter, F., Cynader, M. and Singer, W. (1975a) The cat parastriate cortex, a primary or secondary visual area? *J. Neurophysiol.*, 38: 1099–1113.

Tretter, F., Cynader, M. and Singer, W. (1975b) Modification of direction selectivity of neurons in the visual cortex in kittens. *Brain Res.*, 84: 143–149.

Wiesel, T. N. and Hubel, D. H. (1963a) Effects of visual deprivation on morphology and physiology of cells in the cat's lateral geniculate body. *J. Neurophysiol.*, 26: 978–993.

Wiesel, T. N. and Hubel, D. H. (1963b) Single-cell responses in striate cortex of kittens deprived of vision in one eye. *J. Neurophysiol.*, 26: 1003–1017.

Wiesel, T. N. and Hubel, D. H. (1965) Comparison of the effects of unilateral and bilateral eye closure on cortical unit responses in kittens. *J. Neurophysiol.*, 28: 1029–1040.

Two Types of Brain Plasticity?

G. M. INNOCENTI

Institute of Anatomy, University of Lausanne, Rue du Bugnon 9, CH-1011 Lausanne CHUV (Switzerland)

INTRODUCTION

Fortunately or not, the brain is neither rigidly built during ontogenesis nor rigidly preserved in adulthood. The modifiability of brain structure (plasticity) is usually identified from its final outcomes, mostly deviations of brain connectivity from "normality". However, the initial conditions which allow for those changes are mostly unknown. It is also largely unknown how these initial conditions evolve according to internal (in a broad sense genetic) necessities or to external (epigenetic) contingencies.

An interesting substrate for plastic changes in brain structure was recently discovered in the way callosal connections between visual and somatosensory areas develop postnatally (Innocenti et al., 1977; Caminiti et al., 1978, 1979; Innocenti, 1978; Innocenti and Frost, 1978, 1979). The results of these experiments will be briefly summarized here. They seem to indicate that, besides the changes affecting the distribution of axons and of their terminations, another type of brain plasticity may exist. This involves the temporary occurrence in the developing brain of exuberant populations of projection neurones and their stabilization by extraordinary morphogenetic conditions.

THE ADULT CALLOSAL ZONES IN VISUAL AND SOMATOSENSORY CORTICES

In normal adult cats (Innocenti and Fiore, 1976, and unpublished) after multiple injections of horseradish peroxidase (HRP) into the postlateral and lateral gyri, which fill most of areas 17, 18 (visual areas V1 and V2) and part of area 19, callosal neurones are found in the contralateral V1 and V2, but only in a limited region on each side of the boundary between the two areas. In particular, very few, if any, callosal neurones are found in the medial bank of area 17, and these only near the crest of the postlateral and lateral gyri (Fig. 1). In some animals, however, at the rostralmost end of area 17 they can be found as medially as the fundus of the suprasplenial sulcus. Laterally, in area 18, they commonly extend, as far as the medial bank and sometimes up to the fundus of the lateral and postlateral sulci (Fig. 1). Rostrocaudal and individual differences in the location of this lateral boundary are probably due to the heterogeneity and individual variability of the retinotopic representation in area 18 (Donaldson and Whitteridge, 1977). The restricted tangential distribution (parallel to the pial surface) of callosal neurones contralateral to the injections contrasts with the presence of retrogradely filled neurones in almost the entire mediolateral extent of the lateral geniculate nucleus ipsilateral to the injections. This indicates that HRP was available for uptake over a much larger part of the injected areas 17 and 18 than that over which, in the contralateral cortical field, callosal neurones were found. Radially (normally to the pial surface), the callosal neurones are restricted to the layers 3 and 4; the latter mainly in its upper part and in area 18. A few callosal neurones are found also in layer 6, but they are very rare or absent in layers 1, 2 and 5.

By their radial and tangential locations, the callosal neurones define, within the cortex, an anatomical entity which we call the callosal (efferent) zone (CZ). We believe that this morphological entity corresponds to a functional one. Indeed, the CZ performs the transmission of messages from V1, V2 to the corresponding contralateral cortices. The format of the messages (the set of receptive field properties of the whole population of callosal efferent neurones) is determined by the tangential and radial distributions of the callosal efferent neurones: the distributions determine the morphological type of the neurones, the set of intrinsic and extrinsic afferents that they receive, and hence their receptive field properties. From their radial and tangential locations, in other words, the callosal neurones in areas 17 and 18 derive their characteristically small receptive fields (up to 3° within 8° from area centralis) of either the simple, complex or hypercomplex types but limited to a small portion of the visual field (Choudhoury et al., 1965; Berlucchi et al., 1967; Hubel and Wiesel, 1967; Innocenti and Fiore, 1976, and unpublished) near the vertical meridian of the visual field.

A filtering of the cortical representation of the sensory periphery to some extent similar to that observed in the visual cortex takes place also in the first somatosensory cortex (S1) of the cat (Caminiti et al., 1979). HRP injections in S1 show in contralateral S1 a CZ limited to the trunk representation. Injections in the second somatosensory cortex (S2) show, in contralateral S1 a second, substantial group of callosal neurones in the rostromedial bank of the coronal sulcus, in a region containing a part of the forepaw representation. Thus, in S1, two different partially overlapping CZs exist, each providing the contralateral hemisphere with an incomplete and different replica of the cortical representation of the somatosensory periphery.

There are reasons to believe that the particular relationship between structure and function observed in the CZ is by no means limited to the latter. The neurones of origin of various corticofugal tracts appear, in general, to be radially separated from each other (Gilbert and Kelly, 1975) and, on the other hand, radial changes in receptive field properties of cortical neurones have been described (Gilbert, 1977; Leventhal and Hirsch, 1978). In the visual system, the corticopontine (Sanides et al., 1978) and various association (Zeki, 1978) projections originate from parts of the cortical representation of the retina in V1 differing from each other and from those in which callosal fibres originate. In the somatosensory system, callosal and association (Manzoni et al., 1979) projections originate from different parts of the somatosensory representation in S1. Thus, in general, neurones efferent to the various structures impinged upon by the cortex define efferent zones whose radial and tangential locations differ from each other. The various efferent zones perform different transformations of the cortical representations of the sensory periphery (cf., Innocenti, 1978) and different selections of receptive field properties. In this way, the format of each corticofugal message from a cortical area acquires its unique identity. The next section will deal with how the morphology of the CZ and, therefore, probably the particular format of the message sent through the corpus callosum come about in ontogenesis.

POSTNATAL DEVELOPMENT OF THE CALLOSAL ZONES IN THE VISUAL AND SOMATOSENSORY CORTICES

In both the visual and somatosensory cortices of the cat, the callosal efferent neurones are, at birth, much more widespread than in the adult.

In the visual cortex, during the first postnatal week (Fig. 1), the CZ in areas 17 and 18

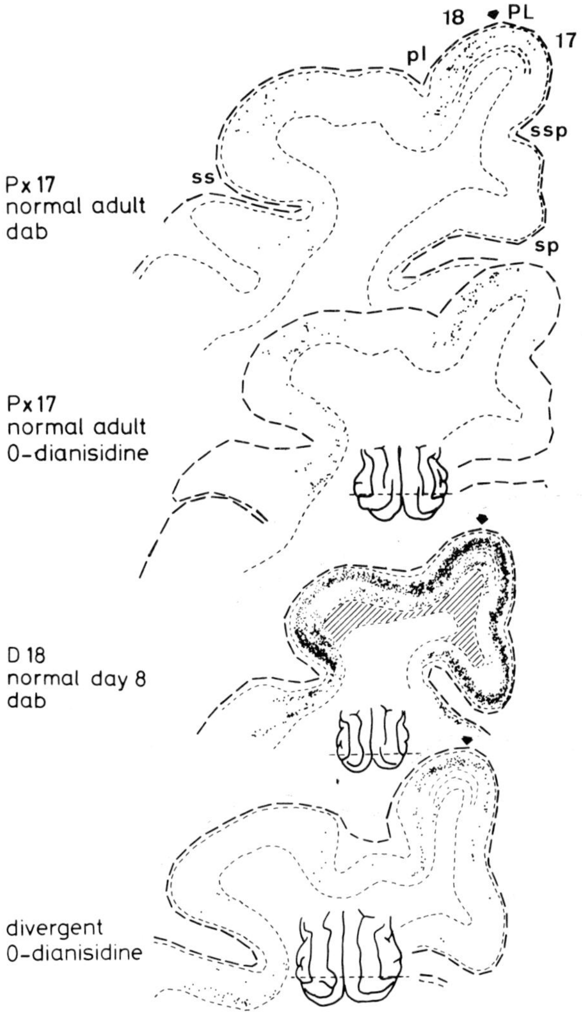

Fig. 1. Computer microscope (Glaser and Van der Loos, 1965) reconstructions of the distribution of HRP-labeled callosal neurones in 80 μm thick coronal sections at comparable rostrocaudal levels in a normal adult cat (Px 17), a cat injected on postnatal day 8 (D 18) and a cat raised with divergent strabismus. The level of sections is indicated in each brain figurine. Two sections 80 μm apart are shown for the normal animal Px 17. They were reacted with different substrates for HRP: diaminobenzidine (dab) and *o*-dianisidine, respectively. In each section, the thin, interrupted line marks the lower boundary of layer 1, 4, 5 and 6. In the Px 17, *o*-dianisidine section only the lower boundary of layer 6 is marked. Dashes in D 18 outline a region of displaced (migrating?) neuronal cell bodies. Abbreviations: ss, suprasylvian; pl, postlateral; ssp, suprasplenial; sp, splenial sulci; PL, postlateral gyrus. The arrow points to the boundary between areas 17 and 18.

differs from the adult in 3 major ways (Innocenti et al., 1977):

(i) The packing density of the callosal neurones is higher. It has not yet been calculated whether this corresponds to a higher total number of callosal neurones at birth or whether it simply reflects the overall crowding of cortical cells due to an incomplete development of the neuropile (Cragg, 1975);

(ii) Near the 17/18 boundary, neurones in layer 6 make a much larger contribution to the callosum. Layer 5 is free of callosal neurones and the CZ in this region appears, at this age, clearly bilaminar.

(iii) The callosal neurones extend throughout the mediolateral extent of areas 17 and 18 and continue without interruption to areas 19, 21 and to the lateral suprasylvian areas.

At the end of the second week (i.e., after about 1 week of visual experience), the number of neurones outside the adult boundaries of the CZ in areas 17 and 18 has decreased (Innocenti, 1978). Quite a few neurones can still be seen in the medial bank of area 17, below the suprasplenial sulcus. Laterally, there are now clear-cut strips of cortex free of callosal neurones between the CZ in area 18 and the CZs in areas 19 or 21, as well as between these and the CZ in the lateral suprasylvian cortex.

At the end of the first postnatal month (Innocenti, 1978) the tangential decrease of the CZ has progressed further. Callosal neurones are found in area 17 only as far as the suprasplenial sulcus although more abundantly than in the adult.

The final tangential distribution of the callosal neurones is acquired during the second and the beginning of the third postnatal month.

In parallel with the tangential diminution of the CZ, the callosal neurones in layer 6 decrease in both packing density and absolute number.

Simultaneously, a similar course of events takes place in the somatosensory cortex (Caminiti et al., 1978). In S1, the CZ for contralateral S2 extends at birth over the entire representation of the periphery and it includes, therefore, the part of the paw representation that is, in the adult, free of callosal neurones. As in the visual cortex, the callosal neurones in layer 6 are more numerous and more densely packed than in the adult. Owing to the lack of neurones in layers 5 and lower 4, the CZ is bilaminar. Gradually, during the first postnatal month the CZ acquires an adult-like morphology.

Thus, it appears that the messages that the visual and somatosensory cortices send through the corpus callosum must be, at birth, very different than in adulthood. However, it is unknown where the fibres of the neonatal callosal neurones terminate and whether they form functioning synapses. The fate of the callosal neurones which disappear during development is also unknown. The next section will report on our first attempts to identify the factors involved in the maturation of the CZ.

PLASTICITY OF THE CALLOSAL ZONE IN AREAS 17 AND 18

A further series of experiments on the visual system (Innocenti and Frost, 1978, 1979) addressed itself to two questions: (i) Does visual information affect the normal shrinkage of the CZ? (ii) Can the neonatal exuberance of the CZ be the substrate for "plastic" modifications of interhemispheric connectivity?

Nine kittens were used: (a) two were deprived of pattern vision in both eyes; (b) two in one eye, by eyelid suture maintained from postnatal day 6–8 (i.e., prior to spontaneous eye opening; day of birth = day 0) onward; (c) convergent strabismus was provoked in 2 animals; (d) divergent strabismus in 2 others, by bilateral sectioning of either both the medial or lateral recti muscles performed on day 6–9; (e) one kitten was monocularly enucleated on day 1.

All these animals were injected with HRP in their visual cortices between 124 and 349 days postnatally. In the monocularly deprived and monocularly enucleated cats the cortex contralateral to the open eye was injected.

In all the animals, as in normal cats, the heaviest packing density of callosal neurones in areas 17 and 18 was found near the 17/18 boundary and gradually decreased away from it.

In the *binocularly deprived animals,* the CZ appeared to have decreased at least to its normal adult size and perhaps slightly further (quantitative analysis of the data is needed on this point). As in normal cats, only very few callosal neurones were found in area 17 medially to the crest of the lateral and postlateral gyri; none as far as the suprasplenial sulcus.

In the strabismic (Fig. 1), monocularly deprived and monocularly enucleated cats the CZ extended further into area 17 than normally. Callosal neurones were found as far as the suprasplenial sulcus or, caudally, where this sulcus does not exist, at comparable distances from the crown of the postlateral gyrus. In one of the divergent strabismic animals and in one of the convergent strabismic ones, a few callosal neurones were found also below the suprasplenial sulcus. Assuming unaltered cortical retinotopicity, the part of visual field in area 17 "seen" through the corpus callosum must have at least doubled in all these animals. The radial location of the callosal neurones seemed not affected, except in the monocularly enucleated cat, in which far more neurones than normal were found in layer 6.

These results indicate that visual experience plays a role in the shaping of callosal connections of the visual cortex. Visual experience seems to be capable of stabilizing juvenile callosal neurones, although with two limitations: (i) None of the conditions of abnormal visual experience succeeded in stabilizing the full-size neonatal CZ. The tangential diminution of the CZ can start and continue (to some extent) in spite of visual experience. (ii) The deprivation of vision achieved by binocular lid suture does not provoke (in the range of survival tested: 128 and 141 days) the disappearance of the callosal neurones, although it may decrease their number.

Thus, other factors (broadly speaking of genetic origin) enter in the shaping of the CZ although they allow some degree of freedom to non-genetic factors.

CONCLUSIONS

The series of experiments reported above lead to an interesting consideration. Brain plasticity seems to have two aspects: on the one hand abnormal distribution of axon terminals in their target structures can take place (afferent plasticity). It can be based on collateral sprouting, rerouting of axons or on the stabilization of transitorily widespread axonal terminations at early developmental stages (Schneider, 1973; Frost and Schneider, 1976; Rakic, 1976, 1977; Hubel et al., 1977; Raisman, 1977). This kind of plasticity can still occur, to some extent, in the adult brain.

On the other hand, deviations from the normal selection of projection neurones from transitorily exuberant populations can occur (efferent plasticity). In the cortex, they result in abnormal (i.e., for size, location, distribution of neurones) efferent zones possibly accompanied by changes in the terminal territories to which the normal efferent zones would have projected. This kind of plasticity is limited to the immature brain.

As it is shown schematically in Fig. 2, when the connection between two structures is considered, afferent (Fig. 2B) and efferent (Fig. 2C and D) plasticity appear to have different

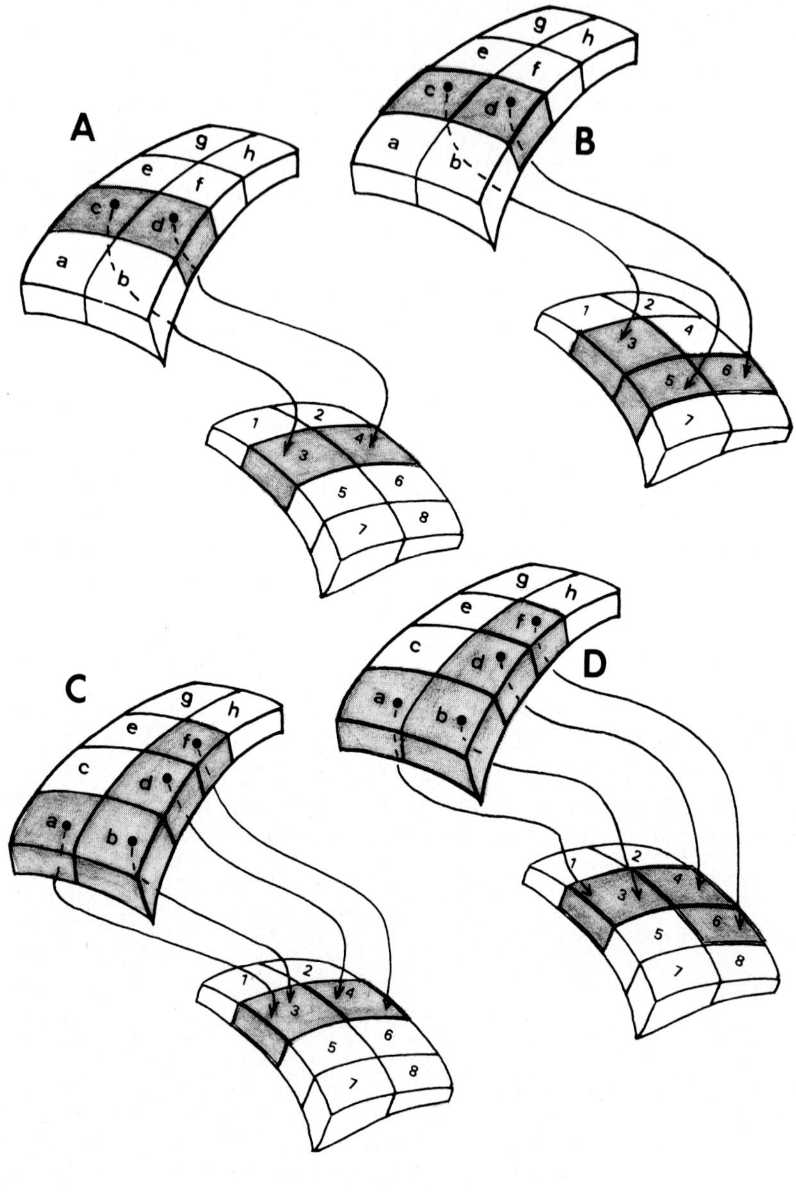

Fig. 2. Different aspects of plasticity. A: normal; a nervous structure containing a functional map (i.e. representation of the sensory or motor periphery, or of differences in receptive field properties of neurones) projects from a limited efferent zone to another structure. B: afferent plasticity; shift or sprouting (or failure in withdrawing) of terminal axons has occurred. A normal efferent zone now relates a message of a normal format to a partially shifted and enlarged terminal territory. C and D: efferent plasticity; the efferent zone has enlarged because of partial stabilization of a juvenile state. The efferent message acquires a new format and it is received by either the normal terminal territory or by an enlarged one.

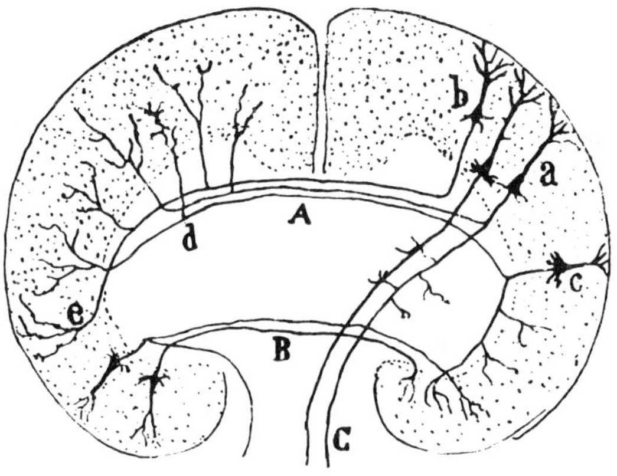

Fig. 3. "Likely" disposition of commissural and projection fibres in the rat. Taken from Fig. 15 of Cajal (1894). A, corpus callosum; B, anterior commissure; C, pyramidal tract (projection fibres). In the text, Cajal describes, at least partially from observations with the silver chromate method on newborn rats, two interesting characteristics of the callosal system: (i) some callosal fibres appear to terminate with widely distributed axonal ramification in contralateral cortex (i.e., e and d); (ii) a number of association and projection axons give off a collateral to the corpus callosum.

consequences. The first can redistribute the messages that a structure sends out, although the format of the messages is not affected. The second can change the format of the messages.

To what extent are efferent and efferent plasticity separable events? The distinction between the two appears to require in a number of cases informations about the connectivity and the fate of the juvenile neurones. For instance, while very appealing as an example of efferent plasticity based on the stabilization of neurones which would have otherwise died, the enlargement of the CZ provoked by abnormal visual experience can still, at this stage, be interpreted otherwise. The callosal neurones which were stabilized outside the normal boundaries of the CZ could have had during development, beside the callosal axon, a second, main axonal branch (cf., Fig. 3; Cajal, 1894). This would have allowed the neurones to survive in spite of the loss of the callosal axons. In this case the enlargement of the CZ provoked by abnormal visual experience would be the secondary effect of a rather new and bizarre, extreme case of (depending on the fate of the non-callosal axon) either rerouting of axons or of stabilization of transitorily widespread axonal arbors. In most of the situations in which deviations from normal connectivity have resulted from experimental manipulations during ontogenesis, the type of plasticity involved remains to be clarified. For instance, either afferent or efferent plasticity could explain the dramatic preservations of function and of thalamic morphology after embryonic lesions of the frontal lobes in the monkey (Goldman and Galkin, 1978).

SUMMARY

In both the visual and somatosensory systems, the set of connections established through the corpus callosum shows one main feature: the neurones of origin of the corpus callosum (callosal neurones) are unevenly distributed within limited portions (callosal zones) of the main visual (V1, V2) and somatosensory (S1) representations. The main consequence of this distribution is that, in the messages that sensory areas send through the corpus callosum the cortical sensory maps are incomplete. At birth, in the cat, the callosal neurones are ubiquitous in V1, V2, S1. The adult distribution is reached postnatally through gradual, selective disappearance of callosal neurones. In order to define the nature of this phenomenon we have studied with anatomical techniques the effects of visual deprivation of various kinds on the development of the callosal zone in V1, V2. It appears that visual experience can stabilize the juvenile callosal neurones. These results suggest the existence of modifications of the efferent neuronal populations (efferent plasticity), possibly different from the modifications which involve changes in the axonal terminations (afferent plasticity).

ACKNOWLEDGEMENTS

I am very grateful to P. Clarke, D. Frost and H. Van der Loos for their merciless criticisms. The drawing from Cajal was given to me by H.V.d.L.

Supported by the Swiss National Science Foundation (3.492.0.75).

REFERENCES

Berlucchi, G., Gazzaniga, M. S. and Rizzolatti, G. (1967) Microelectrode analysis of transfer of visual information by the corpus callosum. *Arch. ital. Biol.*, 105: 583–596.

Cajal, S. Ramón y (1894) *Les Nouvelles Idées sur la Structure du Système Nerveux chez l'Homme et chez les Vertébrés.* Reinwald, Paris.

Caminiti, R., Barbaresi, P. and Innocenti, G. M. (1978) Callosal neurones in SI and SII of the kitten. *Neurosci. Lett.*, Suppl. 1: S342.

Caminiti, R., Innocenti, G. M. and Manzoni, T. (1979) The anatomical substrate of callosal messages from SI and SII in the cat. *Exp. Brain Res.*, 35: 295–314.

Choudhury, B. P., Whitteridge, D. and Wilson, M. E. (1965) The function of the callosal connections of the visual cortex. *Quart. J. exp. Physiol.*, 50: 214–219.

Cragg, B. G. (1975) The development of synapses in the visual system of the cat. *J. comp. Neurol.*, 160: 147–166.

Donaldson, I. M. L. and Whitteridge, D. (1977) The nature of the boundary between cortical visual areas II and III in the cat. *Proc. roy. Soc. B*, 199: 445–462.

Frost, D. O. and Schneider, G. E. (1976) Normal and abnormal uncrossed retinal projections in Syrian hamsters as demonstrated by Fink-Heimer and autoradiographic techniques. *Neurosci. Abstr.*, 2: 812.

Gilbert, C. D. (1977) Laminar differences in receptive field properties of cells in cat primary visual cortex. *J. Physiol. (Lond.)*, 268: 391–421.

Gilbert, C. D. and Kelly, J. P. (1975) The projection of cells in different layers of the cat's visual cortex. *J. comp. Neurol.*, 163: 81–106.

Glaser, E. M. and Van der Loos, H. (1965) A semi-automatic computer-microscope for the analysis of neuronal morphology. *IEEE Trans. bio-med. Engng*, BME-12: 22–31.

Goldman, P. S. and Galkin, T. W. (1978) Prenatal removal of frontal association cortex in the fetal rhesus monkey: anatomical and functional consequences in postnatal life. *Brain Res.*, 152:451–485.

Hubel, D. H. and Wiesel, T. N. (1967) Cortical and callosal connections concerned with the vertical meridian of visual fields in the cat. *J. Neurophysiol.*, 30: 1561–1573.

Hubel, D. H., Wiesel, T. N. and LeVay, S. (1977) Plasticity of ocular dominance columns in monkey striate cortex. *Phil. Trans. B*, 278: 377–409.

Innocenti, G. M. (1978) Postnatal development of interhemispheric connections of the visual cortex. In: *Maturation, Plasticity and Degeneration in the Visual System. Arch. ital. Biol.*, 116: 463–470.

Innocenti, G. M. and Fiore, L. (1976) Morphological correlates of visual field transformation in the corpus callosum. *Neurosci. Lett.*, 2: 245–252.

Innocenti, G. M. and Frost, D. O. (1978) Visual experience and the development of the efferent system to the corpus callosum. *Neurosci. Abstr.*, 4: 1513.

Innocenti, G. M. and Frost, D. O. (1979) Effects of visual experience on the maturation of the efferent system to the corpus callosum. *Nature (Lond.)*, in press.

Innocenti, G. M., Fiore, L. and Caminiti, R. (1977) Exuberant projection into the corpus callosum from the visual cortex of newborn cats. *Neurosci. Lett.*, 4: 237–242.

Leventhal, A. G. and Hirsch, H. V. B. (1978) Receptive-field properties of neurons in different laminae of visual cortex of the cat. *J. Neurophysiol.*, 41: 948–962.

Manzoni, T., Caminiti, R., Spidalieri, G. and Morelli, E. (1979) Anatomical and functional aspects of the associative SI-SII connections. *Exp. Brain Res.*, 34: 453–470.

Raisman, G. (1977) What hope for repair of the brain? *Ann. Neurol.*, 3: 101–106.

Rakic, P. (1976) Prenatal genesis of connections subserving ocular dominance in the rhesus monkey. *Nature (Lond.)*, 261: 467–471.

Rakic, P. (1977) Effect of prenatal unilateral eye enucleation on the formation of layers and retinal connections in the dorsal lateral geniculate nucleus (LGd) of the rhesus monkey. *Neurosci. Abstr.*, 3: 1831.

Sanides, D., Fries, W. and Albus, K. (1978) The corticopontine projection from the visual cortex of the cat: an autoradiographic investigation. *J. comp. Neurol.*, 179: 77–88.

Schneider, G. E. (1973) Early lesions of superior colliculus: factors affecting the formation of abnormal retinal projections. *Brain Behav. Evol.*, 8: 73–109.

Zeki, S. M. (1978) The cortical projections of foveal striate cortex in the rhesus monkey. *J. Physiol. (Lond.)*, 277: 227–244.

Transmitter-Specific Retrograde Tracing of Pathways?

P. STREIT, J. C. REUBI, M. WOLFENSBERGER, H. HENKE and M. CUÉNOD

Brain Research Institute, University of Zurich, Zurich (Switzerland)

The transmitter-related chemospecificity of neurons can be determined by means of a multidisciplinary approach combining a variety of electrophysiological, pharmacological, biochemical and histochemical methods. In the present contribution the phenomenon of transmitter-specific retrograde perikaryal labeling is discussed – proposing its use as a new histochemical method, which indicates both the connectivity and the transmitter of labeled neurons. This method is based on specific terminal uptake of labeled transmitter, on retrograde axonal migration and on perikaryal accumulation and retention of labeled material.

Transmitter-specific retrograde tracing will first be described in some detail in a partly glycinergic pathway of the pigeon visual system; additional results obtained in the rat in connection with known GABA-, serotonin- or dopamine-mediated transmission will be discussed.

PIGEON OPTIC LOBE

After topical application of [^{3}H]glycine in the caudal part of the pigeon optic tectum neural perikarya in a restricted area of the subtectal nucleus isthmi, pars parvocellularis (Ipc) are covered by autoradiographic silver grains with survival times ranging from 30 min to 24 hr (Fig. 1a) (Hunt et al., 1977). The labeled perikarya form a small radially arranged column in Ipc about 4 mm from the center of the injection site. The reciprocal connection between the tectum and Ipc is topographically organized (Cajal, 1899; Hunt and Künzle, 1976a; Hunt et al., 1977; Cuénod and Streit, 1979).

There are 3 possibilities to explain this perikaryal labeling: (i) local uptake from a diffusion gradient spreading from the injection site, (ii) anterograde transport in the reciprocal tecto-isthmic projection and subsequent transneuronal transfer of radioactivity to Ipc neurons, and (iii) retrograde labeling in the isthmo-tectal pathway. The first possibility can be excluded because the localization and the restricted columnar arrangement of labeled perikarya fit the topography of the reciprocal Ipc-tectal connection but not the diffusion gradient. After small injections of horseradish peroxidase (HRP) into the tectum a very similar columnar arrangement of retrogradely labeled cell bodies is observed in Ipc; Golgi-like HRP labeling demonstrates the multipolar nature of Ipc neurons, which spread their dendrites radially into the vicinity (Streit, unpublished observations). High resolution autoradiography on material from animals perfused with glutaraldehyde 30 min after the onset of the [^{3}H]glycine injection (0.05–0.2 μl [2-^{3}H]glycine, 20 μCi, 3.8 Ci/mmol, Radiochemical Centre, Amersham) shows a column of heavily labeled perikarya in Ipc confirming the results of Hunt et al. (1977) (Figs. 1a and 2A). These perikarya are surrounded in a restricted area by cross-sectioned dendrites – the most abundant labeled element in electron microscopic autoradiographs of Ipc (Fig. 2B). Some labeled profiles can be identified as initial axon segments. Labeled axon terminals which might belong to the tecto-isthmic pathway are rare and only exceptionally found on a labeled postsynaptic structure. These observations provide strong arguments against transneuronal and for retrograde labeling via intraaxonal migration of radioactivity in Ipc neurons projecting to the tectum (Streit et al., 1980). Golgi-like tectal labeling after HRP injection into Ipc shows both the superficial termination in boutons en passage of the isthmo-tectal pathway and the deep origin of the tecto-isthmic projection (Hunt et al., 1977; Cuénod and Streit, 1979). This differential arrangement can be utilized for lamina labeling experiments (Hunt et al., 1977). Even after prolonged survival times (26 hr) [^{3}H]glycine administration in the depth of the tectum leads only to neuropile labeling in Ipc. Thus, radioactivity transported anterogradely in the tecto-isthmic projection is not transferred transneuronally in sufficient amounts to label Ipc perikarya. Thirty minutes after the application of [^{3}H]glycine on the tectal surface, however, perikaryal labeling is observed indicating terminal uptake of [^{3}H]glycine, followed by retrograde axonal migration and perikaryal accumulation of labeled material. No neuronal cell bodies are labeled in other tectal afferents or efferents. The speed of the retrograde migration (about 10 mm/hr) hardly fits passive intracellular diffusion, but active axonal transport is not yet demonstrated. Little is known about the chemical nature of the migrating labeled material. Fixation experiments suggest that it is a small molecule (Cuénod and Streit, 1979), because most of the label is lost after formaldehyde perfusion, which is known to retain (mainly) macromolecules but, e.g., to wash out most free amino acids (Price et al., 1978). Is the isthmo-tectal pathway glycinergic? Exogenous radioactive glycine is released upon electrical stimulation of Ipc into the perfusate of a push-pull cannula placed in the tectum (Reubi and Cuénod, 1976). The stimulation evoked release of endogenous glycine into the perfusate analyzed by combined gas chromatography and mass fragmentography (Wolfensberger et al., 1979) provides strong evidence for the glycinergic nature of at least part of the isthmo-tectal pathway. It cannot be excluded, however, that glycine is released transsynaptically, nor that glycine is a metabolite of another related substance. There exists additional electrophysiological and biochemical evidence for a role of glycine as transmitter in the optic tectum. Strychnine-sensitive glycine induced inhibition is found in a large number of tectal units (Barth and Felix, 1974). Glycine-specific strychnine binding indicates glycine receptors in membranes prepared from chick (Zukin et al., 1975) and pigeon optic tectum (Le Fort et al., 1978). Tectal synaptosomes have a high affinity uptake system for glycine (Henke et al., 1976; Henke and Cuénod, 1978). Thus, if one accepts the evidence presented that Ipc-tectal fibers use glycine as transmitter, their selective retrograde labeling after tectal injection of [^{3}H]glycine would be transmitter-specific.

Inhibition experiments suggest two compartments of the glycine high affinity uptake system: one for glycine only and a second mixed one accessible to both serine and α-alanine too (Henke and Cuénod, 1978). It is tempting to relate these observations to the fact that perikaryal labeling in Ipc is found also after tectal injection of [^{3}H]serine and [^{3}H]α-alanine (Hunt et al., 1977). It is at present unclear whether these findings indicate a certain nonspecificity of the uptake system or several neuronal populations with different specificities and possibly different transmitters. The same is true for the perikaryal labeling in Ipc obtained

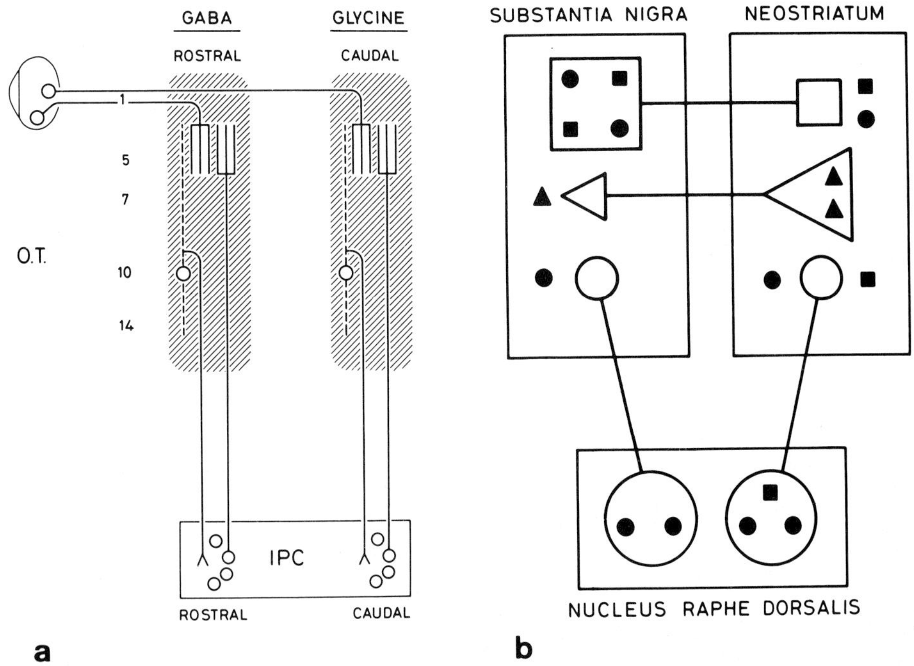

Fig. 1. Schematic representation of experiments in which retrograde labeling was obtained after application of tritiated transmitter substances in the terminal area of the following pathways: a: the projection of the nucleus isthmi, pars parvocellularis (IPC) upon the optic tectum (O.T.) of the pigeon; b: the striato-nigral, nigro-striatal, raphe-striatal and raphe-nigral connections in the rat. Labeling observed after application of [^{3}H]serotonin (circle), [^{3}H]dopamine (square) or [^{3}H]GABA (triangle).

after injection of [^{3}H]choline. No perikaryal labeling is observed after application of [^{3}H]GABA and 8 other amino acids in the *caudal* tectum showing a certain degree of chemospecificity of the system. Following [^{3}H]GABA but not [^{3}H]glycine administration in the *rostral* tectum, however, some labeled cell bodies are seen in the topographically related part of Ipc (Fig. 1a) (Hunt and Künzle, 1976b; Hunt et al., 1977). Although histologically uniform, Ipc seems to contain neuronal populations with regionally different chemospecificities, as judged by retrograde labeling.

RAT NEO-STRIATUM, SUBSTANTIA NIGRA AND RAPHE NUCLEUS

Can the phenomenon of transmitter-specific retrograde perikaryal labeling be generalized to other pathways? Is it found, e.g., in the rat striato-nigral, raphe-nigral, nigro-striatal or raphe-striatal projections (Fig. 1b) (Streit, 1980)? GABA- (and substance P-) mediated transmission is known for the striato-nigral pathway (Kim et al., 1971; Fonnum et al., 1974; Kataoka et al., 1974; Kanazawa et al., 1977; Mroz et al., 1977). The raphe-nigral and the raphe-striatal projections are serotoninergic (Brodal et al., 1960; Kanazawa et al., 1976; Taber-Pierce et al., 1976; Dray et al., 1978; Reubi and Emson, 1978), whereas the nigro-striatal pathway is dopaminergic (Falck et al., 1962; Lindvall and Björklund, 1974).

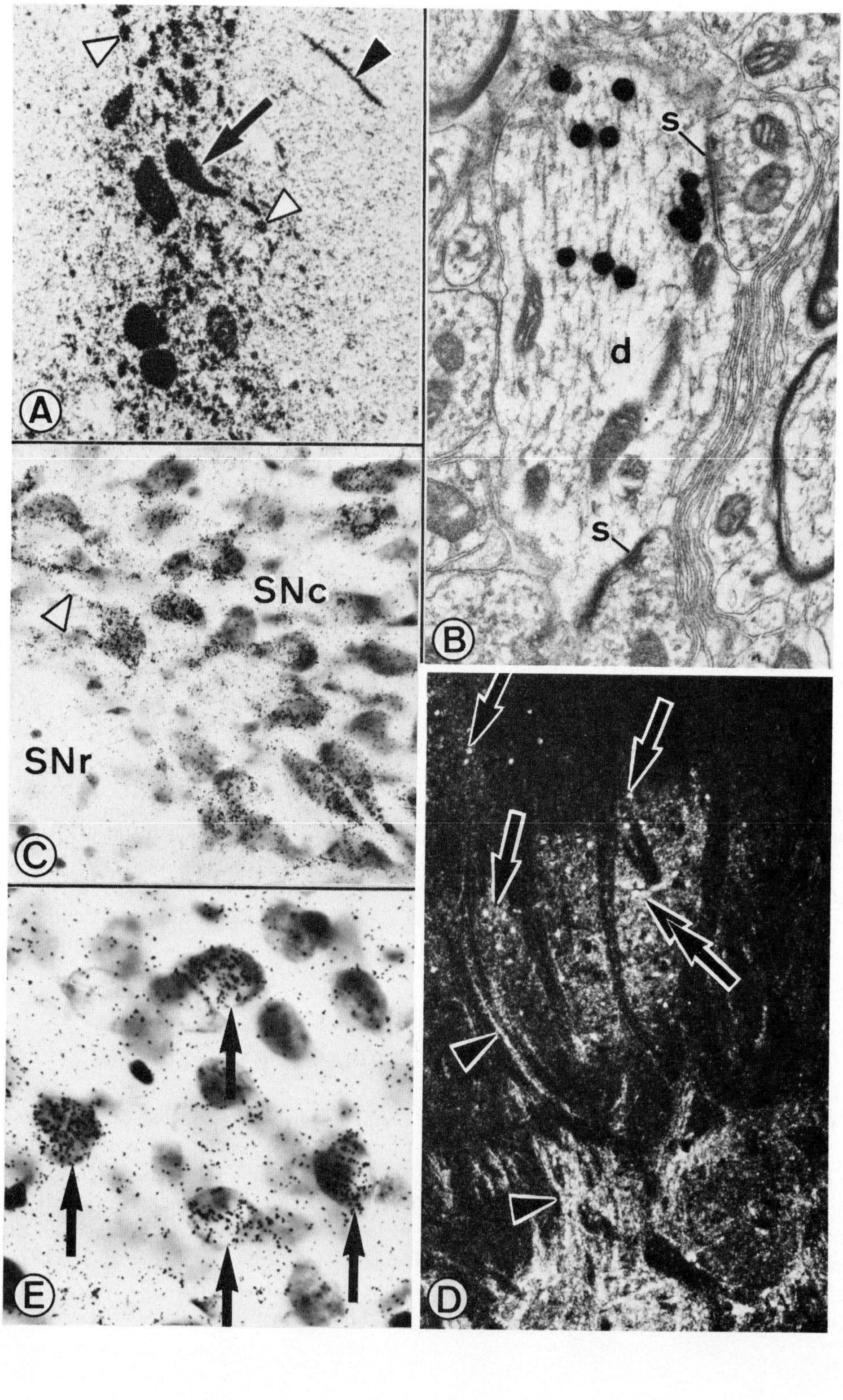
A
s
d
s
B
SNc
SNr
C
E
D

Heavily labeled clusters of relatively small sized neuronal perikarya are observed in a restricted area of the caudo-putamen's body following nigral [^{3}H]GABA application (0.05 resp. 0.1 μl 4-amino-*n*[2,3-^{3}H]butyric acid, 15 resp. 10 μCi, 54 Ci/mmol, Radiochemical Centre, Amersham) Fig. 2D, E) (Streit et al., 1979). As substance P neurons are reported to be situated mainly in more rostral regions (Brownstein et al., 1977; Jessell et al., 1978) it is reasonable to assume that this labeling is in GABA neurons.

Striatal [^{3}H]dopamine injection (0.05–0.2 μl [ethylamine-1,2-^{3}H]dopamine hydrochloride, 10–20 μCi, 7 Ci/mmol, Radiochemical Centre, Amersham) results in heavy labeling in the nigra (Fig. 2C) and in neurons probably corresponding to the dopaminergic cell groups A8 and A10 (Palkovits and Jacobowitz, 1974). Some weakly labeled neurons in the raphe nucleus are also found. No perikaryal labeling can be detected in other striatal inputs and in dopamine cell groups not projecting to the striatum.

Confirming the results of Leger et al. (1977) perikaryal labeling in the nucleus raphe dorsalis after striatal [^{3}H]serotonin injection (0.05 μl 5-hydroxy [G-^{3}H]tryptamine creatinine sulphate, 13–18.5 μCi, 10.7 Ci/mmol, Radiochemical Centre, Amersham) is observed. Heavy labeling of presumably dopaminergic neurons in the substantia nigra and in A8 and A10 has to be noticed too. Other afferent systems to the striatum are unlabeled. Only in 1 out of 5 experiments – in an animal without pretreatment with a monoaminoxidase inhibitor – an occasionally labeled perikaryon has been detected in the cortex (layers 3–5) and in the parafascicular nucleus. After nigral [^{3}H]serotonin administration (0.05 μl; 16 μCi) labeling is confined to some neurons in the nucleus raphe dorsalis, with the exception of a single labeled neuron detected in the cortex (Streit et al., 1979).

The crossed specificity between dopamine and serotonin in serotoninergic resp. dopaminergic afferents to the striatum can easily be explained by the inability of the uptake systems to distinguish between these biogenic amines even at much lower concentrations (Shaskan and Snyder, 1970; Berger and Glowinski, 1978).

In all the pigeon and rat experiments mentioned so far these concentrations were in the range for low affinity uptake. Low affinity uptake, however, should have no transmitter specificity. It is therefore reasonable to postulate that the chemospecificity seen in retrograde labeling is generally determined by the high affinity uptake system which operates at these concentrations under conditions of saturation. Preferentially part of the material taken up by the high affinity system seems to have access to the axon – possibly to a compartment for retrograde axonal transport. Because of the relatively low specific activities of the labeled compounds and the relatively small capacity of the terminal high affinity systems, however, high concentrations of transmitter have to be applied in order to ensure enough radioactivity to be taken up, partly transferred to the axon and moved to the perikaryon, where the label should be accumulated in sufficient amounts to be detected by autoradiography.

◀ Fig. 2. A: labeling over semithin section from part of the nucleus isthmi, pars parvocellularis (Ipc), 30 min after onset of [^{3}H]glycine injection into pigeon optic tectum. Note restricted area with perikaryal (arrow) and probably dendritic (open arrowheads) labeling. Axonal labeling between Ipc and tectum (filled arrowhead). × 330. B: electron microscopic autoradiograph of labeled dendrite (d) in Ipc neuropile (same case as in A). The two axon terminals synapsing (s) on this dendrite are typically not labeled. × 22,500. C: perikaryal labeling in substantia nigra, pars compacta (SNc), 6 hr after injection of [^{3}H]dopamine into rat neostriatum. Note labeled process – probably a dendrite (arrowhead). Labeling over pars reticulata (SNr) is much weaker, × 350. D and E: autoradiographs showing labeling of perikarya (arrows) in body of rat neostriatum 6 hr after injection of [^{3}H]GABA into substantia nigra. Labeled cell bodies often occur in clusters (double arrow). Note probably retrograde labeling of certain fiber bundles between striatum and nigra (arrowheads). Dark-field illumination in D, × 57. Bright-field illumination in E, × 680.

After administration of tritiated precursors like tyrosine (0.05 resp. 0.08 μl L-[3,5-^{3}H]-tyrosine, 16 resp. 19 μCi, 44 Ci/mmol, Radiochemical Centre, Amersham) for dopamine, tryptophan (0.05 μl L-[G-^{3}H]tryptophan 17.5 μCi, 5.96 Ci/mmol, New England Nuclear, Boston) for serotonin, glutamine (0.05–0.1 μl L-[G-^{3}H]glutamine, 15–20 μCi, 21 Ci/mmol, Radiochemical Centre, Amersham) for glutamate and for GABA (Reubi et al., 1978) and glutamate (0.05 μl L-[G-^{3}H]glutamic acid, 10–16 μCi, 28 Ci/mmol, Radiochemical Centre, Amersham) for GABA no retrograde perikaryal labeling has been noticed. These negative findings may indicate that the newly synthetized transmitter has only an insignificant if any access to the axon. No labeled perikarya have been observed in the cortex after striatal application of [^{3}H]glutamate (0.05–0.2 μl L-[G-^{3}H]glutamic acid, 10–16 μCi, 28 Ci/mmol, Radiochemical Centre, Amersham) although the cortico-striatal pathway has been claimed to use glutamate-mediated transmission (Divac et al., 1977; Kim et al., 1977; McGeer et al., 1977).

The method of transmitter-specific retrograde tracing can possibly only be used for certain and not for all transmitters. It is quite probable that the method does not work, e.g., for peptides like substance P for which no uptake has been observed (Iversen et al., 1976). On the other hand, when retrograde labeling after application of a compound occurs the question of its transmitter-related role could be raised. Künzle (1977) described such a case in the cortico- and rubro-spinal pathways after [^{3}H]proline injection. Although proline is by no means an established neurotransmitter, there are some indications for such a role (Künzle and Cuénod, 1973; Felix and Künzle, 1976).

Transmitter-specific retrograde tracing has been described in relatively short pathways; it should now definitely be tried in longer pathways with known transmitter. Transmitters in combination with other retrograde tracers like, e.g., horseradish peroxidase could be used for the demonstration of projections with collateral axonal branching. Transmitter-specific retrograde tracing of pathways may become a useful tool based on phenomena and mechanisms which await further investigation.

Transmitter-specific retrograde labeling may be based on the "error" of some transmitter molecules (or their metabolites) which instead of getting, e.g., into release compartments are shifted into a compartment for axonal migration. This artificial translocation might be caused by an "overflow" due to the application of large amounts of exogenous transmitter. The whole phenomenon could, however, also be based on a physiological process. In this case the transmitter or a metabolite might be used as a signal in the perikaryon and in the dendrites – informing the metabolic machinery and the "input-integrator" about physiological events taking place in the axon terminals.

SUMMARY

In the present contribution the hypothesis is discussed that transmitter specificity in neuronal pathways may be detected morphologically by means of retrograde perikaryal labeling after application of a transmitter in the terminal area. This hypothesis originated from observations made in the connection between the subtectal nucleus isthmi pars parvocellularis (Ipc) and the tectum after injection of [^{3}H]glycine into the pigeon optic tectum. In this Ipc-tectal pathway a retrograde axonal migration of soluble labeled material was found. This pathway is likely to be glycinergic.

The hypothesis of transmitter-specific retrograde labeling of pathways was further tested in some rat central connections with known transmitter. After nigral injection of [^{3}H]GABA perikaryal labeling was observed in the striatum, whereas injection of [^{3}H]serotonin resulted in labeled cell bodies in the nucleus raphe dorsalis. After striatal injections of [^{3}H]dopamine or [^{3}H]serotonin, perikaryal labeling was obtained in the substantia nigra, the dopaminergic groups A8 and A10 and in the nucleus raphe dorsalis.

ACKNOWLEDGEMENTS

The authors are grateful to E. Knecht, D. Savini, E. Schneider and M. Jäckli for excellent technical assistance. The help of Prof. H.-Ch. Curtius and Mr. U. Redweik from the University Pediatric Department of Zurich for the GC-MS determination of glycine is gratefully acknowledged.

This work was supported by Grants 3.744.76 and 3.636.75 from the Swiss National Science Foundation, the Dr. Eric Slack-Gyr Foundation, the Emil Barell Foundation, the "Jubiläumsspende für die Universität Zürich" and the "Stiftung für wissenschaftliche Forschung der Universität Zürich".

REFERENCES

Barth, R. and Felix, D. (1974) Influence of GABA and glycine and their antagonists on inhibitory mechanisms of pigeon's optic tectum. *Brain Res.*, 80: 532–537.

Berger, B. and Glowinski, J. (1978) Dopamine uptake in serotoninergic terminals in vitro: a valuable tool for the histochemical differentiation of catecholaminergic and serotoninergic terminals in rat cerebral structures. *Brain Res.*, 147: 29–45.

Brodal, A., Taber, E. and Walberg, F. (1960) The raphe nuclei of the brain stem in the cat. II. Efferent connections. *J. comp. Neurol.*, 114: 239–259.

Brownstein, M. J., Mroz, E. A., Kizer, J. S., Palkovits, M. and Leeman, S. E. (1976) Regional distribution of substance P in the brain of the rat. *Brain Res.*, 116: 299–305.

Cajal, S. Ramón y (1899) Adiciones a nuestros trabajos sobre los centros opticos de las aves. *Rev. trimest. Microgr.*, 4: 77–86.

Cuénod, M. and Streit, P. (1979) Amino acid transmitters and local circuitry in optic tectum. In: *The Neurosciences, Fourth Study Program*, F. O. Schmitt and F. G. Worden (Eds.), MIT Press, Cambridge, Mass., pp. 989–1004.

Divac, I., Fonnum, F. and Storm-Mathisen, J. (1977) High affinity uptake of glutamate in terminals of corticostriatal axons. *Nature (Lond.)*, 266: 377–378.

Dray, A., Davies, J., Oakley, N. R., Tongroach, P. and Vellucci, S. (1978) The dorsal and medial raphe projections to the substantia nigra in the rat: electrophysiological, biochemical and behavioural observations. *Brain Res.*, 151: 431–442.

Falck, B., Hillarp, N. A., Thieme, G. and Ford, A. (1962) Fluorescence of catecholamines and related compounds condensated with formaldehyde. *J. Histochem. Cytochem.*, 10: 348–354.

Felix, D. and Künzle, H. (1976) The role of proline in nervous transmission. *Advanc. Biochem. Psychopharmacol.*, 15: 165–173.

Fonnum, F., Grofová, I., Rinvik, E., Storm-Mathisen, J. and Walberg, F. (1974) Origin and distribution of glutamate decarboxylase in substantia nigra of the cat. *Brain Res.*, 71: 77–92.

Henke, H. and Cuénod, M. (1978) Uptake of L-alanine, glycine and L-serine in the pigeon central nervous system. *Brain Res.*, 152: 105–119.

Henke, H., Schenker, T. M. and Cuénod, M. (1976) Uptake of neurotransmitter candidates by pigeon optic tectum. *J. Neurochem.*, 26: 125–130.

Hong, J. S., Yang, H.-Y. T., Racagni, G. and Costa, I. (1977) Projections of substance P containing neurons from neostriatum to substantia nigra. *Brain Res.*, 122: 541–544.

Hunt, S. P. and Künzle, H. (1976a) Observations on the projections and intrinsic organization of the pigeon optic tectum: an autoradiographic study based on anterograde and retrograde, axonal and dendritic flow. *J. comp. Neurol.*, 170: 153–172.

Hunt, S. P. and Künzle, H. (1976b) Selective uptake and transport of label within three identified neuronal systems after injection of [^{3}H]GABA into the pigeon optic tectum: an autoradiographic and Golgi study. *J. comp. Neurol.*, 170: 173–190.

Hunt, S. P., Streit, P., Künzle, H. and Cuénod, M. (1977) Characterization of the pigeon isthmo-tectal pathway by selective uptake and retrograde movement of radioactive compounds and by Golgi-like horseradish peroxidase labelling. *Brain Res.*, 129: 197–212.

Iversen, L. L., Jessell, T. and Kanazawa, I. (1976) Release and metabolism of substance P in rat hypothalamus. *Nature (Lond.)*, 264: 81–83.

Jessell, T. M., Emson, P. C., Paxinos, G. and Cuello, A. C. (1978) Topographic projections of substance P and GABA pathways in the striato- and pallido-nigral system: a biochemical and immunohistochemical study. *Brain Res.*, 152: 487–498.

Kanazawa, I., Marshall, G. R. and Kelly, J. S. (1976) Afferents to the rat substantia nigra studied with horseradish peroxidase, with special reference to fibres from the subthalamic nucleus. *Brain Res.*, 115: 485–491.

Kanazawa, I., Emson, P. C. and Cuello, A. C. (1977) Evidence for the existence of substance P-containing fibres in the strio-nigral and pallido-nigral pathways in rat brain. *Brain Res.*, 119: 447–453.

Kataoka, K., Bak, I. J., Hassler, R., Kim, J. G. and Wagner, A. (1974) L-Glutamate decarboxylase and choline acetyltransferase activity in the substantia nigra and the striatum after surgical interruption of the strio-nigral fibres of the baboon. *Exp. Brain Res.*, 19: 217–227.

Kim, J. S., Bak, I. J., Hassler, R. and Okada, Y. (1971) Role of gamma-aminobutyric acid in the extrapyramidal motor system. 2. Some evidence for the existence of a type of GABA strio-nigral neurons. *Exp. Brain Res.*, 14: 95–104.

Kim, J. S., Hassler, R., Haug, P. and Paik, K. S. (1977) Effect of frontal cortex ablation on striatal glutamic acid level in rat. *Brain Res.*, 132: 370–374.

Künzle, H. (1977) Evidence for selective axon-terminal uptake and retrograde transport of label in cortico- and rubrospinal systems after injection of [^{3}H]proline. *Exp. Brain Res.*, 28: 125–132.

Künzle, H. and Cuénod, M. (1973) Differential uptake of [^{3}H]proline and [^{3}H]leucine by neurons: its importance for the autoradiographic tracing of pathways. *Brain Res.*, 62: 213–217.

Le Fort, D., Henke, H. and Cuénod, M. (1978) Glycine specific [^{3}H]strychnine binding in the pigeon CNS. *J. Neurochem.*, 30: 1281–1291.

Leger, L., Pujol, J. F., Bobillier, P. et Jouvet, M. (1977) Transport axoplasmique de la sérotonine par voie rétrograde dans les neurones monoaminergiques centraux. *C.R. Acad. Sci. (Paris)*, 285: 1179–1182.

Lindvall, O. and Björklund, A. (1974) The organization of the ascending catecholamine neuron systems in the rat brain as revealed by the glyoxylic acid fluorescence method. *Acta physiol. scand.*, Suppl. 412: 1–48.

McGeer, P. L., McGeer, E. G., Scherer, U. and Singh, K. (1977) A glutamatergic corticostriatal path? *Brain Res.*, 128: 369–373.

Mroz, E. A., Brownstein, M. J. and Leeman, S. E. (1977) Evidence for substance P in the striato-nigral tract. *Brain Res.*, 125: 305–311.

Palkovits, M. and Jacobowitz, D. M. (1974) Topographic atlas of catecholamine and acetylcholinesterase-containing neurons in the rat brain. II. Hindbrain (mesencephalon, rhombencephalon). *J. comp. Neurol.*, 157: 29–42.

Price, C. H., Coggeshall, R. E. and McAdoo, D. J. (1978) Specific glycine uptake by identified neurons of *Aplysia californica.* I. Autoradiography. *Brain Res.*, 154: 25–40.

Reubi, J. C. and Cuénod, M. (1976) Release of exogenous glycine in the pigeon optic tectum during stimulation of a midbrain nucleus. *Brain Res.*, 112: 347–361.

Reubi, J. C. and Emson, P. C. (1978) Release and distribution of endogenous 5-HT in rat substantia nigra. *Brain Res.*, 139: 164–168.

Reubi, J. C., Van den Berg, C. and Cuénod, M. (1978) Glutamine as precursor for the GABA and glutamate transmitter pools. *Neurosci. Lett.*, 10: 171–174.

Shaskan, E. and Snyder, S. H. (1970) Kinetics of serotonin accumulation into slices from rat brain: relationship to catecholamine uptake. *J. Pharmacol. exp. Ther.*, 175: 404–418.

Streit, P. (1980) Selective retrograde labeling indicating the transmitter of neuronal pathways. Submitted for publication.

Streit, P., Knecht, E. and Cuénod, M. (1979) Transmitter specific retrograde labelling in the striato-nigral and raphe-nigral pathways, *Science*, 205: 306–308.

Streit, P., Knecht, E. and Cuénod, M. (1980) Transmitter related retrograde labeling in the pigeon optic lobe: a high resolution autoradiographic study. *Brain Res.*, in press.

Taber-Pierce, E., Foote, W. E. and Hobson, J. A. (1976) The efferent connection of the nucleus raphe dorsalis. *Brain Res.*, 107: 137–144.

Wolfensberger, M., Reubi, J. C. and Cuénod, M. (1979) Mass fragmentographic determination of endogenous glycine released upon electrical stimulation of a neural pathway. *Neurosci. Lett.*, Suppl. 3: 345.

Zukin, S. R., Young, A. B. and Snyder, S. H. (1975) Development of the synaptic glycine receptor in chick embryo spinal cord. *Brain Res.*, 83: 525–530.

Kainic Acid Toxicity and Binding in the Optic Tectum

H. HENKE, P. STREIT, J. C. REUBI and M. CUÉNOD

Brain Research Institute, University of Zurich, Zurich (Switzerland)

There is some evidence that glutamate is used as neurotransmitter in the pigeon optic tectum. This stucture has a high glutamate content (Beart, 1976) and a sodium-dependent high affinity uptake system for L-glutamate is present (Henke et al., 1976a). A calcium-dependent, potassium-stimulated release of L-[^{3}H]glutamate, newly synthesized from L-[^{3}H]glutamine, has been demonstrated (Reubi et al., 1978). Iontophoretically applied L-glutamate excites tectal neurons, this effect is specifically antagonized by L-nuciferine and glutamic acid diethylester (Wang et al., 1978). In particular, the retino-tectal pathway may use glutamate as neurotransmitter. This is indicated by data obtained after retinal ablation. Unilateral retinal ablation leads to a degeneration of the optic nerve terminals in the contralateral tectum. Since the optic nerves are completely crossed in the pigeon, the ipsilateral tectum can serve as control (Cuénod et al., 1970). Seven weeks after retinal ablation, the glutamate pool is reduced by 30–70% in the superficial layers of the tectum which receive the retinal input. The pool in the deeper layers, which contain no retinal endings, remains unchanged (Fonnum and Henke, 1979). At the same time, the glutamate high affinity uptake by crude synaptosomal fractions, prepared from degenerated tecta, is reduced by 60% when compared to the control side (Henke et al., 1976b).

Kainic acid, a conformationally restricted glutamate derivative, may be helpful to further characterize neurons using glutamate as neurotransmitter. Biochemical (Simon et al., 1976), histological (Biziere and Coyle, 1978; Olney et al., 1978) and physiological (Johnston et al., 1974) evidence in the CNS indicate a close relation between the neuronal effects of glutamate and kainic acid. However, the precise mechanism by which kainic acid acts is not known. In the present study we have examined the L-glutamate-sensitive binding and the neurotoxic effects of kainic acid in the pigeon optic tectum in order to further elucidate the relation between glutamate and kainic acid.

The binding was determined by a centrifugation technique using crude tectal membrane preparations (Henke and Cuénod, 1979). L-Glutamate-specific [^{3}H]kainic acid binding had an apparent dissociation constant (K_d) of 30 ± 18 nM and a maximal binding (B_{max}) of 227 ± 58 fmol/mg protein (Fig. 1). The binding was maximal between pH 6.8 and 7.8 and located predominantly in the crude synaptosomal fraction. The displacement of bound [^{3}H]kainic acid by various chemicals was studied (Table I). The displacing potencies of the substances examined did not parallel their potency when applied iontophoretically. D-Glutamate, almost as effective in exciting neurons as L-glutamate (Curtis and Johnston, 1974), and the glutamate antagonists L-nuciferine (Ben-Ari and Kelly, 1975; Felix and Frangi, 1977) and glutamic acid diethylester (Haldeman and McLennan, 1972) were only weak

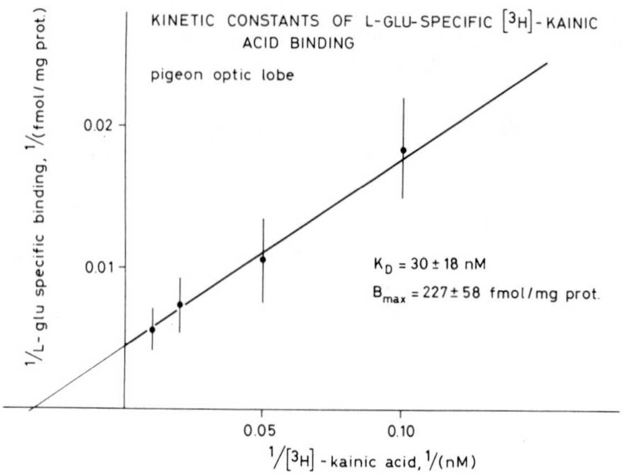

Fig. 1. Double reciprocal plot of [^{3}H]kainic acid binding. The points are the mean ± S.E.M. of 5 separate experiments with a crude membrane preparation.

TABLE I

L-GLUTAMATE-SPECIFIC [^{3}H]KAINIC ACID BINDING IN THE PIGEON OPTIC LOBE, IC_{50} VALUES OF VARIOUS SUBSTANCES

IC_{50} values give the amount of substance needed to displace 50% of the specific [^{3}H]kainic acid binding at 20 nM [^{3}H]kainic acid concentration. The values were obtained from log-probit plots of at least 4 different inhibitor concentrations.

Kainic acid	$6.0 \cdot 10^{-9}$
L-Glutamate	$5.2 \cdot 10^{-7}$
Ibotenic acid	$1.0 \cdot 10^{-5}$
L-Glutamic acid γ-monoethylester	$4.0 \cdot 10^{-5}$
L-Glutamic acid γ-monomethylester	$4.4 \cdot 10^{-5}$
L-Glutamic acid γ-benzylester	$5.2 \cdot 10^{-5}$
α-Aminoadipic acid	$1.4 \cdot 10^{-4}$
L-Glutamic acid di-*t*-butylester-HCl	$1.4 \cdot 10^{-4}$
D-Glutamic acid	$1.5 \cdot 10^{-4}$
L-Glutamic acid dimethylester-HCl	$7.6 \cdot 10^{-4}$
L-Glutamic acid diethylester-HCl	$9.0 \cdot 10^{-4}$
γ-Aminobutyric acid	$> 10^{-3}$
L-Aspartate	$> 10^{-3}$
Bicuculline	$> 10^{-3}$
Glycine	$> 10^{-3}$
Nuciferine	$> 10^{-3}$
L-Proline	$> 10^{-3}$
Strychnine	$> 10^{-3}$

displacers as were some other glutamate derivatives and some putative neurotransmitters and their antagonists. Ibotenic acid, another rigid glutamate derivative with strong excitatory effects (Johnston et al., 1968) on central neurons, was a weak displacer too. One to 4 weeks after retinal ablation the specific binding remained unchanged when compared per mg protein (Table II).

TABLE II

EFFECT OF RETINAL ABLATION ON THE L-GLUTAMATE-SPECIFIC [^{3}H[KAINIC ACID BINDING IN THE PIGEON OPTIC TECTUM

The [^{3}H]kainic acid concentration used was 50 nM.

Survival time	*% Control*		*n*
	Per tectum	*Per mg protein*	
1 week	100 ± 10	97 ± 7	3
2 weeks	102 ± 8	106 ± 12	3
4 weeks	82 ± 17	97 ± 16	6
3 months	80 ± 9	89 ± 4	3

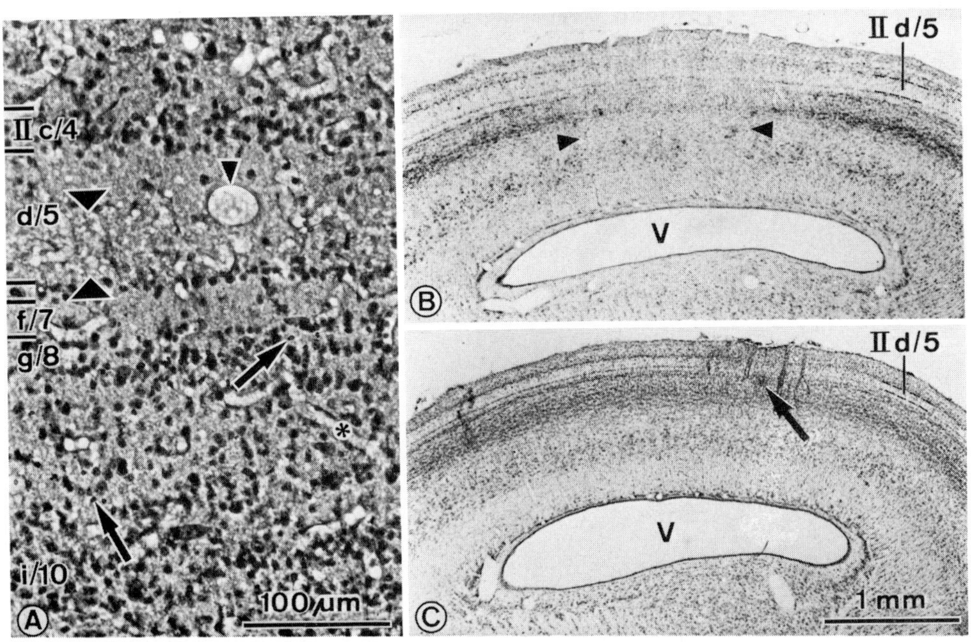

Fig. 2. Light micrographs showing parts of the pigeon optic tectum after injection of 0.5 µl of 20 mM buffered kainic acid solution. Frozen sections, cresylecht violet staining. A: phase contrast micrograph 2 days after kainate injection into normal tectum. Accumulation of many small vacuoles in lower half of sublayer IId/5 (indicated by triangles). The huge vacuole (arrowhead) at the border between upper and lower subdivisions of IId/5 probably represents a destroyed perikaryon. Mainly in sublayer IIg/8 but also IIi/10 small intensely stained "dense bodies" are visible (arrow) – remnants of dying neurons. B: normal light micrograph 7 days after kainate injection into intact tectum. Subtotal destruction of neurons in all layers within region indicated by arrowheads. V, ventricle. Same magnification as in C. C: normal light micrograph 7 days after kainate injection into tectum 5 weeks after contralateral retinal ablation. Arrow points at gliosis around cross-section of needle tract. Some additional gliosis and other changes are found in the area of the injection site. The neurons in all layers are more or less intact. IId/5 is shrunken when compared to the one in B as a consequence of retinal ablation.

Four hours to 21 days after tectal injections of kainic acid (0.5–2.0 μg in 0.5 μl Krebs-Ringer solution, pH 7.4) the tissue was examined microscopically for neurotoxic effects. Already after 4 hr an impressive vacuolization, mainly restricted to the lower part of the neuropil of sublayer IId (Cowan et al., 1961) or 5 (Cajal, 1891), which receives dense retinal terminations, was detected by phase contrast microscopy (Fig. 2A). Later the pattern of neuronal cell loss appeared progressively in the superficial and then in the deeper layers of the tectum (Fig. 2B). Two to 12 weeks after contralateral retinal ablation this type of cell destruction could no longer be induced by kainate injections (Fig. 2C). Only a slight gliosis and some occasional destroyed neuronal perikarya were observed in the area of the needle tract. The neurotoxicity of kainic acid in the tectum, therefore, seems to depend on the presence of an intact retino-tectal pathway and the terminals in sublayer IId may be particularly important (Streit et al., 1979).

Taken together, these results show that in the pigeon optic lobe the kainic acid binding is quite specific for L-glutamate. The binding site for kainic acid, however, is probably not identical with the iontophoretically active binding site for glutamate because the iontophoretic and displacing properties of a series of chemicals do not parallel each other. The

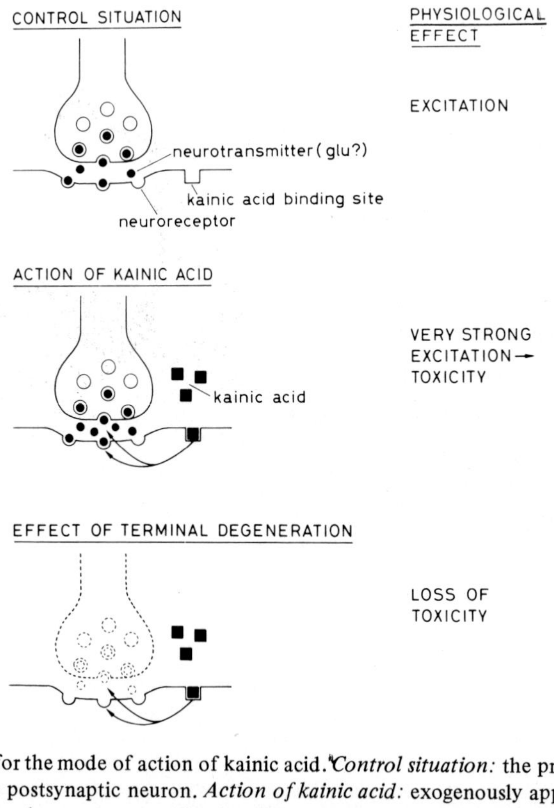

Fig. 3. Possible model for the mode of action of kainic acid. *Control situation:* the presynaptically released transmitter excites the postsynaptic neuron. *Action of kainic acid:* exogenously applied kainic acid binds to the postsynaptic membrane at a specific site. This causes an increased sensitivity of the transmitter receptor and/or leads to an increased transmitter concentration in the synaptic cleft by way of a postsynaptically mediated factor. *Effect of terminal degeneration:* after terminal degeneration no transmitter can be released any more and the toxic effect of kainic acid is abolished. It is in this situation where glutamate can partially restore the kainic acid toxicity. This indicates that glutamate is or can mimic the endogenously released transmitter.

neurotoxicity of kainic acid is abolished 2 weeks after retinal ablation but the number of binding sites is not changed. Assuming that at least some of the specific kainic acid binding sites are essential for the neurotoxic effect of kainic acid, this means that they cannot be located on the optic nerve fibers and terminals. The reduction in binding sites per tectum observed at longer survival times is probably due to some transneuronal degeneration.

Two more results must be taken into consideration regards the possible mode of action of kainic acid. The neurotoxicity of kainic acid in the degenerated tectum can be restored when L-glutamate is injected simultaneously with kainic acid (Streit et al., 1979). In iontophoretic experiments, kainic acid can potentiate the excitatory action of L-glutamate on tectal neurons without having any effect by itself alone (D. Felix, pers. communication). These results indicate a close relation between L-glutamate and kainic acid. A possible model for the action of kainic acid is shown in Fig. 3. Here, kainic acid binds to a postsynaptic site and thereby increases the efficiency of the presynaptically released neurotransmitter, which may be glutamate, to excite the cell. This leads to an "overexcitation" and the subsequent cell destruction. If the presynaptic part is destroyed, no transmitter can be released any more and the neurotoxicity of kainic acid is lost while the binding sites remain unchanged.

The results in the optic tectum are very similar to those obtained in the rat neostriatum. It has been suggested that the cortico-striatal fibers use glutamate as neurotransmitter (Curtis and Johnston, 1974; Spencer, 1976). After degeneration of these fibers, the glutamate pool (Kim et al., 1977) and the high affinity uptake (Divac et al., 1977) are reduced. As in the tectum, the neurotoxicity of kainic acid depends on an intact afferent pathway (McGeer et al., 1977, 1978; Biziere and Coyle, 1978) and after degeneration of the cortico-striatal endings the neurotoxicity of kainic acid can be restored with L-glutamate (Biziere and Coyle, 1978). The binding of [^{3}H]kainic acid is reduced by only 20% 4 weeks after cortex ablation (Henke and Cuénod, 1979).

All these data, and others from the hippocampus (Köhler et al., 1978; Nadler et al., 1978) and the cerebellum (Herndon and Coyle, 1978), show a close relation between L-glutamate and kainic acid. Is it therefore possible to use L-glutamate-specific [^{3}H]kainic acid binding as a marker for glutamate mediated neurotransmission? Experiments with tectal and striatal slices show that this assumption cannot yet be drawn. One month after retinal ablation the calcium-dependent potassium-stimulated release of [^{3}H]glutamate, newly synthesized from [^{3}H]glutamine (Reubi et al., 1978), had not changed (Fig. 4). In contrast, in the rat striatum the same kind of release was reduced by 65% 18 days after cortex ablation (Reubi and Cuénod, 1979). Whether this is due to a principal difference in the function of L-glutamate in the two structures, e.g. a different metabolism or a more rapid re-uptake of glutamate in the tectum, remains to be investigated.

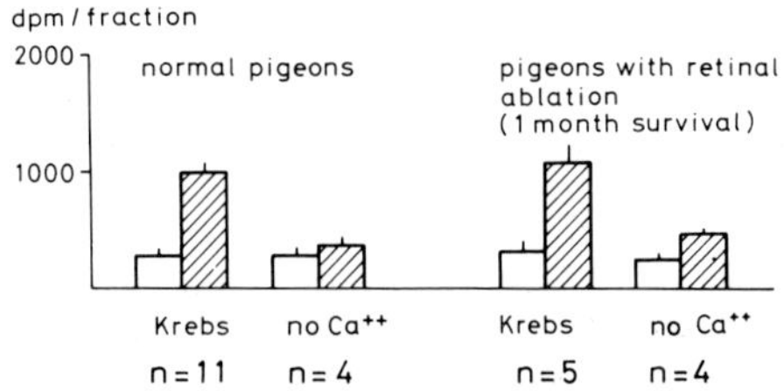

Fig. 4. Release of [^{3}H]glutamate, newly synthesized from [^{3}H]glutamine, from tectal slices. Spontaneous release (white columns) and release evoked by 47 mM potassium chloride (hatched columns). Points are mean ± S.E.M., n gives the number of experiments performed.

ACKNOWLEDGEMENTS

The authors thank R. Grieder, M. Stella, E. Knecht, Ch. Ramseier and A. Fäh for excellent technical assistance.

This work was supported by Grants 3.744.76 and 3.636.75 from the Swiss National Science Foundation, the Dr. Eric Slack-Gyr-Foundation and the Emil Barell-Foundation.

REFERENCES

Beart, P. M. (1976) An evaluation of L-glutamate as the transmitter released from optic nerve terminals of the pigeon. *Brain Res.*, 110: 99-114.

Ben-Ari, Y. and Kelly, J. S. (1975) Specificity of nuciferine as an antagonist of amino acid and synaptically evoked activity in cells of the feline thalamus. *J. Physiol. (Lond.)*, 251: 25–27.

Biziere, K. and Coyle, J. T. (1978) Influence of cortico-striatal afferents on striatal kainic acid neurotoxicity. *Neurosci. Lett.*, 8: 303–310.

Cajal, S. Ramón y (1891) Sur la fine structure du lobe optique des oiseaux et sur l'origine réelle des nerfs optiques. *Int. Mschr. Anat. Physiol.*, 8: 337–366.

Cowan, W. M., Adamson, L. and Powell, T. P. S. (1961) An experimental study of the avian visual system. *J. Anat. (Lond.)*, 95: 545–563.

Cuénod, M., Sandri, C. and Akert, K. (1970) Enlarged synaptic vesicles as an early sign of secondary degeneration in the optic nerve terminals of the pigeon. *J. Cell Sci.*, 6: 605–613.

Curtis, D. R. and Johnston, G. A. R. (1974) Amino acid transmitters in mammalian central nervous system. *Ergebn. Physiol.*, 69: 97–188.

Curtis, D. R. and Watkins, J. C. (1960) The excitation and depression of spinal neurones by structurally related amino acids. *J. Neurochem.*, 6: 117–141.

Divac, I., Fonnum, F. and Storm-Mathisen, J. (1977) High affinity uptake of glutamate in terminals of corticostriatal axons. *Nature (Lond.)*, 266: 377–378.

Felix, D. and Frangi, U. (1977) Dimethoxyaporphine as an antagonist of chemical excitation in the pigeon optic tectum. *Neurosci. Lett.*, 4: 347–350.

Fonnum, F. and Henke, H. (1979) Effect of retinal ablation on the pool of some amino acids in different layers of the pigeon tectum. *Experientia (Basel)*, 35: 121.

Haldeman, S. and McLennan, H. (1972) The antagonistic action of glutamic acid diethylester towards amino acid-induced and synaptic excitations of central neurones. *Brain Res.*, 45: 393–400.

Henke, H. and Cuénod, M. (1979) L-glutamate specific [^{3}H]kainic acid binding in the rat neostriatum after degeneration of the cortico-striatal pathway. *Neurosci. Lett.*, 11: 341–345.

Henke, H., Schenker, T. M. and Cuénod, M. (1976a) Uptake of neurotransmitter candidates by pigeon optic tectum. *J. Neurochem.*, 26: 125–130.

Henke, H., Schenker, T. M. and Cuénod, M. (1976b) Effects of retinal ablation on uptake of glutamate, glycine, GABA, proline and choline in pigeon tectum. *J. Neurochem.*, 26: 131–134.

Herndon, R. M. and Coyle, J. T. (1978) Glutamergic innervation, kainic acid, and selective vulnerability in the cerebellum. In *Kainic Acid as a Tool in Neurobiology*, E. G. McGeer et al. (Eds.), Raven Press, New York, pp. 187–200.

Johnston, G. A. R., Curtis, D. R., DeGroat, W. C. and Duggan, A. W. (1968) Central actions of ibotenic acid and muscimol. *Biochem. Pharmacol.*, 17: 2488–2489.

Johnston, G. A. R., Curtis, D. R., Davies, J. and McCulloch, R. M. (1974) Spinal interneurone excitation by conformationally restricted analogues of L-glutamic acid. *Nature (Lond.)*, 248: 804–805.

Kim, J. S., Hassler, R., Haug, P. and Pasik, K. S. (1977) Effect on frontal cortex ablation on striatal glutamic acid level in rat. *Brain Res.*, 132: 370–374.

Köhler, C., Schwarz, R. and Fuxe, K. (1978) Perforant path transections protect hippocampal granule cells from kainate lesion. *Neurosci. Lett.*, 10: 241–246.

McGeer, E. G., McGeer, P. L. and Singh, K. (1978) Kainate-induced degeneration of neostriatal neurons: dependency upon cortico-striatal tract. *Brain Res.*, 139: 381–383.

McGeer, P. L., McGeer, E. G., Scherer, U. and Singh, K. (1977) A glutamatergic corticostriatal path? *Brain Res.*, 128: 369–373.

Nadler, J. V., Perry, B. W. and Cotman, C. W. (1978) Preferential vulnerability of hippocampus to intraventricular kainic acid. In *Kainic Acid as a Tool in Neurobiology*, E. G. McGeer et al. (Eds.), Raven Press, New York, pp. 219–237.

Olney, J. W., Rhee, V. and Ho, O. L. (1978) Kainic acid: a powerful neurotoxic analogue of glutamate. *Brain Res.*, 77: 507–512.

Reubi, J. C. and Cuénod, M. (1979) Glutamate release in vitro from corticostriatal terminals. *Brain Res.*, 175: in press.

Reubi, J. C., Van den Berg, C. and Cuénod, M. (1978) Glutamine as precursor for the GABA and glutamate transmitter pools. *Neurosci. Lett.*, 10: 171–174.

Simon, J. R., Contrera, J. F. and Kuhar, M. J. (1976) Binding of [^{3}H]kainic acid, an analogue of L-glutamate, to brain membranes. *J. Neurochem.*, 26: 141–147.

Spencer, H. J. (1976) Antagonism of cortical excitation of striatal neurones by glutamic acid diethyl ester: evidence for glutamic acid as an excitatory transmitter in the rat striatum. *Brain Res.*, 102: 91–101.

Streit, P., Stella, M. and Cuénod, M. (1979) Kainate induced lesion in the optic tectum: dependence upon optic nerve afferents or glutamate. *Brain Res.*, in press.

Wang, S. J., Felix, D. and Frangi, U. (1978) The role of glutamate in pigeon optic tectum. *Brain Res.*, 157: 360–368.

Subject Index